Patient
Education
and
Preventive
Medicine

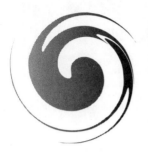

Patient Education and Preventive Medicine

James Brox Labus, PA-C
Bachelor of Science, Health Education
President, Mid-Level Medical Services
Lecturer, Emory University Physician
  Assistant Program
Atlanta, Georgia

Alison Ann Lauber, MD
Emory University School of Medicine
Department of Family and Preventive Medicine
Director of Clinical Operations
Medical Director, Physician Assistant Program
Director of Procedural Education Center
Atlanta, Georgia

W.B. SAUNDERS COMPANY
A Harcourt Health Sciences Company
Philadelphia London New York St. Louis Sydney Toronto

W.B. SAUNDERS COMPANY
A Harcourt Health Sciences Company

The Curtis Center
Independence Square West
Philadelphia, Pennsylvania 19106

Library of Congress Cataloging-in-Publication Data

Labus, James B.

Patient education and preventive medicine/James B. Labus, and Alison Lauber.—1st ed.

p. cm.

ISBN 0–7216–8437–8

1. Medicine, Preventive.   2. Patient education. I. Lauber, Alison. II. Title.

RA427.L33   2001

615.5′071—dc21   00–066126

Editor-in-Chief: Andrew M. Allen
Editor, Health-Related Professions: Shirley A. Kuhn
Senior Editorial Assistant: Katherine A. Macciocca
Manuscript Editor: Jeffrey L. Scheib
Illustration Specialist: John S. Needles, Jr.
Book Designer: Steven Stave

PATIENT EDUCATION AND
PREVENTIVE MEDICINE   ISBN 0–7216–8437–8

Printed in the United States of America.

Last digit is the print number: 9   8   7   6   5   4   3   2   1

I would like to dedicate this book to my wife Louise, who provided me with much needed support during this project. This is also for Brox and Elise, and the future generation of which you are a part, to utilize to become happier, healthier people. I would like to thank Frances Hardin with her help in transcription.

James Brox Labus

Special thanks to my husband, Eric, and my boys, Cameron and Spencer, for all their help and support throughout this project. I would also like to thank my extended "family," especially my mom for proofreading and my co-workers at Emory University, especially Yan, Anne, and Patience. Without all your efforts, I would be lost.

Alison Ann Lauber

"*Here is Edward Bear, coming downstairs now, Bump, Bump, Bump, on the back of his head, behind Christopher Robin. It is, as far as he knows, the only way of coming downstairs, but sometimes he feels that there really is another way, if only he could stop bumping for a moment and think of it.*"

A. A. Milne
Winnie the Pooh

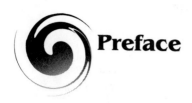 **Preface**

The Purpose of This Book

The purpose of *Patient Education and Preventive Medicine* is to provide a comprehensive reference book to clinicians at all levels of training or clinical practice. Designed both to educate the clinician and to facilitate patient education, the book addresses both general techniques and guidelines for providing effective patient education that will enhance practice style.

For the most part, the role of clinicians in our current system of health care has been primarily defined by the ability to appropriately diagnose, treat, and prevent disease. Professional training programs, which rely on the traditional disease-based education paradigm, often do not adequately address how preventive medicine can be integrated into the clinical practice environment. As a result, many clinicians have not been trained to provide effective patient education and do not approach the patient with prevention strategies in mind.

Patients pose questions regarding their medical condition and care not only to their primary medical caregivers, such as physicians, physician assistants (PAs), and nurse practitioners (NPs), but also to many other traditional and alternative caregivers. Frequently clinicians find themselves in unfamiliar territory, counseling a patient while lacking the skills to effectively communicate about the common treatment plans or to answer basic questions. It is extremely difficult to keep pace with the rapid advances being made in all fields of medicine, especially those outside of one's usual scope of practice.

This text was created to help educate clinicians about the importance of incorporating preventive health messages into all patient encounters. Readers will be provided with reliable information about various conditions commonly encountered in clinical practice, and with practical advice with which they can more effectively educate patients.

Recent literature suggests that understanding the essentials of fostering effective patient-provider communication and being able to provide appropriate patient education messages are paramount to empower patients to assume greater responsibility for their own care.[1] The first chapter, General Preventive Strategies, aims to provide readers with an overview of important concepts and general preventive strategies that can work in any medical or nursing care discipline. Throughout this book, readers will be presented with new knowledge and practice tools that will enable them to make prevention and patient education a more important part of clinical encounters.

1. Post DM, Gegla DJ, Welker MJ, Miser WF. Patient communication training: Implications for physicians. Family Practice Recertification 1999;21:45–58.

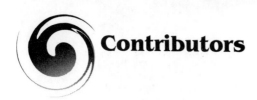

Contributors

Mark Abramson, MD
Assistant Clinical Professor of Family Medicine, University of New Mexico, Albuquerque; Faculty, Southern New Mexico Family Practice Residency Program, Memorial Medical Center, Las Cruces, New Mexico
Nutrition Education in the Clinical Setting

Louise Acheson, MD, MS
Associate Professor of Family Medicine, Assistant Professor of Reproductive Biology, Case Western Reserve University School of Medicine, University Hospitals of Cleveland, Cleveland, Ohio
Clinical Genetics

Jacquelyn B. Admire-Borgelt, MSPH
Assistant Director—Scientific Activities Division, American Academy of Family Physicians, Leawood, Kansas
Safety Precautions In and Around the Home

Joseph J. Altieri, MD
Medical Director, Center for Emotional and Behavioral Health, Vero Beach, Florida
Substance Abuse

Annette Bairan, PhD, RN, CS, FNP
Professor of Nursing, Department of Primary Care Nursing, Kennesaw State University, Kennesaw, Georgia
Bone and Joint Disorders

Sunnie Bell, RN, CDE
Consultant, Southern New Mexico Family Practice Residency Program; Health Education Supervisor, Memorial Medical Center, Las Cruces, New Mexico
Nutrition Education in the Clinical Setting

Larry Borgelt, BS, MS, PE, CSP, SET
Professor Emeritus, School of Fire Protection and
  Safety Engineering Technology, Oklahoma State
  University, Stillwater, Oklahoma; (PE) Registered
  Professional Engineer—Fire Protection (California),
  (SP) Certified Safety Professional, (SET) Senior
  Engineering Technician—Fire Protection
  Safety Precautions In and Around the Home

Kathryn Boyer, MS, PA-C
Assistant Director, Special Medical Education Programs;
  Physician Assistant, Leukemia Department, The
  University of Texas M.D. Anderson Cancer Center,
  Houston, Texas
  Neoplastic Conditions

Carolyn M. Brown, MLS, AHIP
Reference Librarian, Health Sciences Center Library,
  Emory University School of Medicine, Atlanta,
  Georgia
  Resources Appendix

Mary Byam-Smith, MS, PA-C
Physician Assistant, Mainland Family Clinic, Dickinson,
  Texas
  Metabolic Conditions

Amy J. Cofer, PA-C, MMSc
Marietta, Georgia
  Gastrointestinal Disorders; Neurologic Disease

Deborah M. Connor, MDiv
Pastor, Peachtree Presbyterian Church, PCUSA, Atlanta,
  Georgia
  General Preventive Strategies

Frank David Curvin, MD
Fellow, Department of Family and Preventive Medicine,
  Emory University School of Medicine, Atlanta,
  Georgia
  Safety Precautions In and Around the Home

Genie E. Dorman, RN, PhD, CS, FNP
Associate Professor, Department of Primary Care
  Nursing, Kennesaw State University, Kennesaw,
  Georgia
  Gastrointestinal Disorders

Rebecca R. Fehrenbach, MLIS, SLIS
Head of Library Information Center, Robert B.
Greenblatt M.D. Library, Medical College of Georgia,
Augusta, Georgia
Resources Appendix

Mary Fielder, MLS, AHIP
Outreach Librarian, Three Rivers Area Health
Education Center, Columbus, Georgia
Resources Appendix

Francine Fields, MD
Eagle's Landing Family Practice, Atlanta, Georgia
Cultural Influences

Emil J. Freireich, MD, DSc (Hon)
Professor of Medicine, Director, Special Medical
Education Programs, Director of Adult Leukemia
Research Program, The University of Texas M.D.
Anderson Cancer Center, Houston, Texas
Neoplastic Conditions

Kim Gadsden, MS, MPH
Atlanta, Georgia
Epidemiology

Donna Gamero, PA-C
Instructor, Physician Assistant Program, St. Louis
University, St. Louis, Missouri
Men's Health; Infectious Disease

Tomas B. Garcia, MD, FACEP
President, www.heartstuff.com, Miami, Florida
Trauma

James W. Gordon, PA-C, EMT-P, BSM, BBA
Assistant Professor, South College Physician Assistant
Program, Savannah; Midlevel Provider Coordinator,
Emergency Medicine Education Coordinator,
Emergency Care Center, Grady Health System,
Atlanta, Georgia
Trauma

Carol Hamilton, PA-C, EdD
Assistant Professor, Department of Family and
Preventive Medicine, Emory University School of
Medicine, Atlanta, Georgia
Mental Health

Sharne Hampton, MD
Assistant Professor, Emory University School of
Medicine, Atlanta, Georgia
Infectious Disease

Alan M. Harben, MD, PhD, PC
Private Practice, Physical Medicine and Rehabilitation,
Atlanta, Georgia
Exercise

Mark I. Harris, MD
Chief of Staff, Emory Dunwoody Medical Center,
Atlanta, Georgia
Neurologic Disease

Pat Herndon, MLIS
Librarian, Noble Learning Resource Center, Shepherd
Center, Atlanta, Georgia
Resources Appendix

Jennifer Huddleston, PA-C
Minority Women's Health Project Grant Facilitator,
Obstetrics and Gynecology Curriculum Coordinator/
Instructor, Riverside Community College Primary
Care Physician Assistant Program, Moreno Valley,
California
Women's Health

Leslie Irvine, PA-C, MMSc
Atlanta, Georgia
Exercise

Jan LaBeause, MLS, AHIP
Interim Director, Medical Library and Peyton Anderson
Learning Resources Center, Mercer University School
of Medicine, Macon, Georgia
Resources Appendix

James B. Labus, BS, PA-C

Lecturer, Emory University Physician Assistant Program;
President, Mid-Level Medical Services, Atlanta,
Georgia
General Preventive Strategies; Neurologic Disease

Lyle W. Larson, PhD, PA-C

Chief Physician Assistant, Division of Cardiothoracic
Surgery, University of Washington Medical Center,
Seattle, Washington
Cardiology

Alison Ann Lauber, MD

Director of Clinical Operations; Medical Director,
Physician Assistant Program; Director of Procedural
Education Center, Department of Family and
Preventive Medicine, Emory University School of
Medicine, Atlanta, Georgia
*General Preventive Strategies; Geriatrics; Women's Health; Gastrointestinal
Disorders; Infectious Disease*

Erin Fitzpatrick Lepp, PA-C, CDE, MMSc

Advanced Didactic Coordinator, Physician Assistant
Program, Department of Family and Preventive
Medicine, Emory University School of Medicine,
Atlanta, Georgia
General Preventive Strategies

Charles C. Lewis, MPH, PA-C

Assistant Professor, Health Professions Division,
Physician Assistant Program, Nova Southeastern
University, Ft. Lauderdale, Florida
*Environmental Health and Sanitation; Health Planning and
Illness Prevention for International Travel*

Joyce Lewis, MD

Clinical Assistant Professor, Department of Family and
Preventive Medicine, Emory University School of
Medicine, Atlanta, Georgia
Alternative Medicine

Gerónimo Lluberas, MD, FACP

Associate Professor, College of Health and Human
Services, Kennesaw State University, Kennesaw,
Georgia
Bone and Joint Disorders

Lee Lu, MD

Assistant Professor, Baylor College of Medicine; Prime Care Staff, Veterans Affairs Medical Center, Houston, Texas
Metabolic Conditions

Lee R. McCarley, MLIS, AHIP

Systems Librarian, Medical Library and Peyton Anderson Learning Resources Center, Mercer University School of Medicine, Macon, Georgia
Resources Appendix

Charles E. McManus, MPH, RS

Registered Sanitarian, National Environmental Health Association; District Emergency Preparedness Coordinator, District Environmental Health Support Manager, Palmetto Health District, South Carolina Department of Health and Environmental Control, Columbia, South Carolina
Environmental Health and Sanitation

Heidi R. Meyer, MSN, C-FNP, CNRN

Adjunct Faculty–Preceptor, Emory University; Nurse Practitioner, Georgia Neurology Associates, Atlanta, Georgia
Neurologic Disease

Major William A. Mosier, EdD, PA-C, USAFR

Assistant Professor of Health Care Sciences, Associate Director of Academic Curriculum (PA Program), Department of Health Care Sciences, George Washington University School of Medicine and Health Sciences, Washington, DC; Major, United States Air Force (Reserve)
Substance Abuse

Betty R. Nally, RN, MN, CS, ANP

Clinical Supervisor for Collaborative Solutions by Evercare, Atlanta, Georgia
Bone and Joint Disorders

Roxanne M. Nelson, RN, MSLIS

Head of Public Services, Medical Library and Peyton Anderson Learning Resources Center, Mercer University School of Medicine, Macon, Georgia
Resources Appendix

Bich Nguyen, MD
Assistant Clinical Professor, University of Texas Medical
  Branch, University of Texas Medical School of
  Galveston, Galveston; Internist, Mainland Columbia
  Hospital, Texas City, Texas
  Metabolic Conditions

O. Michael Obiekwe, MD
Resident, Department of Family and Preventive
  Medicine, Emory University School of Medicine,
  Atlanta, Georgia; Fellow of the International College
  of Surgeons; Fellow of the West African College of
  Surgeons; Member, Nigerian Urological Association;
  Former Faculty Member, Nnamdi Azikiwe University
  Teaching Hospital, Nnewi, Anambra State, Nigeria
  Men's Health

Christopher A. Ohl, MD, FACP
Assistant Professor of Medicine, Infectious Diseases
  Section, Department of Medicine, Wake Forest
  University School of Medicine; Medical Director,
  Center for Antimicrobial Utilization, Stewardship, and
  Epidemiology, Wake Forest University Baptist
  Medical Center, Winston-Salem, North Carolina
  Health Planning and Illness Prevention for International Travel

Emmanuella Paul, MD
Private Practice, Stone Mountain, Georgia
  Domestic Violence

Pamela L. Plotner, MD
Lecturer, Course Developer, Physician Assistant
  Program, Department of Family Medicine, Baylor
  College of Medicine; Fellow, Medical Genetics,
  Department of Pediatrics, Division of Medical
  Genetics, The University of Texas Houston Medical
  School, Houston, Texas
  Metabolic Conditions

Beth C. Poisson, MSLS
Branch Librarian, Multi-Media Center, Morehouse
  School of Medicine, Atlanta, Georgia
  Resources Appendix

Susan Root, MD, MPH
Assistant Professor, Department of Pediatrics, University
of New Mexico School of Medicine, Albuquerque,
New Mexico
Clinical Genetics

Annette J. Sheppard, MLIS
Health Sciences Librarian, Candler Campus of the St.
Joseph's-Candler Health System, Savannah, Georgia
Resources Appendix

Fred Shessel, MD, FACS
Chair, Department of Surgery, Medical Director,
Urodiagnostic Laboratory, Northside Hospital, Atlanta,
Georgia
Men's Health

Lisa P. Smith, MLS
Outreach Librarian, Magnolia Coastlands Area Health
Education Center, Statesboro, Georgia
Resources Appendix

Rita B. Smith, MLIS
Rural Health Information Clearinghouse (RHIC)
Librarian, Medical Library and Peyton Anderson
Learning Resources Center, Mercer University School
of Medicine, Macon, Georgia
Resources Appendix

Sandra A. Smith, MPH
Clinical Faculty, University of Washington School of
Public Health and Community Medicine, Health
Services Department; Health Education Specialist,
University of Washington Center for Health
Education and Research, Seattle, Washington
Patient Education and Literacy

Troy Spicer, RN, MS, CS, FNP
Assistant Professor, Department of Primary Care
Nursing, Kennesaw State University, Kennesaw,
Georgia
Gastrointestinal Disorders

Linda C. Summers, FNP, MA, MSN
Assistant Clinical Professor of Behavioral Science,
University of New Mexico, Albuquerque; Behavioral

Science Faculty, Southern New Mexico Family
Practice Residency Program, Memorial Medical
Center, Las Cruces, New Mexico
Nutrition Education in the Clinical Setting

Barbara Supanich, RSM, MD

Associate Professor, Family Practice, Michigan State
University/Munson Family Practice Residency; Chair,
Ethics Committee, Munson Medical Center, Michigan
State University/Munson Family Practice Residency,
Traverse City, Michigan
Immunizations

Bradley T. Thomason, PhD

Center for HIV–AIDS Educational Studies and
Training, New York, New York
Mental Health

Kathy Torrente, MLS, AHIP

Head of Reference and Instructional Services, Health
Sciences Center Library, Emory University School of
Medicine, Atlanta, Georgia
Resources Appendix

Carl V. Tyler, Jr., MD

Clinical Assistant Professor of Family Medicine,
Department of Family Medicine, Case Western
Reserve University School of Medicine; Coordinator
of Geriatric Education, Fairview Family Practice
Residency, Fairview Hospital/Cleveland Clinic Health
System, Cleveland, Ohio
Clinical Genetics

Valerie Van Dam, LCSW

Jewish Community Services, Atlanta, Georgia
Domestic Violence

Linda Venis, AS

Library Services Manager, Kennestone Hospital Health
Sciences Library and Cobb Hospital Medical Library,
WellStar Health System, Marietta, Georgia
Resources Appendix

Dorothy White, MD

Private Practice, Atlanta, Georgia
Domestic Violence

Mia Sohn White, MILS, AHIP
Reference Librarian, Health Sciences Center Library,
    Emory University School of Medicine, Atlanta,
    Georgia
    Resources Appendix

Joseph S. Wilson, Jr., MD
Director, Cardiac Catheterization Laboratory, Northside
    Hospital; Cardiology Staff, St. Joseph Hospital,
    Atlanta, Georgia
    Cardiology

Cathy Woolbright, MS/LIS
Director, Simon Schwob Medical Library, Columbus
    Regional Healthcare System, Columbus, Georgia
    Resources Appendix

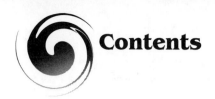

Contents

PART I
General Preventive Strategies 1

CHAPTER 1
General Preventive Strategies 2
James B. Labus, BS, PA-C, Alison Ann Lauber, MD,
Erin Fitzpatrick Lepp, PA-C, CDE, MMSc, and Deborah M.
Conner, MDiv

CHAPTER 2
Alternative Medicine 23
Joyce Lewis, MD

CHAPTER 3
Cultural Influences 46
Francine Fields, MD

CHAPTER 4
Domestic Violence 67
Emmanuella Paul, MD,
Dorothy White, MD,
and Valerie Van Dam, LCSW

CHAPTER 5
Environmental Health and Sanitation 80
Charles C. Lewis, MPH, PA-C,
and Charles E. McManus, MPH, RS

CHAPTER 6
Epidemiology 115
Kim Gadsden, MS, MPH

CHAPTER 7
Exercise 146
Leslie Irvine, PA-C, MMSc, and Alan M. Harben, MD, PhD, PC

CHAPTER 8
Clinical Genetics   163
Louise Acheson, MD, MS, Susan Root, MD, MPH, and Carl V. Tyler, Jr., MD

CHAPTER 9
Geriatrics   190
Alison Ann Lauber, MD

CHAPTER 10
Safety Precautions In and Around the Home   217
Jacquelyn B. Admire-Borgelt, MSPH,
Larry Borgelt, BS, MS, PE, CSP, SET,
and Frank David Curvin, MD

CHAPTER 11
Immunizations   239
Barb Supanich, RSM, MD

CHAPTER 12
Patient Education and Literacy   266
Sandra Smith, MPH

CHAPTER 13
Nutrition Education in the Clinical Setting   291
Mark Abramson, MD,
Linda C. Summers, FNP, MA, MSN,
and Sunnie Bell, RN, CDE

CHAPTER 14
Trauma   317
James W. Gordon, PA-C, EMT-P, BSM, BBA,
and Tomas B. Garcia, MD, FACEP

CHAPTER 15
Health Planning and Illness Prevention for International Travel   343
Christopher A. Ohl, MD, FACP,
and Charles C. Lewis, MPH, PA-C

CHAPTER 16
Women's Health   366
Jennifer Huddleston, PA-C, and Alison Ann Lauber, MD

CHAPTER 17
Men's Health   397
*Donna Gamero, PA-C, O. Michael Obiekwe, MD,
and Fred Shessel, MD*

PART II
Clinical Conditions   423

CHAPTER 18
Cardiology   424
Lyle W. Larson, PhD, PA-C, and Joseph S. Wilson, Jr., MD

CHAPTER 19
Bone and Joint Disorders   453
*Gerónimo Lluberas, MD, FACP,
Annette Bairan, PhD, RN, CS, FNP,
and Betty R. Nally, RN, MN, CS, ANP*

CHAPTER 20
Gastrointestinal Disorders   472
*Amy J. Cofer, PA-C, MMSc, Alison Ann Lauber, MD,
Genie E. Dorman, RN, PhD, CS, FNP,
and Troy Spicer, RN, MS, CS, FNP*

CHAPTER 21
Infectious Disease   505
*Donna Gamero, PA-C, Alison Ann Lauber, MD,
and Sharne Hampton, MD*

CHAPTER 22
Mental Health   569
*Carol Hamilton, PA-C, EdD,
and Bradley Thomason, PhD*

CHAPTER 23
Metabolic Conditions   593
*Mary Byam-Smith, MS, PA-C,
Pamela L. Plotner, MD, Lee Lu, MD,
and Bich Nguyen, MD*

CHAPTER 24
Neoplastic Conditions   624
Kathryn Boyer, MS, PA-C,
and Emil J. Freireich, MD, DSc (Hon)

CHAPTER 25
Neurologic Disease   661
Mark I. Harris, MD, James B. Labus, BS, PA-C,
Heidi R. Meyer, MSN, C-FNP, CNRN,
and Amy J. Cofer, PA-C, MMSc

CHAPTER 26
Substance Abuse   693
Major William A. Mosier, EdD, PA-C, USAFR,
and Joseph J. Altieri, MD

Resources Appendix   715
The Consumer Health Committee of the Georgia Health
Sciences Library Association

Index   771

NOTICE

Medicine is an ever-changing field. Standard safety precautions must be followed, but as new research and clinical experience broaden our knowledge, changes in treatment and drug therapy may become necessary or appropriate. Readers are advised to check the most current product information provided by the manufacturer of each drug to be administered to verify the recommended dose, the method and duration of administration, and contraindications. It is the responsibility of the licensed prescriber, relying on experience and knowledge of the patient, to determine dosages and the best treatment for each individual patient. Neither the Publisher nor the editor assumes any liability for any injury and/or damage to persons or property arising from this publication.

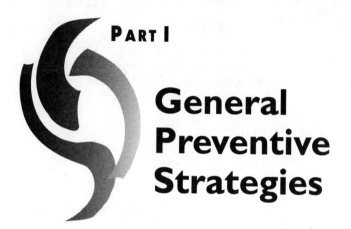

PART I

General Preventive Strategies

CHAPTER 1

General Preventive Strategies

James B. Labus, BS, PA-C,
Alison Ann Lauber, MD,
Erin Fitzpatrick Lepp, PA-C, CDE, MMSc,
and Deborah M. Conner, MDiv

■ INTRODUCTION

Patient education and preventive medicine efforts are means by which clinicians can improve an individual's or an entire community's health. These efforts can be incorporated before, during, or after a disorder has been diagnosed. The ultimate goal is to prevent disease, assure compliance, and promote wellness. The responsibility for behavior change ultimately resides with the patient.

The concept of "empowering" patients has become a "buzzword" of sorts, perhaps brought on by the increased consumerism of health, the availability of health information and products, and the influence of the growing managed care environment. Today, patients and providers alike are expected to be able to maneuver through a health care system that has imposed numerous challenges to traditional continuity of care and placed restrictions on how health care is accessed and utilized. Consider, as examples, patients who are ultimately responsible for ensuring that they have preauthorization for certain tests or treatments and health care providers who are now required to choose from a formulary when selecting certain prescription medications for patients. Bombarded by increased media coverage on health issues, aided by a growing use of the Internet to find health information, and motivated, perhaps, by a certain level of discontent with "traditional" medicine, many patients are, in fact, assuming a more active role in their own health care. All patients should be encouraged to accept a greater role in their own health care, especially because life expectancy and the prevalence of chronic diseases are increasing.

Despite this seemingly greater health consciousness on the part of the public, approximately half of the nearly 700,000 annual deaths due to heart disease, the 500,000 deaths due to cancer, the 140,000 deaths due to stroke, and the 90,000 deaths due to chronic obstructive pulmonary disease remain potentially preventable.[1] Many of these deaths are caused by relatively few modifiable risk factors such as tobacco use, poor diet, and physical inactivity.[2] The morbidity and mortality of certain diseases are disproportionately higher among disadvantaged and minority populations. These groups tend to receive preventive services and counseling at a disproportionately lower rate.[2]

Simple office interventions that help patients take care of themselves can reduce total medical visits by 17% and visits for minor illnesses by 35%. By some estimates, at least 25% of physician office visits are for problems that patients could actually treat themselves.[3]

For many providers, the concepts of preventing disease or preventing complications due to disease may be simpler to grasp than the idea of promoting wellness. One reason for this may be that the medical system has historically focused on providing acute care within a reactive health care paradigm. Today's prevention efforts have changed largely from the traditional public health concerns over which the individual had little personal control (such as having drinkable water) to emphasizing healthy behaviors (such as avoiding tobacco, fatty foods, and a sedentary lifestyle). In the past century, medical historians cite the eradication of smallpox, improved sanitation, and immunization programs resulting in increased longevity as examples of public health successes.[4] Despite the inherent logic found in promoting preventive health measures, much of the medical care delivery and financing systems, provider training, and even patient expectations center on *treating* acute problems or illness rather than *preventing* disease by promoting health.

It was not until the 1970s that health promotion and disease prevention emerged as a national health policy priority.[5] The 1974 Lalonde Report, commissioned by Health Canada to assess priorities for improving the health status of Canadians, called for an integrated health promotion policy. The report also accurately forecast the need for research on how to reduce health risks through modification of health-related behaviors.[6] The Canadian Task Force on Periodic Health Examination Report of 1979 set national priorities for the delivery of clinical preventive services. By systematic review of medical evidence, the report identified those conditions or risk factors that most required or were amenable to preventive interventions.[7] Utilizing an evidence-based decision-making approach to set national priorities for the delivery of clinical preventive services, the report became a template of sorts for the United States Preventive Services Task Force (USPSTF). The recommendations of the USPSTF were first published in 1989, and revised in 1996, as the Guide to Clinical Preventive Services.[8] U.S. national health policy was formalized in 1979–1980 with publication of *Healthy People: The Surgeon General's Report on Health Promotion and Disease Prevention* and *Promoting Health/Preventing Disease: Objectives for the Nation,* which outlined specific national goals for improving national health outcomes by 1990. New objectives to by obtained by the year 2000 came to be known as Healthy People 2000.[9]

In May 1999, the U.S. Surgeon General unveiled Healthy People 2010, the nation's current health care agenda. The goals of Healthy People 2010 are aimed at developing partnerships between public health and private medical caregivers by

* Increasing the longevity and quality of life
* Eliminating health disparities based on race and ethnicity
* Developing community-based partnerships that seek to balance health promotion with efforts to provide universal access to care [www.health.gov/healthypeople/].[10]

Basic clinical knowledge can be employed when beginning a program of patient education and preventive medicine. Patients and health care providers realize that regular exercise, good nutrition, stable family life, spiritual health, stable mental health, and avoidance of excessive stress, alcohol, drugs, tobacco products, or other risky behaviors all contribute to optimal health. However, the means by which these goals are met are much more complex. For instance, depression brought on by an event outside a person's control or due to genetic factors may lead to a feeling of helplessness, poor nutrition, use of tobacco, a sedentary lifestyle, and/or risk-taking behaviors. The results of these behaviors may be disorders such as emphysema, obesity, hypertension, or trauma. By addressing only the results of the behavior, the primary etiologic event may never be addressed. Even when the underlying behavior is addressed by the clinician, it is difficult for patients to initiate and maintain positive or healthier behaviors. Behavioral changes do not necessarily occur immediately.

If prevention is common sense, why is it so difficult to convince patients to adopt healthier lifestyles? If prevention works, why for example, do clinicians fall short of national goals to recommend preventive screening examinations or to counsel patients to stop smoking?[11] Before considering techniques and strategies, keep in mind that no matter how idealistic the intentions of the caregivers and healers, every patient cannot be reached. Patients are, to a large degree, already aware of the health and behavioral changes that need to be made in order to optimize health. The goal of the clinician should be to become a positive influence on patients, to provide education regarding a specific condition or behavioral change that will enhance their health, and to provide patients with the knowledge, attitudes, and skills necessary to improve their quality of life. The ultimate responsibility for personal health resides with the patient; clinicians are but the purveyors of health information and influence.

Patient and societal views must also change. It is not possible to "save life," only to preserve and maximize the potential of the life remaining. Saving life, as coined in the media, denotes an end point after which the clinician is no longer involved. Clinicians must be involved with a patient throughout life to guide healthy behaviors and treat conditions that will inevitably become manifest.

▬▬ UNDERSTANDING PREVENTION

Prevention consists of three types, primary, secondary, and tertiary. Primary prevention encompasses efforts to prevent the initial onset of a condition in those at risk for a disease or illness (e.g., childhood immunization programs). Secondary prevention refers to efforts to identify known risk factors for a disease and to use those efforts to halt or delay progression of an active condition (e.g., an annual Papanicolaou test [Pap smear] to screen for cervical cancer). Even among patients at whom secondary preventive efforts are aimed, primary prevention is also important to revisit as new conditions and issues develop. Tertiary prevention should be included in patient education messages and can be thought of as efforts to "optimize" a patient's health and function once disease is already present (e.g., a cardiac rehabilitation program designed to prevent a second heart attack and restore a patient's level of function).[12]

Five tenets of patient management lend themselves well to the initial discussion of preventive medicine strategies:

* Managing terminal disease
* Maintaining chronic disease
* Diagnosing and treating new (active) disease
* Preventing potential disease
* Improving overall health

Although health care providers are encouraged to identify and discuss risk factors for potential disease with patients, most are consumed by the urgent requirements of secondary prevention and tertiary prevention or active treatment.

MANAGING TERMINAL DISEASE

Terminal disease obviously does not lend itself well to long-term preventive strategies. At this point it is not possible to "save life." Therefore, improving the quality of the remaining life takes precedence. Comfort measures, emotional health, and advanced directives should become the focus. Improved pain management benefits patients, families, and society as a whole. Three decades of research document the inadequacy of pain management. A patient's predicament arising from undermedication for pain is more likely to lead to addiction than is appropriate pain management in terminal, acute, and chronic pain disorder patients.

Realistic expectations based on the patient's understanding should be encouraged. Unresolved issues should be addressed among the patient and the family to avoid unrealistic efforts or guilt at life's end.

MAINTAINING CHRONIC DISEASE

Health care professionals are most likely to encounter patients who seek treatment for a new problem or who are regular users of the health care system because of chronic disease. In these instances, secondary prevention becomes the overriding concern for the provider. Disorders such as asthma, diabetes mellitus, and hypertension need to be efficiently maintained in order to prevent complications. During visits with these patients it is important to periodically revisit the initial history to determine whether there are any additional contributing factors that may worsen the chronic disorder, to identify new behaviors that can be modified, to screen for other potential diseases, and to provide the patient with appropriate health promotion messages.

DIAGNOSING AND TREATING NEW (ACTIVE) DISEASE

A new diagnosis may be reached as a result of screening, history of risk, subjective symptoms, or physical examination. Conditions that are transient may respond well to initial treatment. These situations may require patient education to prevent recurrence or avoid complications. Some conditions, although newly diagnosed, are life-long and will require regular patient follow-up. Secondary and tertiary preventive counseling is important at this stage as well.

PREVENTING POTENTIAL DISEASE

Each patient encounter provides the setting to evaluate potential risk. Even in the tertiary care setting, new and pertinent information can be elicited from the patient that may have a significant impact on his or her health. The patient's comprehensive history should include a listing of past medical/surgical problems, a review of systems, a list of allergies and current medications, and a family and social history. In addition to these "standard" topics, it is also important to ascertain life satisfaction, social support network, educational level, occupation, and spiritual support. Also important is an assessment of behaviors (e.g., tobacco, alcohol, and drug use), nutrition, sexual identity or lifestyle, and exercise habits. Such an all-encompassing approach helps the clinician to view the patient as a total person in order to customize treatment and effectively address health issues. In an effort to increase efficiency, a comprehensive checklist may be used initially. However, additional open-ended questioning may be necessary if the patient does not appear to be completely forthcoming or does not seem to understand the importance of the questions, or if there is little established rapport between the provider and the patient. Although complete physical examinations on otherwise healthy individuals have been routinely performed as part of a "comprehensive screening," the existing medical literature does not support this practice. Instead, a periodic health examination tailored to the age, sex, and individual health risks of each patient is recommended. These focused examinations are more time-efficient for the patient for the patient and provider alike.[13, 15]

IMPROVING OVERALL HEALTH

Health promotion, defined by O'Donnell as "the science and art of helping people change their lifestyle to move toward a state of optimal health,"[14] is a goal to which all primary health care practices should aspire. Improving health in an otherwise healthy individual has not traditionally been the focus of modern medicine. Instead, this task has been deferred to the mass media, an ever-expanding Internet, fitness operations, athletic coaches and trainers, alternative medicine providers, health educators, school teachers, and nutritional supplement manufacturers, to name a few. Although these various sources of health information may be well-intentioned, false or conflicting information may be disseminated to the unsuspecting patient and health consumer. Ulterior motives, such as improved ratings for a news program on a tantalizing health topic, can make information less than objective. According to the U.S. Public Health Service, "Health promotion seeks the development of community and individual means which can help to develop lifestyles that can maintain and enhance the state of well being." With this in mind, health care providers should become involved in community-based programs and work wherever possible to "educate the educators." Any individual who rarely utilizes the traditional health care system many only be reached by such outreach programs. Community involvement of a family medicine practice, for example, has been shown to increase rates of utilization of preventive services. Such services included Pap smears, mammography, and childhood immunizations. In addition to utilization of preventive services, an increased number of patients took steps to stop smoking, and improvements were measured in glycosylated hemoglobin levels among the community's diabetic patient population.[15]

■■■WELLNESS

Health and wellness have been defined in a variety of ways. The World Health Organization (WHO) definition of health as "physical, mental, and social well-being, not merely the absence of disease or infirmity,"[4] seems congruent to the six "dimensions" of wellness that have been proposed by the National Wellness Institute. These aspects of wellness include
1. Physical
2. Emotional

3. Social
4. Intellectual
5. Occupational
6. Spiritual[16]

Promotion of health means, at a minimum, facilitating the maintenance of a person's current position on a spectrum of optimal health.
Ideally, all should work toward advancing the goal of optimal health.
Both behavior and social networks are increasingly recognized as being
related to health.[4] Some wellness guidelines to incorporate into patient
encounters include:

* Actively choose life-enhancing attitudes (rather than passively re-
  acting to external circumstances).
* Live primarily in the present (avoid excessive dwelling on the past
  or anxiously anticipating the future).
* Observe one's thoughts, attitudes, and actions, modifying them as
  necessary.
* Avoid fear-related states such as anger, guilt, resentment, and anxiety.
* Give freely from a sense of abundance (including money, time,
  or talent).
* Recognize and draw support from one's connection to others, to
  nature, and to whatever higher power in whom one believes.

Physical health is the focus of traditional medicine. Focusing on
the physical dimension of wellness at the expense of the others is both
incomplete and potentially counterproductive. A patient's *emotional
health* (mental health) is often overlooked during a typical office visit.
Depression, anger, and/or organic mental illness significantly affect
health behaviors of patients and influence patient/provider interaction
(see Chapter 22, Mental Health).

The social dimension of wellness, or *social health,* can be divided
into two separate categories, individual and societal. Individual social
behavior is an area that needs to be addressed by the clinician as a
means to assess total health. Is the patient satisfied or withdrawn? Is
there a support network of family and friends? Obviously, social health
is intertwined with mental health, but it also differs from mental
health in that it is a measure of an individual's function within the
external structure of society. Societal health refers to the absence of
war and to sound environmental and public health policies and public
safety. These are areas outside an individual's control, but they may
significantly affect individual and societal health. Media influences
that promote unhealthy behaviors include tobacco advertising and
glamorization of alcohol or casual sex, which may directly or indirectly
promote cancer, liver disease, unwanted pregnancy, and sexually transmitted diseases. Society, government, and municipalities are also responsible for health. Correctly motivated, these institutions can have
a tremendous positive impact on societal and individual health. For

example, when the state of Oregon increased taxes on cigarettes and earmarked proceeds for smoking prevention programs, the result was a decline in cigarette consumption at approximately eight times the rate of the decline in the general U.S. population.[17] Interventions targeted at school-age children have been shown to have long-term positive effects on dietary and physical activity behaviors.[18]

Intellectual health is arguably more important in today's society than it was in the past. Much of occupational success in the modern era hinges on intellectual ability. Routine activities require a rudimentary computer literacy. The basics of reading and writing are often taken for granted. Many patients hide illiteracy or low literacy skills from health care providers. Organic problems such as dyslexia can be identified and treated in order to make life more enjoyable for the patient. To a large degree, an individual's self-respect, identity, and interaction with others are governed by his or her occupation. Certain professions command more respect by the community at large. In addition, there is a higher age-adjusted mortality rate for those with lower levels of education (2.4 times higher in those with less than 12 years of education compared with those with 13 or more years of education).[19]

Occupational health can also be thought of as economic health. Economic security or the lack thereof can affect health. This is especially true when a patient is confronted with an unexpected and potentially costly medical condition. A patient's occupation can also be the source of poor health. Coal miners, police officers, firefighters, health care workers, and others who work in high-risk jobs can develop health concerns as a direct result of their chosen occupation.

Spiritual health is important in that it gives the individual a sense of purpose in life. People often compartmentalize their lives into "work," "family," and "faith," as if they could separate themselves into discrete parts. Spirituality is concerned with faith and a belief in things that are unseen. When a person is hospitalized, "illness" may become another compartment. However, the whole person enters into every situation in life. Thus, illness provides another opportunity to integrate the spiritual part of a patient's life into the clinical experience. Questions of mortality may naturally lead into issues of faith. To some patients, faith issues are more important than mere medical issues. This is especially true in patients facing terminal illness. Discussing a patient's feelings regarding spirituality or faith can strengthen the patient/provider bond. Patients, overall, welcome an inquiry regarding spiritual matters from their physicians.[20] In recent years, there has been a greater acknowledgment by the medical community of the restorative and healing power of faith. Belief in something greater than human capacity affects the emotions, the will, and the body. A person with faith or belief in something greater than the self may do better both emotionally and physically in the clinical setting than a patient without such a belief. Faith is a great comfort in the midst of the chaos that illness creates in a person's life. Healing involves more than successful surgery or prescribed medication. It is more than following a specific protocol in a specific order. Healing may defy predicted outcomes. Belief can be as powerful as medicine in creating a healing environment.

Attempts have been made to scientifically measure the benefits of intercessory (third party) prayer and have shown positive results.[21, 22] However, the existence of a higher power cannot be proved. In fact, if scientific proof existed, one would have knowledge rather than faith. "Faith is knowing in your heart what the mind cannot know."[23] Significant strength in any of the other five dimensions of wellness can adversely affect one or more of the other dimensions. The spiritual dimension is probably the only one that will strengthen the other five.

Hospital and private chaplains, pastoral counselors, ministers, rabbis, and priests are an integral part of the health and wellness care team. It is important for the clinician to validate their work and to include them in care whenever agreeable to the patient. Equally, however, illness should not be a time for the caring clinician to proselytize or attempt to "convert" a patient but rather to support the patient's chosen faith.

RATIONALE AND BARRIERS FOR PATIENT EDUCATION

The rationale for providing patient education may be more closely related to personal theories of how medicine should be practiced than to the reality of the current health care system. Empathy for patients, a desire to view the patient as a whole person rather than as a disease, and the desire to make a difference in a person's life may be all that some providers require to allocate time for preventive efforts or patient education. This empathy may be the reason for choosing a career in health care. Other clinicians may require evidence of lives "saved" or specific tools to help them make prevention a part of clinical practice. Primary motivators for physicians providing preventive services are more connected to perceived self-efficacy and effectiveness than to a concern for time and reimbursement.[24] Often, however, the content of the patient education is based on the provider's feelings of necessity rather than on the patient's perception of need.[25] Much of the frustration in medicine today stems from the fact that there is invariably less time to spend with patients. Some providers complain that this equates to a decreased ability to practice "good medicine." Reality often obstructs the idealistic view of health care. Consider, for example, that when a health care provider earns a good reputation for caring for patients and spending time with them, patient load increases. As patient load increases, there is less time to spend with each patient. Demands of managed care require increased productivity. The length of visits dictated by a health maintenance organization may be shorter than traditional visits. Patients value preventive services, but demands for increased productivity may compromise these efforts.[26] Justification of care and demands for documentation also cut into time spent with patients. Corporatization of medical practices has turned many clinicians into employees with less independence. Balancing obligatory constraints and patient desires can strain a provider's resources.

TIME COMMITMENT

A provider's opinions and advice are valued by patients. Patient education can be quite time consuming, especially when dealing with the patient who has unlimited time available or has either limited education and/or limited understanding. However, it is important to build rapport with patients. The adage, "To a patient it does not matter how much you know until he knows how much you care," is certainly true. Because many managed care plan patients often switch primary care provider panels, there may be less opportunity for the serial visits that in the past have allowed for rapport to build. While additional time spent with a patient may not always be directly reimbursable, the realization that there has been a positive impact on a patient's life will offset any direct lack of monetary gain.

TRADITIONAL AND ALTERNATIVE MEDICINE KNOWLEDGE BASE

Patients have high expectations for the knowledge base of their health care provider. With the amount of information that is now available to both patients and providers, meeting these expectations often seems impossible. Knowing the details of an experimental surgical therapy for a rare disorder or the latest alternative therapy is not an efficient use of most providers' limited time. Instead, develop a resource list of organizations, pharmaceutical companies, support groups, reputable web sites, and patient education CD-ROMs to which the patient can be referred for additional information and self-directed education.

FOLLOW-UP

Having mechanisms in place that help to follow up patient comprehension and compliance is important for overall patient care. Revisit issues previously discussed and determine the patient's long-term comprehension of the education efforts. The patient may not have been able to grasp the concept of the educational effort at the first visit, or new questions may have arisen in the interim.

Charting the educational strategies provided at a visit will help recollection on subsequent visits. A staff member can provide telephone follow-up to note progression of behavioral changes and provide redirection. Attempt to obtain realistic information from patients and involve them in setting goals. Work to develop a partnership rather than "parent" the patient. Create a database to document what is effective. If one can be flexible and fluid with strategies, frustrations will decrease while practice satisfaction will increase.

UNDERSTANDING THE IMPORTANCE OF IDENTIFYING RISK FACTORS

A complete, formal risk assessment in clinical practice offers a way to gather important information about a patient's risk factors. However, reliance on an "illness-based thinking process," in an effort to gather information to explain the patient's current symptoms, frequently results in an incomplete risk assessment of limited usefulness for preventive care.[5] Helping patients explore their personal health-related behaviors and identify risk is an important component in the patient education process. However, one barrier to effective preventive screening and risk assessment is confusion among providers as to which screening tests to recommend to patients. The establishment of the Agency for Healthcare Research and Quality (AHRQ) and National Guideline Clearinghouse (www.guideline.gov) in December 1999 was an attempt to provide providers and patients alike with the ability to compare preventive screening guidelines and preventive care recommendations made by various medical specialty societies, government agencies, and private health care organizations.

Another tool that may help clinicians to perform patient risk assessments more adequately is the Health Risk Appraisal (HRA). Initially introduced in the 1970s for use in clinical settings as a means to collect individual epidemiologically-based risk data from which to make a risk prediction for future illness, the HRA is now widely available through numerous commercial vendors. The HRA is utilized by large practice groups and managed care organizations, who often have contractual responsibilities to provide preventive care, to monitor the effectiveness of health promotion programs and products.[5]

UNDERSTANDING THE THEORY OF BEHAVIOR CHANGE

Most physicians (and this likely applies to other providers as well) have traditionally seen their role primarily as a diagnostician or treatment provider and not as a health educator.[27] However, clinicians may spend up to 25% of their time giving information and counseling patients.[28] Although the history collected contributes 60–80% of the data needed to make a diagnosis,[29–31] an important function of the medical interview is to carry out patient education and to implement appropriate treatment plans. Unfortunately, education or information-giving is the most overlooked and inadequately performed function of the time spent with patients.

The goal of patient education is to change behavior.[32] Although health education research has demonstrated that patients will change unhealthy behaviors such as smoking if they are specifically instructed to do so by their health care provider,[33] many clinicians have not been formally taught how to communicate effectively with patients and may lack the knowledge or self-confidence needed to teach patients how to change health behaviors.[34] Health behavior theory is frequently not included in medical school curricula, and a recent survey of physician assistant educational programs reported similar findings.[35]

Health behavior theories can be viewed as a set of basic professional tools that health care providers use in their roles as health educators. These tools can be applied to practice situations in much the same way as other tools of medicine, such as a microscope. Just as medical students first learning to work with a microscope receive an explanation of its purpose, use, and care, look through the lens, and begin focusing on familiar objects, practitioners need to learn about health behavior theories and their use as professional tools.[36]

Perhaps the most effective means of promoting health is convincing patients to change personal behaviors. But this cannot be accomplished if the patient lacks the motivation to change or has insufficient resources and support to change. Voluntarily changing health behavior is difficult.[37] Although providing good patient education requires the clinician to possess a thorough knowledge of the subject, the health care provider must also address the patient's readiness and motivation to learn. Additional factors that contribute to patient education include the patient's ability to learn (which may correlate to educational level), need to learn, age, economic status, and level of self-confidence.[38, 39] Recognizing these factors is only part of a health education strategy. Clinicians should have a working knowledge of some of the most widely utilized concepts of health promotion and patient education theory. Knowledge of these concepts may help the clinician to better understand why patients resist adopting patient education plans and may help him or her to work more effectively with patients to successfully facilitate change.

Although a complete overview of the most widely utilized theories relating to health behavior is beyond the scope of this book, a few key concepts and models deserve mention. First is the Health Belief Model (HBM). Originally developed in the 1950s in an effort to understand why people would participate in preventive health programs, the HBM has been expanded to encompass several key concepts with which the clinician should be familiar. These include perceived susceptibility, perceived severity, perceived benefits, and perceived barriers.[40]

* *Perceived susceptibility:* Patients will likely take action to prevent, screen for, or control a disease if they believe they are susceptible to the condition.
* *Perceived severity:* Patients are likely to take action to improve their health if they perceive the illness or condition has potentially serious consequences.
* *Perceived benefits:* Patients are likely to take steps if they believe in the efficacy of the advised action to reduce the risk or seriousness of the impact of the disease process.
* *Perceived barriers:* Patients are likely to take action as long as they believe that the potential costs or other negative barriers are outweighed by the benefits of doing so.

Perhaps the most important element of the HBM is the concept of *self-efficacy*, which can be defined as the belief that an individual can carry out a health behavior necessary to reach a desired goal.[41] This concept of self-efficacy plays a significant role in helping patients adopt new, healthier lifestyles and behaviors.

Another important health behavior theory clinicians should recognize is the Transtheoretical Model or Stages of Change Theory. Developed in 1983 as a study in participation in a smoking cessation program.[42] The Stages of Change Theory has been applied to a wide range of health behaviors, including alcohol and substance abuse, eating disorders and obesity, HIV/AIDS prevention, and the use of preventive health screening examinations, among other areas. Consisting of six discrete "stages" or steps, the theory uses the analogy of a revolving door to describe how patients often work through various phases of understanding their health problem, making a conscious effort to change, maintaining the new health behavior, and sometimes relapsing back to certain behavioral stages. At each stage, a patient has specific learning needs that, in turn, require an appropriate, stage-specific approach toward counseling and motivation. Visualize the picture of a patient leaving the office's revolving lobby door as you read through a description of each behavioral stage.[43]

1. *Precontemplation:* The patient is unaware of the health problem and may be either uninformed or underinformed of the consequences of his/her health behaviors. Generally, the patient has no intention of changing the unhealthy behavior in the foreseeable future (e.g., within the next 6 months), although he/she may have previously tried to change and failed. Providers tend to label their precontemplative patients as "noncompliant" or "unmotivated" when, in fact, most pre-existing health promotion programs target

individuals who have progressed further along the continuum of readiness for change and who are actually "ready for action."

2. *Contemplation:* Patients develop an awareness of the health behavior and have intentions of changing (usually within the next 6 months). Patients are more aware of the difficulties they will face when they change, which may lead to procrastination.

3. *Preparation* (also referred to as the "Ready for Action" stage): Patients begin to experiment with change and typically make a plan such as buying a self-help book, joining a health club, or talking to their health care provider. They are ready and willing to participate in action-oriented programs such as group smoking cessation programs or exercise classes.

4. *Action:* This stage includes patients who have made specific behavior modifications in the past 6 months. However, these actions must be measured by acceptable measures of risk reduction. For example, among smokers, those truly in the action stage are those who are abstaining altogether from cigarettes and would not include those who are "smoking less than I used to." Taking such action, in turn, creates a sense of pride in their accomplishment and empowers patients to continue their efforts.

5. *Maintenance:* In this stage, patients integrate the new, healthier behaviors into their daily routines and typically need assistance developing coping skills that will help to avoid relapse. Researchers estimate that this stage may last anywhere from 6 months to 5 years.

6. *Termination:* The final stage in the original model may be relevant for those behaviors where patients have been successful in avoiding temptation and have no concerns of relapsing. In this stage, despite feeling bored, depressed, or otherwise emotionally stressed, patients do not return to previously unhealthy habits. However, this stage of change cannot readily be applied to health behaviors such as following cancer screening recommendations for cervical cancer and mammography or modifying dietary fat intake because these behaviors must be on-going. Typically, patients and providers alike view relapse as a failure—either failure of the patient to be "compliant" or on the part of the clinician to "convince" the patient to do what is asked of them. According to the Stages of Change model; however, relapse can be viewed as a valuable and expected learning experience.

For example, when faced with the challenge of trying to convince a 20-year-old female to stop smoking or a 55-year male executive to incorporate exercise into his daily routine, first attempt to determine the patient's stage of change. Then target the educational intervention to the patient's specific needs within the framework of his or her particular stage of change.

One method of providing patient education and counseling is a three-part patient-centered framework that incorporates the Stages of Change model. A few key, "trigger" open-ended questions are recommended at both the first patient visit and all subsequent follow-up visits to ensure that the provider is assessing the appropriate stage and tailoring the intervention and health education messages according to the patient's need for knowledge, skills, and support. According to this approach, five specific levels in the patient education and counseling process can be identified: cognitive, attitudinal, instrumental, coping behaviors and social support.[44]

1. *Cognitive:* Patients must gain an awareness of the health problem and increase their knowledge of it in order to understand key concepts. To enable patients to do this, clinicians can offer nondirected readings or patient education handouts, or allow the patient to listen to audio tapes or watch a videotape on the topic.

2. *Attitudinal:* The health care provider must be aware of and clarify any beliefs and/or concerns the patient has, should attempt to understand the patient's motivations for keeping the behavior, and must assess the patient's readiness to change. The provider must also attempt to build on a patient's initial commitment to change through the use of discussion, negotiation, or confrontation.

3. *Instrumental:* At this level patients must learn new skills that are necessary to effectively manage their health problem, for example, learning how to use a peak flow meter or how to perform home glucose monitoring. Health care providers should demonstrate these skills to the patient and provide on-going opportunities for the patient to practice and demonstrate competency in using these skills or devices.

4. *Coping Behavior:* Patients must learn to incorporate new behaviors into their daily lives by using or creating incentives or reminders for themselves. Health care providers can support these efforts as well.

5. *Social Support:* Patients must be encouraged and assisted to identify sources of support (friends, family members, or support groups) that are capable of providing feedback and encouragement.

According to this framework, there are specific ways to frame patient education messages at each stage in the Transtheoretical Model. At the first patient encounter, the role of the clinician is to help move the patient from the Precontemplation to the Action stage. For this movement to occur, the health care provider must try to raise the patient's own awareness of the unhealthy behavior, define the problem in terms the patient can understand, induce the patient to agree that a problem exists, enlist the patient to make a commitment to change, and negotiate a trial intervention. Certainly no small task!

In order to move a patient along the readiness-for-change continuum from Action to Maintenance, the health care provider should ask the patient to repeat or summarize the main points of the agreed-upon plan. The provider and the patient should set up a return visit date that is far enough in the future as to give the patient sufficient time for trial and error, yet not too far in the future that the patient will be unable to receive important feedback or will become too frustrated in the event of "failure." At follow-up visits, patients may still need to focus on increasing their knowledge or coping skills but should be moving into the Maintenance stage of change. During these visits, the health care provider should be sure to discuss important coping strategies and address how to avoid relapses. The first goal should be to build on patients' skills and enhance their ability to maintain the new behaviors. Asking open-ended questions such as, "Tell me what has happened with your diet plan and goal to lose 10 pounds since our last visit?" encourages the patients to share their successes and allows them to also discuss what has not worked for them. Having this clear understanding of what is and is not working for the patient will allow the health care provider to negotiate new plans with the patient that can be better tailored to the patient's specific situation. The health care providers should spend time helping the patient anticipate problems that might arise within the treatment plan and talk through possible solutions or actions the patient can take if a problem develops. This type of shared decision making increases the patient's ability to cope with his or her disease or health problem and also fosters in the patient a sense of autonomy and increased skill in self-managing the illness.

Another important point to cover with patients at follow-up visits is what the patient can do to prevent relapse or to cope with relapse if it occurs. For example, asking, "Until we meet next month, what will you do for exercise if it is too cold to walk around your neighborhood as you have been doing?" may help the patient to view a setback as temporary and "fixable" and not as a reason to abandon his or her efforts entirely.

Perhaps it is most important to remember that behavior change is a long-term process that requires significant effort on the part of both the health care provider and the patient, increasing the patient's self-confidence that the changes suggested can be successfully made. The clinician's role is not to "fix" everything or provide patients with solutions to every conceivable setback, but to gently support the patient's efforts to become increasingly successful in terms of modifying habits. Support for the patient's efforts has, in turn, been shown to provide patients with a sense of empowerment that ultimately allows them to tackle future health problems with increased confidence. Clinician efforts to become expert patient educators also take time, energy, and commitment.

TARGET THE MESSAGE

A key concept in the patient education process is the ability to adapt health messages to the patient audience. Teaching the adult patient differs from teaching an adolescent or a child. Adult learning theory can easily be applied to the tasks of health educators and clinicians. These tasks include:[45]

* Helping patients diagnose their needs for learning within a clinical setting
* Planning with the patient a sequence of learning experiences that will produce a desired outcome
* Creating conditions that will cause patients to want to learn
* Selecting the most effective materials and techniques for encouraging learning
* Providing resources (human and material) that will help patients learn
* Helping patients measure the outcomes of their patient education learning experiences

When giving patients information, recognize that adults are self-directed, lifelong learners. Patients want practical, meaningful advice and messages; they want to learn at their own pace and on their own time schedules; and they will look to their clinician as the health expert for the support and resources needed to learn. Offer a variety of patient education materials to patients that illustrate the key concepts covered during the encounter. Keep in mind that patients have different learning styles. One patient may have a preference for auditory learning and may be more likely to listen to an audiocassette tape on her way home from the office. Another might be more of a visual learner and more likely to watch a brief videotape in the office at the conclusion of the visit. Adult patients must have "ownership" of the problem in order for educational efforts to be effective. Ensure that patient education materials are written at an appropriate reading level and reflect the cultural and ethnic diversity of the clinic patient population. Written pamphlets or handouts should present one to three distinct messages that are clear and easy to remember. Do not try to cover everything conceivable in one patient encounter, but do try to provide a verbal or written summary of the key points for the patient to understand. (See also Chapter 12, Patient Education and Literacy).

■ PATIENT EDUCATION AND THE INTERNET

The Internet contains an ever-expanding amount of health-related information that patients may access or refer to. To date, however, no consensus guidelines exist as to what constitutes a "good web site" for patient education. Noting that it is increasingly difficult to determine which sites are accurate or appropriate for users, researchers at the

U.S. Department of Health and Human Services' Office of Disease Prevention and Health Promotion recently conducted a review of web and peer-reviewed health-related information. The study was an attempt to evaluate what published criteria currently exist to evaluate health information. Over 165 criteria were revealed during a search using Medline and the Lexis-Nexis databases and popular search engines including Yahoo!, Excite, Altavista, WebCrawler, HotBot, Infoseek, Magellan Internet Guide, and Lycos. The most frequently cited criteria for assessing health-related web sites were the content and design aesthetic of the site, disclosure of site sponsor, developer and authors, currency of the information (defined in the study as frequency of update, site maintenance, and "freshness" of content), authority of the source, ease of use, accessibility, and availability. The authors concluded that a clear, simple set of consensus criteria that the general public can use is much needed.[46] The Internet industry has established its own voluntary "Code of Ethics" to which sites may adhere. The Health on the Net Foundation Code of Conduct (HON code) identifies sites that agree to adhere voluntarily to a defined set of principles (www. hon.ch/HON code/).

CONCLUSION

An initial office visit, even with appropriate patient counseling, is probably not going to alter behavior significantly in most cases. But with continued support, regular patient contact and follow-up, and a concerted effort on the part of the health care provider to make prevention a more integral part of every care plan, clinicians are able to help patients live better, healthier lives. Many providers miss opportunities to provide preventive care services and counseling to patients. Understanding the essentials of fostering effective patient-provider communication and providing appropriate patient education messages are paramount to empowering patients to assume a greater responsibility for their own care.

As health care providers, we are still the best source of patient advocacy, resources, and prevention messages for our patients.

REFERENCES

1. Kochanek KD, Hudson BL. Advance report of final mortality statistics, 1992. Monthly vital statistics report, Vol. 43, no. 6, suppl. Hyattsville, MD, National Center for Health Statistics, 1995.
2. Healthy People: The Surgeon General's Report on Health Promotion and Disease Prevention. HEW Publication No. 79–55071. Washington, DC, U.S. Department of Health, Education, and Welfare, 1979.

3. Grandinetti D. Teaching patients to take care of themselves. Med Econ 1996;73:83–92.

4. Braslow L. From disease prevention to health promotion. JAMA 1999;281:1030–1033.

5. Woolf SH, Jonas S, Lawrence RS, eds. Health Promotion and Disease Prevention in Clinical Practice. Baltimore, Williams & Wilkins, 1996.

6. Lalonde M. A New Perspective on the Health of Canadians. Ottawa, Information Canada, 1974.

7. Canadian Task Force on the Periodic Health Examination. The Canadian Guide to Preventive Health Care. Ottawa, Canada Communication Group, 1994.

8. U.S. Preventive Services Task Force. Guide to Clinical Preventive Services, 2nd ed. Baltimore, Williams & Wilkins, 1996.

9. U.S. Public Health Service. Healthy People 2000: National Health Promotion and Disease Prevention Objectives. Publication (PHS) 91–50212. Washington, DC, U.S. Department of Health and Human Services, 1991.

10. Satcher D. Address to 27th Annual Physician Assistant Conference of the American Academy of Physician Assistants, May 27, 1999. Quote adapted from Advance for Physician Assistants, July 1999, p 42.

11. Counseling to Prevent Tobacco Abuse. Guide to Clinical Preventive Services, 2nd ed. Baltimore, Williams & Wilkins, 1996.

12. Curtis D, Goldstein AO. Helping your patients stay healthy. *In* Sloan PD, Slatt LM, Curtis P, Ebell MH, eds. Essentials of Family Medicine, 3rd ed. Baltimore, Williams & Wilkins, 1998, pp 80–83.

13. Gordon PR, Senf J, Campos-Outcalt D. Commentary. Is the annual complete physical examination necessary? Arch Intern Med 1999;159:909–910.

14. O'Donnell MP. Definition of health promotion. Part III: Expanding the definition. Am J Health Promotion 1989;3:3–5.

15. Bayer WH, Fiscella K. Patients and community together: A family medicine community oriented primary care project in an urban private practice. Arch Fam Med 1999;8:546–549.

16. Hettler B. Wellness: Encouraging a lifetime pursuit of excellence. Health Values. 1984; 8:13–17.

17. Decline in cigarette consumption following implementation of a comprehensive tobacco prevention and education program—Oregon, 1996–1998. MMWR Morb Mortal Wkly Rep 1999;48:140–143; JAMA 1999;281:1483–1484.

18. Nader PR, Stone EJ, Lytle LA, et al. Three-year maintenance of improvement in diet and physical activity. The CATCH cohort. Arch Pediatr Adolesc Med 1999;153:695–704.

19. National Vital Statistics Reports, Vol. 47, No. 19, June 30, 1999.

20. Ehman JW, Ott BB, Short TH, et al. Do patients want physicians to inquire about their spiritual or religious beliefs if they become gravely ill? Arch Intern Med 1999;159:1803–1806.

21. Harris WS, Gowda M, Kolb JW, et al. A randomized, controlled trial of the effects of remote, intercessory prayer on outcomes in patients admitted to the coronary care unit, Arch Intern Med 1999;159:2273–2278.

22. Byrd RC. Positive therapeutic effects of intercessory prayer in a coronary care unit population. South Med J 1988;81:826–829.

23. Geiderman JM. A Piece of My Mind. Faith and doubt. JAMA 2000;283:1661–1662.

24. Cheng TL, DeWitt TG, Savageau JA, O'Connor KJ. Determinants of

counseling in a primary care pediatric practice: Physician attitudes about time, money, and health issues. Arch Pediatr Adolesc Med 1999;153:629–635.

25. Falvo DR. Effective Patient Education: A Guide to Increased Compliance, 2nd ed. Gaithersburg, MD, Aspen Publications, 1994.

26. Stafford RS, Soglam D, Causino N, et al. Trends in adult visits to primary care physicians in the United States. Arch Fam Med 1999;8:26–32.

27. Lipkin M, Putnam SM, Lazare A, eds. The Medical Interview: Clinical Care, Education, and Research. New York, Springer-Verlag, 1995.

28. Orleans CT, George LK, Houpt JL, Brokie HK. Health promotion in primary care: A survey of U.S. family practitioners. Prev Med 1985;14:636–647.

29. Hampton JR, Harrison MJ, Mitchell JR, et al. Relative contributions of history-taking, physical examination, and laboratory investigation to diagnosis and management of medical outpatients. BMJ 1975;2:486–489.

30. Sandler G. The importance of the history in the medical clinic and the cost of unnecessary tests. Am Heart J 1980;100:928–931.

31. Kassirer JP. Teaching clinical medicine by iterative hypothesis testing. N Engl J Med 1983;309:921–923.

32. Mullen PD, Green LW. Educating and counseling for prevention: From theory and research to principles. *In* Goldbloom RB, Lawrence RS (eds), Preventing Disease: Beyond the Rhetoric. New York, Springer, 1990, pp 474–479.

33. Frank E, Kunovich-Frieze T. Physicians' prevention counseling behaviors: Current status and future directions. Prev Med 1995;24:543–545.

34. Jason H. Influencing health behavior: Physicians as agents of change. Cleve Clin J Med. 1994;61:147–152.

35. Scott RL. Physician Assistant Preparation in Patient Education, 1998 Association of Physician Assistant Programs, October 1998 [unpublished data.].

36. D'Onofrio CN. Theory and the empowerment of health education practitioners. Health Educ Q 1992;3:385–403.

37. Westberg J, Jason H. Fostering healthy behaviors. *In* Woolf SH, Jonas S, Lawrence RS (eds), Health Promotion and Disease Prevention in Clinical Practice. Baltimore, williams & Wilkins, 1996, pp 145–162.

38. Hafstad L. Outcome factors in patient education. Physician Assistant 1992;116:37–40.

39. Muma, RD. Factors influencing patient education. *In* Muma RD, Lyons B, Newman TA, Carnes BA (eds); Patient Education: A Practical Approach. Stamford, CT, Appleton & Lange, 1996, pp 11–13.

40. Stretcher VJ, Rosenstock IM. The health belief model. *In* Glanz K, Lewis FM, Rimer B (eds), Health Behavior and Health Education, 2nd ed. San Francisco, Jossey-Bass Publishers, 1997, pp 41–59.

41. Bandura A. Self-efficacy: Towad a unifying theory of behavior change. Psychol Rev 1977a;84:191–255.

42. Prochaska JO, DiClemente CC. Stages and processes of self-change of smoking: Toward an integrative model of change. J Consult Clin Psychol 1983;51:390–395.

43. Prochaska JO, Redding CA, Evans KE. The transtheoretical model and stages of change. *In* Glanz K, Lewis FM, Rimer B (eds); Health Behavior and Health Education, 2nd ed. San Francisco, Jossey-Bass Publishers, 1997, pp 61–84.

44. Grueninger UL, Duffy FD, Goldstein MG. Patient education in the medi-

cal encounter: How to facilitate learning, behavior change and coping. *In* Lipkin M, Putman S, Lazare A (eds), The Medical Interview: Clinical Care, Education and Research. New York, Springer-Verlag, 1995, pp 122–133.

45. Knowles MS. The modern practice of adult education: From pedagogy to androgogy. (Revised) Englewood Cliffs, NJ: Cambridge Adult Education; 1980, pp 26–27.

46. Kim P, Eng TR, Deering MJ, Maxfield A. Published criteria for evaluating health related web sites: Review BMJ 1999;318:647–649.

RESOURCE

The Healthier People Network, Inc.
3114 Mercer University Drive
Suite #200
Atlanta, Georgia 30341
(770) 458–1593
hpnhra@juno.com
The Healthier People Network, Inc., is a not-for-profit organization whose founder, Edwin B. Hutchins, Ph. D., was a member of the team that developed a computerized health risk appraisal (HRA) instrument for the Centers for Disease Control and Prevention. Subsequently, for five years he directed the continuing development and dissemination of the HRA as director of the program at the Carter Center of Emory University. Clinicians can contact The Healthier People Network, Inc., to become members and receive the latest version of the HRA computer program which includes both the "Midlife" and "Older Adult" risk appraisal tools, camera ready questionnaires, participant's guides, and supplemental materials, all for a nominal membership fee.

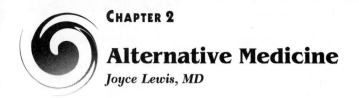

CHAPTER 2

Alternative Medicine

Joyce Lewis, MD

INTRODUCTION

The use of complementary and alternative medicine in the United States is increasing exponentially each year. Acceptance of complementary and alternative medicine by Americans is especially evident in the increased marketing by traditional pharmaceutical companies of their own herbal preparations and by health insurance companies' broadening their coverage to include some alternative therapies. The U.S. government first officially recognized the arena of complementary and alternative medicine by congressional mandate in 1992. The National Center for Complementary and Alternative Medicine (NCCAM), established in 1998, is dedicated to facilitating the evaluation of alternative medical treatment modalities and to determining their effectiveness. This same mandate has also provided for a public information clearinghouse and a research training program.

According to the NCCAM, *complementary and alternative medicine* (CAM) is defined as "those treatments and health care practices not taught widely in medical schools, not generally used in hospitals, and not usually reimbursed by medical insurance companies."[1] CAM covers a broad range of healing philosophies, approaches, and therapies. Alternative medicine systems have been placed into a classification system of seven major categories by the NCCAM:

1. Mind-body medicine
2. Alternative medical systems
3. Lifestyle and disease prevention
4. Biologically based therapies
5. Manipulative and body-based systems
6. Biofield systems
7. Bioelectromagnetics

MAJOR CATEGORIES OF COMPLEMENTARY MEDICAL PRACTICES

Mind-Body Medicine. Mind-body medicine involves behavioral, psychological, social, and spiritual approaches to health. It is further divided into four subcategories:

* Mind-body systems
* Mind-body methods

* Religion and spirituality
* Social and contextual

The average layperson may be most familiar with mind-body methods. Systems that fall into this subcategory are yoga, *tai chi*, psychotherapy, meditation, hypnosis, and biofeedback.

Alternative Medical Systems. Alternative medical systems are complete systems of theory and practice that have been developed outside the Western biomedical approach. The four subcategories in this classification are

* Acupuncture and Oriental medicine
* Traditional indigenous systems
* Unconventional Western systems
* Naturopathy

Acupuncture, sweat lodges, homeopathy, and New Age philosophies are examples of care falling into this broad category.

Lifestyle and Disease Prevention. This category includes theories and practices designed to prevent the development of illness, identify and treat risk factors, and support the healing and recovery process. These theories and practices also seek to integrate approaches to the prevention and management of chronic disease in general, or their common determinants, such as high-risk behaviors like smoking or unprotected sex. Subcategories include

* Clinical preventive practices
* Lifestyle therapies
* Health promotion

Biologically Based Therapies. These include natural and biologically based practices, interventions, and products. This category overlaps with conventional Western medicine's use of dietary supplements, including

* Phytotherapy or herbalism
* Special diet therapies
* Orthomolecular medicine
* Pharmacologic, biologic, and instrumental interventions

Phytotherapy entails the use of plant-derived preparations for therapeutic and preventive purposes. Special diet therapies include plans that are applied as alternative therapies for chronic disease in general or for the reduction of risk factors. Examples in this subcategory are the Atkins diet, vegetarianism, fasting, macrobiotic diets, and the Pritikin diet. The orthomolecular medicine subcategory includes nutritional and food supplements that do not fall into any other category. The main system in this subcategory is single nutrients, such as the use of vitamin C.

Manipulative and Body-Based Systems. This term refers to systems that are based on manipulation and/or movement of the body and include

* Chiropractic medicine
* Massage and body work

❋ Unconventional physical therapies

Examples of the subcategory of massage and body work include reflexology, Swedish massage, rolfing, and acupressure. Osteopathic manipulation also falls into this category.

Biofield Systems. Biofield systems are ones that use subtle energy fields in and around the body for medical purposes. This includes modalities such as Reiki, Shen, therapeutic touch and healing touch.

Bioelectromagnetics. Bioelectromagnetics refers to the unconventional use of electromagnetic fields for medical purposes.

Because of the vastness of CAM, this chapter deals with only a few of the more common alternative systems in use today. This is by no means an exhaustive look, but rather an introduction to CAM. While a brief introduction to each of the eight systems listed immediately following is provided, an annotated reference guide is presented at the end of this chapter for those requiring additional information.

❋ Acupuncture
❋ Homeopathy
❋ Herbal medicine
❋ Single nutrients
❋ Aromatherapy
❋ Reflexology
❋ Biofeedback

ACUPUNCTURE

Acupuncture is the insertion of fine stainless steel needles into specific points in the body to re-establish health and/or relieve pain or other dysphoric symptoms such as nausea. Acupuncture is based on the traditional Chinese concept of life energy, referred to as *chi*. Chi is divided into two opposite and complementary forms of energy, referred to as *yin* and *yang*. When *yin* and *yang* are unbalanced, illness ensues. *Chi* travels along the body by meandering pathways called meridians. Meridians are felt to pass close to skin surfaces at specific points (*hsueh*). The placement of pressure along the specific points of the skin is felt to unblock the *chi*, thus allowing energy to flow freely and health to be re-established. Acupuncture sessions may also include heat therapy, called *moxibustion*. *Moxibustion* involves the burning of cigar- or cone-shaped powdered mugwort (*Artemisia vulgaris*) over the acupuncture needle. Fresh ginger may also be used to help provide a sense of internal warmth.

Generally there is little or no pain with acupuncture. Needles are usually inserted from ¼ to 3 in, depending on the patient's build, and may be left in place for a few seconds or as long as an hour. The length of time a needle is left in place is dependent on the condition that is being treated and on the practitioner's preference. Individuals undergoing acupuncture may experience a temporary increase in the adverse symptoms being treated. The few side effects that have been associated with acupuncture include dizziness, fainting, minor bleeding, or difficulty in withdrawing needles. When the practitioner uses sterile needles, there is little risk of infection; the safest needles are both sterile and disposable. Individuals should also be advised to refrain from strenuous exercise immediately after treatment.

Acupuncture is effective in treatment of pain and analgesic addictions. Other conditions commonly treated include acne, allergies, anxiety, asthma, Bell's palsy, bronchitis, bursitis, colds and flu, colitis, depression, eczema, hay fever, and insomnia.

An individual may be certified by the National Commission for the Certification of Acupuncturists (NCCA), which was established in 1985. NCCA certification requires candidates to take an examination after 3 years of training and 3 years of apprenticeship with an approved acupuncturist (or for an immigrant acupuncturist who was trained abroad to practice acupuncture for 4 years). NCCA certification is the basis for licensure by the states that currently license acupuncturists.

HOMEOPATHY

Homeopathy is based on the concept that large amounts of a substance cause an illness, while very small doses of the same substance will cure it. Homeopathy looks at symptoms as the body's attempt to heal itself; therefore, homeopathic treatments encourage symptoms to run their course by

1. Stimulating the immune system
2. Accelerating healing
3. Strengthening the body

The father of homeopathy is Dr. Samuel Hahnemann (1755–1843). Hahnemann observed that quinine would cause symptoms similar to those of malaria. He concluded that if quinine caused symptoms similar to those of malaria in healthy patients, then small amounts of the drug would help to potentiate the body's natural immune response to the disease in those ill with malaria.

Homeopathy can be used to treat both transient and chronic diseases, including asthma, colds, flu, allergies, and arthritis. Although some practitioners may advocate the use of homeopathy to treat and cure cancer and diabetes, they are in the minority. Homeopathic medicines are formulated by diluting minerals, plants, chemicals, and animal products in either alcohol or water. *Potentization*, or sequential dilution, is the method by which homeopathic medicines are produced. A substance may be diluted 1:100, vigorously shaken, and rediluted 1:100. This process may be repeated 20 to 30 more times. Because homeopathic medications are so dilute, they are generally considered to be quite safe and to have little chance of adversely interacting with mainstream prescriptions. How a substance that is so dilute can still be effective is debated. Homeopathic practitioners state that treatments work by the original substance releasing its healing life force in the dilution process, or by the concept of "trace memory" in the form of electromagnetic frequencies of the active ingredient. Some scientists believe that homeopathy simply works because of the placebo effect, the ability to self-treat with nontoxic and nonaddicting medications, and/or the mind-body interface.

Homeopathic medications are usually in the form of tablets or drops that can be administered sublingually. The dilution of the medication is indicated on the package either by the decimal system (x system) or by the centissimal system (c system). The c system is used mostly in Europe whereas the x system is predominantly used in the U.S. In the x system, potency is given by a number that indicates the number of zeros, followed by an x, while in the c system, the number indicates half the number of zeros. For example, 6x equals 3c, which indicates a dilution of 1:1,000,000. Homeopathic medications should be stored away from direct sunlight and at room temperature. Also, the medications should be handled as little as possible so the minute amounts of active ingredient are not absorbed or altered. Homeopathic medications are known by their Latin names or Latin abbreviations; for example, onion is referred to as *Allium cepa*.

In homeopathy the job is to match a remedy to the individual's symptoms. The steps to doing this are

1. Taking the case: Obtaining a picture of the disease in the person. The two elements in this are observation and objectivity.
2. Analyzing the case: Evaluating the symptoms of the disease in the person by three factors. The three factors are the depth of the symptom, the strength of the symptom, and how uniquely characteristic the symptom is of the patient's state.
3. Selecting the remedy: Matching the symptoms to a remedy picture. By taking the main symptom and going to a remedy chart, the practitioner can refine the treatment by looking for other symptoms.
4. Giving the remedy: Determining the potency and frequency.
5. Results and reactions: Evaluating whether the patient is improving, stable, or deteriorating, and making adjustments to the remedy.

The art and science of homeopathy are more involved than this brief introduction; however, published charts and low potential for toxicity lead many toward self-treatment (rather than consulting a homeopathic provider), especially in the U.S., where supplies abound and providers are few.[2]

HERBAL MEDICINE

Primary care providers can benefit from a knowledge of herbals to help their patients; indications, methods of use, and contraindications.

An excellent source of information on herbal medicine can be found in the German Commission E Monographs.[3] In 1978, an expert committee established by the German government began an evaluation of the safety and efficacy of herbs and herb combinations sold in Germany. The resulting information was published as a series of monographs that provide therapeutic information on over 300 herbs or herb combinations. In 1998 the German Commission E Monographs were compiled and translated into English for health care clinicians and alternative medicine practitioners. The following seven herbals represent some of the preparations used more commonly in the U.S.

ST. JOHN'S WORT

St. John's wort is generally used for mild depression or anxiety. The active ingredient in *Hypericum perforatum* is taken from the above-ground part of the plant obtained during the flowering season. St. John's wort can be used both internally and externally. An oral dosage is approximately 0.2–1 mg of hypericin a day. It appears to have a mode of action similar to that of monoamine oxidase (MAO) inhibitors. Certain sources suggest a possible linkage between St. John's wort and serotonin syndrome when used with MAO inhibitors and selective serotonin reuptake inhibitors (SSRIs), and therefore combinations of these substances should generally be avoided.

GARLIC

Garlic is used for age-dependent vascular changes and lowering of elevated lipid levels in the blood. Fresh garlic bulbs or carefully dried bulbs containing *Allium sativum* can be administered orally. The minced bulb is usually dosed at an average daily dosage of 4 g. There are no known contraindications or interactions. Rare instances of changes to flora of the intestinal tract (sometimes useful in treating thrush), gastrointestinal symptoms, or allergic reactions have been documented.

ECHINACEA

There are two commonly used types of echinacea, *Echinacea pallida* and *Echinacea purpurea*. They are both used for supportive therapy for viral infections of the upper respiratory tract. *E. purpurea* can also be used for lower urinary tract infections. Echinacea is taken orally; the average daily dosage is 6–9 mL of expressed juice for *E. purpurea* or approximately 900 mg of *E. pallida*. The *Echinacea pallida* is usually administered as a tincture. It should not be used with patients with progressive systemic disease such as tuberculosis, AIDS, and multiple sclerosis (reasons were not given in the Commission E Monographs). There are no documented side effects for either form of echinacea when used internally and no known interactions with other drugs. *E. pallida* has no known effects on pregnancy and lactation. It is recommended that echinacea not be used internally for more than 8 weeks in any given treatment course, to avoid lessening its beneficial effects.

GINKGO BILOBA

Ginkgo biloba is usually administered in a dried extract of the dried leaf of *Ginkgo biloba L.* It is used for symptomatic treatment of cerebral function (memory deficits, disturbances in concentration, depressive emotional conditions, primary degenerative dementia, and vascular dementia, to name a few); vertigo and tinnitus of vascular origin; and intermittent claudication. Hypersensitivity is the only listed contraindication. Side effects may include headaches, stomach or intestinal upset, or rashes. The dosage range for cerebral function is 20–240 mg daily, provided as two or three divided doses. The dose for claudication and tinnitus is generally 120–160 mg daily. There are no known restrictions to use in pregnancy or lactation.

SAW PALMETTO BERRY

The ripe dried fruit of *Serenoa repens* is used for urinary problems associated with benign prostatic hypoplasia grades I and II. The herb is given orally, 1–2 g saw palmetto berry, or 320 mg lipophilic extraction. Saw palmetto berry's mode of action is thought to be both antiandrogenic and antiexudative. It relieves the symptoms of benign prostatic hyperplasia, without reducing the actual tissue enlargement. There are no documented contraindications or interactions, and it rarely causes stomach disturbances.

BLACK COHOSH

Cimicifuga racemosa is prepared from fresh or dried rhizomes. Black cohosh is used for premenstrual syndrome, dysmenorrhea, and menopause. Patients may have some gastric discomfort with its use, but there are no known drug interactions or contraindications. It should not be used longer than 6 months and is given internally. The daily dosage is 40 mg of extract. Black cohosh works through estrogen-like actions, binding to estrogen receptors and producing luteinizing hormone suppression.

GINSENG

Patients complaining of fatigue and declining capacity for work and concentration may benefit from use of the dried main and lateral root and root hairs of *Panax ginseng*. The root contains at least 1.5% ginsenosides. There are no contraindications, side effects, or interactions noted in the Commission E Monographs. Internal use of ginseng for up to 3 months with 1–2 g of the root is recommended. A repeated course of ginseng is feasible.

Other Common Herbals Used

Aloe vera applied topically relieves superficial burns.

Chamomile tea steeped for 15 min is very soothing to the upset stomach. One caution is that persons very allergic to ragweed and chrysanthemums may also be allergic to this flower.

Feverfew may reduce frequency of migraines but is commonly associated with stomach upset and fever blisters and may be associated with blood thinning properties that should be avoided when surgery is planned or the patient is taking warfarin.

Valerian in a dose of 400–450 mg at bedtime is not addictive and improves chronic sleep problems when taken regularly.

Herbal medications are not presently under U.S. Food and Drug Administration jurisdiction. As a result, herbal medications may not have labels that give information about side effects or harmful interactions. Herbal products may contain impurities or have huge variations in the quantities of the listed active ingredients. The consumer should choose preparations that are labeled, "standardized extract" and display an expiration date on the label, as these are more likely to contain effective dosages. Users of herbal medicines will increase their chances of good outcomes by selecting herbs from reputable companies (such as Warner Lambert, American Home Products, and PhytoPharmicia). Also review the product's label for the phrase or initials "GMP" (good manufacturing practices), which indicates that the pills are of pharmaceutical-grade quality. Several organizations listed in the Resource section of this chapter allow individuals to obtain detailed information about individual herbal preparations.

Table 2–1 is a list of herbal medicines that can be considered dangerous. While this list should not be considered exhaustive, it does provide the basis to quickly screen a patient's supplies for common offenders.

■■■SINGLE NUTRIENTS

Many vitamins and minerals are on the market today. In the past, it was felt that a healthy diet would provide all the vitamins and

Table 2–1. Dangerous Herbal Medicines

Latin Name	Herb	Potential Toxicity
Aconitine	Larkspur, monkshood	Bradycardia, tachydysrhythmias, paresthesias, seizures, ataxia, respiratory muscle weakness, nausea, vomiting, diarrhea
Adonis vernalis	Pheasant's eye	Sudden heart paralysis
Anemone pulsatilla	Pasque flower	Heart and nervous system damage
Arnica montana	Arnica	Damage to stomach and muscles (safe for external use)
Atropa belladonna	Deadly nightshade	Nervous system depression, respiratory depression
Bryonia dioica	Bryony	Damage to stomach and lungs
Cephaelis ipecacuanha	Ipecac	Violent vomiting
Convallaria majalis	Lily of the valley	Heart and nervous system damage
Symphytum officinale	Comfrey	Veno-occlusive disease
Datura starmonium	Thorn apple	Nervous system damage, liver damage
Digitalis purpurea	Foxglove	Heart and central nervous system damage; potentially lethal
Dryopteris filix-mas	Male fern	Central nervous system, eye, and heart damage
Gelsemium sempervirens	Yellow jasmine	Impaired breathing and heart function, loss of consciousness
Hedeoma pulegioides	Pennyroyal	Stomach toxicity, hepatotoxicity, shock; fetal toxicity
Hyoscyamus niger	Henbane	Central nervous system depression, respiratory depression
Pausinystalia yohimbe	Yohimbe	Hypertension, heart damage, central nervous system damage
Podophyllum peltatum	American mandrake or mayapple	Stomach damage, immune system damage; teratogenic
Rauwolfia serpentina	Indian snakeroot, rauwolfia	Depression, sedation, stomach damage, central nervous system damage
Urginea maritima	Squill	Stomach and kidney damage, central nervous system damage
Veratrum viride	False hellebore	Impaired heart and lung function, central nervous system damage
Viscum album	European mistletoe	Gastrointestinal bleeding, central nervous system and heart damage

Adapted from Yarnell E, Meserole L. Toxic botanicals: Is the poison in the plant or its regulation? J Altern Complement Med 1997;3:13–19, with permission.

31

minerals an individual would need. Extensive research has, however, shown the benefits of supplementing to help prevent or to help manage disease. Although supplementation is advocated by many, one should caution patients regarding exceeding recommended dosages, especially of the fat-soluble vitamins, A, D, E, and K. A few of these single nutrients are discussed briefly.

VITAMIN A

Vitamin A has become popular because of its antioxidant properties. Antioxidants help decrease the number of free oxygen radicals in the body. Free oxygen radicals can cause oxidative damage, which has been shown to alter DNA and play a role in the formation of atherosclerotic plaques. By donating an electron to the free oxygen radicals, vitamin A helps to reduce oxidative damage. When supplementing with vitamin A, individuals should use it in the form of beta carotene. Beta carotene is metabolized by the body into vitamin A. High doses of vitamin A have been found to have detrimental effects, while high doses of beta carotene have not. Vitamin A has been shown to help in wound healing. It helps to maintain vision, bones, hair, teeth, glands, skin, and the reproductive system.

VITAMIN C

Vitamin C is also an antioxidant. It is used to help reduce symptoms of colds, but generally, it does not affect the duration of the colds. Vitamin C helps bones and teeth grow; binds cells together; helps heal cuts and wounds; and is needed for blood clotting. It has been shown in studies by Linus Pauling, Ph.D., that 10 g daily of vitamin C can increase life expectancy of patients with cancer and improve cardiovascular disease risk factors. Vitamin C increases resistance to stress, lessens allergic reactions, helps arthritic conditions, slows down the aging process, and improves energy production.

VITAMIN E

Vitamin E is an antioxidant. Studies have shown that it helps form muscles and red blood cells and ensures function of the immune and endocrine systems, especially the sex glands. It is thought that it may deter atherosclerotic plaque formation by decreasing the amount of oxidized low-density lipoproteins in the blood, thereby lowering risk of heart attacks. Proponents of vitamin E supplementation also feel that it can help with the pain of arthritis. Excess vitamin E, above 1080 IU/day, may be harmful; a documented side effect is headache.

CALCIUM

Calcium is used for the growth and maintenance of bones and teeth, and it enables the heart and other muscles to contract. Calcium supplementation is one mainstay of osteoporosis risk reduction and treatment. Patients supplementing with calcium benefit the most from calcium carbonate preparations, as these preparations are highly bio-available and inexpensive. Vitamin D enhances the absorption of calcium in the gastrointestinal tract. Calcium supplementation may cause bloating and constipation, but in most patients this is only temporary. Calcium supplementation of up to 2 g per day can be safe and effective. Patients should be counseled about the possibility of milk-alkali syndrome increasing the risk of kidney stone formation. The importance of decreasing alcohol intake, smoking cessation, exercise, and appropriate use of hormone replacement therapy should also be stressed.

CHROMIUM

Chromium is in most multinutrient supplements. It is not well absorbed. Chromium may reduce the risk of heart disease. It helps to regulate the body's use of sugar by increasing the effectiveness of insulin. Chromium was initially identified in yeast. The most utilized form of chromium is chromium picolinate. Chromium is touted as a supplement that can aid in weight loss, and, while there are no good studies supporting this at present, most Americans are deficient in chromium intake. Some individuals may note a decrease in craving for sweets when supplementation is used. In animal studies chromium has been shown to increase lean muscle mass and decrease fat body mass. When consumed by pregnant women, chromium has also been shown to pass to the fetus. It has been postulated that the maternal drain of chromium is a cause of gestational diabetes. Supplementation with chromium is usually recommended at 50–200 µg a day.

GLUCOSAMINE SULFATE AND CHONDROITIN SULFATE

Glucosamine sulfate is a mucopolysaccharide that provides structure to the bone, cartilage, skin, nails, hair, and other tissues. It also is a major cushioning ingredient of the synovial fluids of the joints and surrounding tissues. Supplementation with glucosamine sulfate can be a remedy for osteoarthritis by increasing the production of cartilage. It has also been shown to help reduce pain and improve joint function. Chondroitin facilitates lubrication in the joints. The lubrication can increase movement in joints. Glucosamine and chondroitin act synergistically in joint health. Additional benefits of chondroitin sulfate are acceleration of wound and ulcer healing and promotion of cardiovascular health by activating lipoprotein, a fat-digesting enzyme on the inner surface of the capillaries. This prevents fat from accumulating and blocking the blood flow through the capillaries. Dosing of glucosamine sulfate is approximately 1000 mg a day. Approximately 600 mg of chondroitin sulfate a day is recommended.

AROMATHERAPY

Aromatherapy is the use of essential oils for treatment. It is thought that essential oils were first used by the Egyptians for many purposes, including beauty, massage, and mummification. In the early 1920s a French cosmetic chemist, René-Maurice Gattefosse, accidentally discovered the ability of lavender oil to lessen pain and the inflammatory reaction. He dedicated the rest of his life to studying the healing properties of essential oils and coined the term aromatherapy in 1928.

Essential oils are the distilled liquids from the leaves, stems, flowers, bark, roots, or other elements of a plant. The liquid may be distilled by several methods, including steam distillation, carbon dioxide gas extraction, cold expulsion, mechanical pressing, maceration, and solvent extraction. Remember the following rules when using essential oils:

1. Essential oils are very concentrated and should generally be diluted before use on the skin to prevent irritation. They can be diluted with carrier oils or in water.
2. They should be used carefully around the eyes.
3. *Most essential and carrier oils are not safe in pregnancy* because of possible stimulating effects on the uterus. Essential oils that are safe in pregnancy include bergamot, cananga, coriander, cypress, frankincense, geranium, ginger, grapefruit, lavandin, lavender, lemon, lime, mandarin, neroli, orange, patchouli, petitgrain, sandalwood, spearmint, tangel, tangerine, tea tree, temple orange, and ylang-ylang. Carrier oils that are safe in pregnancy are sesame oil and sweet almond oil.
4. Caution should also be used during lactation because the oils could possibly have an effect on the baby.
5. A patch test with carrier oil and then essential oil diluted in carrier oil should be performed to determine skin sensitivity to each essential oil.

6. Individuals should drink plenty of water and consume no alcohol while using essential oils.
7. Essential oils can interfere with some medications.
8. Some essential oils can remove the finish from furniture.
9. Essential oils should be stored in airtight, brown, or cobalt blue glass bottles in cool and dark places. They can deteriorate when exposed to light and oxygen.
10. Glass droppers should be used when measuring drops of essential oils. *Rubber bulbs can be turned into a gum.* A bottle with an orifice reducer will allow drop measurement of oils and ease of dispensing.

It is important to read labels when purchasing essential oils to determine whether the oil has substances added to it to stretch it. This may be done to make an "expensive" essential oil cheaper. One way to ensure high-quality essential oils *is to look for the Latin name of the plant on the label.* This may take some research on the part of the user, before venturing out to purchase oils. It is common to find essential oil blends in stores; several essential oils may be blended with carrier oils and other adulterants. Again, remember to read labels.

There are many methods of use for essential oils. Application is actually placing the oil on the skin (remember that most essential oils should be diluted and not used neat); an example of application would be topically in massage. Aroma lamps make use of a small container with a heating element below. An essential oil is mixed with water, and, as the container is heated, the vapors from the heated water release the aroma in the air. The same concept is used with the light bulb ring method, where the essential oil is placed in a ring that is then placed on a cool light bulb. When the light bulb is turned on, the heat it produces causes the essential oil to disperse into aromatic vapors. Other methods include baths, diffusers, mist sprays, and steam inhalation.

Carrier oils, as mentioned previously, are used to dilute essential oils. If unsure how much to dilute, a good "recipe" would be 12 to 30 drops of essential oil in one ounce of carrier oil. Most carrier oils are made from seeds, nuts, fruits, and vegetables. They can have some therapeutic potentials in and of themselves. Examples of carrier oils include sweet almond oil, apricot kernel oil, grapeseed oil, and jojoba.

Clary Sage (Salvia sclarea)

Clary sage is a colorless or pale yellow-green liquid with a pervading nutty, sweet, heady aroma. Uses of clary sage include easing feelings of depression, anxiety, and tension, and emotional or physical fatigue. The calming and anti-inflammatory qualities can help to relieve sore throats and hoarseness. The anti-inflammatory qualities can be useful in skin inflammations or to help preserve moisture in dry skin, including dandruff. Clary sage's calming effects can help to relieve high blood pressure, premenstrual syndrome, and menstrual pain, and help to establish menstrual regularity. Clary sage can have a calming influence on colic, cramp, and dyspepsia. This essential oil can be used in baths, massage, inhalations, aroma lamps, diffusers, light bulb rings, and mist sprays. *It should NOT be used in pregnancy.*

EUCALYPTUS *(EUCALYPTUS GLOBULUS)*

This essential oil is obtained from leaves and twigs of the tree. Uses of eucalyptus include cooling, stimulation of the nervous system, as a disinfectant, and as an insect repellant. Vapors open sinuses and breathing passages. Eucalyptus also improves circulation, refreshes, revives, and energizes, which can relieve pain and help to improve mental clarity and alertness. *Eucalyptus can be toxic, so it should be used in small doses* (no more than 5–10 drops mixed into 1 oz carrier oil). The oil has a well-known camphoraceous odor and is a penetrating bactericidal and antiviral oil for sickrooms. Methods of use include application, aroma lamp, bath diffuser, inhaler, light bulb ring, massage, mist spray, steam inhalation, and in steam or sauna rooms. Patients using homeopathic treatments and/or who have high blood pressure should not use eucalyptus oil. Individuals with sensitive skin should use with caution.

LAVENDER *(LAVANDULA ANGUSTIFOLIA, L. OFFICINALIS, L. VERA)*

Lavender is a good beginner oil. It is produced mainly in France and is obtained from the flowers of the plant. The clear, light, flowery aroma helps to make it a versatile oil. Lavender is relaxing and balancing for mind and body, aids sleep, soothes tired muscles, benefits the immune system, and encourages stillness and tranquility. Lavender has some antiseptic qualities and is also useful for the skin. It is a relatively safe essential oil; it can be used in pregnancy. Lavender is also one of the few oils that can be used neat (without diluting) on the skin. Aroma therapy methods include application, bath, diffuser, light bulb ring, aroma lamp, massage, mist spray, steam inhalation, and steam or sauna room.

TEA TREE *(MELALEUCA ALTERNIFOLIA, M. LINARIIFOLIA, M. UNCINATA)*

Tea tree oil is made from the leaves and twigs of the tree, which is native to Australia. The steam- or water-distilled oil is a pale yellowy-green or water-white mobile liquid with a warm, fresh, spicy-campho-raceous odor. The oil has powerful antiseptic properties (felt to be active against bacteria, virus, and fungi). It also benefits the immune system, disinfects, and deodorizes. Tea tree oil has been found to be very helpful in skin care and currently can be found as the main ingredient of soaps, toothpastes, deodorants, disinfectants, gargles, and shampoos. In general, it is nontoxic and nonirritative, but it should be used cautiously in individuals with sensitive skin. Large amounts of the oil should not be used neat on the skin. It can be used in aroma lamps, baths, diffusers, massage, light bulb rings, mist sprays, steam and sauna rooms, and in steam inhalation.

YLANG-YLANG (CANANGA ODORATA VAR. GENUINA, UNONA ODORANTISSIMUM)

Ylang-ylang is made from the flowers of the plant and has a sweet, heady, floral aroma. It is an exotic and sensual oil with relaxing qualities that soothe and uplift. The essential oil has a regulating effect on excited and nervous conditions. Ylang-ylang is good for both oily and dry skin, lessening pain, and loosening tight muscles. It is considered to be an aphrodisiac. Methods of use include inhalers, application, aroma lamps, light bulb rings, diffusers, fragrancing, massage, and mist sprays.

REFLEXOLOGY

Two of the pioneers of reflexology in the United States in the early 1900s were Dr. William Fitzgerald, an otolaryngologist, and Eunice Ingham, a physical therapist. They developed and began refining a type of reflexology known as zone therapy. Reflexology is a system of applying pressure to the foot to diagnose and treat illness in other parts of the body. Each part of the foot relates to its own part of the body, and, by applying pressure to the reflex point, that corresponding area or organ is affected. The right foot corresponds to the right side of the body and the left foot to the left side. Reflex points are on the tops, sides, and soles of the foot. Reflexologists feel that treatment helps to increase energy flow to corresponding organs and increase the vitality of the organs. The claims for reflexology include stress reduction, circulation improvement, elimination of toxins, and balancing of the body. Reflexology has a lot of similarities with acupuncture and acupressure by dealing with the body's energy fields (Fig. 2–1).

Foot Reflexology Chart

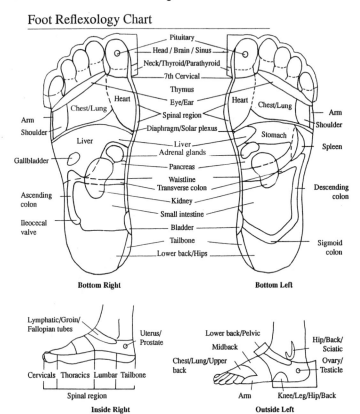

Figure 2–1. Foot reflexology chart. (From Kunz K, Kunz B. The Complete Guide to Foot Reflexology. Revised ed., 1980, with permission.)

■ MASSAGE

The practice of kneading or manipulating a person's soft tissues, including muscles, is called massage. The intent is usually to improve the person's well-being. Touch is one of the ways of demonstrating care and providing comfort to an individual. Ancient cultures, including Chinese, Roman, and Greek, employed massage as therapy. Massage has been shown to have many beneficial effects on the body: increase in blood flow, increase in the oxygen-carrying capacity of the blood, increase in body secretions and excretions, and enhancement of skin condition. Massage affects the nervous system and the muscles. There are many types or systems of massage; many possess similar components, and some examples are

* Therapeutic
* Holistic
* Swedish
* Sports
* Neuromuscular
* Bodywork
* Oriental
* Shiatsu
* Esalen
* Reichian
* Polarity
* Lymphatic

Individuals who have acute infectious diseases, aneurysms, bruises, cancer, hematoma, or phlebitis may not be good candidates for massage therapy.

Sports massage uses techniques to increase blood flow to injured muscles and tendons. It is hoped that the increased blood flow will increase oxygen and nutrients to the injured area that will result in accelerated healing. It is also thought that massage will help break down scar tissue and spread fibers. Sports massage includes deep stroking (pressure along the muscles), deep cross-fiber friction (pressure at a 90-degree angle to separate muscle fibers and break down adhesions), and jostling (loosely grabbing muscle groups, then shaking and squeezing to relieve tension).

Swedish massage was developed in Sweden during the 1800s. It combines principles of anatomy and physiology with Oriental practices of massage. Swedish massage attempts to improve circulation and release endorphins. The increased circulation allows greater amounts of oxygen to reach cells and also aids in washing away toxins. The methods used by practitioners include effleurage, petrissage, friction, vibration, and tapotement. Effleurage is massage that glides along the skin to increase blood flow; it can be either superficial or deep. Petrissage is rolling, kneading, and gently pinching to increase blood flow to muscles. Friction is a technique similar to petrissage except it involves stroking. The strokes of friction produce heat, which is useful for the breakdown of scar tissue. Vibration is steady and quick shaking motions with the fingertips or the flat of the hand. Tapotement is a technique of light tapping movement that aids in toning muscles.

BIOFEEDBACK

Biofeedback is a technique that teaches the patient to detect the body's reaction to stimuli. With the use of electrodes that monitor various organ systems, a patient can learn how to "control" his or her body's responses. Electrodes adhere to the skin and can be used to monitor heart rate, blood pressure, muscle tension, brain wave activity, and skin temperature. By assessing the feedback, the patient and the practitioner can use the information to teach the patient appropriate relaxation skills. The goal is eventually to allow the patient to be able to use psychological control over physiologic activities without the use of feedback instruments. The five most common forms of geometric biofeedback are

* *EMG* (electromyelography) measures muscle tension.
* *Thermal biofeedback* indirectly provides an index of blood-flow changes by measuring the temperature of the skin.
* *Electrodermal activity (EDA)* measures perspiration changes.
* *Finger pulse feedback* measures the amount of blood in each pulse and pulse rate.
* *Respiration feedback* measures the volume, rate, and rhythm of the patient's breathing, and can also be used to determine if the patient is performing abdominal or chest breathing.

Biofeedback is performed by attaching electrodes to the skin adjacent to the system that is being evaluated. The monitoring device gives variable pitched tones or visible readouts that show the activity the electrode is detecting. While monitoring the electrode's information, the therapist can guide the patient through mental and physical exercises. The exercises will attempt to produce desired changes in the monitored system. The process may be repeated several times, but eventually the patient learns to connect alterations in posture, breathing, muscle tension, and thought with the desired results. Biofeedback can also produce a greater body awareness for the patient. The increase in body awareness can help replace feelings of helplessness with feelings of renewed control over personal health.

Biofeedback can be used to treat many diseases. Many of the diseases are psychophysiologic in nature and include attention deficit hyperactivity disorder, depression, bruxism, premenstrual syndrome, conduct disorders, and headaches (migraine and tension). EMG can be used to treat incontinence, muscle stiffness, and chronic muscular pain. Thermal biofeedback has been used to treat migraine headaches, anxiety, Raynaud's disease, and hypertension. EDA is used to treat anxiety. Finger pulse biofeedback has been used in the treatment of hypertension and anxiety. Respiration feedback can be used to treat asthma, anxiety, and hyperventilation. Most importantly, biofeedback can help the patient learn relaxation and stress reduction techniques. For those patients who do not desire formal biofeedback training, simple relaxation techniques may provide some relief (see Box 2-1).

CONCLUSION

Health care professionals daily encounter patients using complementary and alternative medicine, both acknowleged and denied. This

---

Box 2-1–RELAXATION TECHNIQUE

- Set aside a quiet time, free of distractions, for 15 min each day.
- Choose a quiet place to sit or recline comfortably. Remove shoes and loosen any tight clothing
- Begin with slow deep-breathing exercises. Sometimes saying a short prayer or phrase while exhaling will be even more soothing and keep the mind from wandering back to stressful subjects.
- Then begin tightening up all muscles; inhale deeply, then relax while slowly exhaling.
- Repeat this exercise, focusing on different parts of the body. Begin with the feet and work toward the head.
- Repeat the deep-breathing exercises.
- Finally, take a minute to just enjoy the relaxation before returning to work

---

chapter provides only a starting place for the acquisition of information necessary to both the provider and the patient using different CAM methods. Keeping an open mind is the first step that clinicians must take to understand and separate what is a helpful adjunct to care from what is a deadly mistake. Basic knowledge of CAM also helps providers advise patients of different treatment methods and reduce pharmaceutical dependence and antibiotic overuse.

REFERENCES

1. National Center for Complementary and Alternative Medicine web site (http://nccam.nih.gov/).
2. Hammond C. The Complete Family Guide to Homeopathy. New York, NY: Penguin Books USA Inc., 1995.
3. Blumenthal M. The Complete German Commission E Monographs: Therapeutic Guide to Herbal Medicines, 1998.
4. Yarnell E, Meserole L. Toxic botanicals: Is the poison in the plant or its regulation? J Altern Complement Med 1997;3:13–19.

RESOURCES

INTERNET

The Internet has several resources for information on CAM. There are web sites for organizations, sites for a particular system, and sites where items for personal use can be purchased. Some of the web sites used for research for this chapter are:

Herbal Medicine
  http://www.wellweb.com
  http://www.herbalalternatives.com
  http://www.naturopathic.org
  http://www.healthy.net/clinic/therapy
  http://altmed.od.nih.gov
  http://www.aryc.com
  http://www.people.virignia.edu/~pjb3e/Complementary_Practices.html
  http://www.altmedicine.com/app/registeruser.cfm

Aromatherapy
  http://www.geocities.com/~aromaweb/
  http://www.eclipse.co.uk/iys/

Massage
  http://www.amtamassage.org

Reflexology
  http://www.reflexology-research.com

Single Nutrients
  http://www.vitamincfoundation.org/mega_1_1.html
  http://www.calciuminfo.com/
  http://www.arthritisaid.com/FAQ.html
  http://www.chromiuminfo.org/http://www.chromiuminfo.org/
  http://www.healthyideas.com/healing/vitamin/

Biofeedback
  http://www.aapb.org/public/
  http://users.aol.com/eegspectrm/articles/faq.htm
  http://www.athealth.com/AndersonArne_1.html
  http://www.users.cts.com/crash/d/deohair/psychoph.html

It is important to research any information obtained from the Internet, since web page content is unregulated. Some Internet pages are also more testimonial in nature, so that writers frequently include their biases.

ORGANIZATIONS

Acupuncture
  National Acupuncture and Oriental Medicine Alliance
  14637 Starr Road, S.E.
  Olalla, WA 98359
  253–851–6896
  www.acuall.org

  The Acupuncture Institute of America
  1533 Shattuck Ave.
  Berkeley, CA 94709
  510–845–1059
  www.acupressure.com

  American Academy of Medical Acupuncture (AAMA)
  5820 Wilshire Blvd., Suite 500
  Los Angeles, CA 90036
  800–521–2262
  http://www.medicalacupuncture.org

American Acupuncture Academy
20121 Ventura Blvd.
Woodland Hills, CA 91364
818–592–0357

Herbal Medicine
NAPRALERT (Natural Products Alert)
College of Pharmacy–UIC
833 South Wood Street
Chicago, IL 60612
312–996–2246

HerbalGram
American Botanical Council
P.O. Box 144345
Austin, TX 78714–4345
512–331–8868
http://www.herbalgram.org

Herb Research Foundation
1007 Pearl Street, Suite 200
Boulder, CO 80302
303–449–2265
http://www.herbs.org

Single Nutrients
Harvard Health Letter
P.O. Box 420300
Palm Coast, FL 32142
800–829–9045

Mayo Clinic Health Letter
P.O. Box 53889
Boulder, CO 80322
800–333–9037

Tufts University Health and Nutrition Letter
P.O. Box 420235
11 Commerce Blvd
Palm Coast, FL 32142–0235
800–274–7581

Environmental Nutrition
52 Riverside Drive 15A
New York, NY 01124
800–829–5384

Reflexology
International Insitute of Reflexology
5650 First Avenue, North
St. Petersburg, FL 33710
727–343–4811
www.reflexology-usa.net

Reflexology Research
P.O. Box 35820
Albuquerque, NM 87176–5820
505–344–9392

Aromatherapy
National Association for Holistic Aromatherapy
836 Hanley Industrial Court
St. Louis, MO 63144
888–ASK–NAHA/888–275–6242
http://www.naha.org

Homeopathy
National Center for Homeopathy
801 N. Fairfax Street, Suite 306
Alexandria, VA 22314
703–548–7790
http://homeopathic.org

Massage
American Massage Therapy Association
820 Davis Street, Suite 100
Evanston, IL 60201–4464
847–864–0123
http://www.amtamassage.org

National Certification Board for Therapeutic Massage and Bodywork
8201 Greensboro Drive, Suite 300
McLean, VA 22102
703–610–9015
http://www.ncbtmb.com

Biofeedback
Association for Applied Psychophysiology and Biofeedback
10200 W. 44th Avenue, Suite 304
Wheat Ridge, CO 80033
303–422–8436
http://www.aapb.org

Biofeedback Certification Institute of America
10200 W. 44th Avenue, Suite 310
Wheat Ridge, CO 80033
303–420–2902
http://www.bcia.org

Mind-Body Medical Institute
Division of Behavioral Medicine
New England Deaconess Hospital
110 Francis Street, Suite 1A
Boston, MA 02215
617–632–9530
617–632–7383
http://www.med.harvard/programs/mindbody

FURTHER READINGS

Bauwens SF, Drinka PJ, Boh LE. Pathogenesis and management of primary osteoporosis. Clin Pharmacol Ther 1986;5:639–659.

Byers D. Better Health with Foot Reflexology. St. Petersburg, FL: Ingham Publishing, 1987.

Carter M, Weber T. Healing Yourself with Foot Reflexolgy: All Natural Relief from Dozens of Ailments. Englewood Cliffs, NJ: Prentice-Hall, 1997.

Cassileth BR. The Alternative Medicine Handbook. New York: WW Norton & Co., 1998.

Castleman M. Nature's Cures. Emmaus, PA.: Rodale Press, Inc. 1996.

Compston JE. The role of vitamin D and calcium supplementation in the prevention of osteoporotic fractures in the elderly. Clin Endocrinol 1995;43:393–405.

Credit, LP, Your Guide to Complementary Medicine. Garden City Park, NY: Avery Publishing Group, 1998.

Damian P, Damian K. Aromatherapy: Scent and Psyche. Healing Arts Press, 1995.

Davis P. Aromatherapy: An A–Z. CW Daniel Company Limited, 1995.

Dietary Reference Intakes for Calcium, Phosphorus, Magnesium, Vitamin D, and Fluoride, Institute of Medicine Food and Nutrition Board. National Academy Press, 1997.

Downing G. The Massage Book. New York: Random House, 1972.

Herbert V. Total Nutrition: The Only Guide You'll Ever Need—From the Mount Sinai School of Medicine. New York: St. Martin's Press, 1994.

Johnson, J. The Healing Art of Sports Massage. Emmaus, PA: Rodale Press, Inc., 1995.

Kaye A, Matchan D. Reflexology for Good Health: Mirror for the Body. Hollywood, CA: Wilshire Book Company, 1980.

Keville K, Green M. Aromatherapy—A Complete Guide to the Healing Art. Crossing Press, 1995.

Krieger D. Accepting Your Power to Heal: The Personal Practice of Therapeutic Touch. Santa Fe, NM: Bear, 1993.

Lawless J. The Illustrated Encyclopedia of Essential Oils. Element, 1995.

Margen S. The Wellness Encyclopedia of Food and Nutrition. New York: Rebus, 1992.

Mill MA, Finando S. Alternatives in Healing. New York: New American Library, 1988.

Mumford S. The Complete Guide to Massage: A Step by Step Approach to Total Body Relaxation. New York: Plume (Penguin Group), 1996.

Optimal Calcium Intake, NIH Consensus Development Panel on Optimal Calcium Intake. JAMA 1994;272:1942–1948.

Schiller C, Schiller D. Aromatherapy Oils: A Complete Guide. Sterling Publishing Co, 1996.

Schiller C, Schiller D. 500 Formulas for Aromatherapy. Sterling Publishing Co, 1994.

The Handbook of Nonprescription Drugs, 10th ed. American Pharmaceutical Association, 1993.

Thomas S. Massage for Common Ailments. New York: Fireside Books, 1984.

Wise, A. The High-Performance Mind: Mastering Brainwaves for Insight, Healing, and Creativity. New York: Jeremy P. Tarcher, 1995.

Worwood, VA. The Complete Book of Essential Oils & Aromatherapy. Novato, CA: New World Library, 1991.

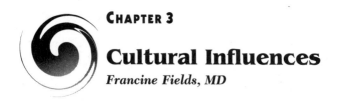

CHAPTER 3

Cultural Influences

Francine Fields, MD

INTRODUCTION

Culture is an integrated pattern of human behavior that includes thoughts, communication, customs, beliefs, values, and institutions of a racial, ethnic, religious, or social group.[1] Culture is a system of shared beliefs, values, customs, behaviors, and artifacts that a society's members use in their interactions with one another and within their worlds. These cultural beliefs are transmitted from generation to generation through learning and patterned behaviors.[2, 3] This learned culture guides action and beliefs as the individual meets both familiar and new life situations. Culture influences how we perceive ourselves and relate to others. Effective health care provision is facilitated first by understanding one's own culture and then by including the patient's cultural beliefs and experiences into assessment and treatment plans.

This chapter discusses the concepts of cross-cultural, holistic health care and some specific cultural examples. Unlike in the past, when the United States was described as a great melting pot, an image that encouraged assimilation, today American society is better likened to a very large, colorful, mixed salad, composed of many distinctively different elements. Each element still possesses its unique identity, but all are enriched when "tossed" together, forming an even richer experience for the palate.

CONCEPTS: CULTURAL COMPETENCE

Cultural competence is a "set of congruent behaviors, attitudes, and policies that come together in a system, agency, or among professionals and enables this system, agency, or those professionals to work effectively in cross-cultural situations.[1] Competence refers to the acquisition of knowledge, skills, and experience that are needed for the development and implementation of interventions that are then adapted to the different groups served.[4]

Culturally competent service necessitates that providers be cognizant of the issues facing the ethnic groups whom they serve. This includes addressing discrimination, immigration, sociopolitical issues (such as racism), and poverty, which then affect a patient's health.

Becoming culturally competent is a process by which one learns to recognize, value, and adapt to diversity by assessing one's own knowledge, attitudes, and beliefs about both one's own and another's culture.

It is important that providers understand their own cultural biases before they can be sensitive to their patients' cultures. The following section includes components of cultural competence as well as tools that are useful for making a culturological assessment. A culturological assessment is a "systematic appraisal or examination of individuals, groups, and communities as to their cultural beliefs, values, and practices to determine explicit needs and intervention practices within the cultural context of the people being evaluated."[4]

COMPONENTS OF CULTURAL COMPETENCE

Cultural Awareness. Health care providers must first become aware of their own culture before they can be sensitive to other cultures.

Cultural Knowledge. Cultural knowledge is a cognitive process of obtaining a solid educational foundation and world view of other cultures through reading, lectures, videos, interviews, and experience.

Cultural Skill. Cultural skill implies learning how to cognitively and *practically* assess a patient's cultural values, beliefs, and practices. This requires conducting a culturological assessment. Assessment of a patient's cultural values, beliefs and practices is a prerequisite to providing culturally responsive care.

Cultural Encounters. The health care provider directly engages in cross-cultural interactions with patients from diverse cultural backgrounds. During this process, the provider applies and refines the skills of conducting a culturological assessment, recommending a culturally responsive treatment plan, and negotiating an agreement. This process is an active, dynamic interaction between provider and patient.

Tools

There are several good tools for making a culturological assessment. The one developed by Berlin and Fowkes is particularly appropriate to primary care. Their tool uses the *LEARN* acronym.[4]

*L*isten with sympathy and understanding to the patient's perception of the problem.

*E*xplain your perceptions of the problem.

*A*cknowledge and discuss the differences and similarities.

*R*ecommend treatment.

*N*egotiate treatment.

The following questions are designed to elicit information about a client's health beliefs.[5]

1. What do you think caused your problem?
2. Why do you think it started when it did?
3. What do you think your sickness does to you?

4. How does it work?
5. How severe is your condition?
6. Will it have a long or short course?
7. What kind of treatment should you receive?
8. What are the most important results you hope to receive from this treatment?
9. What are the chief problems this condition has caused you?
10. What do you fear most about your sickness?

COMMUNICATION STYLES AND INTERPRETERS

Sensitivity and skills can only take a provider so far when the patient is from a distinctly different cultural group and/or speaks

---

Box 3-1–GUIDELINES FOR MONOLINGUAL PROVIDERS IN A CROSS-CULTURAL ENVIRONMENT

1. When you are unsure of a patient's fluency in English as a second language (ESL), ask if he or she needs an interpreter. If the answer is yes, you can be sure one is definitely needed, as many ESL-speaking patients have learned to smile and say yes, to appear polite.
2. Unless you're fluent in the patient's language, always use an interpreter. If one is not physically present, access one through telecommunication resources (see list in text).
3. Avoid using family members as interpreters, unless absolutely necessary. Personal information is closely guarded and difficult to obtain.
4. Learn basic words and sentences in the target language. Become familiar with special terminology used by the patient's community, even if you still require an interpreter.
5. Meet with your interpreters on a regular basis. Evaluate the interpreters' style and approach to patients and match them with problem cases and special situations according to their style. Check the quality of translated materials by having them back-translated.
6. Be patient with your patients.

Adapted from Putsch R. Cross-cultural communication: The special case of interpreters in health care. JAMA 1985;254:3347–3348; Werner O, Campbell DT. Translating, working through interpreters, and the problem of decentering. *In* Naroll R, Cohen R (eds), A Handbook of Method in Cultural Anthropology. Irvington-on-Hudson, NY, Columbia University Press, 1973, pp 398–420; Diaz-Duque OF. Overcoming the language barrier: Advice from an interpreter. Am J Nurs 1982;82:1380–1382.

Box 3-2–GUIDELINES FOR PROVIDER–INTERPRETER–PATIENT INTERACTIONS

1. Address your patients directly, not the interpreter. Observe their body language. Remember that not all mannerisms are interpreted similarly in different cultures. Direct eye contact may establish you as a caring provider to the Western, Euro-American patient, yet may be understood as a sexual overture by a traditional, rural Eskimo.

2. Be certain the interpreter is involved with the patient during the interview. Beware of any interpretation that takes less time than your initial explanation. Translations rarely become abridged, only longer.

3. Invite correction and induce the discussion of alternatives: "Correct me if I'm wrong. I understand it this way.... Do you see it some other way?"

4. Pursue seemingly unconnected issues that the patient raises, which may uncover crucial information.

5. Come back to an issue if you suspect a problem and get a negative response. Be sure the interpreter knows what you want.

6. Provide instructions in the form of a list. Have patients outline their understanding of the plans.

7. If alternatives exist, spell each one out.

8. Emphasize by repetition.

9. Clarify your limitations.

10. Assure the patient of confidentiality. Rumors, jealousy, and reputation are crucial issues in a close-knit community.

Adapted from Putsch R. Cross-cultural communication: The special case of interpreters in health care. JAMA 1985;254:3347–3348; Werner O, Campbell DT. Translating, working through interpreters, and the problem of decentering. *In* Naroll R, Cohen R (eds), A Handbook of Method in Cultural Anthropology. Irvington-on-Hudson, NY, Columbia University Press, 1973, pp 398–420; Diaz-Duque OF. Overcoming the language barrier: Advice from an interpreter. Am J Nurs 1982;82:1380–1382.

another language. Medical interpreters are a vital human resource needed for multiple health-related activities including patient registration, translation of medical records, scheduling appointments, explaining prescriptions, and communicating anticipatory guidance. Interpreters are crucial to obtaining accurate history and explaining treatment options. They may also provide clarity in special circumstances such as those surrounding death and dying issues (see Boxes 3-1 to 3-3).

It is important for the provider to realize that there are a variety

---

Box 3-3–GUIDELINES FOR LANGUAGE USE IN INTERPRETER-DEPENDENT INTERVIEWS

1. Use short questions and comments. Avoid professional jargon.
2. When lengthy explanations are necessary, break them up and have them interpreted piece-by-piece in straightforward terms.
3. Use language and explanations your interpreter can handle.
4. Make allowances for terms that don't exist in the target language.
5. Try to avoid ambiguous statements and questions.
6. Avoid abstractions, idiomatic expressions, similes, and metaphors. For instance, a person is pronounced dead—not *passed on* or *gone on to his reward.*
7. Plan what you want to say ahead of time.
8. Avoid indefinite phrases using "would," "could," and "maybe."
9. Ask the interpreter to comment on the patient's word content and emotions.

Adapted from Putsch R. Cross-cultural communication: The special case of interpreters in health care. JAMA 1985;254:3347–3348; Werner O, Campbell DT. Translating, working through interpreters, and the problem of decentering. *In* Naroll R, Cohen R (eds), A Handbook of Method in Cultural Anthropology. Irvington-on-Hudson, NY, Columbia University Press, 1973, pp 398–420; Diaz-Duque OF. Overcoming the language barrier: Advice from an interpreter. Am J Nurs 1982;82:1380–1382.

of different linguistic services that are often employed when interpretation is required.[6–8]

1. Bilingual and bicultural providers—probably the best interpreters because they speak the same language and have the same cultural background as the patient. Unfortunately they are limited in number.
2. Community health workers—outreach staff hired by community-based programs. Staff represents the cultural diversity of the community, but may have inconsistent health care education or knowledge of medical terminology.
3. Language bank interpreters—employees who speak other languages and are recruited as volunteers. Their primary advantage is one of low cost. However, there can be a problem when a medical emergency interferes with the interpreter's regular job responsibilities.
4. Professional interpreters—rarely used in the medical arena and usually hired when the expense of maintaining such an employee can be justified. However, adverse health outcomes resulting from

inadequate communication can be potentially more expensive than providing well-trained interpreters. Unfortunately, availability, cost, and sporadic need frequently limit an individual practice's ability to hire these professionals.

5. Remote consecutive interpretation—telephone interpretation services are useful for setting up appointments and discussing laboratory results, and for emergencies, particularly when services are infrequently used (e.g., AT&T's Language Line: 800–752–0093, ext. 196, or languageline.com).

6. Nonprofessional interpreters—includes the recruitment of volunteers from the lay community, such as the family and friends of the patient. This should be a provider's last choice since these volunteers may lack appropriate language skills and knowledge of medical terminology and may compromise confidentiality.

7. Written translation materials—can be useful for emergencies and to clarify simple instructions. However, these materials can never take the place of verbal communication between provider and patient.

CULTURE-BOUND SYNDROMES

Culture-bound syndromes are recurring behavioral patterns and experiences that are specific to particular cultures. Formerly used terms include ethnic psychoses, ethnic neuroses, atypical culture-bound syndromes, and exotic psychotic syndromes.[9] The underlying theme is that understanding of these behaviors is influenced by region-specific views held by the patients, their values, their sense of vital essence, their belief in the presence of supernatural beings or power, their perceptions of sickness and health. It is important for primary care providers to be cognizant of these syndromes because they are frequently somatic in nature. Brief descriptions of the more common syndromes follow.[9]

Koro. Also known as *suk-yeong*, Koro is a syndrome found in the Chinese culture. An individual believes his or her genitals are retracting and fears harm will results, including death. Males in early adulthood think that the penis is retracting into the abdomen, and that this will end their lives. Women may believe their breasts or labial folds are retracting into their bodies. In koro, patients usually have panic attacks, and the individual may use clamps, pins, or fellatio to keep his or her genitals from retracting. The condition lasts for days to weeks and is self-limited.

Koro may be associated with social, psychological, or occupational dysfunction, with accompanying depression or suicidal ideation. Precipitating factors include masturbation, sexual identity issues, or sexual intercourse.

The psychiatric differential diagnosis of *koro* includes delusional disorder, schizophrenia, sexual disorders, and substance abuse. Organic causes such as brain tumor, malaria, or epilepsy need to be sought. Treatment, once organic etiologies have been excluded, usually consists of psychotherapy and antipsychotic drugs.

Amok. A culture-bound syndrome seen in Asians, primarily Malays, *amok* generally affects poor, uneducated, young, or middle-aged males who live away from home and have suffered a loss. Individuals tend to be withdrawn and isolated and have a history of being impulsive, immature, emotionally labile, and socially irresponsible.[9]

In *amok*, an individual experiences a period of brooding and preoccupation, followed by outbursts of violent, aggressive behavior that may include indiscriminately attacking and maiming any people or animals that are in their way.[10] The episode may last several hours, leaving the individual exhausted. The affected individual commonly does not remember what happened during the attack and may later attempt suicide. These attacks are believed to be caused by evil spirits and demonic possession. Family members may be at risk for harm owing to the unpredictability of the attacks. The differential diagnosis includes epilepsy, brain tumor, or infections (e.g., malaria, syphilis).

Treatment during an attack includes physical and/or pharmacologic restraint. Subsequent long-term management includes treating any underlying organic disorders, depression, or psychoses.

Hwa-byung. *Hwa-byung* is a culture-bound syndrome that occurs in the Korean population. It is frequently seen in females in their forties and fifties who are less educated and have lower socioeconomic status. The patient may complain of epigastric, abdominal pain due to what he or she believes to be a mass in the throat or upper abdomen, believing it will lead to death. Other complaints include excessive fatigue, insomnia, indigestion, anorexia, dyspnea, palpitations, headaches, dizziness, sexual dysfunction, diplopia, heat intolerance, chest pain, or more generalized aches and pains. Emotional symptoms include depression, anxiety, self-guilt, anxiety, irritability, obsession-compulsion, destructive impulses, panic, and a fear of impending doom. Precipitating factors include family stressors, alcoholism, and domestic violence. The psychiatric differential diagnosis includes major depression, anxiety disorder, dysthymia, phobic disorders, somatization, obsessive-compulsive disorder, and panic states.

The name of this syndrome roughly translates to "anger illness" in English. In many Asian cultures, there is a tendency not to express anger openly in order to preserve harmony in social relationships, and this is believed to be the root cause of *hwa-byung*.

Atraque de Nervios. *Atraque de nervios* is a culture-bound syndrome that is seen in Hispanic cultures, especially in individuals from the Caribbean islands. It is a dissociative condition characterized by a sense of lost control. During an attack the person exhibits uncontrollable verbal outbursts, crying, fainting-like experiences, or seizure-like movements. Physical symptoms include chest palpitations, chest tightness, trembling, shortness of breath, a sensation of heat rising to the head, and occasional striking out at others. After an attack, the patient may not recall the events.

The individual may complain of being possessed by evil spirits. Family stress, such as the death of a family member, divorce, or separation from a spouse, is the usual precipitating factor. Males are usually affected. This disorder is a culturally recognized manner of expressing anger or one's inability to cope. A precipitating factor together with the absence of symptoms of acute fear differentiate this syndrome from panic disorder.

Susto. *Susto* is an illness seen in many Latin American and South American cultures.[11] Local synonyms include *espanto*, *lanti*, *pasmo*, *tripa ida*, *perdida del alma*, or *chihih*. It is believed that the soul leaves the body when a person is startled. The onset of the illness may be days to years after the stressor occurs. It may not occur within the individual who was exposed to the stress but may manifest itself within his or her child.[4, 11] Symptoms include appetite changes, sleep disturbances, depression, lack of motivation, and poor self-esteem. Physical symptoms include diffuse aches and pains, headache, indigestion, anorexia, vomiting, constipation, diarrhea, and stomach bloating. The psychiatric differential diagnosis includes major depression, posttraumatic stress disorder, and somatoform disorder. Traditional treatment focuses on cleansing the person to restore bodily and spiritual harmony by use of an egg, mint tea, or candles.

Brain Fag. Brain fag is a syndrome found in individuals from various regions of Africa.[12] These individuals have problems with concentration, memory, and thought. The patient complains of brain and body fatigue along with anxiety symptoms. Somatic complaints include pain, pressure, or tightness around the head and neck region, blurred vision, and/or feelings of a burning heat. Patients may also report feeling like worms are crawling around in their heads. The psychiatric differential diagnosis includes anxiety, depression, and somatoform disorders.

Falling Out. A disorder found in African Americans, African Caribbean islanders (Bahamians and Haitians), and in the Miami, Florida, area. Falling out is associated with a sudden collapse precipitated by feelings of dizziness.[13] The individual may complain of an inability to see despite the eyes being open. He or she usually is able to hear and understand what is happening, but is powerless to move. There are no convulsions, tongue biting, bladder or bowel incontinence, or symptoms suggestive of a genuine seizure. This disorder is thought to be due to a psychologically traumatic event. The differential diagnosis of falling out includes a conversion and/or dissociative disorder.

Cultural Folk Conditions

Health and Illness in Mexican-Americans

Curanderismo is a Mexican-American form of folk healing. It is practiced in both Mexico and in portions of the southwestern U.S.[14, 15] Major elements include

1. The belief that persons with a special gift (the *curandero*) can heal in God's name
2. A compendium of naturalistic folk conditions such as *empacho* ("blocked intestine") and *caida de mollera* ("fallen fontanelle")
3. The belief in the existence of mystical disease, such as *susto* ("fright" or "lost soul") and *mal puesto* (hexing)
4. The belief in three levels of health and illness—the material, the spiritual, and the mental
5. The use of medicinal herbs and specific rituals, called *barridas*[14] (see also Box 3-4.)

Health and Illness in Native American Communities

Traditionally, Native Americans believe that good health is being in total harmony with nature and surviving difficult circumstances. The earth is considered to be a living organism, the body of a higher individual, with a will and a desire to be well. The earth is periodically healthy and not healthy, just as human beings are. A person should treat his or her body with respect, just as the earth should be treated with respect. In order to maintain health, Indians must maintain their relationship with Nature. "Mother Earth" is the friend of the Indian, and the land belongs to the Indian.[15]

Native Americans practice purification by use of herbs, *moxibustion*, and water immersion to maintain harmony with nature, awaken their senses, and prepare for meditation. Various herbal preparations are an important part of Native American rituals and home remedies (see Table 3–1).

Health and Illness in Asian Americans

In Asian American culture, *yang* represents the male, or a positive energy that produces light, warmth, and fullness. *Yin* represents the female, or a negative energy—the force of darkness, cold, and emptiness. *Yin* and *yang* exert power over the entire universe, and over human beings as well. The theory holds that everything within the universe contains two aspects, both the *yin* and *yang*; while each is in opposition to the other, they are at the same time acting as one whole.

Box 3-4—MEXICAN FOLK ILLNESSES

1. *Empacho* ("blocked intestine") is believed to be caused by a bolus of food that sticks to the wall of the intestine owing to eating improperly cooked food (e.g., cold tortillas or meat) and/or consuming certain foods at the wrong time of day (e.g., bananas late at night).

Major symptoms: Colicky abdominal pain, nausea, and vomiting.

Treatment: Massage of the stomach with olive oil and mint or chamomile tea.

2. *Mal de ojo* ("evil eye") is considered to be an emotional illness in which the person is a victim of circumstances that are out of his or her control. Roughly translated as "evil eye," it is believed to be caused when a person known to have the "evil eye" looks or touches a child with admiration. The condition usually affects children but may affect persons of any age.

Major symptoms: Acute febrile illness, vomiting, irritability, excessive crying, and/or listlessness.

Treatment: Initial treatment is to have the same person with the "evil eye" look admiringly at the child without touching it. If this is unsuccessful, the family will seek the help of a *curandero*. In a healing ritual, an uncooked egg is passed over the child's body and then broken into a dish of water. The appearance of a red or black spot on the egg is diagnostic. The dish is then placed under the head of the child's bed overnight to draw out the evil spirits. When the spot is gone, the child is considered healed.

3. *Caida de mollera* (fallen fontanelle) is believed to be caused by pulling a baby from the breast or bottle too quickly, holding or carrying the baby incorrectly, or letting the baby fall on the floor.

Major symptoms: Diarrhea and vomiting, inability to suck, decreased appetite, restlessness and irritability, sunken eyes, and decreased tears.

Treatment: Push up on the palate. Hold the child upside down and strike its heels. Turn the child upside down and shake. Put foam or soap on the fontanelles.

4. *Aire de oido* ("air in the ear") is believed to be caused by getting air trapped in the ear canal.

Major symptoms: Fullness or popping in the ears, earaches, and pulling at ears in infants.

Treatment: Place cone of paper in the ear and set on fire. Blow smoke in the ear.

Adapted from Marsh W, Hentges K. Mexican folk remedies and conventional medical care. Am Fam Physician 1988;37:257–262.

Table 3–1. Examples of Native American Home Remedies

Native American Group	Condition	Remedy
Yupik Eskimos	Ear infection	Warm seal oil
Oneida Indians	Ear infection	Warm skunk oil
	Mouth sores	Dried raspberry leaves
	Headache	Tansey and sage
	Colds	Witch hazel
	Sore throat	Comfrey
	Diarrhea	Elderberry flowers
Micmac Indians	Diarrhea	Wild strawberry leaves
	Warts	Juice of milkweed plant
	Obesity	Spruce bark and water
	Rheumatism	Juniper bark
	Diabetes	Blueberries and huckleberries
	Insomnia	Lettuce

From informational pamphlet, Boston Indian Council, Boston, MA, 1985; American Association of Indian Physicians, www.aaip.com/tradmed.

Different portions within the body correspond to the *yin* or the *yang*. The interior contents and the anterior aspect of the body, the liver, heart, spleen, lungs, or kidneys, and the diseases of the winter and spring are *yin*, while the skin's surface and the posterior aspect of the body, the gallbladder, stomach, intestines, or bladder, and the diseases of summer and fall are *yang*.

Half of one's *yin* forces are considered to be depleted by age 40. At this age, the body is sluggish, and by age 60 the *yin* is totally depleted, and the body deteriorates. *Yin* stores the vital strength of life. *Yang* protects the body from outside forces, and it, too, must be carefully maintained. If *yang* is not cared for, the viscera are thrown into disorder, and circulation ceases. *Yin* and *yang* cannot be injured by evil influences. When *yin* and *yang* are sound, the person lives within a peaceful interaction, with mind and body in proper order.[17] Acupuncture is the practice of puncturing the body with special metal needles at predetermined points to cure disturbances of the life forces, *chi* (see Chapter 2). The treatment goal is to restore the balance of *yin* and *yang*.[18]

Herbal medicine also plays a part in traditional Chinese medicine (see Table 3–2).

Health and Illness in the African American and African Caribbean Communities

The traditional definition of health in these communities stems from the African belief about life and the nature of "being." Life is a

Table 3–2. Examples of Traditional Chinese Remedies

Treatment	Condition/Indication
Deer antlers, ground	Strengthen bones and sexual potency, dispel nightmares
Lime calcium	Clears excess mucus
Quicksilver (mercury)	Venereal diseases
Rhinoceros horn, powdered	Antitoxin for snake bites, impotence
Turtle shells, ground	Stimulate weak kidneys, remove gallstones
Snake flesh	Keeps vision clear
Seahorse, dried	Gout
Ginseng	Aids digestion, sedative, faintness after childbirth, restorative for weak children

From Wallnofer H, Von Rattauscher A. Chinese Folk Medicine, Trans. M. Palmedo. New York, American Library, 1972, pp 12–16, 19–21.

process, and one can influence others as well as one's destiny through one's behavior, and by intimate knowledge of a person and the world he or she lives in. Health represents harmony with nature. Illness is viewed as a state of disharmony. Traditional beliefs regarding health do not separate the mind, body, and spirit.[19]

In African Caribbean culture, disharmony (illness) is traditionally attributed to a number of sources, primarily demons and evil spirits. Voodoo and spiritual healers are primarily used to dispel the evil spirits. Voodoo is a belief that illness is caused by "a fix" that was placed on a person in anger. *Gris-gris*, the symbols of voodoo, are used to prevent illness or pass an illness onto others. Some examples are listed in Box 3-5.

Essentials to maintaining good health are a balanced diet, rest, and a clean living environment. Laxatives are used to keep the system open. Asafetida (an herb referred to as "devils dung" or "rotten flesh" because of its foul odor) is worn around the neck to prevent the contraction of contagious diseases. Cod liver oil is taken to prevent colds. Copper bracelets are worn by female infants as a form of protection. The wrist turns black as a warning of impending illness. If the bracelet is removed, harm may befall the owner. The precautions against illness include prayer, rest, and a nutritious diet. The most common method of treating illness is prayer. Rooting, a practice derived from voodoo, occurs when a healer is consulted and then prescribes the appropriate treatment. Magic rituals are often employed.

Home remedies are often used for the treatment of disease. Sugar and turpentine are mixed together and taken by mouth to get rid of worms. This combination can also be used to cure a backache and, when rubbed on the skin (from the navel to the back), is used to fight infection and inflammation. Vegetables are frequently used for healing,

---

Box 3-5–SYMBOLS OF VOODOO

1. Good *gris-gris*. Love powder: colored and scented with perfume; Love oil: olive oil to which gardenia perfume has been added; Luck water: ordinary water that is colored. (Red is for success in love, yellow for success in money matters, and blue for protection and friends.)
2. Bad *gris-gris*. Oils and powders have a vile odor; anger powder, war powder, and moving powder are composed of soil, gunpowder, and black pepper, respectively.
3. Flying devil oil is olive oil that has both red coloring and cayenne pepper added to it.
4. Black cat oil is machine oil.
5. Colored candles are also used. White represents peace; red, victory; pink, love; yellow, driving off enemies; brown, attracting money; and black, doing evil work and bringing bad luck.

Adapted from Jacques G. Cultural health traditions: A black perspective. *In* Branch M, Paxtan PP (eds), Providing Safe Nursing Care for Ethnic People of Color. New York, Appleton-Century-Crofts, 1976, p 116.

for instance, the potato. Potatoes are sliced and placed in a bag, which is then placed on the affected part of the body until the potatoes turn black. It is believed that as the potatoes spoil, they produce a "penicillin" mold to cure the illness. Onions are believed to heal infections, and flaxseed poultices are used to treat earaches (Box 3-6 lists further home remedies).

Examples of Religious Cultures

Islam

Many members of the African American community and many immigrants are practicing Muslims. Religious beliefs are an important part of the Muslim lifestyle. Islamic dietary restrictions consist of eating a strictly Halaal, or permissible, diet. Most importantly, this means absolutely no pork, including many "soul foods" that contain pork as seasoning meat (such as legumes or greens seasoned with ham hocks or bacon). Muslims consider such foods to be unclean. Islamic law teaches that certain foods affect the way a person thinks and acts. Practicing Muslims also abstain from the consumption of alcoholic beverages because they feel it dulls the senses. According to Islamic belief, Ishmael, the son of Abraham, was circumcised at 13 years of age; this practice remains an integral part of Islamic culture. Some

Box 3-6–AFRICAN AMERICAN AND CARIBBEAN HOME REMEDIES

1. Placing clay within a dark leaf and wrapping it all around a sprained ankle relieves pain and swelling.
2. Salt pork placed on a rag can be used to treat cuts and wounds.
3. When congestion is present in the chest and the person is coughing, the chest is rubbed with hot camphorated oil and wrapped with warm flannel.
4. An expectorant for colds consists of chopped onion, fresh parsley, and a little water, all mixed in a blender.
5. Hot toddies are used to treat colds and congestion. These drinks consist of hot tea or water mixed with honey, lemon, and peppermint and frequently contain a small amount of an alcoholic beverage, such as brandy or rum.
6. Fever may be broken by placing pieces of raw onions on the person's feet and wrapping them in warm blankets.
7. Garlic can be placed on the ill person or in the sickroom to remove the "evil spirits" that have caused the illness.
8. To treat a "crick" in the neck, two pieces of silverware are crossed over the painful area in the form of an X. Similarly, two crossed knives or a pair of scissors placed under the bed of a woman in labor will "cut the pain in half."
9. Nine drops of turpentine, nine days after intercourse, acts as a contraceptive.

Adapted from Jacques G. Cultural health traditions: A black perspective. *In* Branch M, Paxton PP (eds), Providing Safe Nursing Care for Ethnic People of Color. New York, Appleton-Century-Crofts, 1976, p. 116.

regional Islamic sects also believe in female circumcision as a rite of passage into womanhood and/or to ensure chastity or monogamy.

Orthodox Judaism

The foundation of Jewish life is derived from the Torah (the five books of Moses). From the Torah come the laws that direct a Jew's relationship with God and his fellow man. Laws of purity and *kashruth* (the state of being kosher) are explicitly outlined. Strict religious ritual, including dietary and health regulations, governs the Orthodox Jew's daily life. Keeping a kosher home involves following strict laws concerning diet, hygiene, and sanitation that were enumerated first in the Old Testament. The physician and rabbi Moses Maimonides, who lived in Spain and North Africa, later codified these laws in approximately 1165 C.E. Although Conservative and Reform sects follow much more relaxed standards, it is useful for the health care provider to understand some of Orthodox Judaism's religious requirements.

1. *Bris*—ritual of male circumcision performed on the infant's eighth day of life. The timing predated routine use of vitamin K to prevent neonatal bleeding diathesis, and it was empirically observed that the newborn bled less when the procedure was deferred until the eighth day of life. It is also of interest that early rabbis recognized hemophilia. The Talmud specifically deals with preservation of life as an exception to strict adherence to the law, in this case stating that the sibling of two brothers who had died of bleeding complications may not be circumcised.

2. *Keeping kosher*—All food substances must contain approved foods, in approved combinations, and be inspected and blessed by an approved rabbi or rabbinical council. These restrictions may have implications in certain food supplements, vitamins, and medical treatments, but exceptions can be made in certain cases of protecting or preserving life in an emergency.
   - Scavengers such as pigs, fish without scales, and shellfish may not be eaten.
   - Meat and dairy products must not be served in the same meal, or prepared and/or served using the same set of pots, pans, or dishes.

Mormons, or Latter-Day Saints (LDS)

Traditionally these patients avoid all "stimulants" as identified by Joseph Smith, their founder-prophet. These include alcohol, coffee, tea, and tobacco. Modern soft drinks that contain caffeine are not specifically addressed and therefore are a matter of interpretation. Alcohol is not a true stimulant, but is still abstained from by most LDS members.

Polygamy, illegal within the U.S., may still be practiced by some splinter groups, but is not endorsed by the church's modern leadership.

Other Religions, Cults, and Expressions of Spirituality

It is impossible to reference all the forms of spiritual expression found within communities small and large, both rural and urban. It is sufficient to say that spirituality and religious laws or rituals bring both complementary comfort and conflict to the patient when he or she is interacting with the medical profession. Caring providers must consider carefully the patient's spiritual supports, conflicts, and culture just as they would consider ethnicity. Special care should be taken to avoid global misconceptions. Southern Baptists and Free Will Baptists may have no more in common than individuals from two different tribes in Ghana.

Sexual Diversity

Since gender-preference issues may not be initially acknowledged at the time of a patient's first visit to a new caregiver's office, the provider would do well to use gender-neutral nouns and pronouns when first meeting with a new patient. The simple act of asking about a patient's "partner" can send a signal of openness to discuss many far-reaching health issues going well beyond those of sexuality and sexual identity. (See also Chapters 16 and 17.)

Disabilities

Initially, one might not think of the disabled as a cultural group; however, those challenged by various disabilities may form or benefit from association within a subculture or support group that shares similar issues and challenges.

A string of legal precedents stemming from the Civil Rights Act of 1964 and the Rehabilitation Act of 1973 led to the Americans with Disabilities Act being signed into law in 1988. Equality of opportunity under the law has both improved access to care and simultaneously complicated primary care. Providers today are expected to provide easy access to facilities for the physically disabled, blind, and deaf. Handrails, ramps, raised commode seats, large-print or Braille patient educational materials, and telephone terminals for the deaf (TDD) or personal amplification systems will meet most primary care patients' needs. However, providers are now being increasingly sought out for advice in areas of adaptive technologies and the school-related problems of developmental or learning disabilities and attention-deficit disorder. Although this arena may not be one in which many providers have any real expertise or formal education, they should be minimally familiar with local support groups, resources, or appropriate rehabilitation consultants to expedite patient referrals (see Resources).

Community or Situational Culture

Although many patients have defined their identities through ethnicity or religion, a provider may come across situational cultures that defy definite rationale or roots that have developed into a common community standard. Nowhere else is this more evident than in the myths, rituals, and "old wives' tales" surrounding a woman's labor in childbirth. For instance, a knife or scissors placed under the woman's bed is said to "cut the pain." Although this is common across many cultures, some practices may be more regionally unique. It is a mistake to attempt to undermine or to be unduly critical of the rituals that bring patients comfort, unless those rituals are truly dangerous. Providers must build good rapport before their opinions are likely to impact upon their patients' behaviors. In addition, a critical attitude is much more likely to result in the patient ignoring more important medical issues or keeping silent in the future about alternative therapy or rituals he or she engages in.

■ CONCLUSION

Cultural competence goes beyond mere sensitivity to the plight of the person of another color, race, gender, sexual orientation, national origin, religion, language, or social circumstance. It implies culturally responsive care composed of awareness, knowledge, skills, and the desire to negotiate an agreement as to what really constitutes the best treatment plan for any particular patient.

REFERENCES

1. Cross TL, Bazron BJ, Dennis KW, and Isaacs MR. Towards a Culturally Competent System of Care. Washington, DC, CASSP Technical Assistance Center, Georgetown University Child Development Center, 1989.
2. Bailey E. Sociocultural factors and health care-seeking behavior among black Americans. J Nat Med Assoc 1987;79:389–391.
3. Kramer E, Ivey S, Ying, Y.-W. Immigrant Women's Health: Problems and Solutions. San Francisco, CA, Jossey-Bass Inc., 1999, p 21.
4. Berlin E, Fowkes W. A teaching frame work for cross-cultural health care. West J Med 1983;139:934–938.
5. Kleinman A, Eisenberg L, Good B. Culture, illness and care: Clinical lessons from anthropologic and cross cultural research, Ann Intern Med 1978;88:251–258.
6. Putsch R. Cross-cultural communication: The special case of interpreters in health care. JAMA 1985;254:3347–3398.
7. Werner O, Campbell DT. Translating, working through interpreters, and the problem of decentering. In Naroll R, Cohen R (eds), A Handbook of Method in Cultural Anthropology. Irvington-on-Hudson, NY, Columbia University Press, 1973, pp 398–420.
8. Diaz-Duque OF. Overcoming the language barrier: Advice from an interpreter. A J Nurs 1982;82:1380–1382.
9. Gaw, A. Culture, Ethnicity, and Mental Illness. Washington, DC, American Psychiatric Press, 1993.

10. Carr JE, Tan EK. In search of the true amok: Amok as viewed within the Malay culture. Am J Psychiatry 1976;133:1295–1299.
11. Klein J. Susto—The anthropological study of diseases of adaptation. Soc Sci Med 1978;12:23–38.
12. Morakinyo O. A psychophysiological theory of a psychiatric illness (the brain fag syndrome) associated with study among Africans. J Nerv Men Dis 1980;168:84–89.
13. Weidman HH. Falling out: A diagnostic and treatment problem viewed from a transcultural perspective. Soc Sci Med 1979;13:95–112.
14. Marsh W, Hentges K. Mexican folk remedies and conventional medical care. Am Fam Physician 1988;37:257–262.
15. Spector R. Cultural Diversity in Health and Illness. Stamford, CT, Appleton & Lange, 1996, pp 210–217.
16. Informational pamphlet Boston Indian Council, Boston, MA, 1985.
17. American Association of Indian Physicians; aaip.com/tradmed
18. Wallnofer H, Von Rattauscher A. Chinese Folk Medicine, trans. M. Palmedo. New York, American Library, 1972, pp 12–16, 19–21.
19. Jacques G. Cultural health traditions: A black perspective. *In* Branch M, Paxton PP (eds), Providing Safe Nursing Care for Ethnic People of Color. New York, Appleton-Century-Crofts, 1976, p 116.

RESOURCES

WEB SITES

General

(For ethnic, minority, gay-lesbian, disabled groups)
drkoop.com
ethomed.com
healthanswers.com
healthfinder.org/justforyou/minority/
kzoo.edu
looksmart.com
    Health → Family and Community →
xculture.org

Specific Groups

Asian-American
  healthwave.com
  baylor.edu
African American
  blackhealthnet.com
  library.kent.edu
Spanish-language Prenatal Care
  todobebe.com
Native American
  aaip.com/tradmed
Disabled
  familyeducation.com
  empowermentzone.com

FURTHER READINGS
Cultural Awareness

Borkan JM, Neher JO. A developmental model of ethnosensitivity in family practice training. Fam Med 1991;23:212–217.

Brislin RW, Yoshida T. Improving Intercultural Interactions. Thousand Oaks, CA, Sage Publications, 1994, pp 180–195.

Locke DC. Increasing Multicultural Understanding. Newbury Park, CA, Sage Publications, 1992, pp 1–14.

Paniagua FA. Assessing and Treating Culturally Diverse Clients. Thousand Oaks, CA, Sage Publications, 1994, pp 1–18.

Cultural Skill

Berlin EA, Fowkes WC. A teaching framework for cross-cultural health care. West J Med 1983;139:934–938.

Lajkowicz C. Teaching Cultural Diversity for the Workplace. J Nurs Educ 1993;32:235–236.

Putsch RW. Cross-cultural communication: The special case of interpreters in health care. JAMA 1985;254:3344–3348.

Roberson MH. Folk health beliefs of health professionals. West J Nurs Res 1987;9:257–263.

Counseling

Axelson J. Counseling and Development in a Multicultural Society. Monterey, CA: Brooks-Cole.

Clark A (ed). Cultural, Childbearing, Health Professionals. Philadelphia, FA Davis, 1978.

Asian Americans

Blount BW, Curry A. Caring for the bicultural family. The Korean-American example. J Am Board Fam Pract 1993;6:261–268.

Min PG (Ed). Asian Americans. Thousand Oaks, CA, Sage Publications, 1995.

Yeatman GW, Dang VV. Cao gio (Coin rubbing). JAMA 1980;244:2748–2749.

African Americans

Bailey EJ. Sociocultural factors and health care-seeking behavior among black Americans. J Nat Med Assoc 1987;79:389–392.

Levy DR. White doctors and black patients. Pediatrics 1985;75:639–643.

Cuban Americans

Sandoval M. Afro Cuban concepts of disease and its treatment in Miami. J Operational Psychiatry 1977;8:52–63.

Haitians

Scott C. Haitian blood beliefs and practices in Miami, Florida. Paper presented at the American Anthropological Association Meeting. New Orleans, LA, Nov. 1973.

Latinos

Krajewski-Jaime ER. Folk-healing among Mexican-American families as a consideration in the delivery of child welfare and child health care services. Child Welfare 1991;70:157–167.

Marsh WW, Hentges K. Mexican folk remedies and conventional medical care. Am Fam Physician 1988;37:257–262.

Ripley GD. Mexican-American folk remedies: Their place in health care. Tex Med 1986;82:41–44.

Ruiz R. Cultural and historical perspectives in counseling Hispanics. In Sue D (ed), Counseling the Culturally Different: Theory and Practice. New York, John Wiley & Sons, 1981; pp 186–215.

Schreiber J, Homiak J. Mexican Americans. In Harwood A (ed), Ethnicity and Medical Care. Cambridge, MA, Harvard University Press, 1981, pp 264–335.

Trotter RT. Folk medicine in the Southwest: myths and medical facts. Postgrad Med 1985; 78(8):167–179.

Migrant Health

Resource Catalog, available through the National Center for Farmworker Health, Inc. 1515 Capital of Texas Hwy. South, Suite 220, Austin, TX 78746. Ph.: 512–328–7682.

Puerto Ricans

Harwood A. Mainland Puerto Ricans. In Harwood A (ed), Ethnicity and Medical Care. Cambridge, MA, Harvard University Press, 1981, pp 397–481.

Native Americans

Richardson E. Cultural and historical perspectives in counseling American Indians. In Sue D (ed), Counseling the Culturally Different. New York, John Wiley & Sons, 1981, pp 216–225.

Disabilities

Ablenet, Cerebral Palsy Center, Inc., 360 Hoover Street NE, Minneapolis, MN 55413.

Assistive Device Center, School of Engineering & Computer Science, 6000 J. Street, Sacramento, CA 95819–2694. Ph.: 916–468–6422.

Concepts for Independent Living, 2203 Airport Way, South, Suite 310, Seattle, WA 98134. Ph.: 206–343–0670.

Job Accommodation Network—JAN, The President's Committee on Employment of the Handicapped (PCEH), P.O. Box 468, Morgantown, WV 26505. Ph.: 1–800–JAN–PCEH.

National Brallle Press, Inc., 88 Saint Stephens Street, Boston, MA 02115. Ph.: 617–266–6160.

National Technology Center, American Foundation for the Blind, Inc., 15 West 16th Street, New York, NY 10011. Ph.: 212–620–2080.

Telecommunications for the Deaf, Inc. (TDI), National Association of the Deaf, 814 Thayer Avenue, Silver Spring, MD 20910. Ph.: 301–589–3006.

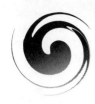

CHAPTER 4

Domestic Violence

Emmanuella Paul, MD,
Dorothy White, MD,
and Valerie Van Dam, LCSW

INTRODUCTION

Domestic violence has many different faces. In the home, various forms of family violence can be found: among intimate partners, siblings, and parent-child units (child or elder abuse). Statistics show that approximately 4 million women are abused annually.[1, 2] A study published in 1998 revealed that one out of five heterosexual couples experienced at least one episode of domestic violence.[3] Research has also demonstrated that 47.5% of lesbians and 29.7% of gay men have been abused by their partners.[4] Approximately 1 out of 25 elders are abused annually, and there are 3 million annual cases of child abuse and neglect in the United States.[5]

This chapter primarily addresses violence between intimate partners (including same-sex partners), child abuse, and elder abuse. Information is provided to assist health care providers to evaluate and direct patients to appropriate resources.

Domestic violence encompasses multiple facets. It can consist of physical assault, resulting in significant morbidity and mortality, or of sexual abuse, including either assault or coercion and psychological abuse. Psychological violence can take the form of threats, attacks against property, isolation, emotional abuse, and the use of children to manipulate the victim. Sole control of the family finances can be a form of both economic and psychological abuse.[5, 6]

Whatever form of abuse or violence is utilized, the ultimate goal of the abuser is to achieve and maintain control of the victim. Studies have shown that the particular abuse tactic is often deliberately chosen to obtain the desired goal, although it may appear that the perpetrator is not in control of his or her actions. Various forms of abuse are used in specific combinations to leave the victim feeling powerless. Intimate violence is characterized by a cycle of abuse with three phases. These are[5, 6]

1. The tension-building phase, in which the victim is systematically demoralized via emotional and economic abuse, which leads to increasing amounts of dependence on the perpetrator
2. The violent stage, in which tension erupts into frank violence. Following an episode of frank violence, the perpetrator may become very apologetic.
3. The honeymoon period, when the perpetrator may be very remorseful, promising never to abuse again. During this period, the

perpetrator may even shower the victim with gifts and indulgences, only to return inevitably to the first phase of the cycle.

ETIOLOGY

Research has not been able to clearly determine the cause of domestic violence, but there are several theories as to its etiology. One of the more popular theories views domestic violence as a learned behavior that begins in childhood. The behavior is learned partly from historical norms of societal behavior and partly from personal experience and/or observation of family violence while a person is still a child. Historically, certain cultures have condoned male-on-female violence. This theory speaks to the belief that people involved in intimate abusive relationships may have observed violence in their families of origin, and that these people may have become violent in turn.

Another perspective focuses on the personality characteristics of the perpetrator. This theory emphasizes the perpetrator's problems with impulse control and unfulfilled dependency needs. However, a primary fault with this theory is that it likens the perpetrator to the mentally ill. Violent acts of the seriously mentally ill tend to be random and disorganized, whereas the actions of the domestic abuse perpetrator exhibit none of these characteristics. Substance abuse, while a common contributor, is not generally thought to be causal, as domestic violence occurs whether or not individuals are under the influence of alcohol or controlled substances, and many addicts are nonviolent.

Finally, another hypothesis promotes the stressing effects of social and environmental factors such as unemployment and poverty. Again, this theory fails to completely explain the origin of domestic violence, which is known to occur in both affluent and impoverished homes. Although there seems to be no one single cause, domestic violence definitely appears to be a learned behavior triggered by multifactorial issues and stresses.[7, 8]

SCREENING

One of the ways that domestic violence can be identified is through screening. One study demonstrates that health care providers asked only six of 364 women about domestic abuse. Abuse victims tend to present with multiple complaints that are difficult to resolve. Not screening patients for domestic violence leads to frustration and disservice to both provider and patient. Although a certain profile may exist that helps to identify victims of abuse who seek help from shelters and public service agencies,[9] it is easy to overlook victims who are of a higher socioeconomic status. Screening for domestic violence meets all the necessary criteria to be established as a standard screening practice because

1. Domestic violence has a significant effect on the quality and quantity of life.
2. Acceptable methods of treatment are available.
3. Domestic violence has an asymptomatic period, during which early detection and treatment can greatly reduce both morbidity and mortality.
4. Treatment in the asymptomatic stage yields a therapeutic result superior to delaying treatment until symptoms appear.
5. Treatment is cost effective.
6. The incidence of domestic violence is sufficient to justify the cost of screening.

Therefore, there is no reason why all patients should not be screened.[8]

Screening patients for domestic abuse and/or violence is a delicate process. The patient should be interviewed alone, without other family

---

Box 4-1–DOMESTIC VIOLENCE SCREENING QUESTIONS

- Many families have difficulties expressing anger. What is that like in your family?
- Has your partner ever destroyed something you care about?
- Has your partner ever forced you to have sex when you did not want to?
- Does your partner ever forbid you to leave your home or to see your friends and family?
- How do you and your partner handle disagreements? Have you ever hit, pushed, or kicked one another when you were angry?
- Domestic violence is a real and growing problem in our community. I'm wondering if anyone you know has hurt you in any way?
- Being in relationships is often very difficult and can cause us lots of pain and suffering. Many people who feel depressed are suffering from violence in their homes. Could this be happening to you?
- People have different ways of showing disagreement or anger; sometimes people talk, other times they make threats. Has your partner ever threatened to use a gun, knife, or other weapon when angry?
- You mentioned that your partner uses drugs/alcohol. Is your partner ever physically or verbally abusive when intoxicated?

Adapted from Levin MD, Carey WB, Crockery AC, Gross R. Family dysfunction, violence, neglect, and sexual misuse. *In* Snyder JC (ed) Developmental Behavioral Pediatrics. Philadelphia, WB Saunders, 1983, pp 256–275; Gremillion DH, Kanoff EP. Overcoming barriers to physician involvement in identifying and referring victims of domestic violence. Ann Emerg Med 1996;27:769–773.

> ### Box 4-2—PREDISPOSING FACTORS FOR ABUSE OF WOMEN
>
> - Youth (ages 17–28)
> - Single status or recent separation or divorce
> - Pregnancy (during which abuse may begin or escalate)
> - Drug or alcohol abuse on the part of the perpetrator
> - Past history of domestic violence within the perpetrator's or victim's family.

From Poirier L. The importance of screening for domestic violence in all women. Nurse Pract 1997;22:105–122.

members present, particularly the suspected perpetrator. Starting with open-ended or broad questions may help introduce the screening process. Asking about intimate partnerships without reference to gender or marital state will enable heterosexual, gay, or lesbian patients to feel comfortable revealing both their sexual orientation and their abusive relationships. Avoid using the terms *battered*, *abused*, or *victim*, as many patients may not identify with these terms.[10] Box 4-1 contains questions that have been suggested to facilitate the screening process.[9, 11]

While ideally every patient should be screened, screening is especially important in the patient with

* Chronic vague complaints
* Poor eye contact
* Pregnancy or history of a spontaneous or elective abortion
* Injuries that are inconsistent with the explanation provided by the patient
* The chief complaint that someone else asked the patient to be examined
* Predisposing risk factors (see Boxes 4-2 and 4-3)
* Suicidal ideation or a history of attempted suicide[9, 11]

> ### Box 4-3—RISK FACTORS FOR ELDER ABUSE
>
> - Living with a family member
> - Prior history of family violence
> - Victim suffering from dementia or other mental disability
> - Drug or alcohol abuse
> - Caregiver resentment/stress

From Life Preservers—A Life Line for Victims of Violence. A Guide for Physicians, Butler R. Warning signs of elder abuse. Geriatrics 1999;59:1319–1320.

Box 4-4–CLINICAL INDICATORS OF ABUSE IN CHILDREN

- Bruises or welts in the shape of articles used to inflict injury
- Burns, lacerations, or rope burns
- Retinal hemorrhages
- Multiple fractures in various stages of healing
- Abrasions or bruises in the genitalia and anus
- Distortion of the hymen or abnormal anorectal tone
- Evidence of a sexually transmitted disease or pregnancy
- Chronic abdominal or anal pain and recurrent urinary tract infections
- Substance abuse

From Ross SM. Risk of physical abuse to children of spouse abusing parents. Child Abuse Negl 1996;20:589–598; Lee WV, Weinstein SP. How far have we come? A critical review of the research of men who batter. *In* Glanger M (ed), Recent Developments in Alcoholism, Vol. 13; Alcoholism and Violence. New York, Plenum Press, 1997, pp 337–356; Gremillion DH, Kanoff EP. Overcoming barriers to physician involvement in identifying and referring victims of domestic violence. Ann Emerg Med 1996;27:769–773.

When abuse potential is detected within the home, it is important to have information readily available to offer help, according to needs identified by the patient screening (see The Resources Appendix at the end of this book for additional resources).

PRESENTATION

Screening should occur at every encounter and with all patients because family violence cuts across all socioeconomic classes and educational backgrounds as well as every age and ethnic group. Because of denial or intimidation and because the patient may be physically unable to report a problem (e.g., child, an elder, or a disabled person), providers need to be aware of some of the "red flag" presentations that can alert them to victims of domestic violence (see Boxes 4-2, 4-3; and 4-4). Suspicion of Münchausen's syndrome by proxy, unusually frequent health care visits for seemingly insignificant or vague complaints, or extremely late night visits to health care providers may also provide the clinician with clues to previously undetected abuse.

Child abuse may be suspected based on such behavioral findings as depression or suicidal tendencies, anxiety, enuresis, sleep disturbances, excessive or public masturbation, poor interpersonal relations, aggressive behavior, poor school performance, and parent-child role reversal.

Abusive intimate relationships may manifest as chronic fatigue syndrome, sexual dysfunction, chronic pain, chronic headaches, posttraumatic stress disorder, and substance abuse. Physical signs of trauma localized to the head, chest, breasts, and abdomen, and recurrent injuries at multiple sites may also provide clues to the existence of domestic violence.[10]

Elderly patients in abusive situations may show signs of dehydration, malnutrition, skin breakdown, poor personal hygiene, bruises, lacerations, bilateral injuries, injuries in various stages of healing, over- or undermedication, unexplained sexually transmitted diseases, and extreme withdrawal, depression, or agitation.[12, 13]

ASSESSMENT

Many barriers exist that prevent health care providers from identifying cases of domestic abuse. Some providers have the mistaken belief that domestic violence is a private family matter rather than a true health care issue, or fear that the patient might become angry at provider "interference." Insufficient time for patient-provider interaction and inadequate provider training and skills also present barriers to both detection and intervention. Providers also fear legal reprisal and poor support from institutional and legal agencies. Clinicians often experience difficulty reconciling their duty and their relationships with both perpetrator and victim when both are patients of the same primary provider. Perhaps more distressing is that many providers still have misconceptions about their patient population, believing that abuse does not occur in their practice. Past personal experience and a desire to remain detached may motivate providers to refrain from asking about violence in the home. Feelings of frustration, scorn, or anger directed toward the victim may arise when the victim refuses to leave the abusive situation (perceived as noncompliance). Many patients may refuse intervention because of a fear of retribution and/or a fear of social ostracism or embarrassment. Victims may feel isolated, or that the partner is their only source of "love" and "support," especially during the honeymoon phase, when victims commonly seek care. There may also be a fear of not being believed or of actually being blamed for the abuse. Recurring cycles of abuse undermine victims' sense of worth and increase their sense of having caused or deserved the abuse. Economic dependence on the perpetrator can influence decisions to stay within the relationship. Religious and cultural beliefs regarding divorce and the fear of losing custody of children may also present barriers to victims leaving an abusive situation.[6, 10, 14] Same-sex partners may additionally fear revealing their sexual orientation if they complain about abusive behaviors to their health care provider.

Suggestions for providers to improve screening and intervention rates include

* Wearing buttons that address domestic violence

* Placing cards with help line numbers in baskets located in examination rooms or bathrooms
* Displaying posters that address domestic violence
* Including domestic violence screening questions on new patient or review of systems questionnaires

When evaluating a relationship for domestic violence, an assessment of all variables should be made, including the risk of imminent violence within the household. Research has shown that the risk of child abuse is significantly increased when domestic violence exists between parents.[15]

Documentation is very important when assessing domestic violence. Detailed, objective, and accurate records need to be kept to assist patients when they finally decide to seek legal help. Records should be kept simple, without extraneous detail, and should include the patient's own words. Body maps, detailed descriptions of physical injuries, and quality color photographs of injuries (taken with patient consent) help to provide an accurate account of physical assault. However, it should be stressed that a good diagnostic examination description and diagram is often far better than a poor Polaroid photograph. Excellent photographs can be taken with a short focal length colposcopic 35 mm, video, or digital camera. If bruising is initially subtle, consider repeating the examination 48–72 h later, when color definition may be more pronounced. Providers should also remember that photo-developing vendors who can ensure confidentiality must process all explicit film. The alternative is to use a digital camera and store images on disks in a locked file in the office. Finally, if the explanation given by the patient is not consistent with the injuries, providers should document their assessment of the inconsistencies.

INTERVENTION

Once screening, identification, and assessment of a patient's situation have occurred, it is important to have resources to provide the patient. State laws requiring reporting vary, depending on the age of the suspected victim. Although there are laws in all states regarding reporting of child abuse, and some states also have laws mandating reporting of suspected abuse of elders or disabled adults, there are no states with laws requiring the reporting of intimate partner abuse.

Safety plans are essential when domestic violence is suspected or identified. Ask patients whether they feel they will be safe and whether the safety of any dependents may be at risk. If safety is an issue, suggestions should be made for the patient to seek sanctuary at a friend's home or at a shelter. In an acute situation, where the patient does not feel safe at home, remind the patient that the police can be contacted by telephoning 911. The patient should be offered information regarding resources for further help, and providers should not be

Table 4-1. National Domestic Violence Organizations

Organization	State	Local Number	Toll-Free Number
Battered Women's Justice Project—Legal Office	PA		(800) 903–0111
Battered Women's Justice Project—Minnesota Program Development	MN	(612) 824–8768	(800) 903–0111
Battered Women's Justice Project—Self Defense for Battered Women	PA	(215) 351–0010	
Center for the Prevention of Sexual and Domestic Violence	WA	(208) 634–1903	
Clearinghouse on Family Violence Information	DC	(703) 385–7565	(800) 394–3366
Family Violence Prevention Fund	CA	(415) 252–8900	(800) 313–1310
National Clearinghouse for the Defense of Battered Women	PA	(215) 351–0010	(800) 537–2238
National Clearinghouse on Marital and Date Rape	CA	(510) 524–1582	
National Coalition Against Domestic Violence	CO	(303) 839–1852	
National Coalition Against Domestic Violence—Policy Office	DC	(202) 544–7358	
National Network to End Domestic Violence	DC	(202) 543–5566	
National Network to End Domestic Violence—Administrative Office	TX	(512) 794–1133	
National Organization for Victim Assistance (NOVA)	DC	(202) 232–NOVA	(800) TRY–NOVA
National Resource Center on Domestic Violence	PA		(800) 537–2238
Resource Center on Child Custody and Child Protection	NV		(800) 527–3223

discouraged if the patient does not accept any help initially. Family therapy should never be recommended until the perpetrator has accepted responsibility for the abuse, has initiated individual therapy, and has stopped the abuse.

■■■CONCLUSION

It is vitally important to screen all patients, without reference to gender or physical appearance, for the possibility of being either a perpetrator or a victim of domestic abuse. Providers need to ask all patients about their approach to disagreements or disputes within their homes, measuring their responses to determine the potential for abuse and/or violence. The majority of batterers do not have any mental illness or a substance abuse problem. If these issues exist, the batterer will need special treatment for these problems in addition to their violent behaviors. Currently most states have a certification process for programs designed to treat persons with battering behavior problems, and programs must meet certain criteria. Before referring a patient to such a program, providers should verify that the program uses a group approach, is at least 24 weeks long, provides education rather than psycho-

Table 4–2. State Domestic Violence Crisis Hotlines*

State	Toll-Free Number
Florida	1–800–500–1119
Georgia	1–800–643–1212
Illinois	1–800–241–8456
Indiana	1–800–332–7385
Iowa	1–800–942–0333
Louisiana	1–800–837–5400
Maryland	1–800–MD–HELPS
Minnesota	1–800–646–0994
Nevada	1–800–500–1556
New Hampshire	1–800–852–3388
New Mexico	1–800–773–3645
New York	1–800–942–6906
North Dakota	1–800–472–2911
Ohio	1–800–934–9840
Oklahoma	1–800–522–9054
Rhode Island	1–800–494–8100
South Carolina	1–800–260–9293
Tennessee	1–800–356–6767
Virginia	1–800–838–VADV
Washington State	1–800–562–6025
Wyoming	1–800–990–3877

*1-800 numbers may work only if dialed from within the specific state.

Table 4-3. State and Regional Domestic Violence Organizations

Organization	Local Number	State
Arkansas Coalition Against Violence to Women & Children	501–663–4668	AR
Arkansas Coalition Against Domestic Violence	501–812–0571	AR
Alaska Network On Domestic Violence and Sexual Assault	907–586–3650	AK
Arizona Coalition Against Domestic Violence	602–279–2900	AZ
Interagency Council Domestic Violence Program	520–453–5800	AZ
California Alliance Against Domestic Violence	916–444–7163	CA
California—National Network on Behalf of Immigrant Battered Women	415–252–8900	CA
Southern California Coalition on Battered Women (**800–978–3600**)	818–787–0072	CA
Colorado Domestic Violence Coalition	303–831–9632	CO
DC—National Network on Behalf of Immigrant Battered Women	202–387–0434	DC
DC Coalition Against Domestic Violence	202–783–5332	DC
Anti-Violence Project—National Gay and Lesbian Task Force	202–332–6483	DC
Delaware Coalition Against Domestic Violence	302–658–2958	DE
Delaware Domestic Violence Coordinating Council	302–782–6111	DE
Delaware Domestic Violence Coordinating Council	302–577–2684	DE
Georgia Coalition on Family Violence Inc.	770–984–0085	GA
Hawaii State Coalition Against Domestic Violence	808–486–5072	HI
Iowa Coalition Against Domestic Violence (**800–942–0333**)	515–244–8028	IA
Illinois Coalition Against Domestic Violence (**800–799–7233**)	217–789–2830	IL
Victim's Services Domestic Violence Program	309–837–6622	IL
Indiana Coalition Against Domestic Violence (**800–332–7385**)	317–543–3908	IN
Kansas Coalition Against Sexual and Domestic Violence	785–232–9784	KS
Louisiana Coalition Against Domestic Violence	225–752–1296	LA
Massachusetts Coalition of Battered Women's Services Groups	617–248–0922	MA
Maryland Network Against Domestic Violence (**800–MD–HELPS**)	301–352–4574	MD

Maine Coalition for Family Crisis Services	207–941–1194	ME
Minnesota Coalition for Battered Women	651–646–1109	MN
Otter Tail County Intervention Project	218–739–0983	MN
Missouri Shores Women's Resource Center	605–224–7187	MO
Mississippi State Coalition Against Domestic Violence (**800–898–3234**)	601–981–9196	MS
Montana Coalition Against Domestic Violence	406–443–7794	MT
North Carolina Coalition Against Domestic Violence	919–956–9124	NC
North Carolina Victim Assistance Network	919–831–2857	NC
North Dakota Council on Abused Women's Services (**800–472–2911**)	701–255–6240	ND
Nebraska Domestic Violence and Sexual Assault Coalition (**800–876–6238**)	402–476–6256	NE
New Hampshire Coalition Against Domestic Violence and Sexual Violence	603–224–8893	NH
New Hampshire Coalition Against Domestic Violence and Sexual Assault	603–584–8107	NH
New Jersey Coalition for Battered Women (**800–224–0211**)	609–584–8107	NJ
New Mexico State Coalition Against Domestic Violence (**800–773–3645**)	505–246–9240	NM
New York State Coalition Against Domestic Violence (**800–942–6906**)	518–432–4864	NY
Long Island Women's Coalition, Inc.	516–666–8833	NY
Ohio Domestic Violence Network (**800–934–9840**)	614–784–0023	OH
Action Ohio Coalition for Battered Women	614–221–1255	OH
Oregon Coalition Against Domestic and Sexual Violence	503–223–7411	OR
Pennsylvania Coalition Against Domestic Violence (**800–932–4632**)	717–545–6400	PA
Rhode Island Coalition Against Domestic Violence (**800–494–8100**)	401–467–9940	RI
(South Dakota) White Buffalo Calf Women's Shelter	605–856–2317	SD
South Dakota Coalition Against Domestic Violence and Sexual Assault	605–945–0869	SD
Tennessee Task Force Against Domestic Violence (**800–356–6767**)	615–386–9406	TN

Table continued on following page

Table 4-3. State and Regional Domestic Violence Organizations *Continued*

Organization	Local Number	State
Texas Council on Family Violence	512–794–1133	TX
Utah—Domestic Violence Advisory Council (**800–897–LINK**)	801–538–4100	UT
Virginians Against Domestic Violence (**800–838–VADV**)	804–221–0990	VA
Vermont Network Against Domestic Violence and Sexual Assault	802–223–1302	VT
Women's Coalition of St. Croix	340–773–9272	VI
Washington State Coalition Against Domestic Violence (**800–562–6025**)	360–407–0756	WA
West Virginia Coalition Against Domestic Violence	304–965–3552	WV
Wisconsin Coalition Against Domestic Violence	608–255–0539	WI
Wyoming Coalition Against Domestic Violence and Sexual Assault	307–755–5481	WY

therapy, avoids couples' counseling, and has consistent procedures for assessing risk of danger and protecting victims from potential disaster.[16]

While Healthy People 2000 and the United States Preventive Services Task Force have made many recommendations regarding the need for an integrated team approach, it remains very clear that there is still a tremendous need for increased awareness and education of individual clinicians in the arena of identifying and treating victims of domestic violence. Tables 4–1 to 4–3 include references, directories of many state, regional, and national domestic violence organizations, and crisis hotline telephone numbers.

REFERENCES

1. Ferris LE, Norton PG, Dunn EV, et al. Guidelines for managing domestic abuse. JAMA 1997;278:851–857.
2. Rodriguez MA, Craig AM, Mooney DR, Bauer HM. Patient attitudes about mandatory reporting of domestic violence: Implication for health care professionals. West J Med 1998;169:337–341.
3. Schafer J, Caetano R, Clark CL. Rates of intimate partner violence in the United States. Am J Public Health 1998;88:1702–1704.
4. Waldner-Haugrud LK, Gratch LV, Magruder B. Victimization and perpetration rates of violence in gay and lesbian relationships: Gender issues explored. Violence Vict 1997;12:173–184.
5. Ross SM. Risk of physical abuse to children of spouse abusing parents. Child Abuse Neglect 1996;20:589–598.
6. Steiner RP, Vansickle K, Lippmann SB. Domestic violence—Do you know when and how to intervene? Postgrad Med 1996;100.
7. Warshaw, Ganley, Salber. Improving the Health Care Response to Domestic Violence: A Resource Manual for Health Care Providers. San Francisco, CA, Family Violence Prevention Fund, 1996.
8. Lee WV, Weinstein SP. How far have we come? A critical review of the research on men who batter. *In* Glanger M (ed), Recent Developments in Alcoholism, Vol. 13: Alcoholism and Violence. New York, Plenum Press, 1997, pp 337–356.
9. Levine MD, Carey WB, Crockery AC, Gross R. Family dysfunction, violence, neglect, and sexual misuse. *In* Snyder JC, Developmental Behavioral Pediatrics. Philadelphia, WB Saunders, 1983, pp 256–275.
10. Poirier L. The importance of screening for domestic violence in all women. Nurse Pract 1997;22:105–122.
11. Gremillion DH, Kanoff EP. Overcoming barriers to physician involvement in identifying and referring victims of domestic violence. Ann Emerg Med 1996;27:769–773.
12. Life Preservers—A Life Line for Victims of Violence. A Guide for Physicians.
13. Butler R. Warning signs of elder abuse. Geriatrics 1999;54:3–4.
14. Wolf R. Suspected abuse in an elderly patient. Am Fam Physician 1999; 59(5):1319–1320.
15. Shea CA, Mahoney M, Lacey JM. Breaking through the barriers to domestic violence intervention. Am J Nurs 1997;97:26–33.
16. Adams D. Guidelines for doctors on identifying and helping their patients who batter. J Am Med Womens Assoc 1996;51:123–126.

CHAPTER 5

Environmental Health and Sanitation

Charles C. Lewis, MPH, PA–C, and Charles E. McManus, MPH, RS

INTRODUCTION

As humans we are intimately bound to the environment by the air we breathe, by the water and food that we consume, and by complex interrelationships with other living organisms. Physical, chemical, and biological processes that occur within the environment constantly affect us.

Humankind's first impact on the environment occurred when people first gathered into loosely organized communities. As societies have become more industrialized and urbanized, they have produced escalating environmental changes, both from the use of numerous chemicals in manufacturing and agriculture, and from sharing space, food, and water supplies.[1] Populations have an increased likelihood of experiencing health problems from exposure to a variety of chemicals and toxins because of industrial mass production and a world market supplying our foods. These foodstuffs are grown, treated with insecticides, fertilized (both organically and inorganically), preserved or transported by a variety of means, and regulated inconsistently. Laborers who are also consumers are especially at risk. The United States alone produces more than 6 billion tons of waste annually. Much of this waste is hazardous to humans and animals, and some of it is frankly toxic. The process of waste disposal often increases the hazard by either concentrating it in large amounts in specified hazardous waste sites or by dispersing it throughout the environment in an effort to dilute the toxic elements. No one wants the hazardous material stored or disposed of in his or her backyard ("NIMBY"). Some of what is known about symptoms has been determined from studies of populations exposed to hazardous waste sites.[2] With the U.S. population reaching approximately 280 million and the world population approximately 6 billion at the close of the 20th century, the problems of the environment can only increase.

The American Public Health Association was founded in 1872 in an attempt to characterize some of the health and hygiene problems of the populace. Shortly thereafter, Congress passed some of the first public health laws in U.S. history to provide care for sailors and to prevent importation of diseases such as smallpox, cholera, and yellow fever. This resulted in the formation of the Marine Hospital Services.

In 1889 the Commissioned Corps was established, and in 1912 its name was changed to the United States Public Health Service (USPHS). These agencies were community-based and directed at addressing some of the health and environmental problems that were affecting the population. The Centers for Disease Control and Prevention (CDC) grew from needs of the USPHS following World War II.[3] Almost 100 years after the USPHS was founded, the Environmental Protection Agency (EPA) was established to quantify risks associated with environmental pollution by conducting studies known as risk assessments. More recently, the Agency for Toxic Substances and Disease Registry (ATSDR) was created by the EPA and charged with the responsibility to conduct human health assessments on target populations associated with hazardous waste exposures. These federal agencies attempt to establish both the risk and its potential for reaching human populations. Ideally, this public information is shared with clinicians treating patients who may have been exposed to toxic substances; however, this communication relies upon a somewhat problematically funded infrastructure.

Exactly who is responsible for conducting investigations into environmental complaints is somewhat vague, owing to the large numbers of agencies, both state and federal, that have overlapping functions. Furthermore, environmental specialists tend to be organized into disciplines that deal with health, engineering, or sanitation. These disciplines are somewhat removed from the practice of medicine and seek to control disease through regulation and by applying methods of prevention. Public concern about the overall problems of environmental exposure to hazardous substances focuses on debates as to whether there is an acceptable standard of exposure other than no exposure at all. Many agencies work through governmental mandates that often overlap in areas of responsibility. All work through various levels of state government to provide technical support and expertise. Each state is charged with supervising the health of its population primarily through local health departments. State health departments are typically separated into divisions based on technical expertise or function. In addition to clinical health services, local health departments provide communicable disease prevention programs and environmental services. Many epidemiologic studies have been commissioned in an attempt to define human health risks in a meaningful way.[4]

ENVIRONMENTAL SERVICES

Environmental services were initially established to prevent the spread of enteric diseases but have expanded to meet the needs of managing toxic exposures due to chemical, radiologic, or biological threats. Local officials are often are called upon to investigate a broad spectrum of citizen complaints of exposure. Typically, complaints are handled within a particular program, such as air quality, water quality, hazardous waste, environmental sanitation, or other specialized areas within federal, state, and municipal agencies. Health department employees in these specialized program areas generally conduct routine inspections of industries and occasionally of private dwellings in which activities occur that may affect the environment. When releases of regulated chemicals occur, the local health department is usually the first to respond. If a health risk to a population exists, other levels of government may be consulted. When an industry releases material into the environment that exceeds guideline standards for that substance the resulting pollution may cause an undesirable effect on humans or the environment itself. Releases or spills that exceed government safety standards generate a response in accordance with requirements set forth in the regulations. The response could range from a single investigator from the local health department to a major effort requiring a team of specialists from the EPA. Depending on the threat to the environment and to human populations, the follow-up could entail anything from a simple cleanup of a spill to an evacuation of people from a threatened area. Regulatory agencies often are empowered to impose penalties such as fines or to close any responsible facility.[5]

Connecting an environmental event to human disease often requires cooperation from scientists working in seemingly nonrelated fields. Sometimes a problem is detected in animal or plant species before it is recognized in human populations. Recently, outbreaks have occurred of diseases that generally have been thought to be confined to animals but are now being detected in humans. Efforts to control these outbreaks on a global basis have led to international conferences on emerging pathogens. Humans are a difficult group to study because of the medical and legal constraints concerning the examination of subjects while actual exposures are occurring. Therefore, effects on human health associated with any given environmental exposure are often estimates.

Environmental epidemiologists attempt to bring together the clinical aspects of exposure with the physical, biological, and chemical factors in the external environment. They must rely on a number of sources to gain the knowledge needed to evaluate the threat from a particular or potential exposure. One such source is the published studies of occupational exposures. Clinical reports of actual cases may also be used when they are available. The EPA also conducts environmental risk assessments on hazardous waste sites (intended to serve as the quantitative basis) for the selection of remedial objectives and strategies for that site. The ATSDR attempts to use qualitative information to inform communities about the potential for adverse human health effects associated with past or present releases from such a site. Both of these processes are time-consuming and are conducted over lengthy periods. Often data collected can be used to predict the health effects of future harmful releases to the environment. The CDC maintains a cadre of health scientists along with specialized laboratories that are dedicated to defining and containing diseases in the population.

Generally when no demonstrable disease exists within a population, it is assumed that all is well within the associated environment. On the other hand, technology has evolved to the extent that many pollutants can be measured in some quantity in the environment, even when no health effect can be demonstrated. Often the public associates the measured presence of a pollutant, even in minuscule quantities, with possible or actual health effects.

Health care providers in a community do not always associate particular symptoms with an environmentally related problem until the number of cases reaches a level sufficient to cause alarm. Not every spontaneous abortion is the result of an environmental chemical exposure. However, when a number of spontaneous abortions occur within an identified locality over a short period, the news media may pick up the story and amplify it. The political structure will often put forth declarations before health agencies even become aware of the complaint. Some problems become sensationalized in this way and may receive even more attention than they deserve. This is more likely to occur when a problem involves a major corporation or has political ramifications. One example was the report of anencephalic babies being born in excessive numbers along the U.S.-Mexican border. Manufacturing plants were known to dispose of toxic solvents in the rivers where Mexican citizens bathed and washed clothing. Media attention can sometimes cause sufficient focus to force needed interventions to ameliorate such a problem.

Laypersons are not always aware that they have been exposed to an environmental agent. They may have symptoms that they attribute to other causes. Patients may also have symptoms that they attribute to exposure when none has occurred. That situation is more likely to occur when a group of citizens does not like having a particular industry close to their neighborhood. Sometimes an environmental release may occur near a population that complains of symptoms that are not caused by the materials released. Those exposed are not likely to accept this explanation. All of these situations may be confusing to a health care practitioner attempting to care for patients with these complaints. One of the more common concerns is fear of cancer. A major part of the education process for both the provider and the patient lies in knowing what environmental hazards exist in the patient's community, and whether the hazard is related to an industrial, agricultural, recreational, or other, as yet unknown, source.

Industries and businesses that deal with production, transportation, or storage of hazardous chemicals and/or hazardous wastes are required by federal regulation to display universal symbols indicating the type and degree of hazards that exist on the site. They are also required to maintain on-site material safety data sheets (MSDS) that describe the material, the hazard potential, and the recommended treatment for exposure. Recent changes in federal regulations also require that certain industries inform community officials of any hazard potential in the advent of a fire, spill, or other release of any toxic material. Industries may be slow to report adverse events because their own response personnel are waiting to determine whether a threat truly exists. Many chemicals in use in industry also have a measurable quantity beyond which reporting is mandatory. If a regulated material has been released, the party responsible faces the possibility of being assessed heavy fines. Some corporations take extra risks by not reporting releases simply to avoid such fines. These businesses must attempt with due diligence to control the release and may become committed to such an activity, thus causing them to delay reporting. The Occupational Safety and Health Administration (OSHA) also has regulations that require supervisors to inform workers of hazards existing in their workplace. Some workers may be required to have periodic medical examinations and screening if they handle certain types of hazardous materials. Not every person is subject to such oversight or regulation, and occasionally problems arise in these areas. In particular, private farms are exempt from a number of regulatory programs that could oversee day-to-day operations.

When patients have dramatic symptoms following a toxic exposure, the likely cause(s) may be readily apparent or at least suspected. However, health care providers must more frequently examine patients who may have been exposed to toxins, pathogens, or chemicals yet relate no history of exposure. When patients do not realize that they have been exposed, clinicians may not initially recognize the true nature of the problem. Once victims begin to arrive in greater numbers, the clinician may then suspect a common exposure. In the 1980s, the U.S. Navy transferred a highly toxic substance to a hazardous waste contractor for disposal. The contractor had his employees bury the material in a landfill. The workers were not informed that the OTTO fuel (a synthetic propellant for torpedoes) could potentially cause severe neurologic problems and required special precautions for handling. Some workers who were exposed developed these symptoms, and subsequently the incident was investigated by a number of agencies, including ATSDR.

Index of suspicion and clinical acumen play a major role in the management of these patients. Employees who are properly trained and informed of the potential hazards may be able to alert the provider. Nevertheless, in some cases, the clinical presentation may be quite perplexing. The medical history may provide few clues if any, and those that are present can be quite subtle. The clinician must explore such issues as:

* Is the patient currently working in a hazardous materials (HazMat) environment?
* Has he or she previously worked in a HazMat environment?

* Does the patient have any family or household member working in such an environment?
* Does the patient live near a farm or a manufacturing or processing plant?
* Do any household members have temporary or part-time employment in or near such activities?
* Does any household member have a hobby or avocation that involves toxic chemicals?

Clinicians generally consider syndromes according to which organ systems are affected. With environmental problems, we often must consider governmental health agency programs in much the same way. Some purists may not appreciate this approach. Clinicians faced with the task of trying to decide which agency to contact for help can easily become confounded. Many situational concerns overlap from environmental health into environmental sanitation. Patients often face a similar dilemma when trying to select a physician or other provider from the telephone directory. Usually the solution is directional. Most problems are best solved at the lowest level possible. Unfortunately, too often departments within the same agency may not know what other services are available.

The remainder of this chapter is confined to the discussion of those areas with the most direct application to the primary care clinical setting.

PROGRAM AREAS

* Control of communicable diseases
* Emerging and re-emerging diseases
* Foodborne infections
* Water and air quality
* Disaster management

CONTROL OF COMMUNICABLE DISEASES

While not a leading cause of death and disability in the U.S., environmentally transmitted infections constitute a cause for concern. These are infections that are transmitted or spread by a common source (such as a community well), or as the result of a source propagated by arthropod or rodent vectors, or by inanimate objects (as with communicable diseases). Responsibility for administering programs of
1. Surveillance and response
2. Prevention and control

Box 5-1–Arthropods as Direct Agents of Disease or Discomfort

- Entomophobia
- Annoyance and blood loss
- Accidental injury to sense organs
- Envenomization
- Dermatosis
- Myiasis and related infestations
- Allergy and related conditions

---

generally rests with the state health departments. World travel has greatly increased the possibility of the spread of organisms that have previously been confined to certain regions. Recent reports indicate that tuberculosis may be a transmittable risk on airline flights lasting longer than 8 h. Trichinosis, while uncommon in the U.S., still occurs in undeveloped regions where pigs and bears feed on garbage and waste.

MEDICALLY IMPORTANT ARTHROPODS AND OTHER VECTORS AND DISEASES THEY TRANSMIT

Arthropods are responsible for much misery and suffering throughout both the developing and the developed world. Even those not known to transmit disease may bite, sting, or otherwise cause discomfort. Some arthropods are responsible for destruction of food stores and crops in the fields. The results can include major economic and nutritional losses and disease in those affected regions (Boxes 5-1 and 5-2). These complex relationships cannot be discussed in detail here.

Many diseases transmitted by arthropods are found in the tropical

---

Box 5-2–Arthropods as Vectors or Intermediate Hosts

- Mechanical carriers (transmission may be accidental); nonbiting flies, cockroaches
- Obligatory vectors (some degree of development or propagation occurs)
- Intermediate host transmission (transmission of a pathogen to the final host)

Table 5–1. Disease Vectors

Vector	Short-Term Effects of Exposure (1–7 days)	Long-Term Disease Effects (30 days or longer)
Flies	Nuisance	Nuisance, diarrheal disease
Mosquitoes	Bites and nuisance	Bites and nuisance, encephalitis, dengue, malaria, filariasis
Lice	Bites and nuisance	Bites and nuisance, epidemic typhus, louse-borne relapsing fever
Fleas	Bites and nuisance	Bites and nuisance, plague, endemic typhus
Mites	Bites and nuisance	Bites and nuisance, scabies, rickettsial pox, scrub typhus
Ticks	Bites and nuisance	Bites and nuisance, tick paralysis, tick-borne relapsing fever, Rocky Mountain spotted fever, Lyme disease, erlichiosis
Bedbugs, kissing bugs	Bites and nuisance	Bites and nuisance, Chagas disease
Rodents	Rat bites	Bites, including rat bite fever, leptospirosis, salmonellosis
Ants, spiders, scorpions, snakes	Bites, stings, envenomization, nuisance	Bites, stings, envenomization, nuisance, allergies

regions of the world. However, recent outbreaks of mosquito-borne encephalitis (arboviruses) in the northern regions of the U.S. have begun to raise concerns among public health officials. Some pathogens are new to the northern U.S. and raise concerns that others will follow. Mosquitoes and other arthropods are common throughout the U.S., and many are capable vectors. Animals other than arthropods may also serve as important disease vectors (see Table 5–1). In addition to carrying diseases such as plague and Hantavirus, rodents are frequently responsible for destruction of food sources.

SNAKEBITE AND RABIES

Snakebite

Snakebites, while much feared, account for fewer than 12 deaths per year in the U.S. Venomous snakes are widely distributed throughout the continental U.S., with virtually all states having one or more venomous species. The highest bite rates occur in the southern states, between April and October each year. Young males and those under the influence of alcohol have the highest rates of envenomation.

Rabies

Rabies is an important disease to consider when treating animal bites. Rabies is a preventable viral disease of mammals, both domestic and wild. Most states require the reporting of all animal bites to the local health department. With the increased emphasis on the inoculation of domestic animals, the incidence of rabies has decreased in these particular species. However, the incidence of rabies has increased in wild animals such as raccoons, skunks, bats, and foxes. The urbanization of land that once was the habitat of wild animals has increased the possibility of an exposure of a pet to the wild animal population, including bats. Although bats have small teeth that may not leave an obvious puncture wound, people usually recognize when a bat has bitten them. Therefore, in the case of a suspected bat bite, many health departments recommend postexposure prophylaxis (PEP) only if

* The bat cannot be tested
* The bat was in the room of an unattended child or a mentally impaired or intoxicated person

A case study can be found at cdc.gov/ncidod/dvrd/rabies/bats%29&%20Rabies/bats&.htm.

Modern rabies prophylaxis has proved nearly 100% successful. Most human fatalities associated with rabies today occur in those people who fail to seek medical assistance (usually because they fail to recognize a risk in the contact leading to the infection). Transmission of rabies virus occurs when the contaminated saliva is passed to a susceptible host. Most rabies vaccine is available only through state health departments, while commercial snakebite antivenins are stocked in most hospital emergency rooms.

▬ EMERGING AND RE-EMERGING DISEASES

Alterations to the environment by humans have created new opportunities for exposures to infections. In some cases the pathogens have been present but have gone undetected. In others, pathogens may be introduced into a human population by an epidemiologic bridge.[6, 7] Changes in land use have had major impacts on wildlife habitats. Deforestation for the development of real estate destroys habitats, causing wildlife either to seek new homes or to remain in close contact with growing human populations. As available habitats continue to shrink, wildlife is pushed closer to human habitation.

On the other hand, reforestation of former farmland to create the "country look" for homesites attracts wildlife that would not ordinarily choose to live so close to humans. In the 1990s, an outbreak of an unknown disease occurred among Native Americans residing in the southwest U.S. that required assistance from the CDC in order to reach the correct diagnosis.[8] People had constructed homes in areas inhabited by *Peromyscus maniculatis*, the rodent vector of Hantavirus. Lyme disease and human erlichiosis are tick-borne diseases that can occur when people move into infested areas. As these trends continue, additional disease emergence is likely.

People and pathogens also encounter each other in nontraditional ways through activities such as "ecotourism," where individuals from various walks of life and regions of the world come together in a tightly concentrated unit. Usually this involves travel to exotic places in order to view, hunt, or photograph wildlife in its natural state, and such excursions have become increasingly popular.

A community's socioeconomic status, geopolitical conflicts (wars), and natural disasters can also play a role in the spread of disease. Flooding can impose the greatest public health risk because it can contaminate water sources, destroy food, cause loss of livestock and crops, and make dwellings uninhabitable. Major fires cause disruptions of the environment and strain the public health programs charged with keeping disease in check. Disasters that are either widespread or protracted may stretch available resources beyond their limits. Mosquito populations that have been in check may explode, bringing with them a host of diseases. Such was the case with a large outbreak of equine encephalitis that occurred in Florida during the mid-1990's. Outbreaks of St. Louis encephalitis and West Nile virus in the fall of 1999 led clinicians to raise new questions when faced with managing a patient with an indolent fever. Flooding in eastern North Carolina following Hurricane Floyd in September 1999 raised concerns that the mosquito population could explode, resulting in an increase in mosquito-borne disease in peak tourist seasons. Occasionally, however, the reverse can occur, with destruction of breeding sites resulting in the lowering of disease rates. Viral encephalitis constitutes the major group of diseases spread by mosquitoes in the U.S. Dengue fever and malaria, in the past, were attributed to imported cases, but foci of infection in the U.S. may now exist or soon re-emerge. World travel from endemic areas is only one contributing factor. The presence of numerous mosquito vectors amplifies the problem. Social pressures also exist beyond the world of medicine, including overpopulation, poverty, and uncontrollable urbanization.

New occupational exposures to *Pfiesteria piscida* and *Cryptoderniopsis* now exist (e.g., commercial fishermen), and a number of studies are under way to determine the extent of human disease that could be caused by these organisms.

FACTORS FAVORING EMERGENCE

Some of the most important weapons against infectious diseases are drugs, vaccines, and pesticides. However, each of these tools has both benefits and risks. Antibiotic resistance is a major factor to be considered in the treatment of microorganisms. Overuse of antibiotics may allow some organisms to proliferate and others, that had not been previously pathogenic, to become virulent. Disease vectors, primarily arthropods, have shown the same kind of resistance to pesticides. Similarly, vaccines have proved effective in many cases but may fail in the future. The race is on to develop more and better vaccines. Ironically, some of the tools that have proved to be most effective in Western medicine have not done as well in developing countries. Often health care providers in less developed countries have neither the technology nor the training to administer health care as practiced in the U.S. Reuse of disposable items and improper sterilization of reusable items are not uncommon. This can result in disease transmission in settings where the balance is already delicate. With travel and commerce expanding into many of these areas, we can no longer assume that these problems will remain problems of other countries (see Box 5-3).

■ FOODBORNE INFECTIONS

Foodborne illnesses result when the host consumes foods or liquids containing infectious organisms or toxins. The United States Food and Drug Administration (FDA) has even labeled ice as dangerous in the transmission of foodborne organisms. Together, food sanitation and management of foodborne illnesses constitute one of the major public health efforts in the U.S. Production, processing, transportation, storage, preparation, and disposal of foods are among the most complex public health regulatory areas. Foods that people consume are located on a spectrum from highly stable to highly perishable. Opportunities

---

Box 5-3–FACTORS FAVORING EMERGING INFECTIONS

- Human demographics and behavior
- Technology and industry
- Economic development and land use
- International travel and commerce
- Microbial adaptation and change
- Breakdown of public health measures

Box 5-4–SOURCES OF FOOD CONTAMINATION

- Improper holding temperatures (foods allowed to remain between 40°–140°F for extended periods of time)
- Inadequately cooked foods
- Contaminated equipment and/or surfaces (cutting boards, counter tops, sinks)
- Infected food handlers
- Food obtained from unsafe or suspect sources, including contaminated hands/gloves—magic gloves syndrome, forgetting to change gloves after touching a contaminated surface

for contamination exist at every step along the way to our tables and increase proportionately to the amount of handling and repackaging. Freezing does not sufficiently destroy all pathogens, and foods that must be held frozen or refrigerated may be rendered unsafe if they remain above proper holding temperatures for an extended period.

Recalls of meats, poultry, and dairy products in the late 1990s indicate that the need for surveillance is increasing. Newly emerging pathogens are cause for concern and heightened awareness. Both sides of the equation from commercially prepared foods to home-cooked meals play roles in foodborne illness. Scrupulous sanitation minimizes but does totally mitigate the problem. Most outbreaks can be traced to a breakdown in handling, as shown in Box 5-4. The food industry has undertaken a number of initiatives in cooperation with federal and state regulatory agencies to minimize health risks from commercial food sources. Restaurants typically require all employees who handle food or work in preparation areas to undergo training in safe handling techniques. However, in spite of efforts to control the spread of disease through handling, outbreaks still occur. The most common organisms responsible for these outbreaks are depicted in Table 5–2. Federal regulations require that all processing plants involved in handling meat or poultry adopt and carry out written Sanitation Standard Operating Procedures (SSOP). In conjunction with this protocol, plants must implement the system of science-based process controls known as HACCP (Hazard Analysis Critical Control Points).

The term *foodborne illness* is applied to any sickness that occurs from the ingestion of foods or beverages that are contaminated with an agent capable of producing the symptom manifested. An outbreak is identified when two or more persons develop the same symptoms after consuming the same foods. Actual occurrences are probably grossly under-reported. In many cases, the symptoms are mild and may go unnoticed by the patient, or are attributed to a 24-h "bug." Many but not all infections are acquired from eating the same contam-

Table 5–2. Organisms Associated with Foodborne Illness

Viruses
Hepatitis A virus
Hepatitis E virus
Rotavirus
Norwalk virus group
Other viral agents

Bacteria
Aeromonas hydrophilia
Bacillus cereus
Campylobacter jejuni
Clostridium botulinum, C. perfringens
Enterovirulent *Escherichia coli*
Listeria monocytogenes
Pleisomonas shigelloides
Salmonella, Shigella
Staphylococcus aureus
Streptococcus
Vibrio cholerae 01 and non-01
Vibrio vulnificus
Yersinia enterocolitica
Parasitic/Protozoa/Worms

Parasitic/Protozoa/Worms
Anasakis spp.
Amoebae
Ascaris lumbricoides
Cryptosporidium parvum
Cyclospora cayetanensis
Diphyllobothrium spp.
Entamoeba histolytica
Giardia lamblia
Eustrongyloides spp.
Nanophyetus spp.
Trichuris trichiura

Natural Toxins
Aflatoxins
Ciguatera poisoning
Grayanotoxin (honey)
Mushroom toxins
Pyrrolizidine alkaloids
Phytohemagglutinin (kidney bean)
Scombroid poisoning
Shellfish toxins
Tetrodotoxin (Pufferfish)

inated food. Some infections such as roundworm, in which the organism is contained in the feces of one victim and passed to another, are transmitted hand-to-mouth. Hepatitis A virus may also be passed in this fashion. As new pathogens emerge, new vehicles of food contamination often emerge with them, frequently occurring earlier rather than later in the production process. Some pathogens have been linked to increased consumption of fresh fruits and vegetables as part of the "eat healthier" pattern that many Americans are adopting. Another trend of combining foods from many countries into single dishes complicates the problem of identifying pathogen sources when outbreaks do inevitably occur.

Investigation of any suspected foodborne outbreak must be conducted swiftly in order to acquire reliable information. People often cannot remember consuming specific food items from a menu. When an outbreak is considered, the clinician must establish a coherent case definition (Box 5-5). Some investigations warrant the inclusion of experts from the public health community, and they should be contacted sooner rather than later. A complicated situation may involve state and federal scientists such as sanitarians and epidemiologists. This situation may occur when potentially exposed persons do not reside in the same community, region, or country. International travel and migration are contributing factors in the spread of foodborne diseases in some parts of the world (Box 5-6).

Box 5-5–CHARACTERISTICS OF FOODBORNE ILLNESS: CASE DEFINITION

- Occurrence of illness within short but variable period of time (2 h to several days)
- A group of individuals who have eaten the same foods from a common source (two or more cases of a similar illness resulting from ingestion of a common food)
- Often associated with a social event such as a concert or family gathering
- Foods usually not adequately heated or refrigerated
- Food handler with illness or exposed skin lesion
- Associated symptoms
1. Viral and bacterial infections typically result in an acute gastroenteritis.
2. Hepatitis A can result in liver damage.
3. *Clostridium botulinum* infection produces neurologic symptoms.
4. Parasitic larvae or trophozoites may migrate to other body sites causing a variety of clinical syndromes.

Box 5-6–FACTORS CONTRIBUTING TO EMERGENCE OF FOODBORNE PATHOGENS

- Genetic variability of some microorganisms
- Environmental factors, such as tropical conditions that favor growth of fungi and production of mycotoxins
- Behavior of people toward food safety (People become vectors as they travel.)
- Urbanization is a major factor; crowding increases contact and opportunity.
- Raw food production involves centralized processing and wide distribution.
- Denial that an outbreak (epidemic) exists is more common in developing countries to avoid trade and travel penalties and restrictions.
- Economic factors, such as warfare and economic decline, provide opportunities for disease outbreaks.
- Technology, in spite of its benefits, brings with it new risks.
- Personal risk factors, such as age, health, and availability of treatment; poverty

The only pathogen that is specifically mentioned in the International Health Regulations is cholera. Outbreaks of this disease are reported to the World Health Organization (WHO), and some international health officials would like to expand reporting to include other organisms. Cholera, while not common in the U.S., does occur. For this reason single confirmed case constitutes an epidemic.

When patients present with complaints or questions regarding foodborne illness, this can provide an excellent opportunity to conduct patient education concerning safe food handling both in the home and when dining out.

* Does the patient use methods that are safe and sanitary when preparing, serving, and storing foods?
* Does the patient use proper hand washing and cleaning of cooking surfaces?
* Does the patient know which foods are associated with foodborne outbreaks?
* Where does the patient acquire information about food preparation and safety?
* Does the information come from reliable health and nutrition sources, or does it come from popular media such as radio and television talk shows or magazines?
* Determining causation in a foodborne outbreak often depends on knowing when suspected foods were consumed in respect to how soon afterward symptoms first appeared (Tables 5–3 to 5–9).

Management of a patient with a suspected foodborne exposure must be based on both the patient's presenting condition and the causative agent. Some patients may appear quite ill, only to fully recover in a few hours without treatment, while others may develop symptoms that become increasingly ominous with time. The general health of the patient prior to the foodborne infection is also a major factor. Even with dreaded diseases such as cholera, fluid replacement is the primary and often the only, treatment consideration (Box 5-7).

Table 5–3. Upper Gastrointestinal Tract Symptoms

Nausea and Vomiting as Presenting or Predominant Complaints

Time of Onset and Symptoms	Causative Agent
Within minutes to 1 h; bad or unusual taste	Metallic salts
1–2 h; weakness or loss of consciousness	Nitrites
1–6 h; retching and abdominal pain	*Staphylococcus aureus*
8–16 h; includes abdominal cramps	*Bacillus cereus*
6–24 h; diarrhea, dilation of pupils, prostration, and coma	Mushroom poisoning (*Amanita* spp.)

Table 5–4. Lower Abdominal Tract Symptoms

Abdominal Cramps or Diarrhea as Presenting or Primary Complaint

Time of Onset and Symptoms	*Causative Agent*
2–36 h with mean of 6–12 h; malodorous diarrhea, and sometimes nausea and vomiting	*Clostridium perfringens, Bacillus cereus, Streptococcus faecalis, S. faecium*
12–74 h with mean of 18–36 h; cramps, vomiting, fever, chills, malaise, occasionally mucoid or bloody diarrhea	*Salmonella/Shigella* spp. enteropathogenic *Escheria coli,* other *Enterobacteriaceae, Vibrio parahaemolyticus, Aeromonas hydrophila, Plesiomonas shigelloides, Campylobacter jejuni,* and many others
3–5 days; abdominal pain and respiratory symptoms	Enteric viruses
1–6 weeks; mucoid diarrhea, abdominal pain, and weight loss	*Giardia lamblia*
1 to several weeks; diarrhea, constipation, headache, drowsiness, ulcers (variable and sometimes asymptomatic)	*Entamoeba histolytica*
3–6 months; nervousness, insomnia, hunger pains, anorexia, weight loss	*Taenia saginata, T. solium*

Box 5-7–PATIENT MANAGEMENT OF SUSPECTED FOODBORNE ILLNESS

- Develop case definition in the event of possible outbreak.
- Obtain careful history (people often cannot remember meal items actually consumed).
- Attempt to obtain complete food diary for at least 72 h prior to onset.
- Seek assistance from public health agencies as soon as diagnosis is suspected (potential patients may have traveled great distances before becoming ill).
- Many foodborne illnesses are benign and self-limiting, while some may be life-threatening.
- Treatment is more often supportive than curative.
- Fluid replacement often provides more relief than all other therapies.

Table 5–5. Neurologic Symptoms

Visual Disturbances, Vertigo, Tingling, or Paralysis

Time of Onset and Symptoms	*Causative Agent*
Less than 1 hour	
Gastroenteritis, nervousness, blurred vision, chest pain, cyanosis, twitching, or convulsions	Shellfish toxin, organic phosphate
Excessive salivation, perspiration, gastroenteritis, irregular pulse, pupillary constriction, and wheezing	Muscaria-type mushrooms
Pallor, hematemesis, desquamation of skin, loss of reflexes, and paralysis	Tetrodotoxins
1–6 hours	
Gastroenteritis, dry mouth, muscular aches, dilated pupils, blurred vision, paralysis	Ciguatera toxin
Nausea, vomiting, weakness, anorexia, weight loss, and confusion	Chlorinated hydrocarbons
2 hours to 6 days (usually 12–36 h)	
Vertigo, blurred or double vision, difficulty in swallowing, speaking, or breathing	*Clostridium botulinum*

FoodNet, a surveillance project of the CDC begun in 1996, augments but does not replace longstanding state and federal efforts to identify, control, and prevent foodborne disease hazards. Nevertheless, this active surveillance of seven bacterial and two parasitic organisms may provide badly needed information that could direct future public policy.

■■■WATER AND AIR QUALITY

POTABLE WATER SUPPLY

Drinking water is regulated by the federal government and managed through a variety of environmental and health agencies at state,

Text continued on page 104

Table 5–6. Allergic Symptoms

Facial Flushing, Itching and Anaphylaxis

Onset Less than 1 hour	*Causative Agent*
Headache, bad taste, nausea, vomiting, burning of throat, facial swelling and flushing, itching of skin	Scombroid poisoning
Numbness around mouth, tingling, flushing, dizziness, headache, and nausea	Monosodium glutamate

Table 5–7. Generalized Symptoms of Infection

Fever, Chills, Malaise, Prostration, Swollen Lymph Glands

Time of Onset and Symptoms	*Causative Agent*
4–28 days (mean 8–10 days); gastroenteritis, periorbital edema, diaphoresis, and labored breathing	*Trichinella spiralis*
7–28 days (mean 4–8 days); headache, cough, vomiting, abdominal pain, rose spots, bloody stools	*Salmonella typhi*
10–13 days; myalgia and rash	*Toxoplasma gondii*
Variable period of time; head or joint aches, prostration, tender lymphadenopathy, and other systemic symptoms, depending on etiologic agent	*Bacillus anthracis, Brucella melitensis, B. abortus, B. suis, Coxiella burnetii, Francisella tularensis, Listeria monocytogenes, Mycobacterium tuberculosis, Mycobacterium* spp., *Pasteurella multocida, Leptospira* spp., and others

Table 5–8. Shellfish Toxins

Gastrointestinal and/or Neurologic Symptoms

Time of Onset and Symptoms	*Causative Agent*
30 min to 2 h; tingling, burning, numbness, drowsiness, incoherent speech, and respiratory paralysis	Paralytic shellfish poisoning (PSP)
2–5 min to 3–4 h; reversal of hot and cold sensations, tingling, numbness of lips, tongue, and throat, muscle aches, dizziness, diarrhea, and vomiting	Neurotoxic shellfish poisoning (NSP), brevetoxins
30 min to 2–3 h; nausea, vomiting, diarrhea, abdominal pain, chills, and fever	Diarrheic shellfish poisoning (DSP), dinophysis toxin, okadaic toxin, pectenotoxin, and others
24 h; gastrointestinal symptoms, followed by neurologic symptoms within 48 h, including memory loss, disorientation, seizure, and coma	Amnesic shellfish poisoning (ASP), domoic acid

Table 5-9. Compendium of Acute Foodborne and Waterborne Gastrointestinal Diseases

I. Diseases Typified by Vomiting After a Short Incubation Period with Little or No Fever

Agent	Incubation Period—Usual (and Range)	Symptoms° (Partial List)	Pathophysiology	Characteristic Foods	Specimens†
Staphylococcus aureus	2–4 h (1–6 h)	N, C, V; D, F may be present	Preformed enterotoxin	Sliced/chopped ham and meats, custards, cream fillings	*Food:* Enterotoxin assay (FDA), culture for quantitation and phage typing of *Staphylococcus*, Gram's stain *Handlers:* Culture nares, skin, skin lesions, and phage type *Staphylococcus* *Cases:* Culture stool and vomitus, phage type *Staphylococcus*
Bacillus cereus	2–4 h (1–6 h)	N, V, D	? Preformed enterotoxin	Fried rice	*Food:* Culture for quantitation *Cases:* Stool culture
Heavy metals 1. Cadmium 2. Copper 3. Tin 4. Zinc	5–15 min (1–60 min)	N, V, C, D		Foods and beverages prepared/stored/cooked in containers coated/lined/contaminated with offending metal	Toxicologic analysis of food container, vomitus, stomach contents, urine, blood, feces

II. Diseases Typified by Diarrhea After a Moderate to Long Incubation Period, Often with Fever

Agent	Incubation Period—Usual (and Range)	Symptoms° (Partial List)	Pathophysiology	Characteristic Foods	Specimens†
Clostridium perfringens	12 h (8–16 h)	C, D (V, F rare)	Enterotoxin formed in vivo	Meat, poultry	*Food:* Enterotoxin assay done as research procedure by FDA, culture for quantitation and serotyping. *Cases:* Culture feces for quantitation and serotyping of *C. perfringens;* test for enterotoxin in stool. *Controls:* Culture feces for quantitation and serotyping of *C. perfringens.*
Bacillus cereus	8–16 h	C, D	? Enterotoxin	Custards, cereals, puddings, sauces, meatloaf	*Food:* Culture. *Cases:* Stool culture
Vibrio parahaemolyticus	12 h (2–48 h)	C, D, N, V, F, H, B	Tissue invasion, ? enterotoxin	Seafood	*Food:* Culture on TCBS, serotype, Kanagawa test. *Cases:* Stool cultures on TCBS, serotype, Kanagawa test
Salmonella (nontyphoid)	12–36 h (6–72 h)	D, C, F, V, H septicemia or enteric fever	Tissue invasion	Poultry, eggs, meat, raw milk (cross-contamination important), fruits, vegetables	*Food:* Culture with serotyping *Case:* Stool culture with serotyping *Handlers:* Stool culture with serotyping as a secondary consideration

Table continued on following page

Table 5–9. Compendium of Acute Foodborne and Waterborne Gastrointestinal Diseases *Continued*

II. Diseases Typified by Diarrhea After a Moderate to Long Incubation Period, Often with Fever *Continued*

Agent	Incubation Period—Usual (and Range)	Symptoms* (Partial List)	Pathophysiology	Characteristic Foods	Specimens†
Parvovirus-like agents (Norwalk, Hawaii, Colorado, cockle agents)	16–48 h	N, V, C, D	Unknown	Shellfish, water	Stool for immune EM and serology by special arrangement
Rotavirus	16–48 h	N, V, C, D	Unknown	Foodborne transmission not well documented	*Cases:* Stool examination by EM or ELISA; serology
Escherichia coli enterotoxigenic	16–48 h	D, C	Enterotoxin	Uncooked vegetables, salads, water, cheese	*Food:* Culture and serotype *Cases:* Stool cultures; serotype and enterotoxin production at FDDB, invasiveness assay *Controls:* Stool cultures; serotype and enterotoxin production. Look for common serotype in food, cases not found in controls; DNA probes
Escherichia coli enteroinvasive	16–48 h	C, D, F, H	Tissue invasion	Same as preceding	Same as preceding
Listeria monocytogenes	20 h (9–32 h)	D, C, F	?	Milk, soft cheeses	*Food:* Culture, serotype *Cases:* Stool/blood cultures, serotype
Vibrio cholerae non–O1	16–72 h	D, V	Enterotoxin formed in vivo, ? tissue invasion	Shellfish	*Food:* Culture on TCBS, serotype *Cases:* Stool cultures on TCBS, serotype

Organism	Incubation	Symptoms	Mechanism	Vehicle	Laboratory
Vibrio cholerae O1	24–72 h	D, V	Enterotoxin formed in vivo	Shellfish, water or foods contaminated by infected person or obtained from contaminated environmental source	*Food*: Culture on TCBS, serotype *Cases*: Stool cultures on TCBS, serotype Send all isolates to CDC for confirmation and toxin assay
Vibrio cholerae O139	24–72 h	D, V	Enterotoxin formed in vivo	Same as preceding	Culture as for O1; serologic test available at state health laboratories
Shigella	24–48 h	C, F, D, B, H, N, V	Tissue invasion	Food contaminated by infected food handler; usually not foodborne	*Food*: Culture and serotype *Cases*: Stool culture and serotype *Handler*: Stool culture and serotype
Escherichia coli enterohemorrhagic (*E. coli* O157:H7 and others)	48–96 h	B, C, D, H F infrequent	Cytotoxin	Beef (especially ground beef), raw milk, water, apple cider, fruits, vegetables (including lettuce, sprouts)	*Cases*: Stool culture on sorbitol-MacConkey, serologic test available at FDDB for epidemiologic investigations; screen stool for toxin (ELISA)
Yersinia enterocolitica	2–7 days (2–14 days)	F, D, C, V, H	Tissue invasion, ? enterotoxin	Pork products, milk, food contaminated by infected human or animal	*Food*: Culture on CIN agar, cold enrichment *Cases*: Stool culture on CIN *Table continued on following page*

Table 5–9. Compendium of Acute Foodborne and Waterborne Gastrointestinal Diseases *Continued*

II. Diseases Typified by Diarrhea After a Moderate to Long Incubation Period, Often with Fever *Continued*

Agent	Incubation Period—Usual (and Range)	Symptoms* (Partial List)	Pathophysiology	Characteristic Foods	Specimens†
Cyclospora cayetanensis	7 days (1–14 days)	D, C, N, V, F (low grade)	Tissue invasion	Raw produce; water	*Food/water:* Consult DPD *Cases:* Stool examination for organisms; PCR (developmental) and testing for oocyst sporulation at DPD
Cryptosporidium parvum	7 days (2–28 days)	D, N, V, F (low grade)	Tissue invasion	Uncooked foods; water	*Food/water:* Consult DPD *Cases:* Stool examination for organisms or antigen; PCR and serologic test developmental (consult DPD)
Giardia lamblia	7–10 days (3–25 days)	D, C, N	?	Uncooked foods; water	*Food/water:* Consult DPD *Cases:* Demonstration of antigen in stool or organisms in stool, duodenal contents, or small bowel biopsy specimen
Entamoeba histolytica	1–3 weeks (days–weeks)	D, B, F	Tissue invasion	Uncooked foods; water	*Food/water:* Consult DPD *Cases:* Demonstration of antigen in stool or organisms in stool or intestinal biopsy specimen; serologic test for antibody

III. Botulism

Agent	Incubation Period—Usual	Symptoms°	Pathophysiology	Characteristic Foods	Specimens†
Clostridium botulinum	12–72 h	V, D, descending paralysis	Preformed toxin	Improperly canned or similarly preserved foods; foods under oil, e.g., garlic	*Food:* Toxin assay *Cases:* Serum and stool for toxin assay by CDC or state laboratory; stool culture for *C. botulinum*

IV. Diseases Most Readily Diagnosed from History of Eating a Particular Type of Food

Agent	Incubation Period—Usual	Symptoms°	Pathophysiology	Characteristic Foods	Specimens
Poisonous mushrooms	Variable	Variable	Variable	Wild mushrooms	*Food:* Speciation by mycetologist
Other poisonous plants	Variable	Variable	Variable	Wild plants	*Cases:* Vomitus, blood, urine *Food:* Speciation by botanist; stool may sometimes be helpful in confirmation.
Scombroid fish poisoning		N, C, D, H, flushing, urticaria	Histamine	Mishandled fish, e.g., tuna	*Food:* Histamine levels
Ciguatera poisoning		D, N, V, paresthesias, reversal of temperature sensation	Ciguatoxin	Large ocean fish, e.g., barracuda, snapper	*Food:* Stick test for ciguatoxin (not widely available)

°B = bloody stools, C = cramps, D = diarrhea, F = fever, H = headache, N = nausea, V = vomiting
†FDA = Food and Drug Administration, TCBS = thiosulfate citrate bile salts sucrose (agar), EM = electron microscopy, ELISA = enzyme-linked immunosorbent assay, FDDB = Centers for Disease Control and Prevention's Foodborne and Diarrheal Diseases Branch, CDC = Centers for Disease Control and Prevention, CIN = Cefsulodin-irgasan-novobiocin agar, DPD = CDC's Division of Parasitic Diseases, PCR = polymerase chain reaction

103

county, and local levels throughout the U.S. Problems vary by region, as do solutions. Contamination can occur at any point along the route from collection through treatment to delivery. In the U.S. chlorine is typically used to sanitize water before it is put into the distribution system for consumption. Chlorine has been associated with formation of toxic residues known as trihalomethanes. These compounds may be carcinogenic and have raised concerns with some about chlorine use. Water obtained from private wells has its own set of problems. If the well is not drilled to bedrock, it may contain surface contamination that normally would not exist in the deeper aquifer. Wells that are not cased and grouted can be contaminated during episodes of flooding. Wells that supply multiple households are subject to overuse, resulting in contamination from siphonage. This occurs when the well cannot recharge sufficiently during periods of use.

Deforestation has contributed to degradation of water sources by increasing the load of sediments from erosion and of toxic chemicals from runoff that reaches flowing surface water. Treatment plants can then become unable to process the increasing amounts of sediments and other materials found in the drinking water sources. The current methods used to treat water have become more and more complex and lend themselves to breakdowns in the system. As a result, diarrheal disease is increasing nationwide.

In the 1970s and 1980s, episodes of the infection primary amebic meningoencephalitis (PAM), caused by a soil ameba, *Naegleria fowleri*, occurred with increasing frequency. Invariably, this organism is found in conjunction with process water that is discharged by manufacturing plants throughout the U.S. that raises the temperature of the body of water receiving the discharge above normal levels for extended time periods. People who swim in these waters may be exposed to this uncommon but potentially fatal infection. Typically, the ameba enters through the nose and passes through the cribriform plate into the brain of the unsuspecting patient. The ameba is quite small, resembling a white blood cell in the view of untrained microscopists.

Other organisms of medical importance that are found in water sources include protozoans such as *Giardia lamblia, Entamoeba histolytica, Cryptosporidium*, and *Cyclospora*. Bacterial diseases such as cholera, thyphoid fever, and others are associated with lack of sanitary facilities or a breakdown in existing ones.

In addition to surface water contamination, chemical leachates eventually reach ground water and contaminate the aquifers. The movement of chemicals through environmental media such as soil, water, air, and biota (food chain) is very complex. Living organisms can be affected in many ways. For this reason, the methyl mercury problem in Minamata Bay, Japan, was not recognized initially. When a large number of residents began developing strange neurologic symptoms, the problem was traced to a methyl mercury compound that had been released into the bay by a manufacturing plant over a long period. The compound became concentrated in the bay's fish and consequently in human tissues (bioaccumulation). Fish that were regularly consumed by residents contained toxic levels of mercury. The mercury release occurred from the 1930s until the 1960s, when the problem was finally recognized. Today a museum in Minamata City stands as a monument to remind Japanese citizens to remain vigilant to environmental contamination and its effects on human populations.

Municipalities obtain drinking water either from deep wells or from surface sources. During periods of drought or flooding, intakes can become contaminated. Water treatment facilities are heavily regulated and inspected; however, errors may still occur. When a problem does occur, it is more likely to be located within the distribution system.

AIR QUALITY

The Clean Air Act was passed by the U.S. Congress in 1970 and amended in 1990. This legislation requires the EPA to monitor air for pollutants that are shown to present a public health risk. Outdoor air contains many naturally occurring pollutants. Among these are soil, dust, pollens, and fungi. Industries that produce pollutants must monitor air concentrations. However, many pollution sources exist for which no safeguards are in place, and people can be exposed to a variety of pollutants in either indoor or outdoor environments. The amount of pollutants released by industry is measured in the billions of pounds annually. Health care costs of persons exposed to outdoor air pollution range in the billions of dollars. Air pollution is a particular problem for patients suffering from asthma or other chronic respiratory diseases.

Health problems related to air quality can be traced to early human history, when people sequestered themselves in tightly enclosed dwellings such as caves.[1] When they began to use fire both for warmth and cooking, they also began to suffer respiratory problems related to polluted air. Migration into cities served to increase the problems of breathable air. Use of coal as a fuel became a two-edged problem that started with miners working in poorly ventilated mineshafts and ended with consumers who used coal in poorly ventilated homes. Other minerals such as asbestos have been associated with human disease through inhalation.

The issue of air quality also includes the presence of infectious agents. Wind currents distribute regional diseases such as histoplasmosis over wide expanses. Other diseases such as tuberculosis are spread from person to person in the form of droplets carried by air currents. Legionnaires' disease was traced to contamination in a cooling tower when it was first described. Industrialization has exponentially increased the magnitude of air-related complaints. At the close of the 20th century, the problems of air pollution seem to be increasing in spite of tremendous strides in technology to improve air quality. Pollutants in the air present unique challenges as a result of dispersion and dilution. Although they tend to be seasonal, regional, and situational, pollutants in the air cause many acute health problems. The factors that increase or mitigate air as an environmental pathway are beyond the scope of this chapter. However, air pollution is an increasingly serious problem throughout the world.

Many methods have been used to classify or categorize air pollution. However, most pollutants fall into one of four categories:

1. Products of sulfur-containing fossil fuels from industry, power plants, and home heating
2. Photochemical smog containing oxidant pollutants and ozone from the action of sunlight on hydrocarbons, nitrogen oxides, and carbon monoxide
3. Toxic pollutants: primarily lead, other metals, and other organic materials
4. Carbon monoxide from various combustion sources

Those who are most likely to suffer acute effects from air pollution are the very young, the very old, and the infirm. People who are exposed to polluted air either indoors or outdoors are at greater risk if they are infants, children, elderly, smokers, or have asthma, chronic obstructive pulmonary disease, or ischemic heart disease. Cities throughout the world with high levels of particulate pollution show an increased rate of chronic cough, bronchitis, and chest illnesses in children. Studies have repeatedly shown an increase in emergency room visits during times of poor air quality due to pollution.

Indoor air pollution presents additional problems for patients. Currently, the health effects of cooking are being studied, and some investigators have already raised concerns about the effects of cooking odors and other indoor air pollutants. The use of kerosene heaters, primarily by lower socioeconomic groups, is a cause for concern, primarily because of the release of carbon monoxide. Tobacco smoke is a major contributor to indoor air pollution, and the effects of passive smoking have long been shown to be both an acute and a long-term hazard to health.[9]

The term *sick building syndrome* (SBS) has been used since the 1980s to encompass a broad range of medically defined symptoms, environmental discomfort, and complaints of odor. In the 1990s the term was expanded to include mucous membrane irritation, central nervous system symptoms, chest tightness, and skin complaints. No clear definition exists from this cluster. The term grew out of documented complaints of office workers in the U.S. who had similar work-related symptoms with associated loss of productivity. The National Institute of Occupational Safety and Health) (NIOSH) conducted a number of studies in an attempt to identify the single most likely cause. A number of factors were identified, but the only characteristic that appeared with any frequency was mechanical ventilation. Canadian studies produced similar results. Other studies have identified building designs that did not allow for adequate outside air supply. Also, these designs did not provide sufficient air circulation throughout the building. Another major factor was inadequate understanding of ventilation systems by persons responsible for operating and maintaining them.[9] Job stress has been linked to likelihood of reporting symptoms.

Along with ventilation deficiencies, researchers have identified volatile organic compounds (VOCs) as a source of problems in buildings. Many building materials emit traces of VOCs, as do work station materials, desk materials, and other items found in the workplace. Wet products such as glues and toners add to the mix. Employee factors such as perfumes, colognes, and other personal items also play a role.

Some specialists in the field of occupational health have advocated that the term sick building syndrome be dropped for lack of compelling evidence that such a syndrome exists.

DISASTER MANAGEMENT

NATURAL DISASTERS

One definition for the term *disaster* is an occurrence that is sudden, catastrophic, disrupts the social structure, threatens the health of the population, and outweighs the ability of the threatened community to provide essential services. It may inflict widespread destruction and discomfort. In contrast, an event such as an airline crash or a train wreck would, instead, be referred to as a *mass casualty incident*. Natural disasters occur commonly throughout the world. However, some regions, such as the Caribbean Islands and Latin America, where tropical storms and hurricanes are commonplace, have taken special care to prepare for these potentially catastrophic events. The Pan-American Health Organization (PAHO) has instituted training in disaster management and distributes a periodic newsletter to interested parties throughout the world. Member countries have established a level of preparedness that is both sophisticated and mobile. However, in the midst of a disaster, mitigation resources can become strained rather quickly, and the costs of relief and recovery are quite high. Economic pressures in these PAHO regions have also taken a heavy toll on resources.

One concern that always arises following a disaster such as, for example, a major flood, is the appearance of communicable diseases. Ecological changes may occur after disasters such as droughts, floods,

Table 5–10. Effects of Natural Disasters on Health

	Earthquake	Hurricane/ Typhoon	Volcanic Eruption	Flooding
Deaths	Many	Few	Varies	Few
Injuries requiring medical care	Overwhelming	Moderate	Varies	Few
Risk of infectious disease outbreak	Moderate	Common	Varies	Common
Food scarcity	Rare	Rare	Common	Common
Population displacement	Rare	Rare	Common	Common

and hurricanes (Table 5–10). Conditions that favor the breeding of vectors may in turn result in significant increases in arthropod-borne diseases. Fortunately, unless a particular disease was present prior to an environmental insult, it is unlikely for it to erupt following a disaster. Conversely, relief workers may on occasion be responsible for importing into the disaster site a disease that was not previously present. In return, relief workers may be exposed to an endemic disease to which they have had little or no previous exposure. When large numbers of displaced persons must be moved from one location to another, risks of new exposures increase. The density of the population also has a direct impact on person-to-person transmission of some diseases. When public utilities, including electricity, potable water, sewage, and refuse collection, are interrupted, breakdowns in basic sanitation occur that facilitate the transmission of both food- and waterborne diseases, proportional to the length of time that services are suspended. Simultaneously, local health and public health facilities may experience a sudden influx of requests, further placing strain on an already compromised system. Disasters may also make for inadequate or absent services and/or facilities, that can further contribute to outbreaks of disease.[10]

The mental health aspects of displacement and shelter living are not inconsequential and must be addressed as well. During the crisis phase of any disaster, most citizens are too consumed by survival to manifest symptoms other than acute shock. However, as the crisis abates and the reality of their situation sets in, people may become severely depressed and otherwise incapacitated.

Some regional disasters, such as tornadoes, occur on a somewhat regular or recurring basis. Communities that have a history of these occurrences should have a formal, written disaster response plan. This plan should be reviewed annually and revised. Agencies that have a formal role in disaster response, such as hospitals, police departments, and rescue squads, should periodically participate in realistic disaster scenario drills. Preplanning allows a community to predetermine how

Box 5-8–POSTDISASTER MANAGEMENT AND RELIEF RECOMMENDATIONS

- Outside help is frequently not needed and may actually hinder local efforts.
- Search and rescue, first aid, and other immediate medical needs are usually short-lived.
- Donations should be appropriate to the needs of the affected community, and agencies should not compete to try to meet these needs. Coordination is essential.
- Emergency assistance should complement local efforts.
- Don't overreact to media reports regarding "urgent" needs. These are frequently based on unreliable accounts by well-intentioned persons.
- Don't send large quantities of used clothing unless requested.
- Don't send household medicines or prescriptions. Considerable space and manpower must be expended to determine the safety and efficacy of these items. Expired medications cannot be used in most cases.
- Medically and other technically trained persons should not assume that their services will be needed. When needs for special types of skills arise, this information will be made available.

it will handle problems such as loss of electric power, contamination of food and water supplies, transportation failures, public safety, structural damage, and communication failures (providing information to both the responding personnel and the public). In an actual disaster occurrence, designated responders and other official personnel implement the plan and define the scope of the disaster. Additional resources may be called in at this time. Rescue and relocation may be prominent features of this phase of the response. The final phase of any disaster response plan involves the postdisaster management period (Box 5-8). Repair, replacement, and cleanup are generally prominent features of this phase. The final phase is likely to be the longest and most arduous for both responders and citizens.

As soon as is practical after a disaster, the community government should thoroughly review the event and its response. Any deficiencies should be addressed and strengthened for the future.

MANMADE DISASTERS

Manmade disasters include warfare, economic or social disruption, and civil unrest. Also included in this category is terrorism, especially

bioterrorism. Public health officials throughout the world have identified a problem labeled weapons of mass destruction (WMD). Response to both traditional and biological terrorism has become a
growing concern to both the public health community and the private
sector. Special attention is being given to the importance of integrating
the health care community into the planning, evaluation, and implementation of a WMD response system.

In addition to WMD, acts of terrorism on a lesser scale are also
creating great concern. The need to improve civilian medical response
to chemical and biological terrorism is becoming more critical. Pre-
incident actions are vital to all disaster operations, but the complex
and unique aspects of WMD occurrences require an even greater
commitment to preparedness. Terrorist acts such as the bombings of
the Alfred P. Murrah Federal Building in Oklahoma City, of the World
Trade Center in New York City, and at Olympic Centennial Park
during the Atlanta Olympic Games are but a few examples. The timely
utilization of protective clothing and equipment by all first responders
is essential to any effective terrorism response plan. Failure to prevent
gross contamination could potentially create caregiver victims and/or
make caregivers inadvertent accomplices in the spread of the terrorist's
sphere of casualties.

Warfare is a specific kind of disaster that may produce many
casualties, both directly from the armed conflict itself, and indirectly
because of economic losses. Civilians may be caught between warring
factions, resulting in large numbers of refugees fleeing from contested
areas without food, water, or shelter. Encampments may lack even the
most basic facilities. Some refugees may arrive sick, while others may
become ill as a consequence of crowding, poor sanitation, and exposure to extremes of weather. Some geopolitical conflicts involve a type
of "indirect" warfare that does not involve the engagement of large
forces. This is referred to as a low-intensity conflict (LIC). Because it
is highly mobile and may not have identifiable objectives, civilians may
not be able to easily escape from an LIC. Guerrilla-type operations or
"peacekeeping" missions are examples of LICs.[11] The Los Angeles
riots (April 1992) were another example of a potential LIC. When
regional or national governments cannot bring such situations under
rapid control, the conflict may persist and escalate.

Lethal chemical weapons including nerve agents are stored at eight
locations within the U.S. and on one island in the central Pacific
Ocean, near Hawaii. In addition, military training exercises have resulted in occasional accidental releases. Concerns have been voiced
regarding the possibility of theft by terrorist groups of these dangerous
materials. Biological weapons are also a concern throughout the world.
Organisms such as anthrax could be introduced into populations by
military units or small terrorist cells.

In addition to military stockpiles, dangerous organisms such as
Ebola virus and smallpox can be found at Level 4 research labora-

tories. These laboratories house both routine organisms that are considered to be dangerous and exotic agents that pose a high individual risk of life-threatening disease.

Environmental spills and releases of various types of chemicals compose yet another category of manmade or technologic disasters. Transportation accidents involving common carriers of all types of chemicals are commonplace on highways, railroads, and waterways. Periodically, these hazardous spills necessitate evacuation of civilian populations. Air releases are particularly hazardous because of the difficulties both in detection and containment. Spills into flowing water pose special dangers to wildlife, domestic animals, and humans. The challenge for the clinician is to recognize signs and symptoms produced by a wide variety of chemicals, occasionally in mixtures, for which no data are available or readily accessible. Nuclear accidents pose one of the greatest threats both to human life and to the environment, primarily because there exists no real intervention beyond primary prevention.

More often than not, the primary disaster is only the tip of the iceberg, the precipitating factor that sets a complex array of events into motion. Hurricane Floyd struck eastern North Carolina in September 1999. This major hurricane caused typical damage to property. The storm passed quickly through the region and left many with the feeling that all was well. However, rivers in the region were well above flood levels even before the hurricane struck. Levels continued to rise over the next 2 to 3 weeks until water was more than 40 ft above flood stage in some areas. People were awakened in the middle of the night by water entering their homes. Water levels exceeded the 500-year flood levels calculated by the U.S. Army Corps of Engineers. Months later, many families were still displaced, living with relatives or in temporary housing. Beyond temporary inconvenience, eastern North Carolina is an agricultural region that has suffered economic loss that may take years to realize. Many farmers were unable to rescue livestock and poultry because of the rapidly rising water. Potential infestations from carcasses and overflowing lagoons, primarily waste-holding ponds on pig farms, added to the devastation. High waters rendered roads impassible and washed out numerous bridges. Many trapped people were rescued by boat and helicopter. Grocery stores, unable to receive supplies, quickly ran out of food and other essential items. U.S. military teams, including units from all branches of service, were pressed into action to conduct rescue missions and ferry in food and water. Local hospitals and clinics had to rely on water brought in from other areas to continue essential operations. Even businesses that remained undamaged had to close because of insufficient water needed for sanitation. The Greenville, North Carolina, water treatment plant (which supplies much of Pitt County) was totally submerged by flood waters, leaving many of the citizens without a safe source of drinking water, with toilets that could not be flushed, and with other basic sanitation needs unmet.

Numerous agencies from other areas of the state provided support; fire, police, and utility workers were among the first to be activated. Local churches, the Red Cross, and the Salvation Army opened centers to provide food, clothing, and shelter. As word reached the media, donations began to arrive from all over the U.S. At one point, warehouses were filled to capacity and closed to further donations. The process of rebuilding and replacing will go on for months and years after all of the emergency response agencies have withdrawn. Ironically, the flooding from Hurricane Floyd arrived on the heels of a relative drought.

Patient education and prevention efforts for disaster situations should be focused on advanced planning. When warnings are issued, stores are quickly depleted of needed items. Patients who have special needs should be counseled to maintain adequate stockpiles of critical medications and supplies. Patients with transportation problems should always maintain food and sanitation supplies in sufficient quantity to carry them through emergencies. Communities not directly affected by a disaster may find themselves the recipients of casualties and refugees. Trained responders will go a long way toward mitigating the effects of many, if not most, disasters. Good communications combined with command and control are absolutely essential for those involved in disaster response.

CONCLUSION

Connecting environmental events to human disease requires excellent communication and cooperation from a wide array of scientists and clinicians, along with a strong infrastructure of seemingly unrelated agencies and public health services. While many state and federal programs share jurisdiction over applied research and the definitive identification of emerging infections, the primary care clinician is the first line of diagnosis, treatment, and preventive education. Excellent history and physical skills, and clinical suspicion, along with access to health department services and/or CDC resources, provide most solutions to environmental health issues.

REFERENCES

1. Lappè M. Evolutionary Medicine: Rethinking the Origins of Disease. San Francisco, Sierra Club Books, 1994.
2. National Research Council. Environmental Epidemiology: Volume 1, Public Health and Hazardous Wastes. Washington, DC, National Academy Press, 1991.

3. Wallace RB, Doebbeling BN. Maxcy-Rossenau-Last Public Health and Preventive Medicine, 14th ed. Stamford, CT, Appleton & Lange, 1998.
4. Blumenthal DS, Ruttenber AJ. Introduction to Environmental Health, 2nd ed. New York, Springer Publishing Co., 1995.
5. Salvato JA. Environmental Engineering and Sanitation, 4th ed. New York, John Wiley & Sons, 1992.
6. Centers for Disease Control and Prevention. Emerging Infections Diseases (EID Journal online) web site.
7. Institute of Medicine. Emerging Infections: Microbial Threats to Health in the United States. Washington, DC, National Academy Press, 1992.
8. McCormick JB, Fisher-Hoch S. Level 4: Virus Hunters of the CDC. Atlanta, GA, Turner Publishing, Inc., 1996.
9. Effects of the indoor environment on health. Occup Med 1995;10.
10. Burkle FM. Disaster Medicine. Medical Examination Publishing Co., 1984.
11. Gallagher JJ. Low Intensity Conflict: A Guide for Tactics and Procedures, Mechanicsburg, PA, Stackpole Books, 1992.

RESOURCES

GENERAL

National Center for Environmental Health Fact Book 1999. Centers for Disease Control and Prevention, June 1999. 72 pp.

CDC FACT SHEETS

CDC's Environmental Hazards Epidemiology Response Program
CDC's Lead Poisoning Prevention Program
Centers for Birth Defect Research and Prevention
The Children's Environmental Health Report Card
Developmental Disabilities Among Children
Exposure of Air Force Veterans to Agent Orange on Vietnam
Food Safety Initiative
Healthy People 2010: A New Chapter on Disability and Secondary Conditions

CDC HEALTH AND SAFETY GUIDELINES

Earthquake: A Prevention Guide to Promote Your Personal Health and Safety (1995). Booklet. 23 pp.
Extreme Cold/Extreme Heat (1995). Booklet. 24 pp.
Flood: A Prevention Guide to Promote Your Personal Health and Safety (1995). Booklet. 12 pp.

Hurricane: A Prevention Guide to Promote Your Personal Health and Safety (1995). Booklet. 19 pp.

Screening Young Children for Lead Poisoning: Guidance for State and Local Public Health Officials. (November 1997). 122 pp.

Carbon Monoxide (CO) Prevention Checklist (1997). Leaflet.

FOODBORNE DISEASES

cdc.gov/ncidod/dbmd/diseaseinfo/foodborneinfections_g.htm
Over twenty patient education (FAQs) online

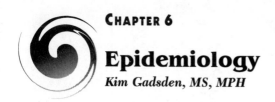

CHAPTER 6

Epidemiology

Kim Gadsden, MS, MPH

INTRODUCTION

Epidemiology is generally regarded as the basic science of public health, and, along with many of the general medical sciences, it tends to be ignored by the clinical provider as something best left to the "ivory tower" researcher. This chapter attempts to disprove this notion and to provide a basic understanding of the most commonly used terms and calculations utilized in this discipline. This, in turn, should permit clinicians to better understand the literature and to use the tools of epidemiology, in combination with their own practical experience, to facilitate health promotion and disease prevention.

The discipline of epidemiology considers many factors that describe disease occurrence in human populations and assumes that there are definite patterns in these occurrences. The basic parameters used in epidemiology to describe populations are person, place, and time. How often a disease occurs over time (incidence), how many cases of a disease exist at a given time (prevalence), where and when a disease occurs, and who is most likely to contract the disease are factors that epidemiologists use in descriptive studies to formulate hypotheses about possible causes of disease. Epidemiologists test these hypotheses using analytic studies to evaluate possible disease etiology. The results of these studies contribute to disease prevention and control.

The scope of epidemiology may be better understood by comparing it to basic sciences and clinical medicine, since these disciplines all contribute to the understanding of the disease process. As an example, Table 6–1 compares how prostate cancer is studied in each discipline.

Suppose a histologist, a physician, and an epidemiologist are all studying prostate cancer. The histologist may obtain a tissue sample, test it to see whether a cell is cancerous, and, after a positive result, conclude that the cell is cancerous. The physician may evaluate the results of a positive-specific antigen (PSA) test from a patient and conclude that the results fall in the range of a possible cancer. However, an epidemiologist may choose a sample from a population, conduct an epidemiologic study, and conclude that men over age 50 are more likely to develop prostate cancer than men under age 50. The epidemiologist in this example used aggregate data on individuals in a population to make inferences about the individual risk of disease. The results of such epidemiologic studies can provide society with new knowledge and positively affect the public's health.

Epidemiology has many applications. The epidemiology of a specific disease can be studied to provide information about the causes

| Table 6–1. The Study of Prostate Cancer in Basic Sciences, Clinical Medicine, and Epidemiology |
Basic Sciences	Clinical Medicine	Epidemiology
What is studied	Tissue	Individual	Population
What is analyzed	Cell	PSA test	Age, race, risk factors
Unit of analysis	Cell	Individual	Individual or population
Study design	Experimental	Experimental and/or observational	Experimental and/or observational
Method of analysis	Laboratory test to see whether cell is cancerous	Evaluation of PSA test results to see whether they indicate cancer	Statistical analysis including incidence rates, prevalence rates, relative risk, odds ratio
Possible conclusion	Cell is cancerous	Results of PSA test are in cancerous range	Men over age 50 are more likely to develop prostate cancer than men under age 50

PSA, prostate-specific antigen

of the diseases and to provide a complete picture of the full spectrum of the disease. It also allows identification of disease-associated syndromes and alternate ways of classifying diseases. The health of entire communities can be studied, which will provide measures of the incidence and prevalence of diseases. A community study can provide information about the prevalence of risk factors, and then help to determine high-risk subgroups within the community. Ecologic epidemiology, which provides information about the health of the environment, allows evaluation of changes in the frequencies of various diseases over time. Epidemiologic principles can be used to prevent and/or control the occurrence of diseases. By means of epidemiologic studies, the effectiveness of prevention strategies and therapeutic interventions can be evaluated. The success of various medical programs and systems can also be determined.

The focus of this chapter is on the correct use and interpretation of epidemiologic findings; it is not intended to teach epidemiologic methods. After completion of this chapter, the reader will be able to critically review findings of various epidemiologic studies and decide whether he or she agrees with the results.

DESCRIPTIVE EPIDEMIOLOGY

Descriptive epidemiology explores the predictable patterns of disease occurrence. These patterns are assumed to be determined by the nature of the cause, by the environment, and by the personal characteristics of the individuals affected. Study populations are analyzed in terms of three basic characteristics: person, place, and time.

* *Person* can be described by demographic and socioeconomic variables such as age, race, ethnicity, gender, religion, education, income, and occupation.
* *Place* can be described as global versus national or rural versus urban.
* *Time* can be described by temporal trends, periodic variation, and endemic versus epidemic diseases.

The results of the analysis are used to differentiate patterns of disease occurrence in populations, to generate hypotheses, or to simply describe study populations by outcome variables before reporting further analyses. Various morbidity and mortality rates and ratios are used to describe variations of disease and deaths in populations.

MEASURES OF DISEASE FREQUENCY

Rates, ratios, and proportions are descriptive statistics us⸗ epidemiology to quantify the occurrence of disease in pop⸴

Epidemiologists need more than the number of individuals who are afflicted with a particular disease to describe its distribution or make causal inferences. They need information about the population at risk for that disease and the time period during which the data were collected. Table 6–2 compares definitions and examples of rates and ratios and proportions in the epidemiologic study of disease.

RATE

Rate measures the frequency of an occurrence of a disease, an outcome, or a vital event. Rates are represented as $(x/y) \times k$, in which x = the number of occurrences, y = the number of persons in the population who are at risk for the occurrence during the specified time period, and k = a constant (always a multiple of 10) that will make the fraction (x/y) a whole number and easier to interpret. For example, a 1-year study is done on 200 people who think they may be susceptible to a back injury. Eight people develop a back injury during the year. The rate of occurrence of the back injury is $8/200 \times 100 = 4$ per 100 per year, or 4% per year.

The following sections provide definitions and examples of rates and ratios commonly used in the epidemiologic literature.

RATIO

A ratio is a measure of the relationship between two distinct and separate values, x and y, represented as $x{:}y$ or x/y. For example, 40 persons out of 100 at a picnic became sick. The ratio of sick persons who ate potato salad at a picnic to sick persons who did not eat potato salad is 32:8, or 32/8, or 4:1, or 4/1.

PROPORTION

A proportion is a ratio in which the denominator represents the total number of persons being considered. Therefore, the numerator is always a portion of the total denominator. For example, at the same picnic the proportion of people who became sick is

$$\frac{40}{40 \text{ sick } + 60 \text{ unsick}} = 100 \text{ total}$$

$$\frac{40}{100} \times 100 = 40\%$$

and the proportion of sick people who ate potato salad is

$$\frac{32}{(32+8)} = \frac{32}{40} \times 100 = 80\%.$$

The following sections provide definitions and examples of rates and ratios commonly used in the epidemiologic literature.

Table 6-2. Rates, Ratios, and Proportions

	Rate	Ratio	Proportion
Definition	A measure of the frequency of occurrence of a particular disease, outcome, or vital event in a defined population over a specified time period	A measure of the relationship between two variables, X and Y, that have separate and distinct values	A ratio where the numerator is always included in the denominator with the result expressed as a percentage
Form	$(X/Y) \times K$	X:Y or X:Y	$(X/Y) \times 100$
Numerator (X)	Number of occurrences of a disease (cases), outcome, or vital event over a specified time period	Number of occurrences of a disease, outcome, or vital event with a certain characteristic that is not always a portion of Y	Number of occurrences of a disease, outcome, or vital event
Denominator (Y)	Number of persons in the population at risk for the occurrence over a specified time period	Number of events with a certain characteristic that does not always represent the population at risk	Number of persons in the population at risk for the disease occurrence of event
Constant (K)	A multiple of 10 (100, 1000, 10,000, 100,000)	One	100
Examples	A 1-year study is done on 200 people who think they may be susceptible to a back injury. 8 people develop a back injury during the year	40 persons out of 100 at a picnic became sick	40 of 100 persons at the picnic became sick 32 of 40 ill persons ate potato salad
Reporting	The rate of occurrence of the back injury is $8/200 \times 100 = 4$ per 100 per year, or 4% per year	The ratio of sick persons who ate potato salad at a picnic to sick persons who did not eat potato salad is 32:8 or 32/8 or 4:1 or 4/1	The proportion of people who became ill is $40/100 \times 100 = 40\%$. The proportion of sick people who ate the potato salad is $32/40 \times 100 = 80\%$

119

Table 6-3. Morbidity Rates

	Incidence Rate	Prevalence Rate	Attack Rate
Definition	The frequency of new occurrences of a nonfatal disease or outcome in a defined population over a specified period of time	The frequency of new and existing cases of a disease or condition in a defined population at a particular point in time or specified time period	The incidence rate of a particular disease, usually with a specific exposure, during an epidemic in a defined population at a specified time; usually expressed as a percentage
X	The number of new cases during a specified time period	The number of current cases (new and existing) at a point in time	The number of new cases due to a specific exposure during an epidemic at a specified time
Y	The population at risk during the specified time period (cumulative incidence) or total person-time units of participation (incidence density)	The total population at that specified time (point prevalence) or time period (period prevalence)	The population at risk for that exposure at that specified time

MORBIDITY RATES

Incidence rates, prevalence rates, and attack rates are commonly used in the epidemiologic literature to quantify the frequency of disease occurrence (see Table 6–3).

INCIDENCE

There are two types of incidence rates, cumulative incidence and incidence density.

Cumulative Incidence

Cumulative incidence (CI) is an estimate of the risk that one person will develop a disease or outcome during a specified time period. For example, a study is done in a hospital outpatient clinic from July 1, 1997, until June 30, 1998. Five thousand pediatric patients are evaluated to see whether any of them develop ringworm in that time period. In order to look for new occurrences of disease, 250 patients who already have ringworm must be eliminated from the study. By the end of the study, we determine that 350 patients have developed ringworm during that year: CI = $[350/(5000 - 250) \times 100]$ = 7.4% per year. The 1-year risk of developing ringworm for this group of patients is 7.4%.

Incidence Density

Incidence density (ID) is a measurement of the "instantaneous rate" for developing an outcome in a specified population. This allows inclusion of study participants who have differing amounts of follow-up time (i.e., differing durations of study participation). In the previous example of ringworm risk, the population was actually quite transient. Many of the 4750 susceptible pediatric patients participated for much less than the full year. When all the months of participation for each person are added up (i.e., perfect participation by all = 4750 × 1 year = 4750 person-years), we actually have only 2180 person-years of participation in this group. By the end of the study, we determine that 350 patients have developed ringworm during that year: ID = $[350/2180 \times 100]$ = 16.16 cases per 100 person-years. The incidence rate for ringworm is 16.16 per 100 participants at risk per year.

PREVALENCE

The prevalence rate (P) is the proportion of the population that has the disease or condition at a specified time. This includes both existing cases and new occurrences during that time. Point prevalence is defined as a specific point in time, such as one day, or the actual time it takes to "count" prevalent cases. Period prevalence is the number of existing cases within a specified time period. For example, if there were 1008 fetal deaths in 1995 in Georgia, with a total number of pregnancies of 112,281, then the prevalence of fetal deaths for 1995 would be P = [10008/112, 281 × 1000] = 8.98 per 1000 per year.

CRUDE AND SPECIFIC RATES

Common statistics used to quantify deaths from disease include crude rates, such as crude death rates, and specific rates, such as age-, race-, gender-, or cause-specific death rates (see Table 6–4).

Crude Death Rate

The crude death rate is a summary rate that describes the frequency of deaths in a population in a given year. For example, a population of 222,000 had a total of 2103 deaths in 1998. The crude death rate for this population would be [(2103/22,000) × 1000] = 9.5 deaths per 1000 persons.

Age-, Race-, Gender-Specific Death Rate

The specific death rate (age, race, or gender) is the rate of the number of deaths in a population subgroup in a given year. For example, a population of 31,000 persons between the ages of 20 and 39 had a total of 217 deaths in 1998. The age-specific death rate in this population would be [(217/31,000) × 1000] = 7 deaths per 1000 persons.

Cause-Specific Death Rate

The cause-specific death rate is the rate of the number of deaths in a population from a specific cause in a given year. For example, a population of 150,000 persons had a total of 194 deaths from septicemia in 1998. The age-specific death rate in this population would be [(194/150,000) × 1000] = 1.3 deaths per 1000 persons.

ADJUSTED RATES

The specific rates described in the preceding sections should only be used to describe a single population and not to compare populations because they obscure or confound other relationships. To compare two populations fairly it is necessary to compare "adjusted" rates.

Table 6-4. Mortality Rates

	Crude Death Rate	Age-, Race-, or Gender-Specific Death Rate	Cause-Specific Death Rate
Definition	The summary rate of the frequency of deaths in a population in a year	The rate of the frequency of deaths in a population subgroup in a year	The rate of the frequency of deaths due to specific cause in a population in a year
X	Total number of deaths to residents of a particular area in a calendar year	Total number of deaths to residents of a particular area in a calendar year for a specific age, race, or gender	Total number of deaths to residents of a particular area in a calendar year due to a specific cause
Y	Estimated mid-year population	Estimated mid-year population for that specific age, race, or gender	Estimated mid-year population

The study population is compared to an external "standard population" in a process called *adjustment*. A single, weighted "adjusted" rate can be calculated to represent the experience of each study population. The standardized rate is used for internal comparison only, since one standard population may vary from study to study. Adjustment can be accomplished by either the direct or the indirect method.

Direct Method

When we use the direct method to age-adjust rates, we ask what the number of events (e.g., diseases, injuries, or deaths) in the standard population would be if they occurred at the same rate as they do in the study population. The first step in the direct method is to select a standard population of known age distribution. A standard population may be obtained by combining the two study populations or by using a United States census population. The next step is to multiply factor-specific rates from study population x and study population y by the standard population to determine the expected number of events for both study populations. Then we add up the expected number of events for study population x and study population y and divide the total expected number of events by the total standard population to get the age-adjusted death rate for each population. For example, the crude death rate of population x is $2103/222,000 = 9.5/1000$, and the crude death rate for population y is $1371/150,000 = 9.1/1000$. After determining the expected number of events for each age group for populations x and y, we can determine their age-adjusted rates.

Population x

Age-adjusted death rate for population x = [1740 expected number of deaths]/[200,000 standard population] = $8.7/1000$

Population y

Age-adjusted death rate for population y = [1845 expected number of deaths]/[200,000 standard population] = $9.2/1000$

When we compare the age-adjusted death rates for population x and population y, we see that the age-adjusted death rate for population y is greater than that for population x, even though the crude death rate for population x is greater than the crude death rate for population y.

Indirect Method

When we use the indirect method, we ask what the number of events in study population y would be if they occurred at the same rate as they do in study population x. Although the direct method is more commonly used, the indirect method may be preferable if age-specific (or other factor-specific) rates in the study population are not known, or if the study population has small numbers in factor-specific subgroups that could cause wide fluctuations in the associated age-specific rates. The first step in indirect adjustment is to compile age-specific rates from study population x and multiply them by population y to determine the expected number of events. The last step is to divide the total number of observed events in population x by the total expected number of events, which results in the standard mortality ratio, or SMR. For example, SMR = [1371 observed deaths]/[1291 expected deaths] = 1.1. Since the SMR > 1, population y has a higher age-adjusted death rate than population x.

If the events were disease cases, the result would be the standardized mortality ratio. These two ratios are compared in Table 6–5. The examples in Table 6–5 illustrate age-adjustment, but adjustment of rates can be done by any known factor, for example, gender, weight, or cigarette smoking.

ANALYTIC EPIDEMIOLOGY

After descriptive studies are used to describe disease distribution by person, place, and time, analytic studies are used to determine why certain populations have a higher rate of disease than other populations, and what etiologic factors contribute to the rate of disease. Analytic studies are usually used to test a hypothesis generated by a descriptive study, but they may also be used to generate a hypothesis. They are used to determine whether there is an association between a specified exposure factor and a specified outcome, and, if so, what

Table 6–5. Standardized Mortality/Morbidity Ratios

	Standard Mortality Ratio	**Standard Morbidity Ratio**
Definition	The ratio of observed deaths to expected deaths	The ratio of observed cases to expected cases
X	The number of observed deaths in the population being studied	The number of observed cases in the population being studied
Y	The number of expected deaths in the population being studied	The number of expected cases in the population being studied

is the strength of that association. These studies may be observational or experimental in nature. In observational studies, the investigator has no control over the groups' exposure and merely observes the outcomes. Types of observational studies include cross-sectional, case-control, and cohort. In experimental studies the investigator creates the groups and controls their exposure. An experimental study used in epidemiology is the randomized clinical trial. All of these studies use a particular measure of effect to describe the association between the disease (the dependent variable) and exposure (the independent variable) that can be demonstrated by formulas derived from the 2 × 2 contingency illustrated in Figure 6–1.

This 2 × 2 illustration is the conventional and convenient way to describe disease and exposure status and calculate measures of effect in study populations. Cell a is the number of diseased individuals who are exposed, cell b is the number of nondiseased individuals who are exposed, cell c is the number of diseased individuals who are not exposed, and cell d is the number of nondiseased individuals who are not exposed. The row and column marginals denote the total number

Disease

	Yes	No
Exposure — **Yes**	a	b
No	c	d

	Disease		
Exposure	Yes	No	Total
Yes	a	b	$a+b$
No	c	d	$c+d$
Total	$a+c$	$b+d$	$a+b+c+d$

Figure 6–1. Association between exposure and disease.

of exposed individuals $(a+b)$, the total number of nonexposed individuals $(c+d)$, the total number of diseased individuals $(a+c)$, and the total number of nondiseased individuals $(b+d)$.

MEASURES OF EFFECT

RELATIVE RISK AND ODDS RATIO

The two most common measures of effect in the epidemiologic literature are the relative risk (RR, rate ratio or risk ratio), and the odds ratio. RR is the incidence rate or risk of disease of the exposed divided by the incidence rate or risk of disease of the unexposed and can be expressed by the following formula:

$$RR = \frac{\left[\dfrac{a}{(a+b)}\right]}{\left[\dfrac{c}{(c+d)}\right]}$$

If RR is equal to 1, then the exposure does not increase the risk of disease. If RR is greater than 1, then the risk of disease is increased in the exposed compared to the unexposed. If RR is less than 1, then the risk of disease is decreased in the exposed compared to the unexposed, denoting a protective effect of the exposure. The odds ratio,

$$OR = \frac{\left[\dfrac{a}{c}\right]}{\left[\dfrac{b}{d}\right]} = \frac{ad}{bc}$$

is the measure of effect and represents the odds of disease among the exposed divided by the odds of disease among the unexposed. If the odds ratio is equal to 1, then the odds of disease among the exposed is no greater than the odds of disease among the unexposed. If the odds ratio is greater than 1, then the odds of disease among the exposed is greater than the odds of disease among the unexposed. If the odds ratio is less than 1, then the odds of disease among the exposed is less than the odds of disease among the unexposed. The odds ratio may approximate RR if the disease being studied is rare and the study groups are representative of corresponding groups in the population.

■■■ARE THE RESULTS DUE TO CHANCE?

HYPOTHESIS TESTING, *P*-VALUES, AND CONFIDENCE INTERVAL

Hypotheses are formulated before an epidemiologic study is begun. For example, surveillance mechanisms indicate that the incidence of leukemia in a particular neighborhood is significantly higher than what would be expected based on U.S. rates in other comparable neighborhoods. It is also noticed that many of the homes in this area are clustered fairly closely to electric power lines and power stations. An epidemiologist would first develop a broad research question such as, "Do electromagnetic fields cause leukemia?" The research question would then be narrowed further into a hypothesis to be tested by an epidemiologic study. A hypothesis is a predictive statement about the relationship between an independent variable (the exposure of interest presumed to be affecting the rate of disease) and a dependent variable (the outcome of interest that includes all possible results that may stem from exposure to the independent variable[s] in the study). A hypothesis, "Electromagnetic fields [independent variable] increase the risk of leukemia [dependent variable]," might be generated from the preceding example. This hypothesis is then expanded to include the following:

Null Hypothesis;   There is no association between the independent and dependent variables.
H_0: RR $=$ 1

Alternative Hypothesis: There is an association between the independent and dependent variables.
HA: RR $=$ 1 (some association, but unsure of exactly what)
HA: RR $>$ 1 (exposure increases risk of disease)
HA: RR $<$ 1 (exposure decreases risk of disease)

An analytic study is performed to test the hypothesis. Epidemiologic studies do not *prove* hypotheses; they can only *support* or *refute* hypotheses with a specific amount of *confidence* or *statistical significance*.

Relative risks and odds ratios are usually presented with measures that explain how likely it is that the results were due to chance. The *P*-value and confidence intervals are two such measures. The *P*-value tells us the probability of obtaining by chance alone, given that there is no association between exposure and disease (H_0 is true), a result as extreme as or more extreme than the one we obtained from the study. If the *P*-value is less than .05 (the convention), we can reject H_0 and conclude that there is probably an association between exposure and disease, and we have statistical significance. However, if the P-value is more than .05, we accept H_0 and conclude that there is no association or statistical significance because the probability that the results occurred by chance alone is greater than .05. However, the P-value is dependent on the sample size and the strength of the association between the exposure and disease.

The confidence interval (CI) represents the range between two values where the true value lies, and to what degree one can be assured that the true value does indeed lie between these two values. If RR is 2.5 and CI is 1.9 to 5.0 with 95% confidence, then we are 95% confident that the true value of the relative risk lies between 1.9 and 5.0, and we can reject H_0. There does appear to be an association between the exposure and the disease, and we know that the P-value is less than .05, since the confidence interval does not include the null value of H_0: RR = 1. If, however, the 95% CI were .8 to 7.3, then the null value of 1 is included, and we cannot reject H_0 because there may be an association between the exposure and disease. We also know that the P-value is greater than .05.

Additionally, the width of the CI is directly related to the variability of the measure of effect and inversely related to the sample size. The wider the CI, the more variable the measure of effect and the smaller the sample size. The narrower the CI, the more precise the estimate.

EPIDEMIOLOGIC STUDY DESIGNS

The following section describes the major types of epidemiologic study designs and provides examples from the published literature.

ECOLOGICAL STUDIES

Ecological (also called correlational) studies are descriptive studies that explore the relationship between specific exposures and diseases in populations. These studies statistically compare morbidity or mortality from a specific disease to some other environmental or lifestyle exposure using the whole population as the unit of analysis. Since the unit of analysis is the population, the results of this type of study cannot be applied to individuals in that population. This is called the *ecological fallacy* and is explained further in the section on critical analysis. A measure of association that is used to describe the relationship between the exposure and the disease in an ecological study is called the correlation coefficient (r). The correlation coefficient is an index, that is, it is the result of analysis of two variables that form one composite measure. The value of the correlation coefficient varies between $+1$ and -1 and describes the strength and direction of the relationship between the exposure and the disease. For example, an r of $-.85$ denotes a strong negative relationship. Other ecological studies may simply compare disease rates among different geographic areas with different levels of some exposure and look for differences in risks.

To explore the possibility that cancer incidence may differ geographically in Costa Rica and be related to pesticide exposure, researchers gathered cancer registry data, population data, and pesticide usage data.[1] A pesticide exposure indicator (PEI) was calculated for each county, and the 27 counties with the lowest population density were categorized into low and high PEIs. Relative risks of specific cancers were calculated separately for men and women, resulting in twice the risk for lung cancer in men and 2.6 times the risk in women in high PEI areas compared with low PEI areas. Cancer of the rectum, skin, and bone in men was increased by 61%, 77%, and 81%, respectively. In women, cancer of the colon, ovaries, and uterus was increased by 65%, 78%, and 78%, respectively.

Care must be taken when interpreting results from ecological studies. The row and column marginals are the only known values in the 2 × 2 table (see Fig. 6–1) in an ecological study. We know the number of diseased, the number of nondiseased, the number of exposed, and the number of unexposed. However, the numbers of exposed diseased, exposed nondiseased, unexposed diseased, or unexposed undiseased are unknown. Therefore, conclusions cannot be drawn about individuals. In the Costa Rican example, it cannot be said that women with high pesticide exposures were more likely to have cancer, and pesticide exposure cannot be causally linked to cancer risk. The risk of cancer can be expressed only by geography, not by individuals.

CROSS-SECTIONAL STUDIES

In cross-sectional studies or surveys, the exposure and disease are ascertained simultaneously at one point in time. A measure of effect for this type of study design is the ratio of prevalences. The ratio of prevalences is defined as the prevalence of the exposed group divided by the prevalence of the unexposed group. According to the 2 × 2 table this would be $[a/(a + b)]/[c/(c + d)]$. If the ratio of prevalences is 5, then it can be said that the prevalence of disease is 5 times greater in the exposed group compared with the unexposed group. The odds ratio is also used in descriptive studies to describe the association between the disease and the exposure.

A cross-sectional study is usually used to generate a hypothesis and has strengths and weaknesses. It can be done quickly, is relatively inexpensive, and can be used to evaluate many diseases and exposures in one study. If the sample is representative, results of cross-sectional studies may be generalized to the larger population. However, causal inferences cannot be made because usually it cannot be determined whether the exposure preceded the disease, unless the exposure was present at birth.

A cross-sectional study design was used to assess the relationship between pain (exposure variable) and functional well-being, as measured by difficulty with activities of daily living (ADL) in a nursing home.[2] The exposure and outcomes were ascertained from the Systematic Assessment of Geriatric drug use via Epidemiology (SAGE) database for 49,971 nursing home residents. Results show that the odds of pain are 2.5 times greater for those with ADL impairment than for those with no ADL impairment. The 95% CI is between 2.3 and 2.6, so we can be 95% confident that the odds ratio lies between 2.3 and 2.6. Note that the small interval width is reflective of the large sample size. The authors of this study caution the audience that the cross-sectional design does not allow the causal inference that pain caused a decrease in functional well-being. The exposure and outcome were measured simultaneously, so it cannot be determined which one was first.

CASE-CONTROL STUDIES

In a case-control study, participants are enrolled based on disease status. Cases are those with the disease of interest, while controls do not have the disease. After these two groups are chosen, the investigator assesses their exposure status. The cases and controls are compared with respect to prior exposure to risk factor(s). If the risk factor is thought to be detrimental, then it is expected to appear more often in the cases than in the controls. A protective exposure, such as vaccination, is expected to appear more often in the controls than in the cases.

Case-control studies are of two types, population-based and hospital-based. Population-based studies have a fixed cohort, that is, once the cohort has been identified, no new members are added. The cohort may be defined based on year of birth or on a specific time interval. Study data are used to determine the odds that a case has been exposed, and whether these odds are higher or lower than what would be expected in the source population. The control group must reflect the source population that is being used as a reference group. The odds that a control has been exposed should reflect the odds of exposure in the source population.

Cases and controls are identified from hospitals in a hospital-based case-control study. The cases have the disease in question, and the controls have a different diagnosis than the outcome being studied.

The controls do not represent a known, well-defined population, and they are not necessarily representative of the source population that gave rise to the cases because of possible referral patterns. Also, cases may not reflect the spectrum of the disease of interest because only the most advanced cases may be hospitalized.

As in cross-sectional studies, many exposures can be studied, and case-control studies are quick and inexpensive to conduct. This study design is useful for studying rare diseases or diseases with long latency periods. There is also efficient sampling of diseased persons. If controls are randomly selected, the results are fairly generalizable, and the length of study time is short. However, since exposure is being retrospectively assessed, it is usually impossible to determine whether the exposure preceded the disease. This type of study design is highly susceptible to bias in selecting cases and controls, and inefficient for rare exposures.

Several important points should be considered when selecting cases and controls:

* Cases should not be unusual, should represent all cases of the disease in the source population, and be incident rather than prevalent cases.
* Controls should reflect all nondiseased persons in the source population.
* The source population should be at risk for both exposure and disease during a specified time period.
* Both cases and controls should be selected without regard to their exposure status.

The measure of effect calculated for a cross-sectional study design is the odds ratio. The odds ratio may approximate the relative risk if three conditions are met:

1. The study used incident cases of disease.
2. Selection of subjects was unbiased, i.e., the prevalence of exposure in the controls is indicative of the experience of nondiseased persons. The prevalence of exposure in the cases is indicative of the experience of all diseased persons.
3. The outcome is rare in the source population.

Familial prostate cancer risk in Sweden was assessed using a population-based case-control study with 356 cases from a registry and 712 controls.[3] The exposure variable, family history of prostate cancer, was ascertained from a questionnaire. A respondent was considered to have a family history of prostate cancer if a father or a brother had the disease. Results showed that with 95% confidence, men with a family history of prostate cancer were 3.2 times more likely to have prostate cancer themselves, with the CI between 2.1 and 5.1. These results are significant at the $P = .05$ level, since the CI does not include the null value of 1.0.

COHORT STUDIES

A cohort study is one in which the study population is chosen based on the presence or absence of an exposure. In prospective cohort studies, the exposure status is assessed, and subjects are followed over time to evaluate their disease status. Retrospective cohort studies are those in which the exposure status is ascertained by gathering information from previous records and assessing the disease status in the present. Both the prospective and the retrospective study designs go forward in time, present to future and past to present, respectively. The measure of effect used for cohort studies is RR.

Prospective Cohort Studies

This study design is the only study design in which incidence rates can be measured directly. The incidence rates can be calculated using either the total number of people (cumulative incidence) or the total amount of person-time (incidence density) as the denominator. RR can be called either a risk ratio (if cumulative incidence is used) or a rate ratio (if incidence density is used).

Advantages of this study design are

* The ability to establish a temporal relationship between the exposure and the disease
* A lack of bias in ascertaining exposure status
* The ability to study rare exposures and additional diseases.

Disadvantages of this design include

* Biases in ascertaining disease status
* High cost
* Long follow-up period
* Problems with attrition
* Difficulty in studying rare diseases

Prospective cohort studies are susceptible to the Hawthorne effect, in which subjects change their behavior after they are in the study, thus possibly changing their exposure status.

The association between early renal function decline and race in African American and white diabetics was studied using the prospective cohort study design.[4] In this study 1434 diabetic participants in the Atherosclerosis Risk in Communities Study from Forsyth County, North Carolina; Jackson, Mississippi, the northwest suburbs of Minneapolis, Minnesota; and Washington County, Maryland, were followed for three years. The incidence density for early renal function decline for African Americans was 28.4 per 1000 person-years, and for whites it was 9.6 per 1000 person-years. Furthermore, after controlling for age, gender, and baseline serum creatine levels, the risk for developing early renal function decline was three times times higher for African Americans than for whites (odds ratio, 3.15; 95% CI, 1.86–5.33). Even though this study is a prospective cohort and the investigators reported incidence densities and could have reported risk ratios, the investigators in this study used the odds ratio. The odds ratio possesses unique statistical properties that allow control for confounding variables. The odds ratio can also approximate RR in a prospective cohort study design.

Retrospective Cohort Studies

The retrospective cohort study is less costly and time-consuming than the prospective cohort study, is not susceptible to the Hawthorne effect, and can be used to study rare exposures and more than one disease. However, the investigator has no control over the quality of earlier measures of exposures, loss of subjects to follow-up may occur, and there may be bias in ascertaining disease status.

A retrospective cohort study was used to examine the relationship between unvaccinated individuals in the U.S. between the ages of 5 and 19 and measles incidence.[5] Measles cases in the U.S. between 1985 and 1992 were identified from the Measles Surveillance System of the Centers for Disease Control and Prevention, the number of unvaccinated individuals was estimated from the CDC's State Immunization Reports, and the number of vaccinated individuals was estimated from a 98% vaccination rate for school-age children reported by the CDC. It was reported with 95% confidence that unvaccinated individuals were 35 times more likely to develop measles during the period 1985–1992. The CI was between 34 and 37.

RANDOMIZED CLINICAL TRIALS

The randomized clinical trial is an experiment in which eligible subjects are randomly assigned either to a treatment group that receives the exposure or to a control group that receives a placebo. The groups are followed over time, and their disease status is measured. Like the prospective cohort study, RR is the measure of effect for this study design and is interpreted as previously stated.

Randomized clinical trials are considered the gold standard for epidemiologic research. However, this is not always the best study design for looking at certain types of exposure-disease relationships. The cohort study is a type of observational study used to try to simulate a clinical trial when a clinical trial is not feasible. A clinical trial reduces many of the biases, such as selection bias (by random assignment) and interviewer bias (by blinding) found in observational studies. Randomization achieves "equality" of baseline characteristics in the treatment groups. Groups are similar with respect to everything

Table 6–6. Types of Error in Randomized Clinical Trials

| | Truth | |
Study Results	Treatments Do Not Differ in Outcome	Treatments Do Differ in Outcome
Treatments do not differ in outcome	Correct answer	Type II error (or false-negative or beta error)
Treatments do differ in outcome	Type I error (or false-positive or alpha error)	Correct answer

except treatment status. Both known and unknown risk factors for disease are distributed equally among the treatment groups. That is, after randomization, the distribution of age, gender, race, and so forth, will be fairly similar in the treatment groups. This process eliminates bias in the allocation of subjects to treatment groups and is a major strength of clinical trials. Each individual in the study has the same chance of receiving each of the possible treatments, independent of the other study subjects.

Ethics, feasibility, and cost are some of the major concerns investigators have before choosing this study design.

* All participants must give informed consent before entering the study.
* Recruitment of study subjects must be done within a reasonable amount of time, and the sample size must be adequate to detect differences among treatment groups.
* Randomized clinical trials are expensive in terms of both time and money to follow and monitor study participants over time.

Also, problems from lack of patient compliance and loss to follow-up may occur. Assessing and monitoring compliance with the treatment regimen is one of the most difficult aspects of a clinical trial. It becomes a problem when participants begin to drop out differentially from the treatment and control groups, that is, more people drop out of the treatment group than out of the control group, or when people begin changing treatment groups. The "Intention to Treat" principle is used in the analysis to deal with problems of noncompliance. All people in the study are evaluated based on which group they were initially randomized to, regardless of whether or not they were compliant with the treatment regimen.

Table 6–6 shows the types of error in a randomized clinical trial design.

* A Type I error is the probability of finding that the treatments differ in outcome when, in fact, there really is no difference in treatment outcomes. This is usually set to .05 by convention, as

the investigator is willing to accept a 5% probability of a false-positive result.

* A Type II error is the probability of finding that the treatments do not differ in outcomes when, in fact, there really is a difference. This is usually set to .20 by convention, as the investigator is willing to accept a 20% probability of a false-negative result.

There is an inverse relationship between the probability of a Type I error and the probability of a Type II error; increasing one will decrease the other. Power (1-beta) is a related measure of the ability of the study to detect a difference in treatment outcomes when, in fact, there really is a difference. Power should ideally be at least 80%. Power is influenced by sample size. Increasing the sample size will increase the power. If a study shows no difference among treatment groups, then perhaps there were not enough people in the study to detect a real difference.

A randomized double-blind, placebo-controlled clinical trial design was used to test the efficacy of zanamivir in preventing influenza infection and disease.[6] In the study 553 subjects received zanamivir, and 554 subjects received a placebo. Recipients of zanamivir were 33% less likely to develop influenza confirmed by a laboratory and 16% less likely to develop symptomatic influenza with fever confirmed by a laboratory. In other words, zanamivir's efficacy in preventing influenza was 67% (efficacy = 1 − RR), and in preventing symptomatic influenza it was 84%.

DESIGN METHODS AND CRITICAL REVIEW OF EPIDEMIOLOGIC STUDIES

There are many issues to consider when planning, interpreting, or critically evaluating an epidemiologic study.

STUDY OBJECTIVE OR HYPOTHESIS

The study should clearly state its objective and hypothesis. The statement should include a clear description of the population from which the investigator intends to generalize the findings.

STUDY DESIGN

The proper study design should be chosen based on the study's objective and hypothesis. Which study design will most effectively test the hypothesis? Or, will this be a hypothesis-generating descriptive study?

The next step is the selection of the study sample and an appropriate control (comparison) group. The population of interest is the group about which conclusions are sought. The *sample frame* is the set of people who actually have a chance to be included in the survey. What is the relationship between the population of interest and the sample frame? A sample survey uses three methodologic fields: sampling theory, designing questions, and interviewing.

SAMPLING

An investigator may choose from various sampling methods to select a study sample. However, it is important that a probability sample be used so that the data are not biased and the subsequent estimates are precise. In a probability sample, everyone in the population has a known, non-zero probability of being selected. The probability need not be the same for all members, but it must be known. This allows computing of valid standard errors for the estimates and evaluation of possible biases. The sampling method and the sample size determine the precision of sample estimates. The choice of sampling method depends on the information available about the population and the relative ease of reaching people by different methods.

Simple Random Sampling

A simple random sample is a probability sample in which everyone in the population has an equal non-zero probability of being selected. The entire population is randomly numbered, and a random number is drawn until the needed sample size has been chosen. This sampling method is easy to understand and uses simple formulas for calculating means, totals, and standard errors. However, it requires not only knowing how many people are in the sample frame but also identifying each individual. This process is laborious for large sample frames.

Systematic Random Sampling

This sampling method requires selection of a random individual from the sampling frame and then every nth individual thereafter. Everyone in the population does not have an equal probability of being selected, but their probability is known and non-zero. This sampling method is usually easier to carry out than a simple random sample. Nevertheless, it is possible to systematically over- or under-sample owing to periodic changes in the sampling frame. For example, if every tenth house is sampled but the standard number of houses or a block is 10 or a multiple of 10, corner homes may never be sampled, or only corner homes may be sampled.

Stratified Sampling

Stratified sampling is a method whereby the population is divided into certain subgroups, or strata, and a sample is randomly drawn from each stratum. If you know the size or proportion of each stratum, you can select subjects to reflect the population structure. Additionally, by sampling a chosen number from each stratum, the sampling error can be greatly reduced. This method can increase the efficiency of the sample, but it requires knowledge of the existence of the strata, the numbers or proportions of people in the sample frame in each stratum, the ability to classify each person unambiguously to his or her proper stratum, and the ability to access people according to their strata.

Cluster Sampling

In cluster sampling, the population is divided into various clusters or natural groupings, and a random sample is drawn from each cluster. Cluster sampling is often not as efficient as simple random sampling, but the ease in obtaining subjects allows for obtaining larger samples to compensate for the lack of efficiency.

BIAS

After the sample is drawn, the investigator must acknowledge any selection bias that might exist and identify strategies to minimize such bias.

Selection Bias

Generally, *bias* is defined as a systematic error introduced into the study design or conduct of a study that results in an incorrect estimate of the association between the exposure and disease. A biased study can result in either overestimation or underestimation of the true measure of effect (RR or odds ratio). Selection bias is the use of noncomparable criteria to enroll study participants in the two study groups that create differences in subject identification, targeting, and participation. For example, investigators want to explore the relationship between oral contraceptive use and thromboembolism with a case-control study design. If the investigators use hospitalized cases, they may overestimate the true relationship between oral contraceptive use and thromboembolism because doctors are more likely to hospitalize women who have symptoms of thromboembolism if the women are currently using oral contraceptives.

Investigators must also be sure that the cases represent the full spectrum of disease under study, and that their sources are clear. The inclusion and exclusion criteria must be specified. Also, they must make sure that any control or comparison group is appropriate. It is also necessary to ensure that the information obtained from the study and control groups is comparable, and that information bias is minimized.

Information Bias

Information bias occurs when noncomparable information is obtained from the different study groups for exposure and/or outcome. Information bias can be caused by interviewer bias, recall bias, or misclassification of subjects with respect to exposure or disease status.

Interviewer Bias

Interviewer bias occurs when investigators elicit and/or interpret information differently from the exposed and the unexposed groups in a cohort study, or from the case and the control groups in a case-control study. For example, if the interviewer knows that the subject has the disease and is aware of the hypothesis under study, he or she may question the subject more closely regarding certain exposures suspected of causing the disease.

Recall Bias

Recall bias occurs when subjects report events differently, depending on whether they are in the exposed or the unexposed group in a cohort study, or in the case or the control group in a case-control study. Recall bias is a primary concern in case-control studies. Subjects are more likely to have thought about different past exposures that might have casued their disease.

STUDY OBSERVATIONS

Investigators should use clear definitions of the study observations, including diagnostic criteria, measurements, and outcome, and the observations should be valid and reliable. The method of classification or measurement should be consistent for all subjects and relevant to the objectives of the investigation. There should be minimal misclassification of subjects with respect to exposure or disease status.

Misclassification

Misclassification of subjects with respect to exposure or disease status may be either differential or nondifferential. In differential misclassification, the proportions of incorrect data are different in the study groups. This may cause an underestimation or overestimation of the true measure of effect. The investigator should try to identify the magnitude and direction of the bias. In nondifferential misclassification, the proportions of incorrect data are the same in both study groups. This random misclassification minimizes the differences between the groups and leads to an underestimation of the true exposure-disease relationship, i.e., the measure of effect is biased toward the null value of 1.0. These biases must be eliminated in the design and conduct of the study because there is no way to control for bias in the analysis of the results.

PRESENTATION OF FINDINGS

Findings should be presented clearly, objectively, and in sufficient detail to enable the reader to judge them. They should be internally consistent, with numbers adding up properly, and with clear and consistent results on all tables.

ANALYSIS

Statistical analysis should be appropriate for the study design and correctly performed and interpreted. Important confounding factors should be controlled for in the study design or in the analysis.

Confounding

Confounding is the mixing of the effect of exposure on disease with the effect of a third factor, which is called a confounding variable. In order for the variable to be a confounder, it must meet certain criteria. First, it must be associated with the exposure. Second, independent of exposure, it must be a risk factor for (or associated with) the disease. It need not be causal. Third, it cannot be only an intermediate step in the causal pathway between exposure and disease. For example, if one looks at the relationship between cancer (outcome) and a diet high in vegetables that are rich in beta carotene (exposure), it appears that diets rich in these vegetables are associated with a decreased risk of cancer. However, this apparent association between exposure and disease may be confounded by several factors. Are consumers of these vegetables different from nonconsumers with respect to age, exercise habits, or smoking habits? Is the fiber in the vegetables rather than the beta carotene really causing the reduction in cancer risk? We can also ask whether the association between oral contraceptive use and coronary heart disease is confounded by religion? Religion may be associated with oral contraceptive use, but, independent of oral contraceptive use, religion is not associated with coronary heart disease, so religion is not a potential confounder. However, an apparent association between increased coffee intake and increased risk of heart attack is probably confounded by cigarette smoking. We know that cigarette smoking is associated with coffee consumption, but, independent of coffee drinking, cigarette smoking increases the risk of heart attack, so smoking fits the criteria for a confounder. We can also look at the relationship between coffee consumption and the risk of death from a heart attack. A history of prior heart attack must be accounted for because it is a confounder. Patients with prior heart attacks are advised to stop drinking coffee; independent of coffee drinking, prior heart attack is certainly a risk factor for death from a heart attack.

Since the investigator is interested in evaluating the relationship between an exposure and a disease, the influence of confounding variables must be eliminated; otherwise the observed relationship between exposure and disease will be incorrect. Confounding can be controlled for either in the design or in the analysis of a study. In the design of a clinical trial, randomization of study participants can be used, the study population can be restricted to a group with certain characteristics, or, in case control studies, cases can be matched to controls based on a particular variable. In the analysis, multivariate methods such as logistic regression can be used. In this procedure, the log of the odds ratio is computed to create a linear relationship between the dependent variable (disease) and various independent variables (exposures or risk factors that may be possible confounders). These possible confounders are then fitted into a mathematical model to test their effects upon the disease or outcome. Confounders can be tested separately or together to estimate their individual or cumulative effects. In the analysis, it is also possible to use stratification, in which separate odds ratios are calculated for each category of the suspected confounding variable, and then an adjusted odds ratio, a summary measure of all of the stratum-specific odds ratios, is calculated. If the adjusted odds ratio is very different from the crude odds ratio, the variable was confounding the relationship, and the adjusted odds ratio must be reported. If, however, the two values are relatively close, then the variable was probably not confounding the relationship between the exposure and the disease. If the stratum-specific odds ratios are very different from each other, a different phenomenon, effect modification, is present.

EFFECT MODIFICATION

Effect modification (also known as interaction) occurs when the magnitude or direction of the exposure-disease association, i.e., the odds ratio, differs for varying levels of the variable that was stratified. There may be very different relationships between the exposure and the disease, depending on which stratum we are observing. If this is the case, do not calculate an adjusted odds ratio for the stratified tables; this would ignore the fact that the odds ratio is different for different levels of the stratified variable. Instead, do separate analyses for the different levels of the stratifed variables to show the interaction.

STUDY CONCLUSIONS

The study conclusions should be justified by the findings and relevant to the questions posed by the investigators. The investigators should also provide a reasonable review of the previous work in the field and present their results in this context. If their conclusions are causal, they should be justified.

The accepted criteria for causation include

* The strength of the association
* A temporal sequence of exposure followed by disease
* A dose-response effect
* Biological plausibility
* Consistency in study findings
* Specificity of effect

In summary, the investigator must

* Develop a research question
* Develop a subsequent null hypothesis
* Perform an analytic study to test the null hypothesis
* Evaluate the role of chance
* Evaluate the roles of bias and effect modification
* Evaluate a causal relationship between the exposure and the disease

INTERPRETING EPIDEMIOLOGIC FINDINGS PRESENTED BY THE MEDIA

Epidemiologic findings presented by the media must be interpreted with caution. It may be reported that only 50,000 people in the U.S. have some type of disease this year compared with 75,000 last year, which does not sound like a large number. The problem is that it is not mentioned that these cases are clustered in the Southeast. The implications of this are far more serious because it is not known whether there is a possibility that environmental factors may be involved. This is the reason that sound results are reported in rates that denote place and time because two numbers cannot simply be compared; the population at risk must be considered. A report of a recent study may mention that a particular variable is a risk factor for some type of cancer in women. However, it is not known whether confounding variables were accounted for in the study design or analysis. It may be reported that a particular variable "causes" a particular disease. But, it is not known whether the proper causal criteria were taken into consideration when this conclusion was drawn.

SCREENING

Screening for the absence or presence of a specific disease is used to identify those who are suspected to have a particular disease or condition. The following concepts may also be applied to diagnostic tests. Two important characteristics of a screening test are *validity* and *reliability*. *Validity* measures whether the test really measures what it is supposed to measure. The two components of validity are sensitivity and specificity. *Reliability* denotes repeatability. Table 6–7 shows the relationship between the outcome of the test result and the presence of disease.

* The sensitivity of a screening test is the ability of the test to identify correctly those who have the disease. The formula for sensitivity is $a/a+c$.
* The specificity of a screening test is the ability of the test to identify correctly those who do not have the disease. The formula for specificity is $d/b+d$.
* The positive predictive value is the proportion of positive test results that are true positives. The formula for positive predictive value is $a/a+b$.
* The negative predictive value is the proportion of negative test results that are true negatives. The formula for negative predictive value is $d/c+d$.

Consider the example in Table 6–8.

Table 6–7. Relationship Between Screening Outcome and Disease Presence

| Test Result | Disease | | |
	Yes	*No*	*Total*
Positive	a	b	$a + b$
Negative	c	d	$c + d$
Total	$a + c$	$b + d$	$a + b + c + d$

Table 6–8. Results of a Screening Test

| Test Result | Disease | | |
	Yes	No	Total
Positive	90	27	117
Negative	10	873	883
Total	100	900	1000

$n = 1000$ Prevalence = 90/1000 = 9%
Sensitivity = 90/100 = 90%   Specificity = 873/900 = 97%
Positive predictive value = 90/117 = 77%
Negative predictive value = 873/883 = 99%

The predictive value reflects the effect the prevalence of the disease has on the sensitivity and specificity of a screening or diagnostic test. Even with a high degree of sensitivity and specificity, if the prevalence of the disease in question is low, the test may have a lower predictive value than would be expected by considering only sensitivity and specificity. For most screening tests, a high negative predictive value with a respectable (15–20%) positive predictive value is needed. For most diagnostic tests, a high positive predictive value (usually more than 75%) is required. As the prevalence of the disease declines, so does the positive predictive value of the screening test.

CONCLUSION

Epidemiology may be considered the basic science of public health. Although it is focused on a working knowledge of statistics, probability, and research methods, epidemiology is also an important tool in advocating health promotion and disease prevention.

Applied epidemiology exists when the principles of epidemiology are applied to answer public health questions and issues. Examples of epidemiology used in this fashion include:

* Analysis of historical trends to project future resource requirements
* Evaluation of the effectiveness of a public education program
* Study of how a lifestyle choice affects a person's risk of developing a particular disease
* Monitoring reports of communicable diseases in the community
* Determining whether a proposed screening strategy is both effective and cost-effective

A good grounding in this public health discipline, based upon science, reasoning, and common sense, provides the practitioner with the tools needed to promote and protect the public's health.

REFERENCES

1. Wesseling C, Antich D, Hogstedt C, et al. Geographical differences of cancer incidence in Costa Rica in relation to environmental and occupational pesticide exposure. Int J Epidemiol 1999;28:365–374.
2. Won A, Lapane K, Gambassi G, et al. Correlates and management of nonmalignant pain in the nursing home. J Am Geriat Soc 1999;47:936–942.
3. Bratt O, Kristoffersson U, Lundgren R, Olsson H. Familial and hereditary prostate cancer in southern Sweden. A population-based case-control study. Eu J Cancer 1999;35:272–277.
4. Krop JS, Coresh J, Chambless LE, et al. A community-based study of explanatory factors for the excess risk for early renal function decline in blacks vs. whites with diabetes. Arch Intern Med 1999;159:1777–1783.
5. Salmon DA, Haber M, Gangarosa EJ, et al. Health consequences of religious and philosophical exemptions from immunization laws. JAMA 1999;282:47–53.
6. Monto AS, Robinson DP, Herlocher ML, et al. Zanamivir in the prevention of influenza among healthy adults. JAMA 1999;282:31–35.

RESOURCES

FURTHER READINGS

Friis RH, Sellers TA. Epidemiology for Public Health Practice, 2nd ed. Gaithersburg, MD: Aspen Publishers, Inc., 1999.

Hirsh RP, Rieglman RK. Statistical First Aid: Interpretation of Health Research Data. Blackwell Scientific Publications, 1992.

FURTHER EDUCATION

U.S. Department of Health and Human Services, Public Health Service, Centers for Disease Control and Prevention, Public Health Program Office, Atlanta, GA 30333

Principles of Epidemiology, a home study course, and Epidemiology in Action, a two-week Continuing Medical Education course, offered in Atlanta, GA, semiannually

CHAPTER 7

Exercise

Leslie Irvine, PA-C, MMSc
and Alan M. Harben, MD, PhD, PC

INTRODUCTION

For years it has been generally accepted that regular physical activity is an important component of a healthy lifestyle. In 1996, the U.S. Surgeon General released a landmark report that reinforced this idea and offered evidence that a moderate amount of daily physical activity provides significant physical and mental health benefits. These benefits include a protective effect in several chronic diseases, including coronary heart disease, hypertension, and non–insulin-dependent diabetes mellitus. Additionally, exercise aids in controlling weight, reduces the risk of colon cancer, helps build and maintain bone integrity, and reduces depression and anxiety.[1, 2] On average, physically active people outlive those who are inactive.[3] Despite this evidence and the public's apparent acceptance of the importance of physical activity, the majority of American adults remain essentially inactive.[4] In order to change our sedentary society, it is imperative that health care providers communicate the types and amounts of physical activity that are needed to promote health. Clinicians may discount the importance of counseling, as the benefits of exercise are common sense. However, intervention by a health care provider can play a significant role in motivating patients to become physically active.

EPIDEMIOLOGY

The 1996 U.S. Surgeon General's report established new guidelines that recommend that all people ages 6 and older participate in 30 min of moderate-intensity physical activity on most (if not all) days of the week. In the United States, it is estimated that 60% of adults do not exercise regularly, and, of that group, 25% are essentially inactive.[4] Among young persons (ages 6–17), 15% are inactive.[1] Such a large degree of physical inactivity creates a significant public health burden of chronic disease and disability. It is estimated that as many as 250,000 deaths (12% of total deaths) per year in the U.S. are attributable to a lack of regular physical activity.[5] This makes lack of physical activity a preventable cause of death second only to smoking.[6]

Patterns of physical activity vary with demographic characteristics. Women tend to be less active than men (1.2–1.7:1). Adults at retirement age tend to increase participation in moderate activity, but, over all, total activity declines with increasing age, with one third to one half of adults over age 74 completely inactive. African Americans, Hispanics, and other minority groups are less active than white Americans. Among different socioeconomic groups, physical inactivity is greater among persons with lower levels of education and income. In households with an annual income of less than $10,000, the level of inactivity is reported at 30–40%, whereas in households with an annual income of $50,000 or more, inactivity is reported at 11–18%.[1]

KEY HEALTH BENEFITS OF PHYSICAL ACTIVITY

Several findings were summarized in the surgeon general's report on physical activity. It was found that routine physical activity reduces the risk of all causes of mortality and can extend life expectancy by 2 years. Specifically, routine physical activity lowers mortality from cardiovascular disease by 40% regardless of other lifestyle habits. Hypertension can be prevented and treated. In non–insulin-dependent diabetes mellitus (NIDDM), physical activity can play a major role in management of blood sugar levels. In osteoporosis, a physically active lifestyle can protect against bone loss. Exercise is associated with decreased colon cancer mortality and is thought to protect against other cancers. Physically active people experience improved mood, reduced stress, and fewer symptoms of depression and anxiety. With regard to weight loss, physical activity is essential and is one of the more effective interventions for maintaining appropriate body weight. Lastly, physical activity was found to enhance activities of daily living (ADL) in elderly populations through improved flexibility and muscular strength.

DEFINITION AND EXAMPLES OF MODERATE PHYSICAL ACTIVITY

In the past it was thought that the benefits of being physically active were only derived through vigorous daily activity, a standard met by only 15% of Americans.[2] In recent years, numerous studies have shown that a moderate amount of activity can provide benefits nearly equal to the benefits of vigorous exercise.[1, 2, 7, 8] Physical activity has been defined as "any bodily movement produced by skeletal muscles that results in energy expenditure." Exercise is a subset of physical activity defined as "planned, structured, and repetitive bodily movement done to improve or maintain one or more components of physical fitness."[9] A moderate amount of physical activity is roughly activity that uses 150–200 calories (kcal) of energy per day, or 1000–2000 calories per week (Table 7–1).[10] Another way to define physical

Table 7–1. Moderate-Intensity Physical Activity*

Activity

Washing and waxing a car for 45–60 min†
Washing windows or floors for 45–60 min
Playing volleyball for 45 min
Playing touch football for 30–45 min
Gardening for 30–45 min
Wheeling self in wheelchair for 30–40 min
Walking 1¾ miles in 35 min (20 min/mile)
Basketball (shooting baskets) for 30 min
Bicycling 5 miles in 30 min
Dancing fast (social) for 30 min
Pushing a stroller 1½ miles in 30 min
Raking leaves for 30 min
Walking 2 miles in 30 min (15 min/mile)
Water aerobics for 30 min
Swimming laps for 20 min
Wheelchair basketball for 20 min
Basketball (playing a game) for 15–20 min
Bicycling 4 miles in 15 min
Jumping rope for 15 min
Running 1½ miles in 15 min (10 min/mile)
Shoveling snow for 15 min
Stairwalking for 15 min

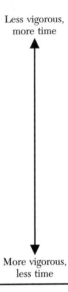

Less vigorous,
more time

More vigorous,
less time

°A moderate amount of physical activity is roughly equivalent to physical activity that uses approximately 150 calories (kcal) of energy per day, or 1000 calories per week.

†Some activities can be performed at various intensities; the suggested durations correspond to expected intensity of effort.

Source: www.cdc.gov/nccdphp/fall96cd.pdf

activity is as a percentage of maximal heart rate. A moderate amount of physical activity is at 50–75% of maximal heart rate for 30 min on most days of the week. As shown in Table 7–1, a moderate amount of physical activity can be achieved in a variety of ways. Since the amount of activity is a function of duration, intensity, and frequency, the same amount of calories burned may be obtained either in longer sessions of moderately intense activity or in shorter sessions of more strenuous activity.

Intermittent bursts of activity as short as 8–10 min but totaling 30 min a day may also provide substantial benefits.[7, 8] For example, in a comparison of people who walked continuously for 30 min a day with a second group who walked 30 min a day in sessions as short as 5 min at a time, at the end of 16 weeks both groups showed improved aerobic fitness, lowered systolic and diastolic blood pressures, and a reduction in body fat.[8] The uniqueness of the 1996 recommendation from the surgeon general is the mounting evidence that the health benefits of physical activity are linked to the total amount of activity performed or to the total amount of calories burned regardless of the type of activity or the length of time the activity is performed. However, it is important to note that while intermittent physical activity is better than no activity, there is a dose-response curve with regard to exercise. There is a significant trend of decreasing risk of death across increasing increments of distance walked, flights of stairs climbed, and degree of intensity of sports played.[11]

▰▰ PHYSIOLOGIC EXPLANATIONS FOR HEALTH BENEFITS OF PHYSICAL ACTIVITY

When engaged in physical activity, the body responds by using many (if not all) of its physiologic systems. The musculoskeletal, cardiovascular, respiratory, endocrine, and immune systems are most notably affected by physical activity. When regular physical activity is performed, these systems undergo changes that increase the body's efficiency and capacity. When training ceases, the result is a loss of the efficiency and capacity that was gained through a process called detraining. All of the effects of physical activity on the body are beyond the scope of this text, but known benefits are addressed.

CARDIOVASCULAR DISEASE

Coronary artery disease (CAD) is the principal cause of death in America, accounting for 41.5% of all deaths annually.[12] Physical inactivity is now recognized as an independent risk factor for CAD. Regular physical activity plays a role in both primary and secondary prevention of cardiovascular disease. Physical activity reduces CAD in a dose-response manner. Moderate physical activity at 40–60% of maximal oxygen uptake on most days of the week is sufficient to relay the majority of health benefits to the cardiovascular system.[7] In addition to preventing CAD, physical activity improves survival rates after myocardial infarction and improves functional capacity in heart failure.[12]

Cardiovascular fitness is measured by maximal oxygen uptake ($\dot{V}O_2max$). The cardiovascular and respiratory systems are responsible for providing the body with oxygen and nutrients, maintaining temperature and acid-base balance, and removing carbon dioxide and other metabolic waste products. The cardiovascular response to exercise is directly proportional to the skeletal oxygen demands for any given rate of work, and to oxygen uptake ($\dot{V}O_2$). Oxygen uptake increases linearly with increasing rates of work, but only until it reaches the individual's maximal capacity ($\dot{V}O_2$max). The percentage of $\dot{V}O_2$max that one is able to achieve increases with regular exercise training.

The improvements seen through training are a direct result of an increase in the body's ability to use oxygen to derive energy for work.[12] Several changes are responsible for this improvement.

1. Cardiac output increases as a product both of hypertrophy of the cardiac muscle fibers, which improves stroke volume, and of elevated heart rate. The improved cardiac output increases blood flow to both skeletal and cardiac muscles.
2. Peripheral resistance to blood flow decreases owing to an increase in the number of capillaries.
3. Oxygenation improves through increases in pulmonary blood flow and tidal volume.

The combined increase in the efficiency of the system allows for a higher level of myocardial oxygenation. The higher level of oxygenation in turn allows for a higher level of physical work to be achieved before the body reaches a point of myocardial oxygen demand that could result in ischemia.[12]

Routine physical activity also plays a role in secondary prevention of CAD through its effects on hypertension, atherosclerosis, obesity, and diabetes mellitus.

HYPERTENSION

Fifty million Americans suffer from hypertension.[1] Hypertension is a well-established risk factor for both CAD and stroke. Less active, less fit persons have a 30–50% greater risk of developing high blood pressure.[12] Routine physical activity has a pronounced effect on decreasing blood pressure and should be highly recommended as a primary prevention method.

Exactly how physical activity improves blood pressure is not clearly understood. During a bout of activity, mean arterial blood pressure increases in response to exercise owing to an increase in systolic blood pressure as diastolic pressure remains at or near resting levels. Like cardiac output, systolic blood pressure also responds linearly to increasing rates of work, reaching peak values of 200–240 mmHg in normotensive persons. This increase in systolic blood pressure is a product of increased cardiac output that outweighs the decrease in total peripheral resistance seen during exercise. It is both normal and desirable because without it one would experience severe arterial hypotension during exercise.[13] Hypertensive persons typically reach much higher systolic pressures for a given rate of work than do normotensive persons. For the first 2–3 h following exercise, blood pressure drops below preactivity levels. The specific reasons for this drop have not been established but are hypothesized to be an important aspect of the role of physical activity in controlling blood pressure.[14] With endurance training, resting arterial blood pressure is lower for all persons, but decreases are greater in people with hypertension. People with normal pressure will experience a systolic/diastolic pressure drop of 3/3 mmHg each, people who are borderline will have a decrease of approximately 6/7 mmHg, and in people with hypertension the drop can be 10/8 mmHg.[15]

ATHEROSCLEROSIS

Atherosclerosis is a result of a complex process that involves deposition of cholesterol on the arterial wall by lipoproteins, especially low-density lipoproteins (LDLs). Deposition usually occurs at sites where injury is present, and a subsequent inflammatory reaction takes place leaving atherosclerotic plaques. Exercise has been shown to reduce atherosclerosis, but exact processes are not known. One important finding is that moderate levels of physical activity have been conclusively shown to increase levels of high-density lipoproteins (HDLs) in the blood.[1] HDLs protect against atherosclerosis by transporting cholesterol to the liver for elimination in the bile. Endurance-trained men and women have HDL levels that are 20–30% higher than sedentary individuals.[1] Additionally, moderate physical activity is known to reduce triglycerides, which are also associated with vascular disease.

NON–INSULIN-DEPENDENT DIABETES MELLITUS (NIDDM)

An estimated 16 million people in the U.S. have diabetes. Annually diabetes directly causes about 200,000 deaths. This number is misleading because diabetes often goes unmentioned on death certificates when someone dies of heart disease, even when diabetes may have been the major contributing factor.[16] The epidemiologic literature strongly supports a protective effect of physical activity against the likelihood of developing NIDDM and also considerable improvement in glycemic control in those with NIDDM. Physical inactivity is strongly associated with NIDDM.[1]

The physiologic explanation for the beneficial effect of physical activity on NIDDM is a consequence of the effect of activity on carbohydrate metabolism and glucose tolerance. During a moderate episode of physical activity, contracting muscle works synergistically with insulin to enhance glucose uptake into the cells. This effect is related to increased blood flow to the muscle during exercise and enhanced glucose transport into the muscle cell. After a meal, glucose and insulin levels are significantly higher in less active people than in more active persons.[1]

With regard to prevention of NIDDM, it is thought that physical activity improves glycemic control primarily by increasing the sensitivity of the muscle cells to insulin.[17] For people with diabetes, this means that physical activity has its most profound effect when the diabetic condition is due to insulin resistance rather than to a general deficiency of circulating insulin.[1] In addition, physical activity also improves the outcome of NIDDM by reducing the risk of CHD and atherosclerosis, which are associated with both micro- and macrovascular disease.

INSULIN-DEPENDENT DIABETES MELLITUS (IDDM)

Exercise programs have not been conclusively shown to improve glycemic control in people with IDDM. However, it is important to note the improved cardiovascular fitness and psychological well-being associated with regular physical activity. The American Diabetes Association recommends regular physical activity for all patients with diabetes with the caveat that health care providers monitor these patients carefully for hypoglycemia, hyperglycemia, ketosis, ischemia, injury due to neuropathy, and progression of retinopathy.[18]

OBESITY

Excess body weight plays an important role in chronic disease and disability. Statistics from the Third National Health and Nutrition Examination Survey, 1988–1994, show that 33% of men, 36% of women, 12% of adolescents 12–17 years old, and 14% of children 6–11 years old are obese. Obesity occurs when energy intake exceeds energy expenditure over a prolonged period of time. Physical activity improves body composition and weight by reducing body fat while preserving or increasing lean tissue.[19, 20] Exercise is most effective as a method of weight loss when it is combined with caloric restriction. There is a dose-response manner to weight loss, with more regular and greater amounts of activity resulting in greater amounts of weight lost.[1]

SKELETAL MUSCLE, OSTEOARTHRITIS, AND ACTIVITIES OF DAILY LIVING

Routine physical activity contributes to improved muscular strength, joint flexibility, and endurance.[1] Improvement in these areas is linked to a reduction in symptoms of back pain and osteoarthritis,[21] to better balance and coordination, resulting in fewer falls, and to improvement in activities of daily living in the elder populations.[2]

Muscle tissue consists of three types, skeletal, cardiac, and smooth. Skeletal muscle is made up of two basic types of fibers distinguished by their speed, slow twitch and fast twitch. Slow-twitch fibers have high oxidative capacity and high fatigue resistance. Fast-twitch fibers tend to have low oxidative capacity and low fatigue resistance combined with fast contractile speed.[1] Performance in certain sports has a direct relationship to the athlete's predominant muscle fiber type. For example, marathon runners have predominantly slow-twitch fibers. A person's predominant muscle fiber type is thought to be genetically driven.[1] With routine endurance training the quantity of both types of skeletal muscle fiber increases, the fibers grow larger, and the number of capillaries to muscle fiber also increases, all of which leads to increased muscle strength.

The threshold for muscle exhaustion is dictated by lactic acid. Lactate is the primary byproduct of the anaerobic glycolic energy system. This system is employed at high rates of work when the muscle cells' demand for oxygen exceeds its supply. As exercise intensity increases, the rate of lactic acid build-up outstrips its rate of removal, and the pH of the muscle cell drops below levels at which adenosine triphosphate (ATP) can be produced, causing exhaustion. People who are regularly physically active have higher lactate thresholds, enabling them to reach a higher percentage of their $\dot{V}O_2max$ and resulting in improved endurance.

Physical activity is essential to maintain healthy joints and appears to relieve symptoms of osteoarthritis.[21] The exact mechanism is not known, but what is clear is that because hyaline cartilage has no blood vessels, it must rely on diffusion of nutrients from joint fluid. Physical activity enhances the process of diffusion.[1] Immobility causes decreased cartilage stiffness and decreased thickness, making cartilage more vulnerable to injury. There is no evidence that physical activity causes osteoarthritis, but injuries sustained during sports activities have been linked to increased risk of developing the condition.[1]

OSTEOPOROSIS

The physiologic impact of exercise on the skeleton is most important in relation to osteoporosis. Osteoporosis is characterized by decreased bone mass and structural deterioration of bone tissue leading to fracture. An estimated 1.5 million fractures are attributable to osteoporosis each year, and of these, 250,000 are hip fractures. Hip fractures are associated with greater morbidity and mortality (15–20%) than any other osteoporotic fracture.[1]

The skeletal response to physical activity is not clearly understood; however, mechanical factors are well documented. Bone cells respond to load-bearing with improved bone formation and bone resorption, which leads to greater bone mass density (BMD). Estrogen replacement therapy has been shown conclusively to decrease bone loss after menopause, and there is evidence that this effect is enhanced by physical activity.[1] Weight-bearing physical activity early in life is more strongly associated with greater BMD than is physical activity in later years.[22] This does not suggest that physical activity in later years has no effect on bones; in fact, physical activity is very important for maintaining BMD, but it does not increase BMD to a significant degree. This fact illustrates the importance of counseling young people on the long-term benefits of a physically active lifestyle.

COLON CANCER

Cancer is the second leading cause of death (one in four deaths) in the U.S., second only to heart disease.[23] Colon cancer is the third leading type of cancer. Physical activity has been shown to have an inverse relationship to the risk of developing colon cancer.[1] Biological explanations for this phenomenon point to changes in prostaglandin synthesis. Exercise increases prostaglandin F_2 synthesis, which increases intestinal motility and has a suppressive effect on prostaglandin E_2, which is known to stimulate tumor growth. It is also thought that regular physical activity may decrease gastrointestinal transit time, thereby reducing the time that colonic mucosa is in contact with potential carcinogens.[1] With regard to other cancers, there is a lack of research pertaining to the effects of physical activity. Many hypothesize that similar benefits will be found (there is some debate regarding exercise and cancer prevention; see Chapter 24, Neoplastic Conditions).

IMMUNE SYSTEM

The immune system appears to be affected in numerous ways by physical activity. Importantly, moderate physical activity bolsters the function of many components of the system, such as natural killer cells, circulating T and B lymphocytes, and cells of the monocyte macrophage system. This effect may decrease the incidence of some infections[24] and possibly of certain types of cancer.[1]

Excessive exercise training is thought to have a dramatically different effect on the immune system as compared with moderate training. Excessive training on a routine basis or even in single episodes results in a marked decline in the functioning of all major cells in the immune system.

MENTAL HEALTH

Mental disorders account for 4 of the 10 leading causes of disability in industrialized countries worldwide. In the U.S., the estimated cost of mental illnesses, including indirect costs of days missed from work, was $148 billion in 1990.[24] Mental health disorders encompass a wide variety of illnesses. The most frequently studied effect of physical activity on mental health is in relation to mood disorders (e.g., depression, anxiety), self-esteem, self-efficacy, and cognitive functioning.[1] Depression affects 19 million Americans ages 18 and over annually, with nearly twice as many women (12%) as men (7%) affected. More than 16 million Americans experience anxiety disorders annually.[25]

Epidemiologic research suggests that physical activity is associated with reduced symptoms of depression, anxiety, and low self-esteem. In general, people who are inactive are twice as likely to have symptoms of depression and anxiety than are more active people.[1] This is true for both clinical and nonclinical levels of depression and anxiety. Though several studies indicate a probable cause and effect relationship, it is not clear whether physical activity can prevent such disorders. It may be the case that people with improved mood are more likely to be physically active. More research in this area is needed.

▬ MAINTENANCE, DETRAINING, AND PROLONGED INACTIVITY

After a person has made gains in $\dot{V}O_2$max through routine daily endurance training, the optimal frequency of training to maintain those gains is at least two to four times a week at the same level of intensity. It appears that the amount of *time* spent being active may be reduced without reducing $\dot{V}O_2$max, but if the *level of intensity* is reduced, $\dot{V}O_2$max will decline. Gains in muscle strength can be maintained through as little as one session per week of resistance training of equal intensity.[1]

Detraining occurs with a complete cessation of activity. A significant reduction in $\dot{V}O_2$max occurs within 2 weeks of the end of training. Over the next 2 to 8 months, all other functional gains previously mentioned begin to decline as well. Prolonged inactivity, such as in a period of bed rest, can be detrimental.

Decreases in cardiorespiratory function are evidenced by a decrease in $\dot{V}O_2$max by as much as 15% in the first 10 days of bed rest.[1] Reversible glucose intolerance and hyperinsulinemia occur. A reduction in skeletal muscle mass and strength, as well as of bone mineral density, occurs in proportion to time spent immobilized.[26] When normal activity is resumed, losses in cardiorespiratory, metabolic, and muscle function can be reversed fairly rapidly. Bone density losses require longer to recover to previous levels.[1]

■■■RISKS OF PHYSICAL ACTIVITY

The risks associated with physical activity must be considered on an individual basis. Most adults do not need to see their health care provider before starting a moderate intensity program. However, men over 40 years of age and women over 50 who have previously been sedentary, or who suffer from a chronic disease, or who have risk factors for a chronic disease should be evaluated by their clinician before beginning an exercise program.[2]

The most common health problems associated with physical activity are musculoskeletal injuries. These injuries occur most often with excessive activity or when someone suddenly begins an activity for which he or she has not been trained. Most of these injuries can be avoided by gradual increases in activity levels.

Sudden cardiac death during exercise is an infrequent but a very frightening possibility. Estimates of rates of sudden cardiac deaths per 100,000 h of exercise range from zero to two per 100,000 h in general populations and from 0.13 to 0.61 per 100,000 h and 0.61 per 100,000 h in participants in cardiac rehabilitation programs.[12] Although there is some increased chance of sudden cardiac death with physical activity, regular participation in moderate activities is associated with an overall reduced risk of sudden death and is therefore recommended.[9] In other words, the benefit of regular activity far outweighs the risk of sudden cardiac death associated with exercise.

A collaborative health care team should evaluate persons with diabetes who plan to be physically active. These individuals should have a pre-exercise evaluation specifically to uncover previously undiagnosed hypertension, neuropathy, retinopathy, nephropathy, and, in particular, silent ischemic heart disease. All patients with diabetes over 35 years of age should have an exercise-stress electrocardiogram before beginning an exercise program. People taking insulin need to self-monitor their glycemic response to exercise.[24]

■■■EFFECTIVENESS OF EXERCISE COUNSELING

Health care providers are in a unique position to encourage people to be more physically active. Despite the opportunity offered by the provider-patient relationship, most health care providers counsel less often about physical activity than they do about smoking or body weight.[27] Only 18–25% of health professionals help patients to formulate an exercise plan.[28] One of the objectives of the Healthy People 2010 program is to increase this percentage to at least 50%.[25] Fully 80% of Americans indicate that their primary source of health information is their health care provider. The average adult makes 2.7 visits to a physician per year, providing a significant degree of contact and opportunities for influence.[6]

A single intervention by a practitioner, taking 5 min or less, has been shown to reduce inactivity.[6, 29] Increases in the time patients spent exercising after a single intervention have been demonstrated to persist up to a year later.[29] This is perhaps the most significant point for a health care provider in this chapter. A few minutes spent with patients on this issue can have an enormous public health impact.

HOW TO COUNSEL A PATIENT

Many modifiable factors explain why some people are more physically active than others. A lack of time is the most commonly cited reason for nonparticipation in activity.[2] Self-efficacy, the confidence that one can achieve activity goals, is consistently associated with participation.[30] A person's awareness of the benefits of activity, support from family and friends, and enjoyment of physical activity are all important factors.[6] Environmental factors such as a lack of walking paths, inclement weather, and unsafe neighborhoods are also barriers to exercise.[2] Any effective approach to a patient needs to include an assessment of the perceived barriers for each individual.

Several effective approaches to counseling patients to increase their levels of activity have been developed. Project PACE (Patient-centered Assessment and Counseling for Exercise) and Fresh Start, an approach created in New Zealand, are just two approaches that have proved successful (see the Resources section at the end of this chapter for additional information). All approaches include a few basic concepts. The main points to convey are:

1. Identify the relevance of exercise as it pertains to benefits for the patient.
2. Provide information on current recommendations for moderate-intensity exercise.
3. Discuss any concerns about barriers to exercise, offering alternatives.

In addition to verbal instructions, providing written instructions that include a list of possible activities (see Table 7–1) is also thought to be very effective.[29]

■ PROMOTING ACTIVITY FOR FUTURE GENERATIONS

Schools and community centers are in a position to help foster lifelong healthy physical activity patterns. Yet, there is a crisis in schools. As previously noted, 15% of U.S. youth ages 6–17 are inactive.[4] Participation in physical activity declines strikingly as age or grade in school increases.[1] In the first half of the 1990s, daily attendance in physical education classes declined from 42% to 25% among high school students. During those physical education classes, only 19% of high school students reported being physically active for 20 min or more.[1]

Much of behavior is learned in the early years.[31] Physical activity must become a priority in schools and communities. Programs should be comprehensive, providing environments that adapt to even the least skilled.[31] The enjoyment of physical activity and the confidence and motor and behavioral skills needed to participate in such activity, if learned in school, could translate into a much more active society in the future.

■ CONCLUSIONS

The proof that physical activity promotes health is indisputable. It is therefore incredible that although knowledge of the benefits of activity increases, societal activity levels continue to decline. If sedentary society would adopt a more active lifestyle, the benefits would be astounding. An active lifestyle does not have to include vigorous activity, and a small increase in activity can lead to a huge improvement in the health of an individual. The few minutes that the health care provider takes to explain preventive measures such as good diet, smoking cessation, and physical activity may in the long run be the most important time spent with a patient.

REFERENCES

1. U.S. Department of Health and Human Services. Physical activity and health: A report of the Surgeon General. Atlanta, GA, U.S. Department of Health and Human Services, Public Health Service, Centers for Disease Control and Prevention National Center for Chronic Disease Prevention and Health Promotion, 1996.
2. Pate RR, Pratt M, Blair SN, et al. Physical activity and public health: A recommendation from the Centers for Disease Control and Prevention and the American College of Sports Medicine. JAMA 1995;273:402–407.
3. Paffenbarger RS, Hyde RT, Wing AL, Hsieh CC. Physical activity, all cause mortality, and longevity of college alumni. N Engl J Med 1986;314:605–613.

4. Centers for Disease Control and Prevention. Prevalence of sedentary lifestyle—behavioral risk factor surveillance system, United States, 1991. MMWR Morb Mortal Wkly Rep 1993;42:576–579.

5. McGinnis JM, Foege WH. Actual causes of death in the United States. JAMA 1993;270:2207–2212.

6. Centers for Disease Control. Project PACE: Physician's Manual: Physician-Based Assessment and Counseling for Exercise. Atlanta, GA, Centers for Disease Control, 1992.

7. Lemaitre RN, Sisovic DS, Raghunathan TE, et al. Leisure-time physical activity and the risk of primary cardiac arrest. Arch Intern Med 1999;159:686–690.

8. Coleman KJ, Raynor HR, Mueller DM, et al. Providing sedentary adults with choices for meeting their walking goals. Prev Med 1999;28:509–510.

9. Caspersen CJ, Powell KE, Christensen GM. Physical activity, exercise and physical fitness. Public Health Rep 1985;100:125–131.

10. U.S. Department of Health and Human Services, Centers for Disease Control and Prevention, National Center for Chronic Disease Prevention and Health Promotion, Division of Nutrition and Physical Activity. 1996.

11. Paffenbarger RS Jr, Hyde RT, Wing AL, et al. The association of changes in physical activity level and other lifestyle characteristics with mortality among men. N Engl J Med 1993;328:538–545.

12. Fletcher GF, Balady, G, Blair SN, et al. Statement on exercise: Benefits and recommendations for physical activity programs for all Americans. Circulation 1996;94:857–862.

13. Rowell LB. Human Cardiovascular Control. New York, Oxford University Press, 1993.

14. Isea JE, Piepoli M, Adamopouplos S, et al. Time course of hemodynamic changes alter maximal exercise. Eur J Clin Invest 1994;24:824–829.

15. Fagard RH, Tipton CM. Physical activity, fitness, and hypertension. In Bouchard C, Shephard RJ, Stephens T (eds), Physical activity, fitness, and health: International proceedings and consensus statement. Champaign, IL, Human Kinetics, 1994, pp 633–655.

16. DiPietro L. Physical activity, body weight, and adiposity: An epidemiologic perspective. Exerc Sport Sci Rev 1995;23:275–303.

17. Ching PL, Willet WC, Rimm RB, et al. Activity level and risk of overweight in male health professionals. Am J Public Health 1996;86:25–30.

18. American Cancer Society. 1999 Facts and figures. American Cancer Society, 1999.

19. Minor MA. Exercise in the treatment of osteoarthritis. Rheum Dis Clin North Am 1999;25:397–415, viii.

20. Ulrich CM, Georgiou CC, Gillis DE, Snow CM. Lifetime physical activity is associated with bone mineral density in premenopausal women. J Womens Health 1999;8:365–375.

21. Pederson BK, Ullum H. NK cell response to physical activity: Possible mechanisms of action. Med Sci Sports Exerc 1994;26:140–146.

22. CDC National Center for Chronic Disease Prevention and Health Promotion. Chronic diseases and their risk factors. Atlanta, GA, Centers for Disease Control and Prevention, 1999, p 23.

23. Regensteiner JG, Shetterly SM, Mayer EJ, et al. Relationship between habitual physical activity and insulin area among individuals with impaired glucose tolerance. Diabetes Care 1995;18:490–497.

24. Position Statement from the American Diabetes Association. Clinical Prac-

tice Recommendation: Diabetes mellitus and exercise. American Diabetes Association, 1996.

25. National Institute of Mental Health. The number count. Bethesda, MD, National Institutes of Health, 1999. NIH publication No. NIH 99-4584.

26. Bloomfield SA, Coyle EF. Bed rest, detraining, and retention of training-induced adaptation. *In* Durstein JL, King AC, Painter PL, et al. (eds), ACSM's Resource Manual for Guidelines for Exercise Testing and Prescription, 2nd ed. Philadelphia, Lea & Febiger, 1993, pp 115–128.

27. Marcus BH, Pinto BM, Clark MM, et al. Physician delivered physical activity and nutrition interventions. Med Exerc Nutr Health 1995;4:24–35.

28. National Center for Health Statistics. Healthy People 2000 Review, 1995–96. Hyattsville, MD, U.S. Department of Health and Human Services, Public Health Service, CDC, National Center for Health Statistics, 1996.

29. Bull FC, Jamrozik K. Advice on exercise from a family physician can help sedentary patients become active. Am J Prev Med 1998;15:85–94.

30. Sallis JF, Howell MF. Determinants of exercise behavior. Exerc Sport Sci Rev 1990;18:307–330.

31. Baranowski T, Bar-OrO, Blair S, et al. Guideline for schools and community programs to promote lifelong physical activity. U.S. Department of Health and Human Services, Public Health Service, CDC National Center for Disease Control and Prevention and Health Promotion.

RESOURCES

American Cancer Society
1599 Clifton Road, NE
Atlanta, GA 30329-4251
(800) 227-2345

American Heart Association
7272 Greenville Avenue
Dallas, TX 75231-4596
(800) 242-8721

American School Health Association
PO Box 708
Kent, OH 44240-0708
(330) 678-1601

National Association for Sport and Physical Education
1900 Association Drive
Reston, VA 20191-1599
(800) 213-7193 ext. 410

National Association of Governors
Council on Physical Fitness and Sports
Hall of States
444 North Capitol Street
Washington, DC 20001–1512
(202) 624-5300
www.nga.org

National Center for Chronic Disease Prevention and Health Promotion
Centers for Disease Control and Prevention
MS K-32
4770 Buford Highway, NE
Atlanta, GA 30341-3724
(888) CDC-4NRG

President's Council on Physical Fitness and Sports
Office of Disease Prevention and Health Promotion
Hubert H. Humphrey Bldg. Rm. 738G
2000 Independence Ave., SW
Washington, DC 20201
(202) 690-9000

Project PACE
5500 Campanile Drive
San Diego, CA 92182-4701
(619) 594-5949

CHAPTER 8

Clinical Genetics

Louise Acheson, MD, MS,
Susan Root, MD, MPH,
and Carl V. Tyler, Jr., MD *

▬▬ INTRODUCTION

As advances in clinical genetics proceed at a dizzying pace, so does the need for family physicians and midlevel providers to keep abreast of innovations in the field of genetics that may affect primary care practice. It is vital for primary care providers not only to recognize the indications for specific genetic tests but also to be able to understand and communicate their limitations. Furthermore, it is critical that the potential benefits of genetic diagnosis and testing be balanced against the complex psychological, ethical, legal, and social ramifications associated with these procedures.[1]

▬▬ THE HUMAN GENOME PROJECT

The Human Genome Project was begun by the United States Department of Energy approximately 50 years ago as a means of studying the health effects of radiation. As the larger implications of the project became clear, the National Institutes of Health (NIH) joined in sponsoring the project. The two agencies now collaborate closely, along with many other organizations throughout the world.

GOALS
Mapping the Human Genome

"Mapping" refers to determining the relative position of genes within a genome. A genome is a complete set of instructions for creating an organism. All living organisms on earth have a genome constructed of DNA or RNA. A gene is a set of instructions for creating a specific protein product. Multiple genes are contained within each DNA or RNA molecule, along with other genetic information that is believed to include special instructions on when to use specific genes. It has been estimated that there are about 100,000 genes in the human genome located on 23 pairs of chromosomes and in the DNA of mitochondria. Each chromosome contains numerous genes along with intervening sections of DNA (called introns) that

---

*This chapter is adapted from Acheson L, Root S, Tyler CV, Jr. Clinical Genetics. Monograph Ed. No. 240. Homestudy Self-Assessment Program. Kansas City, MO: American Academy of Family Physicians, with permission.

appear to provide control functions. A gene map is a schematic representation of the relative position and size of genes.

Sequencing the Human Genome

A gene sequence is a listing of the bases that compose the gene. The standard is to represent each nitrogenous base by its initial letter—for example "A" for adenine, "C" for cytosine (or "U" for uracil, which takes the place of cytosine in RNA), "G" for guanine, and "T" for thymine. As each gene is used, the bases are processed in groups of three (e.g., AAC, GTT, TCA). Each such triplet represents a specific amino acid. Dictionaries listing these amino acids and the triplets that produce them are available.

Sequencing refers to determination of the specific order of nucleotides within the genome. Nucleotides consist of the nitrogenous bases (adenine, guanine, thymine, and cytosine or uracil) linked with a phosphate molecule and a sugar molecule (deoxyribose in DNA, ribose in RNA). Multiple nucleotides linked together in a specific sequence form a molecule of DNA or RNA. The human genome is composed of approximately 3×10^9 base pairs.

Mapping and Sequencing the Genomes of Other Organisms for Comparison

Such studies may be intrinsically significant; for example, by determining points within a bacterial genome that may be susceptible to certain chemical manipulations, new antibiotic therapies can be developed. Alternatively, these studies may demonstrate similarities between organisms. If a gene known to be involved in protein transport is identified in a mouse, and a similar gene is found in a human being, researchers studying this gene may operate under the assumption that the human gene is also involved in protein transport.

Developing Laboratory and Computational Tools

It has become clear that new automated procedures are needed to perform mapping and sequencing operations with speed and accuracy. It is thought that genes make up only about 5% of the total genome. The remainder of the genome is either nonfunctioning or is believed to control sequences that determine when specific genes should be "turned on" (or off), and detect errors or correct sequences that function to maintain information accurately as replication progresses. If gene therapy is on the horizon, then mapping functions must become automated, fast, and accurate to achieve any clinical utility.

Ethical, Legal, and Social Implications

The ethical, legal, and social implications of the Human Genome Project are monumental. Surveys suggest that few primary care providers feel confident when counseling patients about genetics issues or discussing the benefits and dangers of screening for genetically mediated diseases. Issues include

* The duty to warn family members of a potential inherited condition versus the patient's right to confidentiality
* Implications of testing results for the person's living relatives and possible descendants
* Insurance coverage and employability of those who are carriers of a specific gene or possess a mutant gene that could predispose to disease or cancer
* Testing asymptomatic individuals for conditions that may have both genetic and environmental causes
* Changing the genetic instruction set of future generations without fully understanding the consequences of such an action

Legislatures have initiated bills that address issues related to privacy and the use of genetic information, with a focus on prohibiting some forms of discrimination based on a person's genotype. However, it is not yet clear what information is to be considered "genetic," and what degree of protection such laws are capable of providing. In this climate, a person is unlikely to choose genetic testing for a cancer predisposition unless he or she perceives that knowledge of the results will significantly benefit him- or herself or others.

USES OF GENOMIC INFORMATION

POTENTIAL THERAPIES

As gene sequences and functions are identified, alterations to genetic material may be contemplated. Gene therapy attempts to alter genes involved in the etiology or deleterious effects of a disease. Although such therapies are in their early stages, they are already beginning to show promise.

PHARMACOGENETICS

Genomic information may have other therapeutic applications. Knowledge of variations in specific gene sequences may make it possible to tailor therapies to an individual rather than use the same drugs in all patients with a given diagnosis. This process is being applied to chemotherapy, as cancer cells often contain genes that have been altered from those that are contained in noncancerous tissues.

Tailored therapy has been envisioned as a means to select agents to reduce cholesterol in persons at risk for coronary heart disease or to choose postmenopausal drug treatments. The choice of treatment may eventually be based on the individual's genetic profile with respect to a "panel" of genes that code for enzymes, and these panels vary from person to person. Techniques for automated testing of small amounts of DNA from a person's blood to determine whether the individual carries certain mutations in known genes (i.e., a "gene chip") are being developed in conjunction with the Human Genome Project, but clinical application of these techniques has not yet been realized. More importantly, the utility of understanding the role of mutations in the pathogenesis of disease, and the role of mutations in determining individual response to new treatments remains unknown. However, it is thought that by the year 2020, many new therapies will be developed and targeted toward specific subgroups of patients, with goals of improving quality of life and increasing life span.

Multifactorial conditions, such as hypertension, are affected by multiple genes and numerous environmental influences, and the balance between genetic and environmental influences may not be apparent by simply examining the clinical phenotype. Individuals with a genetic predisposition to a condition such as hypertension may never develop the disease if they are subject to favorable environmental influences while others without any genetic predisposition may develop hypertension simply as a result of unfavorable environmental factors. Physicians generally must institute therapy, such as salt restriction in patients with hypertension, without knowing precisely that the therapy will be effective in an individual patient. Unfortunately, it is not yet possible to prospectively identify those individuals likely to respond to such an intervention.

Certain metabolic diseases, such as those in which a single gene that controls the production of an abnormal metabolite has been identified, are clear candidates for the use of gene therapy. Therapy for these conditions may consist of correction of the flawed gene, production of a normal version of the chemical involved, or development of a compound that blocks production of the abnormal metabolite. Even as genetic predilections to disease are revealed, lifestyle modifications remain of paramount importance, and efforts to correct known modifiable risk factors continue to be warranted.

TYPES OF GENE THERAPY

SOMATIC CELL THERAPY

Somatic cell therapy is gene therapy that affects genes in body tissues other than those of the testes or ovaries. Somatic cell therapy might be used to affect the function of skin cells by increasing their resistance to sun damage, or to alter chloride transport activity within the lung cells of a cystic fibrosis patient to improve pulmonary function. However, these genetic changes affect only the tissues of the patient being treated and are not transmitted to offspring.

GERMLINE THERAPY

Germline therapy affects gonadal tissue, altering the genetic structure of eggs, sperm, or the primordial tissues that give rise to eggs or sperm. This type of therapy has a potential to change the genetic makeup of future generations. Such a therapy might be sought by individuals who know that they are carriers for the genetic disorder Tay-Sachs disease, with its inevitable neurologic decline and early death. Patients who received germline therapy for Tay-Sachs disease would thus be able to avoid having children with this lethal disorder.

The functions of most of the human genome have not yet been determined, and unexpected consequences may arise from interfering with the few structures that are understood at this time. In addition, informed consent issues cannot be addressed when providing therapy to "potential persons."

Moreover, researchers have recently highlighted the possibility that gene therapy that is legally and ethically restricted to somatic cell lines may also inadvertently affect germ cells.[2] The NIH has refused to sponsor germline gene therapy amid this important ethical controversy.

DEVELOPMENTAL DISABILITIES

Developmental disabilities remain one of the most challenging areas of genetics in particular and medicine as a whole. Even when the cause of a condition is known and the underlying molecular mechanism is well understood, little treatment or chance of amelioration may be available. Understanding the cause and the risk of recurrence can help alleviate guilt and improve the ability of other family members to make informed reproductive choices.

Several metabolic causes of developmental disabilities have been identified, and plans for their treatment have been developed. Phenylketonuria, an autosomal recessive disorder, can be successfully treated by initiating a phenylalanine-restricted diet soon after birth. Screening for this condition is mandatory in all infants born in hospitals in the United States. Individual states have also mandated screening for various other genetic conditions, including hemoglobinopathies, galactosemia, and biotinidase deficiency. The first step in evaluating an individual with developmental disabilities is to obtain a comprehensive family history.

FRAGILE X SYNDROME

Fragile X syndrome is characterized by learning disabilities, hyperactivity, or autism in the maternal family. Close study of a large pedigree of a family afflicted with fragile X syndrome shows inheritance through females with effects, seen primarily in males, that may worsen over generations. It is rare for families to be aware of fragile X syndrome as a diagnosis, although it is the most common known cause of inherited mental retardation, afflicting about 0.5 per 1000 males.

Physical manifestations include a long, narrow face, large ears, and large testes (recognized after puberty). Affected children often have difficulty interpreting social cues, avoid eye contact, and flap or bite their hands, characteristics that often result in a label of "autistic-like behavior." Speech development is slow during childhood. In adult life, language is often a relative strength. Mathematical and map-reading skills are usually impaired.

Fragile X syndrome is just one of a number of inheritable neurologic disorders that are caused by an excessive number of copies of a particular three-base-pair-sequence within a gene. Although the number of copies of these triplet repeats varies among individuals, it is usually stable as the cell divides and does not increase from one generation to another. However, in families affected by such disorders as fragile X syndrome, myotonic dystrophy, or Huntington's chorea, the area around the repeating sequence is unstable, causing progressive increases in the number of copies from one generation to the next. The clinical term *anticipation* is used to describe an observed increase in severity of symptoms from one generation to the next, a phenomenon that is now known to be related to the increasing number of copies of the triplet sequence in the DNA.[3] DNA testing can quantify the number of repeats and may potentially be used to diagnose carrier status. Gene therapy is not available for these conditions at this time.

MARFAN'S SYNDROME

Marfan's syndrome, a disorder of fibrillin formation, is associated with a number of potential complications, some of which are lifethreatening but preventable with good anticipatory guidance and preventive screening. Fibrillin provides tissue distensibility. All tissues that depend on fibrillin for structural integrity are potentially affected by this condition. Affected areas may include the

* Eye (lens dislocation, myopia, retinal tears)
* Joints (hyperextensible joints, dislocation, and injury)
* Blood vessels (easy bruising, impaired distensibility, dilation and aneurysm formation [most importantly of the proximal aorta, which can cause rupture and premature death])

* Lungs (spontaneous pneumothorax)
* Dura (dural ectasia, or protrusion of the dura through vertebral foramina)
* Skin (stretch marks in areas of growth, poor wound healing)

Current diagnosis requires the use of strict clinical criteria using findings that affect at least two of three body systems:

1. Skeletal: Arm span significantly greater than height, scoliosis, arachnodactyly (spidery fingers), joint laxity, deformed sternum, flatfoot, tall stature relative to family background
2. Cardiac: Aortic root dilation, aortic regurgitation, mitral valve prolapse
3. Ocular: Lens dislocation, severe myopia, corneal abnormalities

The gene for Marfan's syndrome has been identified and localized to chromosome 15q21 (referring to the long arm of chromosome 15, the second band, first sub-band and first marker within the sub-band),[1] but genetic testing for the syndrome remains experimental. This condition is autosomal dominant, and thus having an affected relative is another positive diagnostic clue. Follow-up typically consists of close monitoring of the aortic root with annual echocardiography and of any other medical or surgical treatment instituted. In addition to cardiac follow-up, ophthalmologic monitoring is necessary, with surgery a consideration in cases of dislocated lenses.

It is important to remember that tall, slender individuals deserve close examination, and referral to a geneticist or cardiologist should be considered. Individuals with Marfan's syndrome who are carefully monitored, with interventions provided for cardiac or pulmonary complications should they arise, can have a normal or near-normal life span; without monitoring and treatment, patients typically die in early adulthood.

HEMOCHROMATOSIS

Hemochromatosis, an autosomal recessive liver disease associated with increased iron stores, affects approximately 0.5% of the population. One out of eight Americans has a single copy of the hemochromatosis gene. There does not appear to be a clear ethnic predisposition. Because hemochromatosis is typically clinically silent until end-organ damage has already occurred, many affected individuals are never diagnosed. Hemochromatosis is an abnormality of iron metabolism resulting in accumulation of iron in the body. After red blood cells have reached their full iron-absorption capacity, any remaining iron is deposited in the liver and pancreas. Early symptoms are typically encountered in patients in their 40s but are often subtle and nonspecific. Fatigue and early-onset osteoarthritis are the two most common initial features. Later, Type II diabetes results from iron infiltration of the pancreas, and cirrhosis develops from infiltration of the liver. The patient's skin may attain a bronze hue as a result of deposition of iron pigment. Initial treatment for hemochromatosis involves weekly phlebotomy, during which one to two units of blood are removed at each session until iron stores normalize; this therapy is then repeated every 2 to 4 months for life. Treatment is highly effective and prevents end-organ damage if initiated before symptoms develop. Screening for this condition with a simple blood test, transferrin saturation, is not difficult. The College of American Pathologists has recommended that all adults be screened for hemochromatosis.[4] Although controversial, this recommendation is supported by cost-effectiveness data.

GENETICS AND REPRODUCTION

PRENATAL DIAGNOSIS

Prenatal testing of fetal DNA is feasible and can determine parentage with a high degree of certainty. An invasive procedure such as amniocentesis or chorionic villus sampling is necessary in order to obtain cells that contain fetal genetic material for analysis. Isolation of nucleated fetal cells from the mother's peripheral blood is currently used only in a research context. Initial methods for obtaining fetal DNA and chromosomal material are identical regardless of its intended use. Such a sample may be used for paternity testing, testing for particular inheritable conditions with a known gene sequence (e.g., achondroplasia, sickle cell disease, or cystic fibrosis), or for the identification of an abnormal chromosome number or structure (e.g., trisomy, balanced translocations, missing chromosomes).

Rh-negative women should receive Rh immune globulin when undergoing amniocentesis (50 μg before 12 weeks and 300 μg thereafter).

Generally accepted indications for considering invasive prenatal diagnosis are listed in Box 8-1.

Usually, prenatal fetal genetic testing requires expertise in laboratory as well as in clinical genetic medicine and also patient counseling provided by trained genetic counselors. The family health care provider is in an ideal position to explore the desire and need for prenatal diagnosis and thus make appropriate referrals. Clinicians who wish to learn more about conditions that may be diagnosed with genetic testing can access such information from sources listed in the Resources Appendix at the end of this book.

> **Box 8-1–INDICATIONS FOR CONSIDERING PRENATAL DIAGNOSIS WITH AMNIOCENTESIS OF CHORIONIC VILLUS SAMPLING**
>
> • Maternal age 35 or over at time of birth
> • Previous offspring with chromosomal abnormality
> • Chromosomal abnormality in either parent (e.g., aneuploidy, balanced translocation)
> • Fetus at risk for a detectable prenatal condition (e.g., cystic fibrosis, Tay-Sachs disease, thalassemia)
> • To determine gender of a fetus at risk for an X-linked disorder for which DNA diagnosis is not available
> • Abnormal maternal triple screen results
> • Fetal anatomic abnormalities detected on ultrasonography

From Ross HL, Elias S. Maternal serum screening for fetal genetic disorders. Obstet Gynecol Clin North Am 1997;24:33–47.

TESTING FOR PARENTAGE

Prenatal Testing. Paternity testing has taken a leap forward as techniques for ascertaining personal identity by DNA analysis, or "DNA fingerprinting," have become widespread. Samples of DNA from the fetus are compared with DNA from the mother and from the possible father(s). Fetal DNA sequences that are different from sequences found in the mother must have derived from the biological father of the fetus or have appeared as new mutations. If identical DNA sequences that are different from maternal DNA are present in the fetus and in a particular man, it is highly likely that he is the father. If the putative father's DNA sequences are not similar to sequences in the fetal DNA, he can be excluded as the biological father with high likelihood.

Parentage testing relies on analysis of DNA sequences in regions of the human genome that are highly variable from person to person. Many such sequences consist of multiple repeat regions of DNA between genes. When several highly variable segments of DNA are compared, the chance of two individuals having the same sequence at each location is extremely small.

Restriction fragment length polymorphism (RFLP) analysis uses specific enzymes of bacterial origin (restriction endonucleases) that cleave DNA strands wherever a particular sequence of nucleotides appears. These enzymes break the DNA into hundreds of fragments whose length varies according to the sequence of nucleotides in the original strands. Fragments corresponding to repeat sequences of different lengths can be separated and identified, with each tested

DNA sequence forming a distinct pattern of bands (Southern blot test). When the process is repeated with a series of different enzymes that cleave DNA into different sets of fragments, identity or disparity between two samples of DNA can be established in most cases with virtual certainty. For example, in a published case in which prenatal DNA analysis was used to determine paternity, the pregnant woman's husband was identified as the father of the fetus with only a 1 in 340 trillion chance of error.[6]

More recently, polymerase chain reactions (PCRs) have been used to amplify DNA from "short tandem repeat" loci—that is, places in the genome with multiple base-pair sequence-repeats—and quantify the number of repeats present at each locus, a value that varies from person to person. Because PCR-based techniques use less DNA and are more rapid than RFLP or Southern blot techniques, PCR is now favored for prenatal testing. By using three or more different PCR primers to copy different segments of DNA, probabilities of paternity of greater than 99% are typically achieved.[7] The testing process requires 1 to 4 weeks and costs several hundred dollars. Paternity testing often carries legal implications, and a meticulous "chain of evidence" must be maintained. Therefore, the involvement of legal counsel is usually prudent.

Postnatal Testing. Postnatal parentage testing by DNA fingerprinting is essentially identical to that performed prenatally, except that DNA for analysis is obtained from white blood cells in a sample of blood or epithelial cells from the mouth of the infant, rather than from cells in the amniotic fluid or chorionic villi. If DNA from more than one possible father is available for testing, it is highly likely that many candidates can be excluded, while one may be confirmed with a high probability (unless the possible fathers are close relatives such as father and son or identical twins). DNA-based testing is typically so conclusive that it is accepted as proof of parentage in courts of law.

PRENATAL TRIPLE SCREEN

The prenatal triple screen consists of measurements of alpha-fetoprotein, human chorionic gonadotropin (HCG), and estriol in the maternal serum. Alpha-fetoprotein is a normal protein produced by all fetuses, HCG is a hormone produced by the placenta, and estriol is a form of estrogen that can be used to indirectly assess the health of a pregnancy. An elevated alpha-fetoprotein level may indicate an open neural tube or abdominal wall defect in the fetus. A combination of these three measurements is also used to screen for chromosomal abnormalities, especially trisomy 21 (Down syndrome) and trisomy 18. In many communities, it is now the standard of care to offer this triple screening test to all pregnant women between 15 and 20 weeks of pregnancy (ideally 16–18 weeks). Women who have already been referred for invasive prenatal testing (see Box 8-1) would generally be exempt from screening. The American College of Obstetricians and Gynecologists (ACOG) recommends universal screening of pregnant women with this test.

The triple screen allows pregnant women identified as having an increased risk of having a baby with a neural tube defect or Down syndrome to undergo more definitive prenatal diagnosis and make choices regarding termination of an affected pregnancy. Moreover, if an adverse fetal condition is diagnosed antenatally, the health care provider can better counsel and prepare parents. Appropriate delivery arrangements can be made, including elective cesarean section and delivery at a perinatal center, if warranted (e.g., in cases of open spina bifida).

The health care provider should appropriately counsel the patient about the potential benefits of screening, available treatment options, and the risks of false-positive or false-negative screening results before and after the test is performed.[8, 9, 10] Expected levels of alpha-fetoprotein, HCG, and estriol vary according to gestational age of the fetus and the mother's weight, ethnicity, and presence of diabetes. Information regarding these factors is necessary for valid interpretation of the results.[8, 9, 10] The most common reason for an abnormal triple screen result is inaccurate pregnancy dating or multiple gestations, which may be detected by ultrasonographic examination.

Elevated Maternal Serum Alpha-Fetoprotein. If the maternal serum alpha-fetoprotein level is greater than 2.5 multiples of the median (MoM)—a patient's level divided by the median normal value—for a specific gestational age, further evaluation is indicated. Such evaluation may include comprehensive ultrasonography, repeat serum alpha-fetoprotein measurement, consultation with a maternal-fetal medicine and/or genetics specialist, and amniocentesis.

Alpha-fetoprotein is produced by the fetus. The maternal serum level is likely to be elevated in multiple-gestation pregnancies (in 60% of twin pregnancies, the maternal serum alpha-fetoprotein level is over 2.5 MoM).[5] In the presence of an open neural tube defect, such as anencephaly or spina bifida, abnormal amounts of alpha-fetoprotein enter the amniotic fluid and cross the placenta into the maternal circulation. Abnormally high levels of maternal serum alpha-fetoprotein may also be seen with

* Other birth defects, such as abdominal wall defects, renal anomalies, gastrointestinal atresia, and dermatologic disorders
* Fetal hydrops, occasionally with maternal liver disease
* Abnormalities of placental function that are associated with poor obstetric outcomes, such as intrauterine growth retardation, gestational hypertension, premature birth, or fetal demise.[5]

Neural Tube Defects. Anencephaly is incompatible with life; most persons with open spina bifida have significant neurologic deficits. Seventy percent to 90 percent of persons with severe spina bifida also have hydrocephalus, and about 20% have additional congenital malformations (e.g., cardiac or abdominal wall defects). Ten percent to 15 percent of cases of spina bifida are closed and are not detected by maternal serum alpha-fetoprotein screening, although 70% of closed neural tube defects result in moderate to severe disability.[5]

A personal or family history of neural tube defects increases the risk; the recurrence risk after one affected child is 1 in 40, which is sufficiently high to recommend that these women be referred for genetic counseling and possible amniocentesis rather than triple screening. Folate intake of 0.4–0.8 mg daily for average-risk women and 4.0 mg daily for high-risk women during the first 5 weeks after conception is known to be protective. Hereditary and environmental factors are implicated in the etiology of neural tube defects; only 5% of neural tube defects appear to follow a monogenic inheritance pattern.

The sensitivity of maternal serum alpha-fetoprotein testing in screening for neural tube defects is greater than 85%; closed defects will be missed, but the test is sensitive for open defects. An elevated maternal serum alpha-fetoprotein level will be detected in 5–10% of all pregnancies. However, only 0.5–3% of pregnancies with elevated levels actually prove to have a neural tube defect.[5] If the maternal serum alpha-fetoprotein level is 2.5–2.99 MoM and the pregnancy has not reached 19 weeks' gestation, the serum measurement may be repeated while ordering ultrasonography for confirmation of dating, which reduces the false-positive rate by 40%.[5]

Down Syndrome. Down syndrome is caused by trisomy 21. This abnormality can occur *de novo* or through inheritance from a parent carrying a balanced translocation involving chromosome 21. It results in hypotonia, mental retardation, and growth retardation. Forty percent of children with Down syndrome have congenital heart defects. Approximately 10–25% of infants with Down syndrome die during the first year of life; those who survive typically have a shortened life expectancy.[8] However, 25% of individuals with Down syndrome live to age 65. Families differ in deciding whether they wish to know this diagnosis prenatally; if a pregnancy is determined to be at substantial risk for Down syndrome, genetic counseling can help clarify the family's preferences.

The incidence of Down syndrome (1 per 700 live births overall) increases with maternal age, occurring in 1 in 1250 births in women age 25, 1 in 378 births in women age 35, and 1 in 30 births per women age 45.[8, 9] The incidence of other chromosomal abnormalities also increases with maternal age; their combined incidence can be roughly estimated as equal to that of Down syndrome. Nonetheless, in the U.S., 75% of children with Down syndrome are born to women under age 35 because most births occur in women in that age group.[8, 11]

The triple screening result is abnormal in 58–75% of pregnancies complicated by trisomy 21.[5, 8, 10] In Down syndrome, the maternal serum HCG level tends to be elevated, the alpha-fetoprotein level is decreased, and the estriol level is lower than expected for gestational age. The triple screen result is reported as a probability of Down syndrome (e.g., 1 in 2000) and is compared with the probability based solely on the mother's age. Traditionally, if the probability of Down syndrome based on triple screening is greater than that for a 35-year-old woman (threshold: usually 1 in 190 to 1 in 275), further evaluation is indicated. In this situation, triple screening should not be repeated. Because parents may vary in how they compare the risk of amniocentesis-related pregnancy loss to the risk of having an affected child, some may request amniocentesis when the probability of Down syndrome is less than that seen at age 35.[11] If the probability of a child's being born with a trisomy 21, based on the mother's age and the triple screen result, is 1 in 100 (similar to that seen at maternal age 40), there will still be a 99% probability that the fetus will not have this error. The value of this information varies among patients according to their personal beliefs and the use that they think that they would make of the screening information. Many women who believe that they would decline amniocentesis and/or therapeutic abortion may choose not to undergo triple screening. The ACOG currently does not recommend that triple screen testing be used as a basis for women over age 35 to decide to defer definitive prenatal diagnosis by amniocentesis (fetal chromosomal analysis). However, some parents and providers may choose to use this combination of triple screening and an organ-survey sonographic examination in such a manner.[5-11] In the future, screening for Down syndrome by measuring substances in maternal serum or urine during the first trimester may become feasible.[5]

Trisomy 18. This error causes a lethal pattern of anomalies and occurs in 1 per 8000 births. Estriol, HCG, and alpha-fetoprotein levels in maternal serum are often low with trisomy 18. By using a combination of triple screening and maternal age, 60% of cases of trisomy 18 can be detected, with a false-positive rate of 2 per 1000. Thus, screening would incorrectly identify eight fetuses as at increased risk for trisomy 18 for each case of trisomy 18 detected.[12]

Evaluation of an Abnormal Triple Screen Result. A comprehensive ultrasonographic examination is the first step in evaluating an abnormal triple screen result. Ultrasonography can diagnose multiple gestations and determine gestational age to within 10 days. In cases of revised pregnancy dating, triple screen values can be recalculated. If possible, visualization of the fetal anatomy, especially the spine, skull, and brain in cases of suspected neural tube defect, and the heart, nuchal fold, and limbs in cases of suspected trisomy, can help elucidate the diagnosis. A comprehensive (level 2) ultrasonographic examination (in the presence of an elevated serum alpha-fetoprotein level) has a sensitivity of 90–95% for open neural tube defects (but cannot completely exclude such defects).[1, 13] If the significance of an abnormal triple screen result remains uncertain after ultrasonographic examination, genetic counseling and amniocentesis should be offered. Amniocentesis allows measurement of amniotic fluid alpha-fetoprotein, acetylcholinesterase levels, and chromosomal analysis. If these values are normal in the face of an elevated maternal serum alpha-fetoprotein, increased surveillance of fetal growth and well-being may be warranted during the third trimester because of the increased chance of a poor pregnancy outcome. Although, no definitive action is known to prevent such third-trimester complications, close surveillance allows for more timely interventions. It is important to remember that in most cases in which a chromosomal abnormality is suspected, based on an abnormal triple screen result, chromosomal studies are found to be normal.

CARRIER TESTING FOR CYSTIC FIBROSIS

Indications for prenatal genetic counseling and possible testing are listed in Box 8-2. Cystic fibrosis is the most common serious autosomal recessive disorder in persons of northern European descent, occurring in about 1 in 1600 to 1 in 2500 individuals. As with any autosomal recessive disorder, it is important to identify all potentially affected family members and ask about consanguinity (i.e., whether the parents or their forebears are related to one another).

The appearance of cystic fibrosis in anyone in a family with no previous history of the disorder suggests a recessive pattern of inheritance. Persons of European descent have a 1 in 25 chance of carrying at least one mutant allele for cystic fibrosis; for those of Scandinavian ancestry, the chance is slightly higher.[14]

The "cystic fibrosis gene" codes for a protein involved in chloride transport. Currently, laboratories can test DNA for the 10 to 30 most common mutations in the cystic fibrosis gene, thereby detecting 80–89% of cystic fibrosis carriers in populations of European ancestry, 75% of carriers in African American populations, and 30% of carriers among Asian Americans.[15, 16] Individuals with one normal and one mutant allele (cystic fibrosis carriers) have no health impairment. Individuals with two mutant and no normal alleles have cystic fibrosis. There is a spectrum of severity of both lung and gastrointestinal manifestations, but the causes of variations are unknown. Cystic fibrosis is a disease characterized by normal mental function; a shortened life expectancy (average is age 30); a need for chronic disease management, including several medications and daily chest physical therapy; and a high likelihood of periodic illness throughout life.[13]

If DNA testing reveals that each parent carries a mutant allele for cystic fibrosis, the chance that a child of theirs would have cystic fibrosis is 1 in 4. The severity of disease would be unpredictable. If

---

Box 8-2–INDICATIONS FOR PRENATAL GENETIC COUNSELING

History in either parent or their family members of
- Thalassemia or Italian, Greek, Asian, Philippine, or Mediterranean ancestry with a microcytosis or microcytic anemia
- Neural tube defect (meningomyelocele, spina bifida, anencephaly)
- Down syndrome or other chromosomal abnormality
- Tay-Sachs disease, a known carrier state, or Ashkenazic Jewish, Cajun, or French-Canadian ancestry
- Sickle cell disease, trait, or Mediterranean or African ancestry
- Hemophilia
- Muscular dystrophy
- Cystic fibrosis
- Huntington's chorea
- Mental retardation (if so, has the person been tested for any genetic syndrome?)
- Congenital heart disease
- Other inherited disorder or birth defect
  OR
- Woman's age 35 or over at the expected time of birth
- Frequent miscarriages (three or more)
- A stillbirth or infant death
- Fetal abnormality (e.g., anatomic abnormality) detected on ultrasonography
- Exposure to potentially teratogenic agents or infections

From Milunsky JM, Milunsky A. Genetic counseling in perinatal medicine. Obstet Gynecol Clin North Am 1997;24:1–17.

one parent has no detectable mutation and the other is a carrier, each child has a 50% chance of carrying the mutant allele. However, the chance that the child would have cystic fibrosis would be greater than zero because of the possibility of receiving an uncommon mutant allele that cannot be detected by carrier testing.[13]

In circumstances in which only a single individual in a family carries a mutant allele for cystic fibrosis, a more parsimonious approach to testing, such as "cascade" testing of relatives, is preferred.

A 1997 NIH consensus conference recommended that all adults considering conception should be tested to determine whether they carry a known cystic fibrosis mutant allele.[16] However, this recommendation has proved controversial and has not been endorsed by any other large professional organizations. It is, however, widely agreed that carrier testing should be offered to those with a family history of cystic fibrosis. Preconception counseling may be even more complex. For example, in the case of white parents of French-Canadian ancestry who are considering carrier testing for cystic fibrosis, they may also need to know that their ethnic background may be associated with an even higher frequency of carrying an allele for Tay-Sachs disease. Such patients should also receive counseling about enzyme- and DNA-based carrier testing for this autosomal recessive disorder.[14]

Since carrier testing for Tay-Sachs disease was first introduced and promoted among the Jewish population of the U.S., many individuals have chosen to be tested and have used the information in reproductive decision-making; consequently, the incidence of children born with Tay-Sachs disease has decreased dramatically.[13, 14] A similar effect of preconception counseling has been seen in some Mediterranean populations following the introduction of screening for thalassemia minor. Disorders for which ethnicity-based carrier testing has been advocated are listed in Table 8–1.[13, 14, 17]

Table 8–1. Ethnic Groups Affected by Recessive Disorders for Which Carrier Testing Is Available

Ethnic Groups	Disorder	Carrier Frequency	Test
Northern European	Cystic fibrosis	1 in 25	DNA test for 10–30 of 700 known mutations detects 80–89% of carriers.
Ashkenazic Jew (Eastern European)	Tay-Sachs disease	1 in 25	DNA or enzyme test
	Gaucher's disease	1 in 13	DNA test for 5 mutations detects 98% of carriers.
	Cystic fibrosis	WI 282X mutation is most common	DNA test for common mutations detects 97% of carriers.
French-Canadian	Tay-Sachs disease	Unknown	Enzyme test
	Myotonic dystrophy	Unknown	DNA test
African	Sickle cell anemia	1 in 15	Screen with hemoglobin electrophoresis; DNA test for single codon mutation detects 100% of carriers.
Mediterranean, African, Indian, Southeast Asian	Thalassemias	Variable	Screen with RBC indices (MCH less than 23 ng), Hg electrophoresis, confirm with genetic test

RBC, red blood cell; MCH, mean corpuscular hemoglobin; Hg, hemoglobin.

Box 8-3–KNOWN HUMAN TERATOGENS

Maternal conditions and illnesses:
- Intrauterine infection (e.g., TORCH infections: toxoplasmosis, other [HIV, varicella, parvovirus, syphilis], rubella, cytomegalovirus, herpes)
- Endocrine disorders. (e.g., diabetes mellitus, hyperthyroidism, hypothyroidism)
- Hypertension
- Maternal phenylketonuria
- Hyperthermia (fever, hot tubs, or saunas), radiation, or toluene exposures

Maternal addictions (e.g., tobacco, alcohol, cocaine)

Drugs
- Thalidomide (Synovir, Thalomid)
- Lithium
- Isotretinoin (Accutane)
- Warfarin (Coumadin)
- Anticonvulsants, especially valproic acid (Depakote) and phenytoin (Dilantin)
- Angiotensin-converting enzyme inhibitors
- Antibiotics, such as streptomycin or tetracycline
- Antithyroid medications
- Chemotherapy agents

Procedures (e.g., chorionic villus sampling, dilatation and curettage, amniocentesis)

From Antenatal diagnosis of genetic disorders. ACOG Technical Bulletin, September 1987, No. 108; Gupta GK, Bianchi DW. DNA diagnosis for the practicing obstetrician. Obstet Gynecol Clin North Am 1997; 24:123–142; Online Mendelian inheritance in man. Home page. http://www.ncbi.nlm.nih.gov.Omin. Accessed March 18, 1999; Cohen LS, Friedman JM, Jefferson JW, et al. A reevaluation of risk of in utero exposure to lithium. JAMA 1994; 271:146–150 [published erratum appears in JAMA 1994; 271:1485].

TERATOGENS

Teratogens are environmental influences encountered before and during pregnancy that may induce birth defects.

Drugs, maternal conditions, and other influences that are known to be associated with adverse pregnancy outcomes are listed in Box 8-3.

If an agent is suspected of being teratogenic, the evidence for this suspicion must be carefully assessed. If malformations occur in a fetus, it must be determined whether the mother was exposed to the suspected agent during the embryonic, organogenesis stage, during which such malformations could be expected to develop. For example, exposure to a teratogenic agent during the third trimester cannot be the cause of a malformation, such as a neural tube defect, that can only be produced during the first trimester. Nonetheless, teratogens may still cause other problems after the first trimester (e.g., brain or tissue injury).

It must also be determined whether the rate of the observed malformation in women exposed to the agent exceeds the background rate for the malformation in the general population. Two and a half percent of all infants have a major congenital malformation. Other questions must also be answered: Is the malformation isolated, or is it part of a syndrome? If part of a syndrome, is it one known to be associated with another cause, such as chromosomal aneuploidy? Is an underlying disorder for which the mother is being treated responsible for the malformation, or is the treatment responsible?

Primary care providers should remember that there are risks and benefits of medication use during pregnancy that need to be weighted. While it is true that exposure to a compound, such as phenytoin (Dilantin), during pregnancy has been convincingly associated with congenital defects (growth retardation, a characteristic facial appearance, and fingernail hypoplasia), these effects are seen in only about 5% of exposed infants and are often mild. Therefore, is the low likelihood of malformations in an infant a sufficiently severe concern to justify stopping maternal use of an anticonvulsant that is working well? A hypoxic event associated with an episode of status epilepticus may represent a significantly greater hazard to the unborn child.

Lithium. Lithium use in pregnancy has been definitively associated with Ebstein's anomaly of the heart in infants.[18] The risk of this anomaly is 1 in 20,000 live births among the general population,[18] compared with 1 in 1000 births in women who use lithium. Women taking lithium typically suffer from bipolar disorder, and, if lithium is discontinued, they have at least a 50% chance of relapsing. Acute mania during pregnancy is a medical emergency that may necessitate the use of lithium, antipsychotic medication, and, possibly, electroconvulsive therapy; depression during pregnancy may result in poor self-care and suicide. The provider must carefully evaluate these issues in consultation with the parents before making a recommendation regarding whether to continue any medication.

▬ GENETICS AND CANCER

HEREDITARY BREAST AND OVARIAN CANCER

It is estimated that 5–10% of breast cancers in the U.S. are attributable to mutations of susceptible genes. Specifically, mutations of BRCA1 and BRCA2 appear to be responsible for the majority of hereditary breast cancers.[19]

Determining a need for cancer susceptibility genetic testing begins by taking a thorough family medical history that extends back at least three generations and encompasses aunts, uncles, and cousins. Translation of this information into a pedigree allows certain patterns of disease to be more readily recognized. The presence of cancer in a family pedigree may be characterized as sporadic, familial, or hereditary. Sporadic cancer occurs in only a few scattered cases. Familial cancer clusters in certain lines of a family and may reflect shared environmental or hereditary risks. Hereditary cancer occurs frequently in multiple generations of a family, typically following an autosomal dominant inheritance pattern.[20]

It is important to determine the type of cancer by objective means (charts, death certificates), as primary or metastatic cancers may be misidentified by the family.

Even an accurate and complete family pedigree may fail to show a hereditary pattern if there are few family members, or, as is often the case with breast or ovarian cancer, if there is a lack of females in any given generation. On the other hand, large families may appear to have familial or hereditary cancer simply because breast, prostate, lung, and colorectal cancers are relatively common in any group of individuals who survive to an older age. In general, most women who have a family history of breast cancer do not have a true hereditary breast cancer syndrome.

It is important for the family-focused health care provider to obtain both a paternal and a maternal genetic history, as a genetic mutation predisposing to breast or ovarian cancer is just as likely to be inherited from either father or mother.

A number of features should alert the primary provider to the possibility of hereditary cancer syndromes (Box 8-4).[21]

Box 8-4–ELEMENTS OF THE FAMILY MEDICAL HISTORY THAT SUGGEST A HEREDITARY CANCER SYNDROME

- Cancer in two or more first- or second-degree relatives
- Multiple cancers involving several successive generations
- Bilateral cancers in paired organs
- Multiple primary cancers in the same individual
- Onset of cancer at an atypically early age
- Constellation of rare cancers constituting a known hereditary cancer syndrome

From Burke W, Daly M, Garber J, et al. Recommendations for follow-up care of individuals with an inherited predisposition to cancer. II. BRCA1 and BRCA2. Cancer Genetics Studies Consortium. JAMA 1997;277:997–1003.

BRCA Analysis. BRCA1 was identified through a technique called linkage analysis.[22] The BRCA1 gene appears to act as a tumor suppressor, possibly by preventing errors from occurring during replication and recombination of DNA.[20] A family history characteristic of BRCA1 mutations may include an increased number of relatives with ovarian or breast cancer, early average age of onset of breast or ovarian cancer, or the presence of bilateral breast cancer. The incidence of this type of mutation is higher in Ashkenazic Jews.[23] Early onset of breast cancer in the absence of a family history of breast or ovarian cancer is associated with a low likelihood of BRCA1 mutation.[24] In families with three or more cases of breast or ovarian cancer, the prevalence of BRCA1 mutations may be around 16%.

If BRCA mutation testing is being considered, it is important to first test one or more family members affected by breast or ovarian cancer rather than the unaffected individuals. Subsequent testing of additional family members can then determine whether they also carry the same disease-causing mutation.

The same principles of occurrence and testing apply to the other known breast-cancer–susceptible gene, BRCA2. Lik BRCA1, BRCA2 follows an autosomal dominant pattern with variable expression. Male as well as female breast cancer appears to be associated with BRCA2. The relative risk of ovarian cancer associated with BRCA2, although higher than normal, appears to be less than that associated with BRCA1.[19]

In 1997, the Cancer Genetics Studies Consortium task force published recommendations for follow-up care for individuals with BRCA1 and BRCA2 mutations.[25] To date, no randomized controlled trials have demonstrated efficacy in reducing cancer by enhanced screening protocols in individuals with BRCA1 or BRCA2 mutations. This task force, based solely on expert opinion, recommended annual mammography, transvaginal ultrasonography (with color Doppler), and determination of CA-125 (tumor marker associated with ovarian cancers) levels annually or semiannually beginning at ages 25–35 in this high-risk population. Evidence is insufficient to recommend for or against prophylactic mastectomy or prophylactic oophorectomy. Nevertheless, one decision analysis calculated potential gains in life expectancy in women with BRCA1 or BRCA2 mutations of 2.9–5.3 years in women who undergo prophylactic mastectomy, and of 0.3–1.7 years in women who undergo prophylactic oophorectomy.[26] Therefore, a 1995 NIH consensus conference on ovarian cancer recommended that prophylactic oophorectomy after completion of childbearing or at age 35 should be offered to women with such a mutation who also have two or more first-degree relatives with ovarian cancer.[27] Unfortunately, disseminated peritoneal malignancy can occur despite oophorectomy because of the shared embryonic origin of both the ovaries and the peritoneum.[28]

Additional unanswered questions also remain regarding the use of oral contraceptives, estrogen replacement therapy, and chemoprophy-laxis in BRCA1 and BRCA2 mutation carriers. In the general popula-tion, oral contraceptive use appears to decrease ovarian cancer risk; whether this finding also applies to women with a BRCA mutation is unknown. A recent decision analysis regarding the value of postmeno-pausal estrogen replacement therapy suggested that life expectancy is likely to be increased in all women except those with two first-degree relatives with breast cancer and no risk factors for coronary heart disease or hip fracture.[29] However, the risk-benefit analysis for use of estrogen replacement therapy in women with a BRCA1 or BRCA2 mutation is still unknown.[25] Randomized trials involving the use of tamoxifen (Nolvadex) to prevent breast cancer in at-risk women ac-cording to BRCA mutation status are pending.[30, 31]

Genetic susceptibility testing carries with it enormous psychosocial and economic consequences. Individuals who test negative often expe-rience the expected relief from worry and anxiety about cancer, but they may also experience "survivor guilt." Individuals who test posi-tively may experience anxiety or depression and may also feel "trans-mitter guilt" for passing the mutation on to other family members.[32] Perhaps more worrisome is the finding that some women who perceive their risk for breast cancer to be high may be paradoxically less willing to follow cancer surveillance recommendations. Finally, testing can be quite costly.

HEREDITARY COLON CANCER

Colon cancer may occur in a sporadic, familial, or hereditary fash-ion. About 20% of colorectal cancer occurs in a familial but nonheredi-tary pattern.[33] An estimated 1–5% of colorectal cancer is caused by an autosomal dominant hereditary condition called hereditary nonpolypo-sis colorectal cancer (HNPCC). The other major hereditary colorectal cancer syndrome, familial adenomatous polyposis (FAP), is rarer. It manifests as hundreds of colonic polyps, with virtually a 100% proba-bility of developing colon cancer at a young age. An attenuated variant of FAP, which appears clinically similar to HNPCC but is associated with the same genetic mutation seen in FAP, has also been identified.[34]

Hereditary Nonpolyposis Colorectal Cancer (HNPCC). In some families with HNPCC, there appears to be a predisposition to colorectal cancer only. In others, there is an increased risk for colo-rectal cancer as well as a predisposition for the following extracolonic cancers: endometrial, ovarian, hepatobiliary, pancreatic, gastric, small intestinal, renal, pelvic, and ureteral (Lynch syndrome II). Compared with sporadic colon cancers, those associated with HNPCC occur at an earlier age (mean ages 45) and are predominantly seen in the right colon, proximal to the splenic flexure. In addition, there is an increased likelihood of the patient's developing multiple primary colorectal cancers, both synchronous (simultaneous) and metachronous (subsequent).

The Amsterdam criteria were developed to identify families that are likely to have HNPCC.[35] These criteria follow a "3–2–2–1" mnemonic:

1. At least three relatives are affected by colorectal cancer.
2. One affected person is a first-degree relative of the other two.
3. At least two successive generations are affected.
4. One affected person is diagnosed before age 50.

The criterion of having affected first-degree relatives of either gender in successive generations indicates an autosomal dominant pattern of inheritance, which is typical for most known hereditary cancer syndromes.

HNPCC is caused by mutations of genes involved in DNA mismatch repair. The function of these mismatch-repair genes is to correct errors that occur during normal DNA replication and to replace DNA damaged by mutagens. If these repair genes are themselves mutated and no longer function properly, the DNA becomes increasingly altered with each cell division. Eventually, genes that function as tumor suppressors are mutated and rendered nonfunctional, and tumors emerge.

Geneticists can now test the actual colorectal tumors themselves for replication errors that may occur when DNA repair mechanisms fail.[36] This process requires that patients undergo genetic counseling during a psychologically stressful time, following the initial diagnosis of colorectal cancer but before primary surgical treatment.

Because HNPCC is associated with a nearly 50% risk for metachronous colorectal cancer, many experts recommend that individuals with HNPCC undergo subtotal colectomy with ileorectal anastomosis rather than limited resection of their tumor.[37]

A task force organized by the National Human Genome Research Institute has developed recommendations for follow-up care of individuals with HNPCC.[38] This task force found that the efficacy of cancer surveillance, prophylactic surgery, and chemoprevention in individuals with HNPCC was unproved. However, based on multiple longitudinal series, with and without intervention, colonoscopy beginning at ages 20–25 and repeated every 1 to 3 years was recommended. Also based on expert opinion, annual transvaginal ultrasound or yearly endometrial aspiration beginning at ages 25–35 years was recommended. There is insufficient evidence to recommend for or against prophylactic hysterectomy, oophorectomy, or subtotal colectomy. Although sulindac (Clinoril) appears to reduce the incidence of adenoma formation in individuals with FAP, this agent has not been studied in individuals with HNPCC.[39] Likewise, the effects of aspirin or nutritional interventions, such as dietary fat reduction, are unknown in patients with HNPCC.

ALZHEIMER'S DISEASE

APOLIPOPROTEIN E

As with other common neuropsychiatric disorders such as schizophrenia and the affective disorders, Alzheimer's disease appears to be influenced by genetic as well as environmental factors, with complex interactions between the two. Despite the inherent difficulties of genetic study of a late-onset disorder, including survivor bias, a Norwegian twin study published in 1997 showed a concordance rate for Alzheimer's disease of 78% in monozygotic twins compared with 39% in dizygotic twins.[40]

A small number of families carry specific mutations responsible for early-onset Alzheimer's disease, which occurs before age 60. These rare mutations, involving the amyloid precursor protein or presenilin 1 or 2 genes, account for a small fraction of individuals with Alzheimer's disease.

Over 95% of Alzheimer's disease occurs after age 60 and is termed late-onset disease. The risk for developing this type of Alzheimer's disease appears to be in part associated with a gene for a lipid-carrying protein called apolipoprotein E. There are three major alleles of this gene, identified as apoE2, apoE3, and apoE4. About 30% of the U.S. population has at least one apoE4 allele, and 15% of the population carries at least one apoE2 allele. Individuals homozygous for apoE4 have a severe form of familial hypertriglyceridemia, which is associated with an increased risk for coronary heart disease. It appears that individuals with at least one apoE4 allele also have a higher risk for developing Alzheimer's disease, with an earlier age of onset, compared with individuals with at least one apoE2 or apoE3 allele. Individuals with apoE2 alleles appear to have the lowest risk for developing Alzheimer's disease.

Research has suggested the existence of an interaction between environmental factors and the apoE-associated risk for Alzheimer's disease. In general, head trauma has been identified as an environmental risk factor. It appears that individuals with the apoE4 allele who have sustained head trauma are at a fivefold greater risk for developing Alzheimer's disease, compared with individuals with the apoE4 allele but no trauma history.[41] Similarly, individuals with the apoE4 allele who underwent coronary artery bypass grafting demonstrated greater neuropsychological deficits 6 weeks postoperatively compared with patients with other apoE alleles.[42]

As with many other genetic tests, apoE testing may be easily misused and misinterpreted. At present, there is insufficient support for apoE testing of asymptomatic individuals.[43] Because individuals with two apoE4 alleles represent only 2% of the general population, and because they are subject to other causes of mortality, especially cardiovascular disease, the apoE test has a poor positive predictive value. Many persons with one apoE4 allele live to an old age without manifestation of Alzheimer's disease. Similarly, because 36% of patients with Alzheimer's disease in the U.S. carry no apoE4 alleles, the test has a poor negative predictive value. However, there may be a role for apoE testing in individuals already manifesting dementia to enhance the diagnostic accuracy for Alzheimer's disease. In general, when individuals with dementia who are followed in memory disorder clinics undergo autopsy, the diagnosis of Alzheimer's disease is supported by neuropathologic findings about 85% of the time. However, in individuals with a diagnosis of probable Alzheimer's disease and positive apoE4 testing, nearly 100% have later been found to have Alzheimer's disease confirmed by neuropathology.[42] Better diagnostic accuracy for Alzheimer's disease may assist patients and their families in planning for the future and may aid in testing potential therapies to enhance function or slow progression of the disease.

▬ CONCLUSION

With the completion of the Human Genome Project and the sequencing of the entire complement of human DNA, the practice of medicine is on the verge of changing dramatically. Although scientists' current ability to understand the functional implications of variations in the human genetic makeup is limited and attempts at gene therapy are to date only rudimentary, a solid foundation has been laid for dramatic advances in diagnosis and treatment. The ethical, legal, and social implications of genetics are broad and controversial. Because of the complex interplay among genetics, environment, and personal lifestyle, the family health care provider will no doubt remain an important source of information, motivation, and treatment. This chapter offers a brief introduction to this rapidly advancing field. In the not-too-distant future, it will become imperative for family-centered health care providers, with the aid of appropriate information systems, to know how to obtain and interpret a family pedigree and when to refer patients and their families for genetics services.

REFERENCES

1. Collins FS. Preparing health professionals for the genetic revolution [editorial]. JAMA 1997;278:1285–1286.
2. Anderson WT. Evolution Isn't What It Used to Be: The Augmented Animal and the Whole Wired World. New York, W.H. Freeman, 1996.
3. Milunsky JM, Milunsky A. Genetic counseling in perinatal medicine. Obstet Gynecol Clin North Am 1997;24:1–17.
4. Witte DL, Crosby WH, Edwards CQ, et al. Practice guideline development task force of the College of American Pathologists. Hereditary hemochromatosis. Clin Chim Acta 1996;245:139–200.

5. Ross HL, Elias S. Maternal serum screening for fetal genetic disorders. Obstet Gynecol Clin North Am 1997;24:33–47.

6. Kovacs EW, Shabbabrami B, Medearis AL, et al. Prenatal determinations of paternity by molecular genetic "fingerprinting." Obstet Gynecol 1990;75:474–479.

7. Hammond HA, Redman JB, Caskey CT. In utero paternity testing following alleged sexual assault. A comparison of DNA-based methods. JAMA 1995;273:1774–1777.

8. Dick PT. Periodic health examination, 1996 update: 1. Prenatal screening for and diagnosis of Down syndrome. Canadian Task Force on the Periodic Health Examination. CMAJ 1996;154:465–479.

9. Antenatal diagnosis of genetic disorders. ACOG Technical Bulletin, September 1987, No. 108.

10. ACOG issues educational bulletin on maternal serum screening. Am Fam Physician 1997;55:1454.

11. Pauker SP, Pauker SG. Prenatal diagnosis—Why is 35 a magic number? [editorial]. N Engl J Med 1994; 330(16):1151–1152 [published erratum appears in N Engl J Med 1994;331:415].

12. Palomaki GE, Haddow JE, Knight GJ, et al. Risk-based prenatal screening for trisomy 18 using alpha-fetoprotein, unconjugated oestriol and human chorionic gonadotropin. Prenat Diagn 1995;15:713–723.

13. Beaudet AL. Prenatal screening including cystic fibrosis. Presentation given at the American Medical Association Conference, "Genetic Medicine and the Practicing Physician"; New Orleans, March 13–15, 1998.

14. Gupta GK, Bianchi DW. DNA diagnosis for the practicing obstetrician. Obstet Gynecol Clin North Am 1997;24:123–142.

15. Bernhardt BA, Chase GA, Faden RR, et al. Educating patients about cystic fibrosis carrier screening in a primary care setting. Arch Fam Med 1996;5:336–340.

16. Genetic testing for cystic fibrosis. NIH Consens Statement 1997;15:1–37.

17. Online Mendelian inheritance in man. Home page. http://www.ncbi.nlm.nih.gov.Omim. Accessed March 18, 1999.

18. Cohen LS, Friedman JM, Jefferson JW, et al. A reevaluation of risk of in utero exposure to lithium. JAMA 1994;271:146–150 [published erratum appears in JAMA 1994;271(19):1485].

19. Greene MH. Genetics of breast cancer. Mayo Clin Proc 1997;72:54–65.

20. Brody LC, Biesecker EB. Breast cancer: The high-risk mutations. Hosp Pract (Off Ed) 1997;32:59–63, 67–68, 70–72.

21. "Doctor, do I need genetic testing?" In Gould RL. Cancer and Genetics: Answering Your Patients' Questions, A Manual for Clinicians and Their Patients. Huntington, NY, PRR, Inc., and the American Cancer Society, 1997; pp.55–76.

22. Rennert OM. Clinical Genetics. Monograph, Edition No. 168, Home Study Self-Assessment Program. Kansas City, MO: American Academy of Family Physicians, May 1993.

23. Couch FJ, Hartmann LC. BRCA1 testing—Advances and retreats [editorial]. JAMA 1998;279:955–957.

24. Newman B, Mu H, Butler LM, et al. Frequency of breast cancer attributable to BRCAI in a population-based series of American women. JAMA 1998;279:915–921.

25. Burke W, Daly M, Garber J, et al. Recommendations for follow-up care of

individuals with an inherited predisposition to cancer. II. BRCA1 and BRCA2. Cancer Genetics Studies Consortium. JAMA 1997;277:997–1003.

26. Schrag D, Kuntz KM, Garber JE, et al. Decision analysis—Effects of prophylactic mastectomy and oophorectomy on life expectancy among women with BRCA1 or BRCA2 mutations. N Engl J Med 1997;336:1465–1471 [published erratum appears in N Engl J Med 1997;337:434].

27. NIH consensus conference. Ovarian cancer. Screening, treatment, and follow-up. NIH Consensus Development Panel on Ovarian Cancer. JAMA 1995;273:491–497.

28. Tobaeman JK, Greene MH, Tucker MA, et al. Intra-abdominal carcinomatosis after prophylactic oophorectomy in ovarian-cancer-prone families. Lancet 1982;2:795–797.

29. Col NF, Eckman MH, Karas RH, et al. Patient-specific decisions about hormone replacement therapy in postmenopausal women. JAMA 1997;277:1140–1147.

30. O'Shaughnessy JA. Chemoprevention of breast cancer. JAMA 1996;275:1349–1353.

31. Powles TJ. Status of antiestrogen breast cancer prevention trials. Oncology (Huntingt) 1998;12:28–31.

32. MacDonald DJ. Ethical, legal, and social issues related to predisposition testing for breast cancer risk: What nurses need to know. Quality of Life—A Nursing Challenge 1997;6:8–14.

33. Marra G, Boland CR. Hereditary nonpolyposis colorectal cancer: The syndrome, the genes, and historical perspectives. J Natl Cancer Inst 1995;87:1114–1125.

34. Lynch J. The genetics and natural history of hereditary colon cancer. Semin Oncol Nurs 1997;13:91–98.

35. Vasen HF, Mecklin JP, Khan PM, Lynch HT. The International Collaborative Group on Hereditary Non-polyposis Colorectal Cancer. Dis Colon Rectum 1991;34:424–425.

36. Rodriguez-Bigas MA, Boland CR, Hamilton SR, et al. A National Cancer Institute workshop on hereditary nonpolyposis colorectal cancer syndrome: Meeting highlights and Bethesda guidelines. J Natl Cancer Inst 1997;89:1758–1762.

37. Offit K. Clinical cancer genetics: Risk counseling and management. New York, Wylie-Liss, 1998; pp. 125–149.

38. Burke W, Petersen G, Lynch P, et al. Recommendations for follow-up care of individuals with an inherited predisposition to cancer. I. Hereditary nonpolyposis colon cancer. Cancer Genetics Studies Consortium. JAMA 1997;277:915–919.

39. Giardiello FM, Hamilton SR, Krush AJ, et al. Treatment of colonic and rectal adenomas with sulindac in familial adenomatous polyposis. N Engl J Med 1993;328:1313–1316.

40. Bergem AL, Engedal K, Kringlen E. The role of heredity in late-onset Alzheimer disease and vascular dementia. A twin study. Arch Gen Psychiatry 1997;54:264–270.

41. Mayeux K, Ottman R, Maestre G, et al. Synergistic effects of traumatic head injury and apolipoprotein-epsilon 4 in patients with Alzheimer's disease. Neurology 1995;45:555–557.

42. Roses AD. Alzheimer's disease: The genetics of risk. Hosp Pract (Off Ed) 1997;32:51–55, 58–63, 67–69.

43. Post SG, Whitehouse PJ, Binstock RH, et al. The clinical introduction of genetic testing for Alzheimer disease. An ethical perspective. JAMA 1997;277:832–836.

RESOURCES

Brody LC, Biesecker BB. Breast cancer: The high-risk mutations. Hosp Pract (Off Ed) 1997;32:59–63, 67–68, 70–72.

Couch FJ, Hartmann LC. BRCA testing—advances and Retreats [editorial]. JAMA 1998,279:955–957.

Genetic testing for cystic fibrosis. NIH Consens Statement 1997;15:1–37. Also available at http://odp.od.nih.gov/consensus/cons/106/106_statement.htm.

Gould RL. Cancer and Genetics: Answering Your Patients' Questions, A Manual for Clinicians and Their Patients. Huntington, NY, PRR, Inc., and the American Cancer Society, 1997.

Rosenthal TC, Puck SM. Screening for genetic risk of breast cancer. Am Fam Physician 1999,59:99–106.

Roses AD. Alzheimer's disease: The genetics of risk. Hosp Pract (Off Ed) 1997;32:51–55, 58–63, 67–69.

Ross HL, Elias S. Maternal serum screening for fetal genetic disorders. Obstet Gynecol Clin North Am 1997;24:33–47.

Saenz RB. Primary care of infants and young children with Down syndrome. Am Fam Physician 1999;59:381–396.

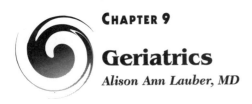

CHAPTER 9

Geriatrics

Alison Ann Lauber, MD

INTRODUCTION

The new millennium is both golden and graying. While the number of Americans over the age of 65 has increased from 3 million in 1900 to 34 million in 1995, this elder group is expected to more than double by 2030. Perhaps more significant is that older Americans composed a mere 4% of the United States population in 1900, but they will represent approximately 22% of the population once the last baby boomer turns 65 in the year 2029. Health care promotion and planning and disease prevention issues targeting the older American will become increasingly demanding in the first 30 years of the 21st century. By 2030, one in five Americans will be receiving Social Security (SS) and Medicare benefits, while those same programs will be supported by the taxes of a much smaller work force.[1, 2]

Even as America is aging, it is also becoming increasingly difficult to define what it means to be older. New membership in the American Association of Retired Persons (AARP) requires an adult to be a mere 50 years old, Medicare uses an age of 65, and the World Health Organization defines a person as older beginning at his or her 75th birthday. If the proportion of the U.S. population over age 65 will double over the next 30 years, more worrisome is the fact that the population over age 85 will triple in that period. Terms such as "frail elderly" and "oldest-old" pepper literature and political debates, but few universal age-limited recommendations have been provided to guide daily health care decisions. The average primary care provider spends little time on health promotion because of lack of reimbursement and/or lack of training. As standards and guidelines for health care become less certain with a patient's advancing age and accumulation of confounding chronic diseases, adherence to health-promoting strategies may grow less and less. Chronic diseases such as arthritis, cardiovascular conditions, diabetes, and diminished special senses increase in prevalence with advancing age. Many elders have more than one chronic condition. Functional status also declines with age. By age 65, 13–18% of Americans have developed difficulties with personal care functions or in performing activities of daily living or instrumental activities of daily living (ADLs and IADLs). Whereas an estimated 9% of the population under age 70 needs assistance in performing personal care, the population needing assistance rises to 50% of the 85 + age group. Younger adults are hospitalized one third as often as the elderly and stay in the hospital only half as long. Almost 50% of all hospital days of care each year are attributed to the elderly, who currently compose somewhat less than 15% of the general population.

Resources are strained by rising costs of prescriptions and personal care assistance that are not commonly covered by Medicare and some supplemental insurance products. Approximately one fifth of the older population lives at or near the poverty level. For this group, paying for medical care is frequently a poor third to paying for food and shelter. Poverty rates are twice as high for older women than for older men and three times higher for ethnic minorities when compared with older whites.[1, 2]

Currently there are *no data* to support several widely held beliefs about health promotion and disease prevention among the elderly:

* Health promotion and disease prevention are cost-effective.
* Community-based long-term care is less expensive than nursing home care.
* All patients should have equal access to high-technology care, regardless of chronological age.

Despite the lack of evidence, these beliefs are widely held and seem to be empirically correct. "Successful aging" is defined by many as being able to live a fulfilling and active life until death. Some would argue that common problems such as Alzheimer's disease and arthritis do not have recognized risk factors that can be modified by lifestyle changes, while high-technology "expensive" care can only prolong life and cannot prevent disease. Instead, an argument can be made for continued and enthusiastic efforts at reducing tobacco abuse, sedentary mental and physical lifestyles, obesity, high cholesterol, and blood pressure. In this way, the prevalence of disease at any age may be reduced, and both the quality and the quantity of life might be extended in tandem, until a natural death occurs.

With all patients but especially with the elderly, health care providers must have a broader concept of health, including

* Encouraging feelings of empowerment
* Fostering positive, supportive, and loving relationships
* Facilitating a sense of meaning and joy in life
* Maximizing independence
* Avoiding focusing on disease as defining "lack of health"
* Strengthening social supports

SCREENING AND HEALTH ASSESSMENTS

Ideally, to prevent or minimize the disabilities and diseases associated with aging, prevention efforts should start earlier in life. The U.S. Preventive Services Task Force (USPSTF) has developed qualifications for evaluating suggested preventive strategies. These USPSTF criteria are largely based on the degree of certainty that any given recommendation is an evidence-based, cost-effective intervention, rather than a simple measure of benefit that might be realized if the recommendation were to be followed.

The annual complete physical examination has been increasingly devalued in favor of more age-targeted interventions, including counseling, screening, and prophylaxis (Table 9–1). However, many older persons have numerous conditions and/or disabilities that will require a minimum of an annual checkup. The domain of the comprehensive, multidimensional geriatric assessment does not have to remain the sole province of a multidisciplinary team. Instead, there is support demonstrating that a single health care provider using a systematic format can arrive at similar recommendations. Practically speaking, there is little economic support for team assessments; however, the use of simple questionnaires and instruments can improve the primary care provider's recognition of significant opportunities and barriers unique to the care of the individual older patient. The multidimensional assessment can include, but need not be restricted to, the following:

* Traditional history (including a complete review of symptoms common in elders) and physical examination
* Assessment of mental status, dementia, and/or depression (Boxes 9–1 and 9–2)
* Functional and Instrumental ADL questionnaires (Boxes 9–3 and 9–4)

Text continued on page 198

Box 9-1–FOLSTEIN MINI-MENTAL STATUS EXAM[5]

Add points for each correct response.

	Score	Points
Orientation		
1. What is the:		
Year?	————	1
Season?	————	1
Date?	————	1
Day?	————	1
Month?	————	1
2. Where are we?		
State?	————	1
County?	————	1
Town or city?	————	1
Hospital?	————	1
Floor?	————	1

Registration
3. Name three objects, taking 1 second
   to say each. Then ask the patient to
   repeat all three after you have said
   them. Give one point for each correct answer. Repeat the answers until
   patient learns all three.   _____ 3

Attention and Calculation
4. Serial sevens. Give one point for each
   correct answer. Stop after five answers. (Alternate test: Spell WORLD
   backwards.)   _____ 5

Recall
5. Ask for names of three objects
   learned in question 3. Give one point
   for each correct answer.   _____ 3

Language
6. Point to a pencil and a watch. Have
   the patient name the object as you
   point to it.   _____ 2

7. Have the patient repeat, "No ifs,
   ands, or buts."   _____ 1

8. Have the patient follow a three-stage
   command: "Take a paper in your
   right hand. Fold the paper in half.
   Put the paper on the floor."   _____ 3

9. Have the patient read and obey the
   following: "CLOSE YOUR EYES."
   (Print it in large letters.)   _____ 1

10. Have the patient write a sentence of
    his or her choice. (The sentence
    should contain a subject and an ob-
    ject and should make sense. Ignore
    spelling errors when scoring.)   _____ 1

11. Have the patient copy the design.
    (Give one point if all sides and
    angles are preserved and if the inter-
    secting sides form a quadrangle.)   _____ 1

                              *_____ = Total

*Scoring: Normal elderly score a mean of 27.6 points (maximum
30 points). Commonly a cut-off score of 23 is used to
differentiate the normal from the impaired; however, allowances
should be made for a history of retardation, limited education,
and/or a history of superior intellect or educational
achievement.

From Folstein MF, Folstein S, McHugh PR. Mini-Mental State—A practical
method for grading the cognitive state of patients for the clinician. J Psych Res
1975;12:189–198, with permission.

Table 9–1. Summary of Preventive Screening, Counseling, and Prophylaxis Recommendations for Older Adults (age 65+)[3, 4]

Screening	Counseling	Prophylaxis
Blood pressure, height, weight annually	Diet	Tetanus-diphtheria booster every 10 years
Breast examination annually	Exercise	Pneumococcal vaccine at least once
Mammogram annually*	Safe sex§	Annual influenza vaccine
Pap smear every 1–3 years†	Avoid drinking and driving	Aspirin
Bimanual pelvic examination once a year	Lap/shoulder seat belts	Discuss hormone replacement therapy with women
Rectal/prostate exam once a year	Motorcycle, bike helmets	Calcium w/ vitamin D
Fecal occult blood test once a year	Fall prevention	? Vitamin E
Test/inquire about hearing impairment periodically	Hot water heater set to <120–135°F	? Multivitamin and mineral (antioxidants) supplement
Vision periodically‡	Smoke/carbon monoxide detectors	? Vitamin B$_{12}$
Fasting blood sugar, cholesterol, thyroid-stimulating hormone: prn	Safe storage of firearms	? Ginkgo biloba
Sigmoidoscopy every 3–5 years	CPR training for caregivers	? St. John's wort
Assess for alcohol problems	Regular dental care	? Saw palmetto
Assess for tobacco use	Avoid excess/midday sun	
Home safety assessment		
Mental status examination and/or depression inventory prn		
Bone densitometry NR/prn		
Chest x-ray, electrocardiogram: NR/prn		

NR=not recommended; prn = at provider's discretion or diagnostically; ? = no official recommendations exist, but initial literature seems to support use in special populations.

*After age 69, continue in willing/appropriate patients only.

†All women who have been sexually active and still have a cervix: Every 1–3 years. Consider discontinuation of testing after age 65, if previous regular screening documented consistently normal results.

‡Various recommendations exist, best done by eye care specialist. Based on maximizing quality of life, author recommends every one to two years. High-risk patients may require retinal screening more frequently.

§If patient is sexually active and not monogamous, consider hepatitis B and A vaccines.

Sources: Goldberg TH, Chavin SI. Preventive medicine and screening in older adults. J Am Geriatr Soc 1997; 45:344–354; Haber D. Health Promotion and Aging. New York, Springer Publishing Co., 1999.

194

Box 9-2–Yesavage-Brink Geriatric Depression Scale[6]

1. Are you basically satisfied with your life? (no)
2. Have you dropped many of your activities and interests? (yes)
3. Do you feel that your life is empty? (yes)
4. Do you often get bored? (yes)
5. Are you hopeful about the future? (no)
6. Are you bothered by thoughts that you just cannot get out of your head? (yes)
7. Are you in good spirits most of the time? (no)
8. Are you afraid that something bad is going to happen to you? (yes)
9. Do you feel happy most of the time? (no)
10. Do you often feel helpless? (yes)
11. Do you often get restless and fidgety? (yes)
12. Do you prefer to stay home at night, rather than go out and do new things? (yes)
13. Do you frequently worry about the future? (yes)
14. Do you feel that you have more problems with memory than most? (yes)
15. Do you think it is wonderful to be alive now? (no)
16. Do you often feel downhearted and blue? (yes)
17. Do you feel pretty worthless the way you are now? (yes)
18. Do you worry a lot about the past? (yes)
19. Do you find life very exciting? (no)
20. Is it hard for you to get started on new projects? (yes)
21. Do you feel full of energy? (no)
22. Do you feel that your situation is hopeless? (yes)
23. Do you think that most persons are better off than you are? (yes)
24. Do you frequently get upset over little things? (yes)
25. Do you frequently feel like crying? (yes)
26. Do you have trouble concentrating? (yes)
27. Do you enjoy getting up in the morning? (no)
28. Do you prefer to avoid social gatherings? (yes)
29. Is it easy for you to make decisions? (no)
30. Is your mind as clear as it used to be? (no)

Score one point for each response that matches the yes or no answer after the question. A score of 8 or more points is 90% sensitive and 80% specific. A score of 11 or more raises the specificity to 95%, but lowers sensitivity to 84%.

From Yesavage JA, Brink TL. Development and validation of geriatric depression screening: A preliminary report. J Psych Res 1983;17:41, with permission from Elsevier Science.

Box 9-3–FUNCTIONAL ACTIVITIES OF DAILY LIVING (ADL) ASSESSMENT: KATZ INDEX[6]

1. *Dressing:*
   - I: Gets clothes and gets completely dressed without assistance
   - A: Gets clothes and gets dressed without assistance except in tying shoes
   - D: Receives assistance in getting clothes or in getting dressed or stays partly or completely undressed

2. *Bathing (sponge, shower, or tub):*
   - I: Receives no assistance (gets in and out of tub if tub is the usual means of bathing)
   - A: Receives assistance in bathing only one part of the body (such as the back or a leg)
   - D: Receives assistance in bathing more than one part of the body (or not bathed)

3. *Feeding:*
   - I: Feeds self without assistance
   - A: Feeds self except for getting assistance in cutting meat or buttering bread
   - D: Receives assistance in feeding or is fed partly or completely by using tubes or intravenous fluids

4. *Continence:*
   - I: Controls urination and bowel movement completely by self
   - A: Has occasional "accidents"
   - D: Supervision helps keep urine or bowel control; catheter is used, or is incontinent

5. *Toileting:*
   - I: Goes to "toilet room," cleans self, and arranges clothes without assistance (may use object for support such as cane, walker, or wheelchair and may manage night bedpan or commode, emptying it in the morning)
   - A: Moves in and out of bed or chair with assistance
   - D: Doesn't go to room termed "toilet" for the elimination process

6. *Transfer:*
   - I: Moves in and out of bed as well as in and out of chair without assistance (may be using object for support such as cane or walker)
   - A: Moves in and out of bed or chair with assistance
   - D: Doesn't get out of bed

   General Rule:
   - I = Independently
   - A = Requires some Assistance
   - D = Dependent

From Katz index of daily living. JAMA 1963;185:915, in Gallo JJ, Reichel W, Andersen L. Handbook of Geriatric Assessment. Rockville, MD, Aspen Publishers, 1999, with permission.

Box 9-4–FILLENBAUM INSTRUMENTAL ADL ASSESSMENT[6]

1. Can you get to places out of walking distance:
   1 Without help (can travel alone on bus, taxi, or drive your own car)
   0 With some help (need someone to help you or go with you when traveling) or are you unable to travel unless emergency arrangements are made for a specialized vehicle such as an ambulance?
   — Not answered

2. Can you go shopping for groceries or clothes (assuming you have transportation):
   1 Without help (taking care of all your shopping needs yourself, assuming you have transportation)
   0 With some help (need someone to go with you on all shopping trips), or are you completely unable to do any shopping?
   — Not answered

3. Can you prepare your own meals:
   1 Without help (plan and cook meals yourself)
   0 With some help (can prepare some things but unable to cook full meals yourself), or are you completely unable to prepare any meals?
   — Not answered

4. Can you do your housework:
   1 Without help (can scrub floors, etc.)
   0 With some help (can do light housework but need help with heavy work), or are you unable to do any housework?
   — Not answered

5. Can you handle your own money:
   1 Without help (write checks, pay bills, etc.)
   0 With some help (manage day-to-day buying but need help with managing your checkbook and paying your bills), or are you completely unable to handle money?
   — Not answered

General Rule: Items in these categories get progressively more difficult; therefore, if patients are still able to manage their finances, they usually are having no significant problems with the previous categories. This can be of special use to follow a patient for change over time.

* Social support, economic, caregiver, and abuse evaluations (Boxes 9–5 and 9–6, and Table 9–2)
* Patient values history regarding chronic care and end-of-life preferences (Box 9–7)
* Laboratory tests (Table 9–3)
* Paper Bag or Shoebox test (Box 9–8)

Text continued on page 204

Box 9-5–SOCIAL RESOURCES SECTION OF DUKE'S OLDER AMERICANS RESOURCES AND SERVICES (OARS) MULTIDIMENSIONAL FUNCTIONAL ASSESSMENT QUESTIONNAIRE[6]

1. Are you single, married, widowed, divorced, or separated?
2. Who lives with you?
3. How many persons do you know well enough to visit with in their homes?
4. About how many times did you talk to someone—friends, relatives, or others—on the telephone in the past week (either you called them or they called you)?
5. How many times, during the past week, did you spend some time with someone who does not live with you? That is, you went to see them or they came to visit you, or you went out to do things together?
6. Do you have someone you can trust and confide in?
7. Do you find yourself feeling lonely quite often, sometimes, or almost never?
8. Do you see your relatives and friends as often as you want to, or are you somewhat unhappy about how little you see them?
9. Is there someone who would give you any help at all if you were sick or disabled, for example your husband/wife, a member of your family, or a friend?
   If "yes," answer a and b:
   a. Is there someone who would take care of you
      • as long as needed
      • only for a short time
      • only now and then (for example taking you to appointment or fixing lunch occasionally)?
   b. Who is this person? (Obtain the name and relationship of this person.*)

*Interestingly, in a study using this instrument, 23% refused to allow the investigator to contact this "contact person."

From Palmore E (ed). Multidimensional Functional Assessment Questionnaire and OARS Social Resources Questionnaire. *In* Normal Aging II: Reports from the Duke Longitudinal Studies, 1970–73. Duke University Press, 1974. All rights reserved. Reprinted by permission of Duke University Press.

Box 9-6–GERONTOLOGICAL SOCIETY OF AMERICA'S CAREGIVER STRAIN INDEX[6]

Instructions given to the caregiver: "I am going to read a list of what other persons have found to be difficult in helping out after somebody comes home from the hospital. Would you tell me whether any of these apply to you? (Give the examples)"

1. Sleep is disturbed (e.g., because _____ is in and out of bed or wanders around at night).
2. It is inconvenient (e.g., because helping takes so much time or it's a long drive over to help).
3. It is a physical strain (e.g., because of lifting in and out of a chair; effort or concentration is required).
4. It is confining (e.g., helping restricts free time or cannot go visiting).
5. There have been family adjustments (e.g., because helping has disrupted routine; there has been no privacy).
6. There have been changes in personal plans (e.g., had to turn down a job; could not go on vacation).
7. There have been other demands on my time (e.g., from other family members).
8. There have been emotional adjustments (e.g., because of severe arguments).
9. Some behavior is upsetting (e.g., because of incontinence; _____ has trouble remembering things; or _____ accuses others of taking things).
10. It is upsetting to find _____ has changed so much from his/her former self (e.g., he/she is different from the person that he/she used to be).
11. There have been work adjustments (e.g., because of having to take time off).
12. It is a financial strain.
13. Feeling completely overwhelmed (e.g., because of worry about _____; concerns about how you will manage).

Scoring (total "yes" responses): The higher the number of points, the more perceived burden or strain on the caregiver is acknowledged, which increases the risk of neglect or abuse. Remember that the competent elder may refuse help. If elder abuse is suspected, the euphemism, *unmet needs*, is less emotionally sensitive and is received by both patient and caregiver better. (Required reporting of suspicions varies by state.)

From Caregiver strain index. J Gerontol 1983;38:345, in Gallo JJ, Reichel W, Andersen L. Handbook of Geriatric Assessment. Rockville, MD, Aspen Publishers, 1999, with permission.

Table 9-2. Elder Abuse Risk Assessment[7]

Situations at Risk	Visible Signs	Abuse Without Physical Signs
Increasing care needs or financial burdens	Bruises and lacerations	Threats
Family history of abuse	Burns	Verbal harassment
Caregiver with history of violent behaviors	Sprains, fractures, and dislocations	Intimidation
Caregiver burnout	Pressure sores	Unreasonable confinement
Alcohol or drug abuse in patient or household	Over- or undermedication or sedation	Financial mismanagement
Sudden increase in caregiver's personal stress	Dehydration and/or malnutrition	Sexual abuse
Depression in patient or caregiver	Poor hygiene	

From Hoffer EP: Emergency Problems in the Elderly. Oradell, NJ, Medical Economics Books, 1985, pp 235–236, with permission.

Box 9-7–Aging With Dignity's "Five Wishes" Document[8]

"Five Wishes" is a combination workbook, communication tool, and advanced directive instrument developed as a project supported by a grant from the Robert Wood Johnson Foundation. More than one million American families are using "Five Wishes," and nearly 2000 organizations are distributing the form. To order a copy of "Five Wishes," call 1-888-5-WISHES, or write to Aging with Dignity, PO Box 1661, Tallahassee, FL 32302. Copies of "Five Wishes" are $5 each, or $1 per copy for orders of 25 or more. For more information, visit www.agingwithdignity.org. Providers must order copies or request permission to reprint. It constitutes a person's wishes for:

1. The person I want to make decisions for me when I can't
2. The kind of medical treatment I want or don't want
3. How comfortable I want to be
4. How I want people to treat me
5. What I want my loved ones to know

Box 9-8–Paper Bag or Shoebox Test

- Ask patient and caregiver(s) to go throughout the house gathering together all prescription medications, over-the-counter medications, herbal or dietary supplements, and home remedies.
- Remind them to include expired or duplicate bottles, topical preparations, and inhalers. Usually these items come to you in a paper or plastic bag or, more distressingly, a shoebox.
- Review all the contents; ask permission to discard those you do not want them to use.
- Rewrite prescriptions and/or label all containers so that accuracy is assured.
- Give patient and caregiver(s) a list of approved "medications" and supplements, and ask them to call before adding to the list. Provide them with your business card, with instructions to notify you if another provider prescribes a new medication or changes doses of an existing medication so that you can keep current.
- Ask for phone number of their pharmacy and underline the importance of using the same one all the time. Explain about drug interactions.
- Ask if enlarged font labeling or easy-open caps would be of assistance.

Table 9-3. Laboratory Tests to Consider When Evaluating the Elder Patient[9]

Laboratory Parameters Unchanged[a]

Blood urea nitrogen
Calcium
Complete blood count (including platelet count and differential white blood cell count)
Electrolytes (sodium, potassium, chloride, bicarbonate)
Liver function tests (transaminases, bilirubin, prothrombin time)
Phosphorus
Thyroid-stimulating hormone, free thyroxine index

Common Abnormal Laboratory Parameters†

Parameter	Clinical Significance
Albumin	Average values decline (<0.5 g/mL) with age, especially in the hospitalized elderly, but generally indicate undernutrition.
Alkaline phosphatase	Mild elevations are common in asymptomatic elderly; liver and Paget's disease should be considered if moderately elevated.
Creatinine	Because lean body mass and daily endogenous creatinine production decline, high-normal and minimally elevated values may indicate substantially reduced renal function.

Chest x-ray	Interstitial changes are a common age-related finding; diffusely diminished bone density generally indicates advanced osteoporosis.
Electrocardiogram	ST-segment and T-wave changes, atrial and ventricular arrhythmias, and various blocks are common in the asymptomatic elderly and may not need specific evaluation or treatment.
Erythrocyte sedimentation rate	Mild elevations (10–20 mm) may be an age-related change.
Glucose	Glucose tolerance decreases. Elevated fasting blood sugar must be used to diagnose diabetes because >50% of elders will have an abnormal glucose tolerance test.
Prostate-specific antigen	May be elevated in patients with benign prostatic hyperplasia. Marked elevation or increasing values when followed over time should prompt consideration of further evaluation in patients for whom specific therapy for prostate cancer is warranted.
Total iron-binding capacity	Decreased values are not an aging change and usually indicate undernutrition and/or gastrointestinal blood loss.
Urinalysis	Asymptomatic pyuria and bacteriuria are common and rarely warrant treatment; hematuria is abnormal and needs further evaluation.

*Aging changes do not occur in these parameters; abnormal values should prompt further evaluation.
†Includes normal aging and other age-related changes.
From Kane R, Ouslander JG, Abrass IB. Essentials of Clinical Geriatrics, 4th ed. New York, McGraw-Hill, Inc., 1999, pp 57–58, with permission of McGraw-Hill, Inc.

Despite the preceding list of additional evaluation instruments available to the health care provider, it is important to realize the economic or physical impracticality of pursuing all of these evaluations within one encounter with the patient. Even the classic history and physical is best broken down into two separate encounters, while questionnaires and other instruments may frequently be administered during nonphysician provider visits in conjunction with laboratory appointments, immunizations, or counseling sessions. While the axiom of geriatric pharmacology may be, "Start low and go slow," the same advice should also be applied to geriatric assessment. Trying to do too much in a single encounter may impress the patient and/or caregiver as convenient, but it is frequently exhausting and nonproductive for both the patient and the health care provider. Although a series of office visits may seem superficially self-serving, taking a more measured approach over time can in fact be more economical and productive.

■■■INTERVENTIONS

Once the patient's initial assessment has been completed, an action plan can be developed to include expanded assessment tools, indicated counseling, screenings, prophylaxis, and specific problem-based interventions. Common issues or problems requiring treatment, modifications, or specific intervention include

* Nutrition and herbal, vitamin, or dietary supplements
* Exercise, independence, and mobility
* Concerns about Alzheimer's disease, "senility," or decision-making capacities
* Falls and fear of falling
* Sensory deficits and swallowing disorders
* Incontinence and urinary retention
* Chronic diseases (e.g., arthritis, diabetes, chronic obstructive pulmonary disease, cardiovascular disease, high blood pressure, congestive heart failure, depression, osteoporosis, and fractures)
* Polypharmacy and/or iatrogenesis
* Assisted living and long-term care
* Quality of life and end-of-life concerns

While the scope of this chapter only permits a general discussion of these topics, references and resources are provided to supplement the health care provider's understanding and patient education efforts.

NUTRITION AND HERBAL, VITAMIN, OR DIETARY SUPPLEMENTS[4, 9, 10]

As we age, our metabolism slows generally, and our fat metabolism processes slow by approximately 30%. At the same time, chronic diseases and conditions such as arthritis impose limitations on mobility and exercise. As a result, people generally gain weight as they age. Although there is evidence that persons over age 70 tend to lose weight, the loss is usually attributable to loss of muscle mass, not loss of fat. Weight management, nutrition, and exercise form the cornerstone of health promotion and disease prevention in any age group (see also Chapter 13, Nutrition Education in the Clinical Setting). General counseling should stress limiting fat and cholesterol in the diet and emphasize the importance of including whole grains, fruits, and vegetables (fiber) along with maintaining caloric balance.

Dietary supplements became increasingly popular throughout the 1990s, becoming a big business that even traditional pharmaceutical manufacturers began to enter in the latter part of the decade. Despite popular enthusiasm, the U.S. Food and Drug Administration (FDA) has reported thousands of side effects and drug interactions (including nearly 100 deaths) associated with dietary supplement use. Before 1994, nutritional supplements were regulated and tested for premarket safety in much the same way foods and drugs were evaluated. However, in 1994 the U.S. Congress passed the Dietary Supplement Health and Education Act. This law eliminated premarket safety testing and permits the FDA to intervene only after consumer complaints, and then only if serious harm can be proved. The legislation also allows advertisers of dietary supplements to make unsubstantiated claims for their products as long as they specifically do not claim to prevent or treat disease. Thus, statements that claim a product "promotes leg vein health" or "reverses aging" are technically legal though often medically misleading. There is also no substantial regulation of purity. Contamination of "all-natural" products has been linked to complications including heavy metal poisoning, arrhythmias, altered mental status, and coagulation disorders, in addition to the more common gastrointestinal complaints.[4]

Nevertheless, there is good evidence that many supplements may offer substantial benefits as well as risks to the elderly (see also Chapter 2, Alternative Medicine).

* 1200–1500 mg of calcium along with 400–600 IU of vitamin D (in divided doses) has been recommended as the daily intake for elders.
* Vitamin E has been shown to improve immune function, reduce the risk of heart disease, reduce mortality in male smokers, reduce the incidence of prostate cancer, and slow the progression of Alzheimer's disease. However, doses indicated are variable in these studies, and ingesting too much of a fat-soluble vitamin can cause problems of toxicity. This is an especially important consideration in elders, as aging tends to increase the fat to lean muscle mass ratio. Vitamin E is also a natural "blood thinner," and supplements should be avoided in persons on anticoagulant therapy. Doses generally should be less than 800 IU/day.

* Vitamin B$_{12}$ deficiencies have been observed in 30% of the older population. Therefore the minimum daily allowance for those over age 50 is 25 μg.
* Antioxidant multivitamin and mineral supplements are commonly recommended because less than 10% of all Americans eat the daily recommended five or more servings of fruits and vegetables.
* Ephedrine compounds (such as ephedra and ma-huang) contained in many "energy-boosting" and weight control preparations have been responsible for stroke, myocardial infarctions, hypertensive urgencies, arrhythmias, seizures, and death.
* The effects of garlic on high blood pressure and cholesterol, purportedly significant, are actually negligible.
* Ginko biloba appears safe and seems to stabilize (although not to improve) cognitive function. It may cause feelings of anxiety and/or restlessness.
* The purity of ginseng products varies widely, and most contain alcohol, while alleged benefits are debatable.
* St. John's wort is more effective than a placebo for mild depression. It costs less than 20% of a monthly brand-name selective serotonin reuptake inhibitor (SSRI). However, the dangers of inadequate treatment and drug interactions, especially with digoxin, monoamine oxidase inhibitors, and SSRIs must be stressed.
* Saw palmetto improves symptoms of urinary urgency and seems to have few side effects. It does not shrink prostate tissue nor replace traditional treatments.
* Glucosamine and chondroitin appear to ease arthralgias (studies have been restricted to osteoarthritis) equal to many medications with fewer side effects, but they are relatively expensive and vary in quality, while the safety of long-term use remains open to question.
* Nutritional drinks designed for the debilitated are currently being promoted to the "young-old." For these persons use of these beverages is expensive and may be ineffective because they are sometimes incompletely absorbed and represent less than 35% of the calories in an average balanced meal.[4]

EXERCISE, INDEPENDENCE, AND MOBILITY[4, 10, 11]

Activity decreases with age. By age 75, a third of all men and half of all women get no physical activity. Ideally, through patient education, health care providers can encourage patients to develop regular exercise as a routine at earlier ages and continue this pattern of behavior beyond retirement. Although older people can continue to learn, statistics demonstrate well that the odds are very much against a person developing new habits, hobbies, or routines after retirement if they never engaged in them earlier in life. The loss of strength and stamina that is associated with aging can be reduced by regular exercise. Support for physical activity from family and friends can increase compliance with exercise programs. Activity does not have to be strenuous to achieve health benefits. Previously sedentary persons should consult their primary care provider before beginning a program of exercise. Many special programs exist for those with special limitations such as obesity, heart disease, and arthritis. New programs should begin with short intervals of activity for 5–10 min every 1 or 2 days until the desired level of activity is reached (see also Chapter 7, Exercise).

The opposite of mobility is immobility, and with immobility come complications such as decubitus ulcers, constipation, and functional incontinence. Physical therapy (PT) and the services of an enterostomal therapist or wound care advanced-care practitioner can be useful in caring for the patient who has already developed many of the problems characteristic of the bedridden. Depression is another enemy of independence. It may also lead to malnutrition, fatigue, lack of interest in activity, and the misdiagnosis of dementia. Depression is especially common following stroke. The signs and symptoms of depression in the elderly may be much more subtle and harder to diagnose. Screening instruments such as the Beck's Depression Inventory or the Geriatric Depression scale (see Box 9–2) can assist the primary provider. Because of the difficulty of diagnosing depression in the elderly, empirical antidepressant medication trials are often initiated during rehabilitation programs. Antidepressants best suited to the geriatric patient include SSRIs, bupropion, trazodone, and the least cholinergic tricyclic antidepressant, nortriptyline. Very small doses should be used in the beginning and increased slowly.

CONCERNS ABOUT ALZHEIMER'S DISEASE, "SENILITY," OR DECISION-MAKING CAPACITIES

Alzheimer's disease (AD) currently affects 2.5–4.0 million Americans, and these numbers will triple or quadruple by the year 2050 if no substantial treatments are found. Currently, if Alzheimer's disease is diagnosed early, several medications have been found to stabilize cognitive function (e.g., donepezil [Aricept] and tacrine [Cognex]), but none have been developed that reverse losses or cure the condition. Most adults fear loss of their mental faculties and decision-making capabilities more than any other loss associated with aging. Dementias also represent a huge burden for both the patient and society. These diseases compromise the quality of life for both the patient and the caregiver, compromise the patient's dignity, diminish society by the loss of productive citizens, and produce tremendous financial costs for both the family and society. Currently, direct and indirect costs due to AD exceed 100 billion dollars annually (see also Chapter 25, Neurologic Disease).

Table 9–4. Causes of Falls[9, 11]

Physical Status (Intrinsic)	Environmental Factors (Extrinsic)
Acute illnesses	Cracked or uneven pavement
Age >75 years	Lack of adequate railings or grab bars
Alcohol excesses	Poor lighting
Amputations	Throw rugs; unsecured carpeting or flooring
Cognitive dysfunction	Uneven stairs
Degenerative arthritis	Unstable or low-lying pieces of furniture
Diseases causing nocturia	Wet or otherwise slippery surfaces
Diseases or deformities of the feet	Poor footwear
Dizziness	
Hip fractures	
Impaired vision and hearing	
Parkinson's disease	
Peripheral neuropathies	
Postural hypotension	
Previous lower extremity fractures	
Sedative-hypnotic medications	
Strokes with residual deficits	

From Kane R, Ouslander JG, Abrass IB. Essentials of Clinical Geriatrics, 4th ed. New York, McGraw-Hill, Inc., 1999; Dial LK. Conditions of Aging. Baltimore, Williams & Wilkins, 1998.

FALLS AND FEAR OF FALLING

In the community-dwelling healthy elderly, most falls are viewed as "trips," or minor in nature. Many are not even reported to a health care provider, and only 5% result in fractures. Nursing home patients fall at a rate of 60% annually, and approximately 25% of these falls end in fractures. Risk factors for falls can be divided into two categories, intrinsic and extrinsic; however, most falls are multifactorial in nature (Table 9–4). A careful history and physical examination should be the initial tool in determining cause(s) and appropriate intervention(s) when evaluating a patient following a fall. "Standard" diagnostic tests are not indicated. The examination should include

* Vital signs, including orthostatics
* Visual and hearing screens
* Mental status testing
* Cardiac examination
* Musculoskeletal examination
* Neurologic examination, including proprioception and cerebellar testing
* Gait and balance evaluation

Most standardized assessment guidelines are too time consuming for the primary care provider's office, but a simple evaluation of the patient's gait and balance is the "Get Up and Go" test.[11] Simply observe the following:

* Getting up from a chair and sitting down
* Bending over
* Ability to withstand a slight push
* Neck movement/range of motion
* Initiation of ambulation
* How legs and feet are used in ambulation
* Symmetry of ambulation
* Ability to turn
* Need for balance support

Primary and secondary fall prevention can include

* Specific treatment of reversible causes
* A household safety and fall-prevention assessment (see Chapter 10, Safety Precautions In and Around the Home)
* Review of all medications (see Box 9–8)
* Improved lighting at home
* Exercise programs
* Use of assistive devices
* Distribution of patient education materials such as those available on the American Academy of Family Physicians web site (aafp.org).

SENSORY DEFICITS AND SWALLOWING DISORDERS

Vision declines with age despite corrective lenses and surgical treatments. The cornea yellows, admits less light, and distorts color perception. Glaucoma and cataracts are common problems. Vision deficits mean better lighting may be needed in the home and may result in an impaired ability to correctly identify and/or describe objects, text, or medications (e.g., a pale blue medication tablet may be recalled as green). Deficits may necessitate adaptives and/or education modifications. High frequency hearing loss is also common, and the usual 512-frequency tuning fork is too low in frequency to be useful for screening purposes. Portable audiometers should be used for periodic screening, as patients frequently will not admit to problems. Visual and auditory deficits both can contribute to safety and compliance problems. Patients who have difficulty with normal conversation or fail a screening should have a more formal test by an audiologist. Taste and swallowing problems also increase with age. Excess sugar and salt should be discouraged. Flavor enhancers and supplemental zinc may aid taste satisfaction and indirectly improve appetite. If a speech and/or swallowing disorder is suspected, assistance from a physical therapist, an occupational therapist, and/or speech-language pathologist is indicated. Aspiration and communication problems are especially a problem following a stroke.[9, 11]

INCONTINENCE AND URINARY RETENTION[9, 11]

Incontinence is a common problem in the elderly. Up to 35% of persons over age 60 have some incontinence problems (urinary and/or fecal), and this percentage increases to almost 50% in hospitalized elders. Men are half as likely to suffer from urinary incontinence as women. Instead, men are much more prone to urinary retention as a result of benign prostatic hypertrophy.

Incontinence should be first divided into temporary or chronic defects. Temporary or easily reversible conditions account for 30–50% of all cases. The differential diagnoses of transient urinary incontinence can best be recalled using the mnemonic DIAPPERS.

D = Delirium
I = Infections
A = Atrophic vaginitis or urethritis
P = Pharmaceuticals
P = Psychological
E = Endocrine disorder or Excess urine production
R = Restricted mobility or Retention
S = Stool (fecal impaction)

Chronic incontinence is best viewed in four categories; however, it is important to note that many persons suffer from more than one type of incontinence. These categories are:

* Functional: Inability to get to the toilet unrelated to genitourinary problems
* Overflow: Leakage from an overdistended bladder, due to anatomic or neurologic retention
* Stress: Involuntary leakage due to increased intra-abdominal pressure, such as in coughing or sneezing
* Urge: Spontaneous and uncontrolled emptying of bladder

Incontinence carries such social stigma with it that patients are frequently too embarrassed to complain of such problems to a provider. Many women also accept it as an "inevitable" consequence of aging and past childbearing. Because of this stigma, a routine review of systems should include at least one of the following questions:

* Do you ever lose urine when you don't want to?
* Do you ever lose urine when you cough, sneeze, or laugh?
* Do you wear a protective pad to catch urine?

If these questions elicit a positive answer, then further history can be sought about volume, circumstances, triggers, medications, daily fluid intake, activities, environment, associated genitourinary symptoms, and bowel habits. The physical examination should focus on overall fluid status and on general abdominal, genitourinary, rectal, vascular, endocrine, and neurologic evaluations. Functional assessment (ADL), mental status, and observed voiding evaluations should also be performed.

Diagnostics can include:

* Pad test: A sanitary napkins is placed between the patient's legs and the patient is asked to perform the Valsalva maneuver.
* Postvoiding residual test: The patient is asked to void completely and then catheterized immediately to determine residual volume. Less than 100 mL is considered normal and more than 200 mL is considered abnormal and sufficient to consider referral.
* Urinalysis and urine culture
* Consider: BUN, creatinine, electrolytes, glucose, urine and serum osmolarity, prostate-specific antigen, thyroid-stimulating hormone, and cortisol levels, and dexamethasone suppression tests, as appropriate.

Treatments can include toileting programs, pelvic floor (Kegel) exercises, vaginal weight training, electrical stimulation, biofeedback, medications (Table 9–5), and surgery.

CHRONIC DISEASES

(e.g., Arthritis, Diabetes, Chronic Obstructive Pulmonary Disease, Cardiovascular Disease, High Blood Pressure, Congestive Heart Failure, Depression, Osteoporosis, and Fractures)

Maximizing control of a chronic disease may improve or compromise a patient's quality of life and have an impact on functional concerns. Careful consideration and a willingness to reconsider treatments and medications are especially important when treating the older adult. For instance, ideal treatment of systolic hypertension yields significant benefits in lowering stroke rate. However, if treatment repeatedly leads to serious complications, such as orthostasis and/or falls, the decision to treat should be modified or reconsidered.

POLYPHARMACY AND/OR IATROGENESIS[4, 9]

Iatrogenesis, and especially the narrow therapeutic window of pharmacologic treatment in the elderly, is a primary issue in rendering thoughtful care for older patients. Polypharmacy may occur simply

Table 9–5. Medications Used to Treat Urinary Incontinence

Class	Mechanism of Action	Adverse Effects	Type of Incontinence
Alpha-adrenergic agonists (e.g., Entex, Sudafed, Tofranil)	Increases urethral muscle contraction and sphincter tone	Headache, high blood pressure, tachycardia	Stress
Estrogen replacement	Strengthens tissues, decreases trauma and infections	May require progestin to prevent endometrial cancer	Stress
Anticholinergics and/or antispasmodics (e.g., Ditropan, Detrol, Pro-Banthīne, Bentyl, Urised, Tofranil)	Increases bladder capacity; decreases involuntary bladder contractions	Constipation, dry mouth, blurred vision, confusion, urinary retention	Urge
Cholinergic agonists (e.g., bethanechol)	Stimulates bladder contractions	Decreased blood pressure, bronchospasm, bradycardia	Overflow
Alpha-adrenergic antagonists (e.g., Hytrin, Cardura)	Relaxes urethral smooth muscle and prostatic capsule	Hypotension	Overflow

because of a patient's many chronic complaints and conditions, multiple providers, and/or the increasing use of over-the-counter medications and dietary supplements. The primary care provider must be ever vigilant to avoid drug-drug interactions and toxicities. Other forms of iatrogenesis common in caring for the older American include

* Hazards of hospitalization, including immobility, risks and errors associated with procedures, falls, nosocomial infections, and medication errors, interactions, or reactions
* Overzealous labeling of the patient and treatment of dementia and incontinence
* Incorrect, under, or overdiagnosis
* Overuse of diagnostic procedures; especially when management is unlikely to be altered

* Transfer trauma and environmental hazards
* Enforced or learned dependency, immobility, and bed rest

ASSISTED LIVING AND LONG-TERM CARE

These terms *assisted living* and *long-term care* do not enjoy uniform definitions from one community to another. What they should imply is a wide range of services that address the holistic needs of the patient who is unable to meet all his or her own needs for self-care. Services may be intermittent or continuous, but all will generally be delivered over a long period of time, with needs being measured by functional incapacity or resources. While the proportion of noninstitutionalized elders requiring daily assistance rises with age (from approximately 6% of those aged 60–69 to 35% of those aged 85 and over), it is important to realize that family and friends commonly provide 80% of this long-term care. Although some patients qualify for Medicaid or are covered by the rare insurance policy that provides for long-term care, most long-term care is informal and represents tremendous physical, emotional, and financial hardships both to the individual and to the caregiver. Non-nursing home, community-based services and/or alternatives include

* Home health, including homemaking assistance, nursing, home hospice, social work/case management, physical therapy, occupational therapy, and speech-language pathology services
* Assistive devices, including grab rails, lifts, scooters, blinking light doorbells, and amplified telephones
* Emergency assistance call button
* Home delivery of meals
* Sheltered housing
* Senior centers and adult day care
* Foster care
* Personal care providers within the patient's own home
* Assisted care facility
* Respite care
* Caregiver support groups and counseling services (e.g., The Alzheimer's Disease Foundation or The Arthritis Foundation)

The primary care provider can greatly assist both the patient and the caregiver by taking time to assess a patient's functional disabilities and making appropriate recommendations for long-term care. Although most patients and families would prefer alternative care, there are times when health care providers must push toward an institutional placement if they are to best serve the needs of the patient, the family, and society. Even in the best case scenario, many elders will continue to require nursing home care. Therefore, all health care providers must be careful that in their zeal to provide alternative care, they not lose sight of the need to improve the quality of the extended-care and skilled-nursing-care facilities within their own communities.

QUALITY OF LIFE AND END-OF-LIFE CONCERNS

Death is the inevitable outcome of life and should not always be viewed as a failure of treatment but rather as the final common pathway. "Perfect healing" may include release from pain and suffering by passage through death's portals. Ideally all patients will discuss and plan in advance for death with dignity. It is the often-uncomfortable responsibility of the health care provider to discuss end-of-life concerns, advanced directives, and comfort care issues with terminally ill patients. Ideally, the concept of advanced directives should be dealt with well before dementia and/or terminal illness becomes an issue, as it is frequently much easier for a patient to decide how he or she would like to be treated. Family members are commonly hindered making appropriate choices because of fear of losing a loved one, guilt, and their own preferences. Discussions about advanced directives should be a routine part of annual preventive care. Tools made available to assist the provider include

* Patient education materials through organizations such as the American Geriatric Association, the American Academy of Family Physicians, and Aging with Dignity.
* Advanced directive instruments, including a living will, a durable power of attorney for health, and Five Wishes.[8]

Comfort care is an area that many providers are poorly trained to deliver. The focus must be on maximizing the quality of life and on relieving the suffering of both the individual and the family in a time of terminal illness. Common comfort care issues include relief from

* Pain
* Anxiety
* Air hunger
* Nausea
* Anorexia
* Constipation
* Urinary retention

Of these complaints, pain is the biggest enemy. While analgesia is an important part of pain management (give enough!), other aggravating factors should also be addressed, including loneliness, anxiety, depression, fatigue, immobilization, inflammation, and fears about suffering or a lingering death. A holistic approach encompassing family, friends, health care providers, and spiritual support all contribute to a patient's sense of well-being throughout this process.[11]

CONCLUSION

Geriatric care is an expanding field of medicine for which many physicians and midlevel health care providers have received little or no formal training and are poorly prepared to provide. The population is aging rapidly, and expectations for care are also climbing exponentially. Older Americans are living longer and doing more, well into advanced age. If we are to provide excellent care, we must focus on early preventive interventions, on maximizing function, and on quality of life issues, and become better prepared to manage terminal comfort care.

REFERENCES

1. Report of the Special Committee on Aging, U.S. Senate. Developments in Aging: 1996. Vol. 1.
2. Administration of Aging. A Profile of Older Americans: 1996. aoa.dhhs.gov/aoa/pages/profil96.html#older
3. Goldberg TH, Chavin SI. Preventive medicine and screening in older adults. J Am Geriatr Soc 1997;45:344–354.
4. Haber D. Health Promotion and Aging. New York, Springer Publishing Co., 1999.
5. Folstein MF, Folstein S, McHugh PR. Mini-Mental State—A practical method for grading the cognitive state of patients for the clinician. J Psych Res 1975;12:189–198.
6. Gallo JJ, Reichel W, Andersen L. Handbook of Geriatric Assessment. Rockville, MD, Aspen Publishers, 1999.
7. Hoffer EP. Emergency Problems in the Elderly. Oradell, NJ, Medical Economics Books, 1985.
8. The Commission on Aging with Dignity. Five Wishes. 1998.
9. Kane R, Ouslander JG, Abrass IB. Essentials of Clinical Geriatrics, 4th ed. New York, McGraw-Hill, Inc., 1999.
10. Allen L. Active Older Adults. Champaign, IL, Human Kinetics, 1999.
11. Dial LK. Conditions of Aging. Baltimore, Williams & Wilkins, 1998.

RESOURCES

Adaptives and assistive devices to make senior living easier: maturemart.com

Aging with Dignity: Best advanced directives tool; agingwithdignity.org

Human Kinetics: Active Older Adults, supported by the Sporting Goods Manufacturers Association, and an excellent resource for elder exercise promotion and programs. Humankinetics.com

Medweb: Geriatrics. The Health Sciences Library at Emory University has created a directory devoted to geriatrics and gerontology, with 47 direct links in six categories.
cc.emory.edu/WHSCL/medweb.geriatrics.html
Aoa.dhhs.gov.webres/craig.htm

Organizations with good provider and patient education resources
aafp.org
ags.org

Roxane Pain Institute: A wide range of educational material on pain management; roxane.com/

"Seven-minute" Screen (for Alzheimer's disease). Developed by Paul R. Solomon, PhD, and William W. Pendlebury, MD, co-directors, The Memory Clinic, Southwestern Vermont Medical Center, Bennington, VT.
This screening instrument is distributed by Janssen Pharmaceutica/Foundation to health care professionals at no charge.

U.S. Administration on Aging: Provides direct links to community services and agencies; over 175 direct links to other web sites about aging.

CHAPTER 10

Safety Precautions In and Around the Home

Jacquelyn B. Admire-Borgelt, MSPH,
Larry Borgelt, BS, MS, PE, CSP, SET,
and Frank David Curvin, MD

INTRODUCTION

Accidents in and around the home represent the most likely traumatic cause of significant morbidity and mortality in both children and adults. Safety precautions in the home and surrounding community are a very important part of prevention and health promotion because most accidents are preventable. Messages about safety come from many different sources and are presented through a variety of media. The health care professional is characteristically identified as the most creditable source of accurate information. Counsel given as part of a health care visit enhances and supports messages from other sources about hazards that threaten the patient or family and may lead to behavior modification that could prevent accidents and/or injuries. In 1996 there were 102,105 visits to health care providers because of accidental injuries. Of those visits, 21% were for falls alone.[1] The goal of counseling patients and families is to provide recommendations that can reduce risks, firstly effectively communicating those recommendations to a receptive audience, and then by reinforcing the importance of prompt corrective action and preventive safety practices. Whenever possible, the health care provider should identify resources that can inform or assist in carrying out these objectives. It is not the role of the health care provider to monitor or police the recommendations but to facilitate safe behaviors in much the same way that other aspects of preventive care are addressed within a medical practice.

The key safety education issues to be considered by the health care provider are listed in Box 10-1. As any patient visit must address a number of disparate topics, it is important that the provider focus on the most important considerations given the ages and lifestyle of the family. Those considerations are

* Safety essentials for every home
* Childproofing the home
* Hazards in the home
* Risks to children in day care and school settings
* Adolescence and associated risks
* Special precautions for older adults
* Personal safety issues

Box 10-1–Key Safety Education Issues
• Accident prevention • Fire prevention, home escape planning, and "Learn not to Burn" • Prevention of carbon monoxide inhalation • Prevention of lead poisoning and other toxic exposures • Safe interaction with pets and other animals • Hazards of toys and play equipment • Risks associated with sports activities, preparticipation examinations, and safety gear recommendations • Personal risk assessment and management • First aid, cardiopulmonary resuscitation (CPR), and 911 calls

SAFETY ESSENTIALS FOR EVERY HOME

A number of checklists and reference materials that can facilitate efforts to increase personal safety awareness, both in and around the home, are identified at the end of this chapter (see the Resources section). Health care providers should also familiarize themselves with local resources appropriate for their unique patient populations. Many resources are also available through the Internet and do not need to be kept on file in the office if they can be easily accessed throughout the working day.

Patients can do a number of things to reduce the risk of accidents in their homes. In "Safety Items No Home Should be Without,"[2] the National Safety Council (NSC) recommends the safety items/actions listed in Box 10-2. The brochure, available from the NSC via its web site, provides a brief description of actions essential to each area listed in Box 10-2.

The National Center for Injury Prevention and Control (NCIPC) reported that burns and fires account for more than 1.4 million injuries, 54,000 hospital admissions, and approximately 4000 deaths each year in the United States, making the category of burns and fires the fourth leading annual cause of unintentional traumatic death. Smoking and its associated paraphernalia around the house are known risk factors for fire and burns. Parents should ensure that all matches, lighters, and flammable materials are kept out of the reach of children. Childproof mechanisms for cook tops and ranges are sold in most hardware stores and can be especially helpful in preventing kitchen fires. Handles of pots and pans should always be turned away from stove edges to reduce accidental scalding injuries to young children when they simply want "to see" or "to help." Home fire extinguishers should be purchased and stationed in any potential fire hazard areas (e.g., kitchen, outdoor grill). Families can also improve fire prevention

---

Box 10-2–NATIONAL SAFETY COUNCIL RECOMMENDED ACTIONS AND ITEMS

- List of emergency telephone numbers
- Working flashlights
- Fire extinguishers
- Emergency evacuation plan
- First-aid kits
- Survival kits
- Working smoke alarms
- Carbon monoxide alarms
- Ground-fault circuit interrupters
- Tagged water and power
- Tested appliances bearing a certification mark (e.g., Underwriters Laboratory)
- Safety glass
- Handrails and gates
- Illumination of entrances, stairwells, and hallways
- Grab bars and slip-resistant mats in showers and bathtubs
- One-step step stools
- Safety goggles

---

safety by mapping out escape routes and a rendezvous in case of fire, and by practicing the evacuation procedures that they will use during an actual fire.

COUNSELING SUGGESTIONS

The single most statistically significant factor that has contributed to a reduction in the loss of life in residential fires over the last quarter century is the use of affordable early-warning smoke detectors with built-in power supplies and dead-battery alarms. Further augmented by carbon monoxide alarms and oxygen depletion sensors, these devices continue to be successful in reducing injury and loss of life. The number, method of detection, and location of these notification appliances vary based on the size and configuration of the home. Basically:

1. Each floor should have at least one smoke-sensing device, located in the intervening space between any sleeping quarters and the principal living area.
2. Both a smoke and a carbon monoxide detector should always be located inside each sleeping room or area.
3. Devices that have been in service for more than 10 years should be replaced.

Next, establish and practice a fire escape plan, and then post it in full view of all family members as a constant reminder of preplanned procedures.

An appropriate fire extinguisher, when used by a trained person, can be very effective in controlling small fires. However, there is an expressed reservation among fire officials that misapplication of a fire extinguisher may delay an expeditious call for help and/or an evacuation. Errors in the use of an extinguisher or application of an inappropriate extinguishing agent may also make a bad situation worse. If a fire extinguisher is purchased or given as a gift, the unit should be a multipurpose, dry-chemical device containing 2½ to 5 lb of agent. Halon agents have proved to be very undesirable environmentally, and any fire extinguisher using bromochlorodifluoromethane (Halon 1211) should be replaced. Every individual in the household expected to use an extinguisher should participate in an educational program and skill-development exercise.

Assistance in setting up a home fire safety program is usually readily available through the local fire department. Other organizations such as the National Fire Protection Association and the NSC also provide information for residential settings (see the Resource section at the end of this chapter).

Finally, families should be encouraged to have a first-aid kit and a list of emergency telephone numbers posted near each telephone (see Box 10-3). Everyone in the family should know when and how to dial the 911 emergency service number. While wireless telephones have revolutionized personal communications, their portability has technologically challenged the ability of emergency reporting systems to automatically trace the location where a call for assistance is initiated. When using a cellular phone, it is even more important that the person reporting the problem be able to provide accurate location information.

Keeping calm is critical when dialing 911 to report an emergency.

Box 10-3–IMPORTANT TELEPHONE NUMBERS

- In an emergency, call 911. State the problem, your name, and your address (have your family name, address, and/or directions posted in case a visitor or baby sitter places the call).
- Primary health care provider's telephone number(s)
- Hospital emergency room or hot line telephone number
- Poison Control telephone number
- Crisis Hot Line telephone number
- For persons taking chronic medications or having advanced directives, indicate where this information may be found.

All members of the family, including children, need to rehearse maintaining composure in an emergency.

▬▬ CHILDPROOFING THE HOME

All families with infants or toddlers need to take specific precautions, as identified in Box 10-4.

Box 10-4–CHILDPROOFING THE HOME

1. Ensure that crib safety meets recognized standards and that cribs are used correctly.
   - Any cutouts in the end panel and corner post should not allow head entrapment.
   - The drop sides of cribs should require two distinct actions, or a minimum force of 10 lb with one action, to release the latch or locks to prevent accidental release by the child.
   - As soon as the child can pull himself or herself to standing position, set and keep the mattress at its lowest position. Stop using the crib once the height of its top rails is less than three-fourths the child's height.
   - The mattress should fit snugly next to the crib so there are no gaps. If two adult fingers can be placed between the mattress and the crib, the mattress should be replaced.
   - Do not use plastic packaging materials (such as dry cleaning bags) as mattress covers.
   - Bumper pads should cover the entire inside perimeter of the crib and tie or snap in place, with excess lengths of ties removed. Pads should be removed from the crib as soon as the child can pull himself or herself to standing position.
   - Teething rails that are damaged should be fixed, replaced, or removed immediately.
   - To prevent possible entanglement, mobiles and crib gyms, which are meant to be hung over or across the crib, should be removed when the child is 5 months old, or when he or she begins to push up onto hands and knees or can pull himself or herself up.
   - Do not place the crib next to windows. Drapery and blind cords pose an entanglement and choking hazard.

Box continued on following page

*Box 10-4–*CHILDPROOFING THE HOME *Continued*

2. Ensure that a child safety seat meets recognized standards and that the car seat is installed correctly.
3. Lock up guns in a gun safe, trigger-lock all weapons, and store hunting and sporting goods in a separate, locked cabinet.
4. Inspect the home to identify and pad any items that have sharp corners or edges.
5. Install safety plugs in all electrical outlets.
6. Install childproof latches on cabinets that contain items that might be dangerous to children.
   - Remove and secure hazardous or poisonous substances and plants.
   - Keep all medications, cleaning products, or chemicals out of reach and sight of children.
   - Remember that medication containers are child-resistant not childproof.
   - Never refer to medication as candy, and do not make a game of taking medication.
   - Discard all old medications by flushing them down the toilet. Never throw pills in a trash can.
   - Never store chemicals in unmarked containers or food and beverage containers. Each year, thousands of children and adults mistake poisonous chemicals for what they thought was a harmless drink of lemonade or juice.
   - Take extra care at times of family stress or celebration. These are common times for poisonings to occur.
   - Keep syrup of ipecac in the home, but always call the local poison control center for advice before using it.
   - Have a poison center sticker posted on each telephone in the home.
7. Have all gas appliances checked regularly for leakage and damage.
8. Install steel window guards in any windows that may be opened and accessible from outside the home.
9. Reduce the temperature on the hot water heater to less than 130°F.
10. Ensure that all swimming pools, creeks, lily ponds, or other bodies of water are appropriately fenced to keep children away, and that all containers of water are emptied immediately after use.
11. Do not leave infants or young children unattended in the bath.
12. Make sure infants or young children have no access to small parts of toys or to toys suspended on a cord around the neck, as these are choking hazards.

COUNSELING SUGGESTIONS

Vehicle safety seats are a specific area where patients frequently request assistance. A list of resources that will offer information about selection and installation is included in the Resources section at the end of this chapter. A safety seat over 10 years old should be discarded. It should be considered no longer safe because of structural deterioration that has naturally occurred in the plastic; also, design of safety seats has improved. A seat that has been involved in an accident is also compromised and should not be used. *Consumer Reports* magazine evaluates almost all seats currently on the market, and that information is available through both the magazine and its web site. The U.S. National Highway Traffic Safety Administration (NHTSA) provides extensive information on safety seats for new parents and caregivers. Two additional important messages must be communicated to all persons who transport children in safety seats.

* ALL SEATS DO NOT FIT ALL CARS.
* NEVER PLACE A SAFETY SEAT IN THE FRONT SEAT OF A VEHICLE WITH A RIGHT FRONT SEAT AIR BAG, EVEN IF THE SAFETY SEAT IS FACING BACKWARD.

Contemporary vehicles may allow for deactivation of the air bag triggering mechanism. One should carefully consider the benefits and risks of deactivation before consulting the owner's manual for the vehicle to identify options for deactivation.

New parents and caregivers should be encouraged to go through the "baby-proofing" process immediately after the birth of a child and before the infant begins to crawl. A number of checklists and resources are available to assist with this process. As children become mobile, it becomes important to "toddler-proof" the yard and outdoor play equipment. (See the Resources section at the end of this chapter.) Strong cautions about small children around bodies of water, especially swimming pools, should be emphasized to parents of toddlers. Early water safety and swim classes are available through many swim clubs and organizations such as the YMCA/YWCA.

Counseling about firearms or weapons in the home is an essential part of safety education.[3] Rather than focus on the appropriateness of weapons in the home (which frequently invites debate), the health care provider should ask whether weapons are stored in a locked gun safe, whether trigger locks are in place, and whether ammunition is stored in a separate, secure location. If not, then strong encouragement to implement these fundamental prevention practices is very important. Do not allow arguments concerning the Bill of Rights or personal adult protection to distract from the purpose of creating a home safe for all family members. Firearm safety is equally important in all homes a child may visit.

▬▬ HAZARDS IN THE HOME

The home itself can be hazardous. Issues that should be considered when doing a home safety audit include

* The presence of lead-based paint
* The presence of asbestos
* The presence of plumbing fixtures fitted with lead components or installed with lead-based solder
* Accumulations of radioactive radon gas released from the soil

An audit should always be done prior to moving into a pre-existing dwelling.

Lead poisoning is a serious threat to children and may lead to mental retardation and irreversible brain damage. The U.S. Task Force on Clinical Preventive Services recommends that all children be screened at 12 months of age.[3] Lead-based paint can be ingested or inhaled as a dust created by scraping, sanding, or heating the paint, or by crushing paint chips. The U.S. Consumer Product Safety Commission recommends having paint in homes constructed before 1980 tested for lead before any renovations are done or if the paint is deteriorating.[4] Older plumbing techniques frequently used lead pipe and/or solder. Water in such homes should be tested for lead content. If the water tests safe and the pipes remain undisturbed, risk is minimal. However, if modifications or repairs are made to the plumbing without totally replacing the system, water should be tested again before its use is resumed. If you think a child has taken in leaded paint or soil, or need help in identifying and/or removing lead paint, call the NSC's National Lead Center at 1–800–424–5323.

Environmental authorities have identified many areas of the country where a hazardous level of radon may be emitted from soil or ground water. Some of these overlapping county/state/federal jurisdictions may enforce testing requirements. Realty boards are a good source of local information. Any home with a crawl space or windowless cellar with a bare earth floor should be tested for radon as a precaution. If the radon is detected, a series of inexpensive corrective actions may be prudent.

COUNSELING SUGGESTIONS

The role of the health care provider is to encourage and reinforce actions to increase safety for the patient and the patient's family. Whenever time permits, pertinent questions should be asked. Also, if, in the course of the visit, it is learned that the patient or family is moving or considering modification or renovation of the present home, the provider should use this opportunity to inquire about home safety in general. More specific questions should be asked when the family has small children or disabled adults living in the home.

RISKS FOR CHILDREN IN DAY CARE AND SCHOOL SETTINGS

The importance of seeking *licensed* day care should be the first communication to families seeking child care. If care is to be provided by a friend or family member, then ensuring the safety of the setting should be the primary consideration. In addition to ensuring the basic aspects of home safety, parents should make certain the caregiver has

1. All pertinent information about the health of the child(ren)
2. Complete contact information for the parents
3. A list of persons authorized by the parents to deliver and remove the child(ren) from the caregiver
4. Authorization to seek medical care for the child(ren) in case of emergency or when the caregiver is unable to contact the parents

Patients who are parents may frequently express concern about the safety of children in school. The health care provider's response needs to be one of encouragement and support. Parents should be encouraged to become involved in their children's school activities and to learn about precautions to ensure student safety. Organized parent groups working with the community can help to create an environment that reduces the risks facing children in schools.[5]

Finally, encourage parents to monitor playground equipment and sports activities to ensure that safe equipment is available and that safety gear is appropriately used for all sports. Playground equipment made from some treated wood may expose children to toxic chemicals. If soil around these play areas is contaminated, simply playing close to the equipment is equally hazardous.

COUNSELING SUGGESTIONS

* Ask parents if they have found safe and supportive day care settings for their children.
* Help parents to identify specific resources in the community to assist them.
* Encourage parents of school-age children to become involved in their children's school.
* Remind parents and children of the importance of using safety equipment when playing sports.

ADOLESCENCE AND ASSOCIATED RISKS

Adolescence is a time when children move toward independence, yet seek reassurance from parents and other significant adults. At the same time, teens are powerfully influenced by their peers and their desire to be accepted. Parents or guardians should be encouraged to consider the specific needs of the child moving through adolescence. Numerous studies and surveys have shown that adolescents experiment with drugs, alcohol, and sexual behavior.[6] At the same time, the adolescent is learning to drive a motor vehicle, is participating in a number of unsupervised activities such as dating, and is often employed outside the home. Developing a routine of interaction and discipline that recognizes and supports appropriate adult behaviors is often an important consideration for families with adolescents. Families who share dinner together an average of five nights per week are much less likely to have teens participate in high-risk activities.

With adolescence, risk increases. High-tempo activities are characteristically linked to more frequent accidents. The consequences of daredevil and copycat behavior can be catastrophic. The trauma of a physical or emotional injury to an adolescent may be overshadowed by the psychological impact suffered by parents, siblings, and peers, all of whom may need posttraumatic stress counseling. Health care providers should be sensitive to this need, recognize the symptoms, and intuitively participate in the process. Health professionals may find themselves counseling a youth for improprieties that appear to be irresponsible, thoughtless, or unnecessarily self-destructive. One should be mindful that substitution frequently delivers better results than prohibition, and prevention produces more positive results than protection. Identifying services and programs available in the school system and the community, such as the Boy or Girl Scouts, Four-H Club, team sports, or clubs, provides resources for a family who seeks assistance in meeting an adolescent's needs.

The teen's right of passage is often heralded by his or her first permit or license to drive a motor vehicle on public roads. Peer dynamics inevitably call for a vehicle of one's own, usually newer, faster, or more powerful than those of friends. Image and status are all-important to this age group. Most states have mandatory seat belt laws while providing absolutely no assurance of compliance. The design features that affect the safety or operation of a motor vehicle, particularly sport utility vehicles (SUVs), pickup trucks, and some vans, are frequently quite seriously compromised by efforts to "customize" the vehicle. Alterations such as changing the suspension system or tire size can shift the center of gravity of the vehicle to the point that the vehicle may no longer be safe to drive. If the adolescent is interested in motorcycles or all-terrain vehicles (ATVs) that do not offer the driver or passenger any impact protection, appropriate certified head gear and personal protective apparel for hands, feet, limbs, and torso should be worn regardless of minimum legal requirements for the area. Not riding barefoot or bareheaded cannot be underscored. Special operator training classes are to be strongly recommended. Casual conversation during the medical visit may provide a critical opportunity to engage the adolescent in a discussion addressing myriad topics about vehicle safety. This may require some "heavy homework." You may even be considered "cool" if you are able to offer the name of a mentor when an opportunity is presented.

Adolescence is also the age of competitive sports. Some of these activities involve substantial physical contact and expenditure of energy, but even activities that are not strenuous are not free from the possibility of serious injury. Physical conditioning and appropriate selection and use of personal protective equipment are fundamental considerations. When the sporting event involves the use of hardware items or special apparatus, such as bars and balance beams in gymnastics or saddles and bridles in equestrian events, these items need equal attention. Safety assurance activities require a collective effort on the part of coaches, equipment managers, parents, and medical professionals.

COUNSELING SUGGESTIONS

Opportunities to counsel adolescents directly are limited because of less frequent visits to health care providers. The sports physical is one unique opportunity. Each visit should provide an opportunity for the adolescent to bring up his or her particular concerns as well as to respond to questions from the provider. Providers should also address health promotion as well as injury prevention. The American Medical Association's Guidelines for Adolescent Preventive Services[6] recommends health guidance for injury prevention as listed in Box 10-5.

Box 10-5–ADOLESCENT INJURY PREVENTION GUIDANCE

All adolescents should receive health guidance annually to promote the reduction of injuries. Health guidance for injury prevention includes the following:

- Counseling to avoid the use of alcohol, drugs, or other substances while using motor or recreational vehicles, or in situations where impaired judgment may lead to injury.
- Counseling to use safety devices including seat belts, motorcycle and bicycle helmets, and appropriate athletic protective devices.
- Counseling to resolve interpersonal conflicts without violence.
- Counseling to avoid the use of weapons and/or promote weapon safety.
- Counseling to promote appropriate physical conditioning before exercise.

Since the health care provider may be viewed as a role model or mentor, each visit should include specific encouragement to the adolescent to make thoughtful, safe choices.

More frequently, parents will seek assistance or reassurance from health care providers. These visits are often for a medical purpose, and the provider's skill in interviewing may uncover a concern about an adolescent child's actions and/or risk-taking behaviors. Care must be taken both to honor a teen's confidences and to ensure a teen's safety. Recommendations must be based on knowledge of the family dynamics, of the available community services or programs, and of professionals who specialize in issues of adolescence.

■ SPECIAL PRECAUTIONS FOR OLDER ADULTS

While aging may be inevitable, each individual ages at a unique rate. Therefore some people at the chronological age of 55 are "old," while some at 75 are still relatively youthful. Even organizations developed to support the aging process dispute specific birthday cut-offs. Nevertheless, older adults have or will have a unique set of needs and are also at increased risk for accidents and injuries. Specific areas of concern for this age group are

* Loss of self-sufficiency—For older adults, the frequent outcome of a physical, emotional, or financial crisis is loss of self-sufficiency. Depending on others for activities they once were very capable of doing independently can lead to many new problems for older adults. Personal freedom is limited and self-esteem is diminished when an individual cannot maintain independence. In this situation, requests are often made by the family to assess whether an older family member can safety maintain an independent existence. The provider is confronted with difficult dialogue with the designated patient if placed in an adversarial role by suggesting eliminating options that are no longer feasible or safe for an older person. Implications for safety include ensuring that the home or apartment of the older adult is, as much as possible, free of hazards, and that systems are in place to assist and monitor the older patient. Intervention could be as simple as a home audit to check for such hazards as loose area rugs, or for the presence or absence of assistive devices such as night-lights and grab bars in a bathtub. If the living environment is found to be overly unsafe, home health care services or an assisted living setting may be an advisable accommodation.
* Reduced mobility—Osteoporotic degeneration can restrict mobility for intermittent periods or permanently. When the ability to move freely and at will is impeded, there can be both emotional and physical consequences. Depression is common among older persons with limited mobility. Falls also reduce mobility, either because of

the physical consequences or out of fear of another fall. Again, ensuring that the home is as safe as possible is important. Rehabilitation can often restore some level of mobility and self-esteem.

* Reduced capacity for quick reaction—Slower reaction time is a problem that must be recognized and appropriate actions taken to ensure the safety of elders who do not react quickly to hazards with the potential for injury. Related safety issues include driving an automobile, using power tools (or other machinery requiring some form of quick reaction in operation), and using a stove for cooking.

* Loss of sensory functions—Impaired vision, deadening of the olfactory sense, and presbycusis also limit self-sufficiency. If indicated, sensory functions should be tested and action taken to accommodate for impairments. If the presence of a flammable gas is the recognized hazard, installation of combustible gas indicators should be considered.

* Acceptance of increasing limitations—Changing ways of conducting personal business, modifying habits of many years, and adhering to new rules become more difficult as we age. Some older adults have difficulties complying with restricted smoking areas or using telebanking services, while others are unwilling to stop driving an automobile even when their reduced reaction time warrants such a step. Assisting in the acceptance of increasing limitations is often an unpopular task for the health care provider. Maintaining a balance between restriction and encouragement can help older adults to make this difficult transition. Helping an older patient to recognize both his or her own limitations and to consider the safety of others requires tact and patience.

COUNSELING SUGGESTIONS

The health care provider's knowledge of both the individual patient and the purpose of the patient's visit drives decisions about the important questions to be asked. Use of a structured set of questions often elicits concerns that would not commonly be offered by the patient, but it may consume more time than more targeted questions. One approach is to ask a general, open-ended question about the patient's emotional health, home environment, comfort with mobility level, and perception of hazards to his or her own safety. The simple screening question originally designed to open dialogue concerning domestic violence is an equally good question in these circumstances: "Do you feel safe at home?"

Because falls are so debilitating, consider asking all elderly patients about grab bars and slip-resistant mats or appliqués in bathtubs, handrails on stairways, and adequate lighting to move safely inside and outside the home at night. The checklist in Box 10-6 lists specific areas that can also be addressed as part of the visit or given to the

Box 10-6–HOME SAFETY CHECKLIST FOR OLDER ADULTS

Ladders and Step Stools
- Do you always use a step stool or ladder that is tall enough for the job?
- Do you always set up your ladder or step stool on a firm, level base that is free of clutter?
- Before you climb a ladder or step stool, do you always make sure it is fully open and that the stepladder spreaders are locked?
- When you use a ladder or step stool, do you face the steps and keep your body between the rails?
- Do you avoid standing on the top step of a step stool or climbing beyond the second step from the top on a stepladder?

Outdoor Areas
- Are walks and driveways in your yard and other areas free of breaks?
- Are lawns and garden free of holes?
- Do you put away garden tools and hoses when they are not in use?
- Are outdoor areas free of rocks, loose boards, and other tripping hazards?
- Do you keep outdoor walkways, steps, and porches free of wet leaves and snow?
- Do you sprinkle icy outdoor areas with de-icers as soon as possible after a snowfall or freeze?
- Do you have mats at doorways for people to wipe their feet?
- Do you know the safest way of walking when you can't avoid walking on a slippery surface?

Footwear
- Do your shoes have soles and heels that provide good traction?
- Do you avoid walking in stocking feet and wear house slippers that fit well and don't fall off?
- Do you wear low-heeled oxfords, loafers, or good quality sneakers when you work in your house or yard?
- Do you replace boots or galoshes when their soles or heels are worn too smooth to keep you from slipping on wet or icy surfaces?

Personal Precautions
- Are you always alert for unexpected hazards, such as out-of-place furniture?

Box 10-6–HOME SAFETY CHECKLIST FOR OLDER ADULTS *Continued*

- If young children visit or live in your home, are you alert for children playing on the floor and toys left in your path?
- If you have pets, are you alert for sudden movements across your path and pets getting underfoot?
- When you carry packages, do you divide them into smaller loads and make sure they do not obstruct your vision?
- When you reach or bend, do you hold on to a firm support and avoid throwing your head back or turning it too far?
- Do you always move deliberately and avoid rushing to answer the telephone or doorbell?
- Do you take time to get your balance when you change position from lying down to sitting and from sitting to standing?
- Do you keep yourself in good condition with moderate exercise, good diet, adequate rest, and regular medical checkups?
- If you wear glasses, is your prescription up-to-date?
- Do you know how to reduce injury in a fall?
- If you live alone, do you have daily contact with a friend or neighbor?

Housekeeping
- Do you clean up spills as soon as they occur?
- Do you keep floors and stairways clean and free of clutter?
- Do you put away books, magazines, sewing supplies, and other objects as soon as you are through with them and never leave them on floors of stairways?
- Do you store frequently used items on shelves that are within easy reach?

Floors
- Do you keep everyone from walking on freshly washed floors before they are dry?
- If you wax floors, do you apply two thin coats and buff each thoroughly or use self-polishing wax?
- Do all area rugs have nonslip backings?
- Have you eliminated small rugs at the tops and bottoms of stairways?
- Are all carpet edges tacked down?
- Are rugs and carpets free of curled edges, worn spots, and tears?
- Have you chosen rugs and carpets with short, dense pile?
- Are rugs and carpets installed over good-quality, medium-thick pads?

Box continued on following page

Box 10-6–HOME SAFETY CHECKLIST FOR OLDER ADULTS *Continued*

Lighting
- Do you have light switches near every doorway?
- Do you have enough good lighting to eliminate shadowy areas?
- Do you have a lamp or light switch within easy reach of every bed?
- Do you have night-lights in your bathrooms and in hallways leading from bedrooms to bathrooms?
- Are all stairways well lighted, with light switches at both top and bottom?

Bathrooms
- Do you use a rubber mat or nonslip decals in tubs and showers?
- Do you have a grab bar securely anchored over each tub and in each shower?
- Do you have a nonslip rug on all bathroom floors?
- Do you keep soap in easy-to-reach receptacles?

Traffic Lanes
- Can you walk across every room in your home, and from one room to another, without detouring around furniture?
- Is the traffic lane from your bedroom to the bathroom free of obstacles?
- Are telephone and appliance cords kept away from areas where people walk?

Stairways
- Do you have securely fastened handrails that extend the full length of the stairs on each side of the stairways?
- Do the handrails stand out from the walls so that you can get a good grip?
- Are handrails distinctly shaped so that you are alerted when you reach the end of a stairway?
- Are all stairways in good condition with no broken, sagging, or sloping steps?
- Are all stairway carpeting and metal edges securely fastened and in good condition?
- Have you replaced any single-level steps with gradually rising ramps or made sure such steps are well lighted?

Adapted from Clinician's Guide and Handbook of Preventive Services, 2nd ed. Baltimore, Lippincott, Williams & Wilkins, 1996.

patient or caregiver for guidance in conducting a home safety audit[1, 3] (see also Chapter 9, Geriatrics).

PERSONAL SAFETY ISSUES

Personal safety is frequently not considered a part of interaction between a health care provider and a patient, yet personal safety issues enter into many of the recommendations made by the primary provider. Whenever the patient expresses any need or concern about safety, the health care provider should respond to the opportunity to explore personal issues. Typical issues are

* Physical security—External doors of the home should be kept locked. Careful attention should be given to sliding patio doors. Ensuring the security of a sliding door may be as simple as cutting a dowel or broomstick to proper length to block the door closed or as complicated as the installation of specifically designed hardware that incorporates a tamper-proof locking mechanism. Consider purchasing electronic home security systems in settings where crime rates are high or if valuable items are kept in the home. The local police department or representatives of a private security firm can offer suggestions about specific situations. Discovering that one's home has been broken into and entered leads to an immediate feeling of being violated followed by an expression of anger. Anyone may thoughtlessly enter his or her residence after finding window glass broken or previously locked doors open, only to be confronted by an intruder. Rather than enter the home, persons should be encouraged to use a cellular phone or to go to a neighbor's home to call and await police.
* Personal safety in case of fire—Beyond smoke alarms, fire escape plans, and rehearsals of exit procedures, persons should be made aware of hazards associated with security bars on doors and windows. All bars and restraining devices should have an interior release to permit escape in case of fire. When staying in hotels or other unfamiliar surroundings, review exit plans posted in the room, corridors, and the elevator lobby, and locate two alternate routes of exit from the room before going to sleep. Never use the elevator as a means of exit if the fire alarm system is activated. Listen carefully for instructions relayed over a public address system. Only the newest buildings are required by the National Fire Protection Association and the National Safety Council to have a standardized audible emergency evacuation signal. The prescribed sound is based on a repetition of three audible pulses separated by brief periods of silence. For buildings built before 1996, there is no standard signal associated with fire alarms, so assume that any loud, repeated noise, pulsed tone, or bell sound could be a fire alarm, and exit the building using the fire exit. Return to your room or apartment only

when advised that it is safe to return by firefighters or staff of the facility. If smoke is identified in the corridor, stay in the room, seal the door with wet towels, and wait for rescue. If using stairs as a fire escape route, do not prop open the door between the corridor and the stairs. Purchase a portable smoke alarm and encourage others who travel to carry one. They are readily available and may save lives. If a disabled person is traveling, make sure to reserve accessible accommodations.

* Safety in the car—Car doors should be kept locked and windows closed when a vehicle is parked. When the car is being driven, the doors should be locked and the windows opened only enough for ventilation, as they allow penetration of the interior of the vehicle if completely open. Before entering a vehicle, always check to make certain no one is crouching behind the front seat. Seat belts should always be worn. If shoulder and lap belts are separate, both should be used. Air bags decrease injury and loss of life, but they are hazardous to children and small adults. Make certain that drivers are at least 10 in away from the steering wheel if it contains an air bag. Children should never ride in the front seat of a vehicle with a right-side air bag.

  Each vehicle should carry a first-aid kit, an ABC (A = trash, wood, paper; B = liquids and grease, C = electrical equipment) multipurpose, dry-chemical fire extinguisher (which will not freeze), a flashlight, an adjustable wrench, pliers with wire cutter, a screwdriver, road flares, a spare windshield wiper blade, duct tape, and a container of water. During the winter, a winter kit should also be added. The winter kit should contain gloves, socks, and stocking caps for the entire family, matches, one or more candles, candy bars, and an assortment of plastic freezer bags (to keep feet dry), all packed in a one-gallon metal can. A lighted candle placed in such a metal can as an improvised source of heat can provide sufficient warmth for a prolonged period in a stalled car.

* Yard and area lighting—Artificial lighting offers enhanced safety and is a deterrent to crime at night. Consideration should be given to the options that exist for lighting: gas versus electric lighting, and timers or photosensitive switches.

* Moving about in the community—Knowing the ins and outs of the community provides the best assurance of working, living, and playing in a safe place. It remains true that safety is always increased in numbers. Walking is often more enjoyable when shared, and two or more persons walking together are always at less personal risk. Being aware of places where an attacker could hide, and staying in lighted areas and away from dark or shadowy areas are important as well. Personal safety devices such as whistles, screamers, mace, or pepper spray may be appropriate in some settings. It is important to contact the police to learn what legal restrictions on such devices may be applicable to your area. The police department can also identify self-defense courses that are offered to enhance personal

safety, some especially intended for women. If you believe that you are being followed or have a sense that a stalker is present, do not lead the person(s) to your home; go directly to the police station or to a location identified as a "safe place" and request an escort home. Finally, it is acceptable to report a person who seems "out of place" in a given setting to the police. Reluctance to make such a report this has allowed many perpetrators the freedom to commit crimes.

COUNSELING SUGGESTIONS

Patient concerns about personal safety should direct any counsel on the part of the provider. Efforts should be focused on identifying resources for assistance and encouraging the development of skills that can increase personal safety.

CONCLUSION

Prevention is a multifaceted intervention challenge, anticipatory guidance in safety precautions being only one small part. Nevertheless safety counseling is relatively cost-effective. During a time when health cost management frequently seems to have superseded the concept of health maintenance, clinicians must provide both advocacy and guidance for those most at risk for unintentional injury, the very young, the very old, and the disabled. (See also Chapters 3 and 9.)

REFERENCES

1. Centers for Disease Control and Prevention, National Center for Injury Prevention and Control. http://www.cdc.gov/ncipc
2. National Safety Council. Items No Home Should Be Without. http://www.nsc.org/pubs/fsh/archive/homesaf.htm
3. U. S. Preventive Services Task Force. Clinician's Guide to Clinical Preventive Services. Baltimore, Lippincott, Williams & Wilkins, 1996.
4. Consumer Products Safety Commission. What You Should Know About Lead Based Paint in Your Home: Safety Alert. Document #5054.
5. American Academy of Pediatrics, Committee on Injury and Poison Prevention. Office-based counseling for injury and prevention. Pediatrics 1994;94:566–567.
6. American Medical Association, Department of Adolescent Health. Guidelines for Adolescent Preventive Services, 1992.

RESOURCES

GENERAL RESOURCES

Centers for Disease Control and Prevention, National Center for Injury Prevention and Control
On the web at http://www.cc.gov/ncipc
The National Safety Council. On the web at www.nsc.org
The Injury Prevention Program (TIPP), American Academy of Pediatrics
PO Box 927
Elk Grove Village, IL 60009–0927;
(800) 433–9016.
Internet address: http://www.aap.org

Patient Education Handouts
American Academy of Family Physicians,
8880 Ward Parkway
Kansas City, MO 64114–2797 (800) 944–0000
Internet address: http://www.aafp.org

The American Red Cross
On the web at htpp://www.americanredcross.com

INFANT, CHILDREN, AND ADOLESCENT SAFETY

American Medical Association
Department of Adolescent Health
515 State Street
Chicago IL 60610
ama-assn.org/adolhlth/adolhlth.htm

Bright Futures Project
National Center for Education in Maternal and Child Health
Georgetown University
2000 15th Street North, Suite 701
Arlington, VA 22201–2617
brightfutures.org

The National SAFE KIDS Campaign
1301 Pennsylvania Ave., NW, Suite 1000
Washington, DC 20004–1707
(202) 662–0600
safekids.org

CHILD SAFETY SEATS

National Highway Traffic Safety Administration
DOT Auto Safety Hotline
1–888–DASH–2–DOT 1–888–327–4236
nhtsa.dot.gov

National Highway Traffic Safety Administration
nhtsa.dot.gov
(click on Buckle Up America icon)

CRIB SAFETY AND RECALL INFORMATION

Consumer Product Safety Commission
CPSC Hotline (1–800) 638–2772
cpsc.gov

PLAY YARD SAFETY

Safe Kids Campaign web site at www.safekids.org

YOUTH SPORTS PROGRAM SAFETY

National Youth Sports Safety Foundation
333 Longwood Avenue, Suite 202
Boston, MA 02115
(617) 277–1171
Provides inexpensive fact sheets, guidelines, and materials about sports played
by youth

POISONING

Shannon M. Ingestion of toxic substances by children. N Engl J Med
2000;342:186–191.
National Lead Center
(800) 424–5323

WORKING TEENS

Rubenstein H, Sternbach M, Pollack SH. Protecting the health and safety of
working teenagers. Am Fam Physician 1999;60:575–580.

FIRE PREVENTION AND SAFETY

National Fire Protection Association, "Fire in Your Home: Prevention and
Survival," NFPA No. SPP–52G, 1999.
This 50-page booklet addresses prevention, protection, survival, special situa-
tions, fire extinguishers, and the "Home Fire Safety Kit."
nfpa.org and sparky.org.
Relevant information and brochures are available at these sites.

Consumer Product Safety Commission
"Your Home Fire Safety Checklist"
CPSC Document #4556 Consumer Product Safety Commission
Washington DC 20207
(800) 638–2772
cpsc.gov/cpscpub/pubs/4556.html

ELDER SAFETY

Consumer Product Safety Commission
"Safety for Older Consumer Home Safety Checklist"
CPSC Document #701
Consumer Product Safety Commission
Washington DC 20207
(800) 638–2772
cpsc.gov/cpscpub/pubs/701.html

Underwriters Laboratory
"Room-by-Room Home Safety Tips"
333 Pfingsten Road
Northbrook, IL 60012
(847) 272–8800
ul.com

Centers for Disease Control and Prevention
"Safe at Home"
cdc./gov/safeusa/home/safehome.htm

MOTORCYCLE SAFETY

Motorcycle Safety Foundation
2 Jenner Street, Suite 150
Irvine, CA 92718
(949) 727–3227

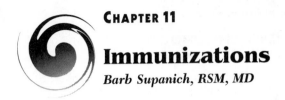

CHAPTER 11

Immunizations

Barb Supanich, RSM, MD

INTRODUCTION

The primary care office that provides immunizations to all patients in a style that honors each patient's educational, cultural, and preventive health care needs, while creating a system and an atmosphere within the office that make prevention and immunization top practice priorities, will be a successful practice. Published studies and my own practice experience demonstrate that both clinicians and patients value preventive services.[1, 2] Thus the major challenges facing clinicians are

* Establishing procedures within our offices that serve as reminders and tracking systems for our patients (to avoid missed opportunities)
* Dispelling myths about when immunizations can be administered
* Assuring that our preventive intervention goals for any individual patient coincide with the patient's own goals

The major challenges for patients frequently vary by ethnic, cultural, and socioeconomic group. Common challenges within all patient groups include

* Ignorance of the current immunization recommendations and schedule sequence
* Lack of knowledge concerning the importance of receiving immunizations in a timely manner within a cost/benefit framework
* Differing expectations and attitudes concerning the need for preventive services

Despite these challenges, it is well established that prevention is "more important to patients than many . . . [providers] . . . realize."[1]

It is clearly the goal of many health care groups and organizations, including the American Academy of Family Physicians (AAFP), the American Academy of Pediatrics (AAP), the Advisory Committee on Immunization Practices (ACIP), most health maintenance organizations (HMOs), and of *Healthy People 2000,* to achieve childhood immunization rates of 90% or higher by the year 2005.[1, 3–5] This chapter discusses the current recommendations for childhood and adult immunizations, including benefits and risks, current strategies for minimizing missed opportunities, and some of the newer immunizations, such as those for rotavirus, varicella, meningococcus, and hepatitis A.

239

CURRENT CHILDHOOD IMMUNIZATION SCHEDULES

The childhood immunization schedule as endorsed by ACIP, the AAFP, and the AAP is summarized in Figure 11–1. Also included in this figure are the newest recommendations for the pediatric pneumococcal conjugate vaccine series.

Figure 11–1 is an easy reference for primary care clinicians and their staff to utilize in the office. This figure can be posted in the clinicians' and nurses' work areas for ready reference and verification of needed vaccinations at the time of the child's visit. The figure can be obtained from any local public health department, or an annual update may be downloaded from the Centers for Disease Control and Prevention (CDC) web site at www.cdc.gov.

EPIDEMIOLOGY AND RATIONALE FOR IMMUNIZATIONS

The bacteria and viruses that cause diphtheria, tetanus, pertussis, varicella, and other vaccine-preventable diseases (VPDs) still exist. Vaccines have dramatically reduced the number of serious associated symptoms, illnesses, and deaths related to VPDs since the 1950s.[6] Other consequences of VPD-related illnesses include much higher health care expenditures (e.g., for office visits, hospitalization, outpatient treatment) in addition to general economy losses of income, work production, or school attendance (see Table 11–1).

POLIO

Before the first polio vaccine was available, there were between 13,000 and 20,000 cases of paralytic poliomyelitis in the United States each year.[6] Table 11–2 provides the data for the polio success story—in 1952 there were 21,269 cases of paralytic poliomyelitis, and in 1993 there were *zero* cases.

Effective implementation of polio vaccination programs in the U.S. and in the Western Hemisphere in general has eliminated cases of paralytic poliomyelitis in these areas of the world. In 1996, as a result of global immunization programs targeting polio, there were only 3500 documented cases of polio in the world.[6] Unfortunately, owing to wide variations in immunization practices in many countries, a case of poliomyelitis may only be a plane ride away. Case in point: In 1994 wild polio virus was imported into Canada from India.[6] However, the excellent vaccination levels among Canadians prevented the spread of the virus into the general population, stopping a potential epidemic before it could start. With careful attention to worldwide immunization, the CDC predicts that we may well achieve polio eradication

Figure 11–1. Recommended childhood immunization schedule, United States, January–December 2000. Approved by the Advisory Committee on Immunization Practices (ACIP), the American Academy of Pediatrics (AAP), and the American Academy of Family Physicians (AAFP).

Vaccines[1] are listed under routinely recommended ages. *Bars* indicate range of recommended ages for immunization. Any dose not given at the recommended age should be given as a "catch-up" immunization at any subsequent visit when indicated and feasible. *Ovals* indicate vaccines to be given if previously recommended doses were missed or given earlier than the recommended minimum age.

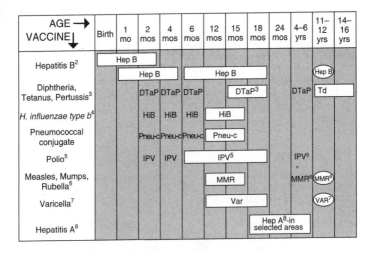

On October 22, 1999, the Advisory Committee on Immunization Practices (ACIP) recommended that Rotashield (RRV-TV), the only U.S.-licensed rotavirus vaccine, no longer be used in the United States (MMWR Morb Mortal Wkly Rep. Nov. 5, 1999;48:1007). Parents should be reassured that their children who received rotavirus vaccine before July are not at increased risk for intussusception now.

[1]This schedule indicates the recommended ages for routine administration of currently licensed childhood vaccines as of November 1, 1999. Additional vaccines may be licensed and recommended during the year. Licensed combination vaccines may be used whenever any components of the combination are indicated and its other components are not contraindicated. Providers should consult the manufacturers' package inserts for detailed recommendations.

[2]*Infants born to HbsAg-negative mothers* should receive the first dose of hepatitis B (Hep B) vaccine by age 2 months. The second dose should be at least 1 month after the first dose. The third dose should be administered at least 4 months after the first dose and at lease 2 months after the second dose, but not before 6 months of age for infants.

Figure 11–1 *Continued. Infants born to HbsAg-positive mothers* should receive hepatitis B vaccine and 0.5 mL hepatitis B immune globulin (HBIG) within 12 h of birth at separate sites. The second dose is recommended at 1 month of age and the third dose at 6 months of age.

Infants born to mothers whose HbsAg status is unknown should receive hepatitis B vaccine within 12 h of birth. Maternal blood should be drawn at the time of delivery to determine the mother's HbsAg status; if the HbsAg test is positive, the infant should receive HBIG as soon as possible (no later than 1 week of age).

All children and adolescents (through 18 years of age) who have not been immunized against hepatitis B may begin the series during any visit. Special efforts should be made to immunize children who were born in, or whose parents were born in, areas of the world with moderate or high endemicity of hepatitis B virus infection.

[3]The fourth dose of DTaP (diphtheria and tetanus toxoids and acellular pertussis vaccine) may be administered as early as 12 months of age, provided 6 months have elapsed since the third dose and the child is unlikely to return at age 15 to 18 months. Td (tetanus and diphtheria toxoids) is recommended at 11 to 12 years of age if at least 5 years have elapsed since the last dose of DTP, DTaP, or DT. Subsequent routine Td boosters are recommended every 10 years.

[4]Three *Haemophilus influenzae* type b (Hib) conjugate vaccines are licensed for infant use. If PRP-OMP (PedvaxHIB or ComVax [Merck]) is administered at 2 and 4 months of age, a dose at 6 months is not required. Because clinical studies in infants have demonstrated that using some combination products may induce a lower immune response to the Hib vaccine component, DTaP/Hib combination products should not be used for primary immunization in infants at 2, 4, or 6 months of age unless FDA-approved for these ages.

[5]To eliminate the risk of vaccine-associated paralytic polio (VAPP), an all-IPV schedule is now recommended for routine childhood polio vaccination in the United States. All children should receive four doses of IPV at 2 months, 4 months, 6 to 18 months, and 4 to 6 years. OPV (if available) may be used only for the following special circumstances.

1. Mass vaccination campaigns to control outbreaks of paralytic polio.
2. Unvaccinated children who will be traveling in <4 weeks to areas where polio is endemic or epidemic.
3. Children of parents who do not accept the recommended number of vaccine injections. These children may receive OPV only for the third or fourth dose or both; in this situation, health care professionals should administer OPV only after discussing the risk for VAPP with parents or caregivers.
4. During the transition to an all-IPV schedule, recommendations for the use of remaining OPV supplies in physicians' offices and clinics have been issued by the American Academy of Pediatrics (see *Pediatrics*, December 1999).

from our planet, much as we did with smallpox, within the next decade. Indigenously acquired polio last occurred in the U.S. in 1979. Over the preceding 15–20 years, there were approximately eight cases of clinical polio reported each year. Of these eight cases per year, six were among immigrants from outside the U.S.; the last known case of imported polio infecting a U.S. citizen occurred in 1986.[7]

Figure 11–1 *Continued.* [6]The second dose of measles, mumps, and rubella (MMR) vaccine is recommended to be given routinely at 4 to 6 years of age but may be administered during any visit, provided at least 4 weeks have elapsed since receipt of the first dose and that both doses are administered beginning at or after 12 months of age. Those who have not previously received the second dose should complete the schedule by the 11- to 12-year-old visit.

[7]Varicella (Var) vaccine is recommended at any visit on or after the first birthday for susceptible children, i.e., those who lack a reliable history of chickenpox (as judged by a health care professional) and who have not been immunized. Susceptible persons 13 years of age or older should receive two doses, given at least 4 weeks apart.

[8]Hepatitis A (Hep A) is recommended for use in selected states and/or regions; consult your local public health authority. (Also see MMWR Morb Mortal Wkly Rep. Oct. 1, 1999;48(RR-12):1–37.)

Table 11–1. Benefit-Cost Analysis of Commonly Used Vaccines (Savings per Dollar Invested)

Vaccine	Direct Medical Savings ($)	Direct + Indirect[*] Savings ($)
DTaP	8.5	27
MMR	10.3[†]	13.5[†]
H. influenzae type b	1.4	2.2
Hepatitis B:		
Perinatal	1.3	14.5
Infant	0.5	3.1
Adolescent	0.5	2.2
Varicella	0.9	5.4
Rotavirus	0.6	1.7

[*]Indirect Savings includes workloss, death, and disability.
[†]Recently revised to include second dose of MMR vaccine.
Source: Centers for Disease Control and Prevention.

Table 11–2. Comparison of Maximum and Current Morbidity from Vaccine-Preventable Diseases

Disease	Maximum Cases (year)	1993	% Change
Diphtheria	206,939 (1921)	0	−100.0
Measles	894,134 (1941)	312	−99.9
Mumps	152,209 (1968)	1692	−98.9
Pertussis	265,269 (1934)	6586	−97.8
Polio[*] (paralytic)	21,269 (1952)	0	−100.0
Rubella	57,686 (1969)	192	−99.7
Congenital rubella syndrome	20,000 (1964–65)	1	−99.3
Tetanus	601 (1948)	48	−97.3

[*]Due to wild poliovirus.
Source: Centers for Disease Control and Prevention.

There have been many reports in the lay press over the last few years concerning use of polio vaccine and vaccine-related or -associated paralytic poliomyelitis (VAPP). According to the CDC, there have been only 8–10 cases of VAPP per year, and it is exclusively associated with oral polio vaccine.[7] About half the cases occur in recipients and half in contacts (all are immunocompromised individuals).[6, 8]

A 1999 article articulated well the current issues surrounding the use of polio vaccines.[7] The main discourse has focused on the use of inactivated polio vaccine (IPV) and oral polio vaccine (OPV), and the risk of VAPP. The AAFP, ACIP, and the AAP all participated in a discussion of these issues in 1996–1997. The initial recommendation was to have the physician discuss with the parent the option of using either IPV or OPV. Since that recommendation, several major issues have been clarified:

* The price of IPV has dropped and is now equivalent to the price of OPV.
* Global near-eradication of polio has continued.
* The U.S. decision in favor of sequential immunization has had no negative impact on developing countries.
* Media attention to opposition to vaccination has grown, and VAPP is the big issue.

Recent health services research has shown that 61% of parents would choose IPV even if more injections were required, and 88% of parents would choose IPV if IPV were combined with other vaccines.[7]

Therefore, in June 1999, the ACIP recommended to the CDC that as of January 2000 the infant polio series be changed to an all-IPV schedule, making oral vaccines acceptable only in special circumstances.[9]

MEASLES-MUMPS-RUBELLA

Rubeola (Big Red Measles or 10-Day Measles)

Before the measles-mumps-rubella (MMR) vaccine was available, nearly everyone in the U.S. personally experienced a case of measles. Approximately 3 to 4 million cases of measles occurred each year, with an average of 450 measles-associated deaths annually between 1963 and 1993.[6] Measles morbidity and mortality statistics included pneumonia, diarrhea, or ear infections in 7–9% of all affected patients, with hospitalization required in almost 20% of these patients.[6] Although less than 1% of patients developed encephalitis from measles, those who did frequently suffered from sequelae that included developmental and special sensory morbidity. Overall mortality rate was approximately 1 death per 1000 cases.[6] Active cases of measles have been reduced by approximately 95% with the consistent and correctly administered use of the MMR vaccine. In fact, during the first three months of 1997, all U.S. cases of measles were imported.[6] Nevertheless, the World Health Organization has indicated that in 1995 measles caused approximately 1.1 million deaths worldwide, and has estimated that approximately 2.7 million annual deaths could be expected if vaccination were to be stopped.[6]

Mumps

Mumps is an infectious illness involving the parotid gland caused by a parvovirus. As of 1998 in Michigan, there were fewer than 2000 cases reported per year, and the highest incidence of mumps was in children between the ages of 5 and 14.[8] Approximately 4–6% of persons who get mumps will develop meningitis.[9] Four to ten percent of adolescent or adult males can develop the complication mumps orchitis.[9] The usual symptoms of mumps are fever, headache, and swelling of one or both parotid glands.

The mumps vaccine is a live attenuated vaccine. A relatively small dose of virus is administered to the recipient; the virus replicates in the body and increases to a volume large enough to stimulate an immune response. The immune response to the vaccine is virtually identical to the response to the natural infection. Therefore, when a child receives the MMR vaccine, the immune system responds to the vaccine by producing adequate levels of antibodies to the viruses. These vaccines ensure adequate antibody levels and offer complete protection to the person when administered according to the CDC guidelines.

Rubella (German Measles or 3-Day Measles)

The greatest risk of rubella in the U.S. is to newborns of mothers whose immunity to rubella is inadequate. It is crucial for the health of pregnant women and their newborns that women who are capable of conception and pregnant women at the time of their first prenatal visit have their rubella immunization status verified. If a fetus is infected congenitally during the first trimester, the infant will develop congenital rubella syndrome (CRS) in up to 90% of cases.[6] An infant born with CRS can have deafness, heart defects, cataracts, and mental retardation.

Rubella is a contagious respiratory illness associated with fever, cough, and coryza lasting up to a week, although its distinctive rash resolves within 3 or 4 days. Rubella can cause ear infections and/or pneumonia in one out of every 12 children. Encephalitis, which can lead to convulsions, deafness, and mental retardation, occurs in about one to two of every 2000 persons affected.[9] The mortality rate of rubella is 2 deaths per 1000 cases.[9]

Before routine use of rubella immunization in the U.S., an epidemic occurred in 1964–1965.[6] This epidemic resulted in approximately 20,000 infants born with CRS, 2100 neonatal deaths, and 11,250 miscarriages. Of the 20,000 infants born with CRS, 11,600 were deaf, 3580 were blind, and 1800 had mental retardation.[6] Routine use of the MMR vaccine could potentially lower the incidence of congenital rubella, measles, and mumps to zero.

PERTUSSIS-DIPHTHERIA-TETANUS

Pertussis

Prior to the availability of the pertussis vaccine in the U.S., many children suffered from pertussis, better known as whooping cough. In the prevaccine era, there were as many as 260,000 cases per year and up to 9000 deaths annually reported in the U.S.[6] Pertussis results in severe coughing spasms punctuated by the distinctive whooping inspiration and associated vomiting. The spasms of coughing can be so severe that they frequently interfere with eating, drinking, and breathing. One out of three cases of pertussis encephalitis will result in permanent brain damage sequelae, while another third of encephalitic patients will die.

The newer acellular pertussis vaccine contained within the diphtheria-tetanus-pertusiss (DTaP) vaccine has been available for use in the U.S. since 1991 and has far fewer side effects than the older, whole-cell diphtheria-tetanus-pertussis (DTP) vaccine. Neurologic side effects such as hypotonic-hyporesponsive episodes (HHEs) and seizures noted with administration of the whole-cell vaccine, although relatively uncommon, have led in the past to immunization refusal and ultimately to the creation of a safer vaccine. The reported incidence of HHE ranges from 8 to 81 per 100,000 doses, while the incidence of seizure was 8–16 per 100,000 doses. By calculated extrapolation, these rates translate to only one seizure and one HHE per study.[10]

DTaP is an acellular pertussis vaccine that contains one or more of five purified antigens derived from *Bordetella pertussis* organisms. All acellular vaccines contain inactivated pertussis toxoid in different concentrations but vary in the inclusion and concentration of the four other antigens.[10] In 1991 and 1992 the National Institutes of Health (NIH) conducted phase 1 and phase 2 trials evaluating 13 acellular pertussis vaccines[10] and found that there were significantly fewer and less severe adverse events with the acellular vaccine compared with the traditional DTP vaccines. In February of 1997, in *Pediatrics*, the AAP's Committee on Infectious Diseases recommended that all doses administered to children under the age of 7 be of the DTaP vaccine.[10]

If administration of this vaccine were stopped, the number of pertussis cases in the U.S. would markedly increase.

Despite current vaccination efforts, about 5000 cases of pertussis still occur in the U.S. each year. A 1999 review of international health data by the CDC[6] showed that in eight countries where immunization coverage was reduced, the incidence rates of pertussis increased up to 100 times the rates in countries where vaccination rates were sustained.

Diphtheria

The diphtheria vaccine is a toxoid type of inactivated vaccine that is composed of fractions of bacterial toxins. Inactivated vaccines are produced by growing the bacterium or virus in culture media and inactivating it with heat or formalin.[11] Inactivated vaccines do not replicate. Although the entire dose of the antigen is administered with each injection, multiple doses of inactivated vaccines are required. The first dose primes the immune system, and a protective immune response occurs after the second or third dose. With inactivated vaccines the immune response is humoral. Since the virus or bacterium has been inactivated, the vaccine is noninfectious and cannot replicate.

Diphtheria is a respiratory illness. Common symptoms include coughing, sneezing, gradual onset of sore throat, and a low-grade fever.[9] Prior to the availability of the DTP vaccine, there were between 100,000 and 200,000 cases of diphtheria reported annually in the U.S. (see Table 11–2). Serious complications associated with diphtheria include heart failure, pneumonia, convulsions, encephalitis, and paralysis. In 1993 there were no cases reported in the U.S. Administration of the DTP or DTaP vaccine has essentially eliminated these illnesses in the U.S.

Tetanus

The tetanus vaccine is also an inactivated toxoid vaccine. Tetanus is caused by bacteria entering the body through a break in the skin. A toxin is produced that attacks the nervous system and can cause lockjaw. Early symptoms include headache, irritability, and stiffness in the jaw and neck.[9] If tetanus progresses, the person can experience severe muscle spasms in the jaw, neck, arms, legs, abdomen, and back. With progression to severe disease symptoms, the person usually requires hospitalization and treatment in the intensive care unit. Most cases in the U.S. occur in adults, and in persons older than 20 years of age there is a 40% mortality rate.[9] In contrast, over 500,000 newborns died from tetanus in developing countries in 1993.[9] The administration of DTaP vaccine eliminates the risk of such serious illness.

If a patient is presumed unimmunized and at acute risk, Hyper-Tet and the initial tetanus-diphtheria (Td) vaccine may be administered, with the primary series completed later according to schedule. Td boosters should be administered every 10 years, routinely. If an acute booster is needed in urgent situations, the Td boosters are also recommended rather than simple tetanus toxoid.

HAEMOPHILUS INFLUENZAE TYPE B (Hib)

Before *Haemophilus influenzae* type B (Hib) immunization was available, infections due to Hib, including otitis media and meningitis, were very common among children under age 2. About 20,000 cases of Hib infection occurred annually; in the prevaccine era (before 1987) two thirds of these were cases of meningitis.[6] Other serious or life-threatening illnesses from Hib infection included epiglottitis, pneumonia, and septicemia.[6] Hib meningitis killed 600 children each year and left many survivors with deafness, seizures, or mental retardation.[6] The mortality rate from Hib meningitis was 5%, and 10–30% of survivors had permanent brain damage.[9]

Since the introduction of the Hib vaccine in 1987, the incidence of serious Hib diseases has declined by close to 99%.[6] Fewer than 10 reported cases of invasive Hib disease were documented in 1995.[6] Many medical, nursing, and physician assistant students and clinicians trained after 1990 have never seen a case of Hib meningitis or pneumonia. This is one of the recent success stories in public health in the U.S.

HEPATITIS B

Hepatitis is a serious disease and is responsible for 5000 to 6000 deaths per year in the U.S. due to cirrhosis or cancer of the liver.[12] The hepatitis B virus (HBV) (DNA type) is the cause of hepatitis B. The virus can cause both acute and chronic forms of hepatitis. Anorexia, myalgias, and abdominal pain, with diarrhea and vomiting and jaundice, are signs of the acute illness. The chronic form of hepatitis B can lead to very serious illnesses, including liver cancer and cirrhosis, and death. Each year in the U.S., approximately 130,000 new cases of HBV infection are diagnosed, of which more than 11,000 require hospitalization. In the U.S., an estimated 1.25 million people have chronic HBV infection.[12]

The hepatitis B vaccine is a safe and effective vaccine for the prevention of hepatitis B infectious illnesses for all age groups—

infants, children, adolescents, and adults. Although some studies have sought to link this vaccine to asthma, diabetes, multiple sclerosis, autism, and sudden infant death syndrome, CDC studies have established no associations. This vaccine is an efficacious tool in the prevention of infection, illness, and death from hepatitis B. More than 20 million persons in the U.S. and more than 500 million persons worldwide have received the vaccine without any adverse effects.[12] There is no confirmed scientific evidence that this vaccine causes chronic illnesses such as multiple sclerosis, chronic fatigue syndrome, rheumatoid arthritis, or autoimmune disorders. There is no risk of HBV infection from the vaccine.[12] Although infants are currently receiving routine immunization, there remains a large pool of unimmunized teens and adults who still need to "catch up."

Some question why immunization of infants is necessary when the majority of cases of hepatitis B are contracted by transmission of body fluids as a result of injecting drugs with contaminated needles, or by sexual contact. Although this is true, of the 1.25 million persons in the U.S. who have chronic liver disease due to hepatitis B, more than one third of them contracted the disease as young children. Even more startling, only 20–50% of children with hepatitis B can be shown to have been born to a hepatitis B–infected mother. Until these statistics can be explained, hepatitis B vaccination should be done in infancy.

Currently Pentacel, a pentavalent vaccine (DaPT/Hib/Hep B) manufactured in Canada, is not licensed in the U.S. However, it is expected that this vaccine, in some form, will become available soon and will greatly decrease the total number of vaccine-related injections that each infant must currently receive. The recent concerns regarding thiomersal as a preservative in some vaccines, although largely theoretical, have been rendered moot owing to reformulations.

PNEUMOCOCCAL VACCINES

There are now two types of pneumococcal vaccines, the polysaccharide vaccine licensed for use in older children and adults and the newer conjugate vaccine indicated for vaccination of infants and young children.

The 23-valent polysaccharide pneumococcal vaccine is recommended for all adults aged 65 years and older, and for persons with asplenia, immunosuppression, chronic renal failure, nephrotic syndrome, or severe pulmonary or cardiac illnesses.[12] About 40,000 deaths occur each year from pneumococcal disease,[7] and the mortality rate from pneumococcal pneumonia in the U.S. is still about 30%.

In 1999 new recommendations for revaccination with Pneumovax were released. Revaccination was recommended only for persons at high risk for pneumococcal illnesses. People at highest risk include children more than 2 years of age and adults with functional or anatomic asplenia (e.g., due to sickle cell disease or splenectomy), HIV infection, leukemia, lymphoma, Hodgkin's disease, multiple myeloma, generalized malignancy, chronic renal failure, nephrotic syndrome, and conditions associated with immunosuppression, and those receiving chemotherapy or long-term corticosteroids. Others who should be revaccinated are those who were previously vaccinated when they were younger than age 65, did not have one of the illnesses in the preceding list, and received the vaccine more than 5 years previously.[12] While the current 23-valent pneumoccoccal polysaccharide vaccine induces poor immune response in those under the age of 2 years, a newer conjugate vaccine became available in 2000. Preliminary testing suggests that pneumococcal vaccination is especially effective in reducing the frequency of serious infections and death due to pneumococcal infections in young children.[9] All healthy infants and toddlers should receive 4 doses of the pneumococcal conjugate vaccine. Doses may be given at 2, 4, and 6 and at 12–15 months of age at the same time as other routine vaccinations. This vaccination series should protect children for at least 3 years when they are most at risk for pneumococcal meningitis, sepsis, pneumonia, and otitis media.[9] It targets the most common seven strains of pneumococcus that account for approximately 90% of invasive disease in infants.

It is estimated that each year in the U.S. there are about 16,000 cases of pneumococcal bacteremia and 1400 cases of pneumococcal meningitis among children under the age of 5 years. Children under the age of 2 are at highest risk for infection. In up to half the cases of meningitis, brain damage and hearing loss occur, and about 10% of patients die.

This vaccine is not indicated for use in adults, or as a substitute for other approved pneumococcal polysaccharide vaccines approved for high-risk children over the age of 2. Side effects in the trials were generally mild and included local injection site reactions, irritability, drowsiness, and decreased appetite.

Children at risk should still receive the 23-valent vaccine after age 2, as this may still provide some additional protection from other serotypes.

Adult booster schedules changed several times in the 1990s and likely will change again. However, all authorities agree that all persons immunized more than 5 years ago and under the age of 65 should receive at least one booster at age 65.

STRATEGIES TO PREVENT MISSED OPPORTUNITIES

We've all been there. Patients come in for routine visits to discuss their hypertension management or the management of their diabetes, or, even worse, for their "annual visits," and after they leave, we look at the flow sheet and realize that they were due for a tetanus shot or Pneumovax. Our stomach flutters as we realize that we missed an opportunity to offer and provide them with their needed immunization update.

A few office strategies, however, can help us to prevent undervaccination and to promote wellness opportunities for our patients.

At least six factors contribute to undervaccination, and they fall under three main categories:

* Parent perceptions/beliefs
* Vaccine-related issues
* Practice barriers

Our patients are bombarded with multiple health messages on a daily basis. The information related to immunizations and their safety comes from a variety of sources, and both the veracity and the reliability of this information are quite variable. It must be a priority of every primary care clinician to ensure that the office staff (receptionists, medical assistants, and nurses) are all properly updated on current and accurate information regarding immunizations for children and adults.

All clinicians in the practice also need to agree upon the importance of preventive activities in the office and particularly the importance of barrier-free immunization practices. We need to ensure that our office practice styles result in ease of vaccination for children and adults.

What is a missed opportunity? A missed opportunity is when a child or adult comes into the office for any type of visit and does not receive all needed updates of their immunizations. The major cause of missed opportunities is office policies that make it difficult for many patients to easily obtain the needed immunization(s). Some examples of barriers include

* Office hours that do not accommodate employed parents
* Office not located on public transportation routes
* Immunizations may only be administered with a doctor's order
* Policy that allows only a licensed nurse to administer the immunization
* Policy that requires an appointment with a clinician for immunization or requires that a physical examination be given before the immunization is administered
* Lack of knowledge concerning the true contraindications to administering a vaccine

Considering these key barriers to timely reception of needed immunizations, what are the strategies that will make an office prevention-friendly and free of barriers to obtaining vaccinations? One of the major barriers is in reality a knowledge barrier. Many clinicians and nursing personnel have a misunderstanding about the true contraindications to administering a vaccine. Only three contraindications are valid:

* The patient had an anaphylactic reaction to a prior vaccine.
* The patient had an anaphylactic reaction to a component of the vaccine.
* Immunocompromised patients should not receive live attenuated vaccines.[1]

Several *invalid* reasons for not administering a vaccine are still strongly held by various segments of the medical population and by parents. Some of the most common are

* Presence of minor illnesses, such as upper respiratory infections ("colds"), otitis media, low-grade fevers, or mild diarrhea
* Concurrent administration of antibiotics
* Recent exposure to a disease or recent convalescence from an illness
* A pregnancy in the household
* Breastfeeding
* Premature newborn (either the patient or another member of the household)
* Allergies to products not in the vaccine
* Family history unrelated to immunosuppression[7]

The family practice office that has a positive attitude toward prevention and is oriented toward promoting good health among its patients will have office policies that reduce barriers and missed opportunities, improve tracking and charting, and facilitate the administration of vaccines. The practice will also place a high priority on educating staff, clinicians, parents, and children about the importance of healthy lifestyles, including the timely reception of vaccines.

Some strategies to promote immunization that are successful and easily implemented in a busy office practice include the following:

* Make "immunization update" a part of the check of vital signs that is obtained by the medical assistant at *each* visit.
* If it is determined that the patient needs an immunization and does not meet any of the true exclusion criteria, make it office policy that the medical assistant or nurse can administer the vaccine at that visit, preferably before the clinician sees the patient.
* Make it office policy that an immunization flow sheet is an integral part of the patient chart. Reward staff who consistently have immunization rates $\geq 90\%$.
* Review the patient's chart in his or her presence and make a positive comment to the patient about the importance of receiving an immunization. Remind patients when immunizations are due for themselves and for other family members.

* Let patients know that they and their family members can receive immunizations whenever the office is open.
* Have office hours that are responsive to patients' schedules, i.e., be open in some combination of early mornings, evenings, and Saturdays.
* Schedule immunizations on a "nurse" schedule, not exclusively on the clinician's schedule.
* Utilize some form of an office reminder system for health maintenance services, including immunization reminders.
* Place health-related messages on the office telephone system, including current information on immunization needs of children and adults, for patients to hear when they call to schedule appointments.

The next step to assure successful office immunization strategies is to utilize a focused, continuous quality improvement (CQI) process:

* Identify the focus for improvement, e.g., what is the present rate of immunizations of all patients ≤ 2 years of age?
* Obtain data through chart review, especially noting the level of documentation of immunizations on the flow sheet or health maintenance list.
* Discuss with staff members the present policies regarding immunizations and their impact on a patient's ease of obtaining an immunization.
* Run a representative sample of immunization data on the patients of each clinician and share the results with the clinicians.
* Brainstorm and discuss new strategies for improving immunization opportunities in the practice with staff, clinicians, and patients.
* Enroll in local and federal public health immunization programs to ensure access for all patients to needed immunizations.

To facilitate patient/parent education about vaccinations the health care provider should use handouts or posters including information in Boxes 11–1, 11–2, and 11–3. In addition, complete Vaccination Information Statements (VISs) for all current vaccines may be downloaded from a CDC-linked web site, Immunization Access Coalition (IAC), in approximately 20 languages (see the Resources section at the end of this chapter).

NEWER VACCINES AND CURRENT ISSUES

This section briefly discusses some of the current issues and controversies surrounding new vaccines, including varicella, rotavirus, meningococcus, and hepatitis vaccines.

VARICELLA

The late 1990s witnessed some discussion and clarification concerning varicella vaccination strategies for children and young adults.[7, 13] Varicella vaccine is licensed for use in children aged 12 months and older and in adults. One dose should be given subcutaneously (SC) to children aged 12 months to 12 years, and two doses should be given SC at least one month apart to persons more than 13 years of age. The vaccine can be given at the same time as other immunizations.

Text continued on page 261

Box 11-1–TEN THINGS YOU NEED TO KNOW ABOUT IMMUNIZATIONS

1. Why should my child be immunized?

Children need immunizations (shots) to protect them from dangerous childhood diseases. These diseases have serious complications and can even kill children.

2. What diseases do vaccines prevent?

- Measles
- Mumps
- Polio
- Rubella (German measles)
- Pertussis
- Diphtheria
- Tetanus
- *Haemophilus influenzae* type b (Hib disease)
- Pneumococcus
- Hepatitis B
- Varicella (chickenpox)

3. How many shots does my child need?

The following vaccinations are recommended by age 2 and can be given in five visits to a doctor or clinic:

- 1 vaccination against measles/mumps/rubella (MMR)
- 4 vaccinations against Hib (a major cause of spinal meningitis)
- 4 vaccinations against pneumococcus (responsible for 200 + deaths in young children each year)
- 3 vaccinations against polio
- 4 vaccinations against diphtheria, tetanus, and pertussis (DTP)
- 3 vaccinations against hepatitis B
- 1 vaccination against varicella

Box 11-1–TEN THINGS YOU NEED TO KNOW ABOUT IMMUNIZATIONS *Continued*

4. Are the vaccines safe?

Serious reactions to vaccines are extremely rare but do occur. However, the risks of serious disease from not vaccinating are far greater than the risks of serious reaction to the vaccination.

5. Do the vaccines have any side effects?

Yes, side effects can occur with vaccination, depending on the vaccine: slight fever, rash, or soreness at the site of injection. Slight discomfort is normal and should not be a cause for alarm. Your health care provider can give you additional information.

6. What do I do if my child has a serious reaction?

If you think your child is experiencing a persistent or severe reaction, call your doctor or get the child to a doctor right away. Write down what happened and the date and time it happened. Ask your doctor, nurse, or health department to file a Vaccine Adverse Event Report form or call 1–800–338–2382.

7. Why can't I wait until school to have my child immunized?

Immunizations must begin at birth and most vaccinations should be completed by age 2. By immunizing on time (by age 2), you can protect your child from being infected and prevent the infection of others at school or at day care centers. Children under age 5 are especially susceptible to disease because their immune systems have not built up the necessary defenses to fight infection.

8. Why is a vaccination health record so important?

A vaccination health record helps you and your health care provider keep your child on schedule. A record should be started at birth, when your child should receive his/her first vaccination, and updated each time your child receives the next scheduled vaccination. This information will help you if you move to a new area or change health care providers, or when your child is enrolled in day care or starts school. Remember to bring this record with you every time your child has a health care visit.

9. Where can I get free vaccines?

The Vaccines for Children Program will provide free vaccines to needy children. Eligible children include those without health insurance coverage, all those who are enrolled in Medicaid, American Indians, and Alaskan Natives.

Box 11-1–TEN THINGS YOU NEED TO KNOW ABOUT IMMUNIZATIONS *Continued*

10. Where can I get more information?

You can call the National Immunization Information Hotline for further immunization information at 1–800–232–2522 (English) or at 1–800–232–0233 (Spanish). Internet address: http://www.cdc.gov/nip

Immunization Hotline
1–800–232–2522, English
1–800–232–0233, Spanish

Source: Centers for Disease Control and Prevention.

Box 11-2–VACCINE-PREVENTABLE CHILDHOOD DISEASES

Polio

- Serious cases cause paralysis and death
- Mild cases cause fever, sore throat, nausea, headaches, and stomach aches; may also cause neck and back pain or stiffness
- Polio vaccine can prevent this disease

Diphtheria

- Respiratory disease spread by coughing and sneezing
- Gradual onset of sore throat, and low-grade fever
- Heart failure or paralysis can result if disease is not treated
- Diphtheria toxoid (contained in DTP, DT, DTaP, and Td vaccines) can prevent this disease

Tetanus

- Neurologic disease also known as lockjaw
- Bacteria enter the body through a break in the skin
- Produces a poison (toxin) that attacks the nervous system
- Early symptoms are headache, irritability, and stiffness in the jaw and neck
- Later, causes severe muscle spasms in the jaw, neck, arms, legs, back, and abdomen
- May require intensive care in hospital
- In the U.S., most cases are in adults; 4 out of every 10 patients with tetanus aged 20 or older will die from the disease
- In developing countries, tetanus frequently affects newborn babies; more than 500,000 babies died from neonatal tetanus in 1993

Box 11-2–VACCINE-PREVENTABLE CHILDHOOD DISEASES *Continued*

- Tetanus toxoid (contained in DTP, DT, DTaP, and Td vaccines) can prevent this disease

Pertussis

- Highly contagious respiratory disease also known as whooping cough
- Causes severe spasms of coughing that can interfere with eating, drinking, and breathing
- Complications include pneumonia, convulsions, and encephalitis
- One out of every three patients with pertussis encephalitis will die, another 1 of 3 will have permanent brain damage
- In the U.S., most cases are in children under age 5, and half of those are in infants under 1 year old
- About 5000 cases are reported in the U.S. each year
- Pertussis vaccine (contained in DTP and DTaP) can prevent this disease

Measles

- Highly contagious respiratory disease
- Causes rash, high fever, cough, runny nose, and red, watery eyes, lasting about a week
- Causes ear infections and pneumonia in 1 out of every 12 children who get it
- Causes encephalitis that can lead to convulsions, deafness, or mental retardation in 1 to 2 of every 2000 people who get it
- Of every 1000 people who get measles, 1 to 2 will die
- Measles vaccine (contained in MMR, MR, and measles-only vaccines) can prevent this disease

Mumps

- Causes fever, headache, and swelling of one or both cheeks or sides of the jaw
- Four to 6 persons out of 100 who get mumps will get meningitis
- Inflammation of the testicles occurs in about 4 of every 10 adult males who get mumps
- May result in hearing loss, which is usually permanent
- Mumps vaccine (contained in MMR vaccine) can prevent this disease

Rubella

- Also known as German measles
- Mild disease in children and young adults, causing rash and fever for 2 to 3 days

Box 11-2–VACCINE-PREVENTABLE CHILDHOOD DISEASES *Continued*

- Causes devastating birth defects if acquired by a pregnant woman; there is at least a 20% chance of damage to the fetus if a woman is infected early in pregnancy
- Rubella vaccine (contained in MMR and MR vaccines) can prevent this disease

Haemophilus influenzae type b (Hib)

- Causes meningitis, pneumonia, sepsis, arthritis, and skin and throat infections
- More serious in children under age 1; after age 5, there is little risk of getting the disease
- Before 1992, Hib was the most common cause of bacterial meningitis in the U.S.
- Before the introduction of infant vaccination, 1 child in 200 was affected before age 5
- One out of 20 children who get Hib meningitis will die, and 10–30% of survivors will have permanent brain damage
- Hib vaccine can prevent this disease

Pneumococcal infection

- Causes meningitis, pneumonia, sepis, ear infections, hearing loss, brain damage, and death
- Children under age 5 highest risk for serious disease
- Vaccine prevents 90% of cases of invasive (serious) disease and spreading of disease from person to person

Varicella

- Also known as chickenpox
- Varicella-zoster is a virus of the herpes family
- Highly contagious, it causes a skin rash of a few or hundreds of blister-like lesions, usually on the face, scalp, or trunk
- Usually more severe in older children (age 13 or older) and adults
- Although complications are rare, annually 9000 hospitalizations for chickenpox occur in the United States, with up to 100 deaths
- Complications include bacterial infection of the skin, swelling of the brain, and pneumonia
- Often leads to quarantine, causing children to miss school and parents to miss work
- Varicella vaccine can prevent this disease

Hepatitis B

- Can destroy the liver (cirrhosis)
- Can lead to liver cancer
- Causes pain in muscles, joints, or stomach
- Hepatitis B vaccine can prevent this disease

Source: Centers for Disease Control and Prevention.

Box 11-3-Are You 11-19 Years Old?

Then you need to be vaccinated against these serious diseases!

Many people between the ages of 11 and 19 think they are done getting immunized against diseases like measles and tetanus. They think shots are just for little kids. But guess what? There are millions of people between the ages of 11 and 19 who need tetanus-diphtheria shots, hepatitis B shots, hepatitis A shots, chickenpox shots, measles-mumps-rubella shots, "flu," and/or pneumococcal shots. Are you one of them?

Getting immunized is a lifelong, life-protecting job. Make sure you and your doctor or nurse keep it up! Don't leave your clinic without making sure you've had all the shots you need.

Hepatitis B (Hep-B)
You need two or three doses of hepatitis B vaccine if you have not already received them.

Measles, Mumps, Rubella (MMR)
Check with your doctor or nurse to make sure you've had your second dose of MMR.

Tetanus, diphtheria (Td) ("tetanus shot")
You need a booster dose of Td between the ages of 11 and 16 (if it has been 5 years or more since your last dose). After that you will need a "tetanus shot" every ten years. A tetanus shot is not just something you get when you step on a nail!

Varicella (Var) ("chickenpox shot")
If you have not been previously vaccinated and have not had chickenpox, you should get vaccinated against this disease. Children 12 years of age and under need one dose. Teens 13 years of age and older need two doses.

Hepatitis A (Hep A)
Many teens need protection from hepatitis A. Do you travel outside the United States?* Do you live in a community with a high rate of hepatitis A? Are you a male who has sex with another male? Do you inject drugs? Do you have a clotting factor disorder or chronic hepatitis? Talk to your doctor or nurse regarding your risk factors.

Box 11-3—Are You 11–19 Years Old? *Continued*

Meningococcal vaccine

Many teens will live in dormatories at boarding school or in college. Talk to your doctor or nurse about this "meningitis shot."

Influenza vaccine ("flu shot")

Do you have a chronic health problem such as asthma, diabetes, heart disease, etc.? "Flu shots" are recommended every fall for many people with chronic diseases. Ask your doctor or nurse if you should have a yearly "flu shot."

Pneumococcal vaccine ("pneumococcal shot")

Do you have a chronic health problem? Talk to your doctor or nurse about whether you should receive a "pneumococcal shot."

*Do you travel outside the United States?

If so, you may need additional vaccines, including hepatitis A vaccine. Consult your clinic or local health department about recommended and/or required vaccines for your destination.

A special message for parents of 11–12 year olds

A visit to the clinic when a child is 11–12 years old is recommended by the American Academy of Pediatrics, the American Academy of Family Physicians, the American Medical Association, and the U.S. Public Health Service. This visit is a good time to make sure your child has had all the shots he or she needs!

Source: Centers for Disease Control and Prevention.

Common side effects include redness, swelling, and soreness at the injection site, low-grade fever (<100°F), rash at the injection site, and, rarely, nausea or a more generalized rash.[7] Although all states do not currently provide free varicella vaccination, it is expected to become part of the universal "package" within the next few years. Meanwhile, most HMOs and Medicaid programs include this immunization as part of their insurance coverage.

Some advice that should be emphasized to parents regarding the risks and benefits of administering the varicella vaccine include

- Administering the vaccine does not guarantee that a child will not contract a varicella infection.
- About 1–3% of children receiving the vaccine will get a breakthrough infection; however, the infection that they may get is much milder than that caused by a natural infection.
- If a child does get a rash after receiving the varicella vaccine, it is highly unlikely that he or she will transmit the virus to others; however, there is good evidence that those who are immunocompromised should be protected from persons who have received this vaccine.[7, 14, 15]
- It is also uncertain whether the immunization offers life-long protection. At this point, experts think that it offers protection for at least 10 years and possibly as long as 20 years. Therefore, it is possible that a second dose may be needed for those immunized in early childhood.

What advice should be offered to older children and adults? If they have had a varicella infection, they do not need to be immunized, since they have natural immunity. If they have not had a varicella infection or are unsure of their status, then they should be serologically tested and immunized if they are seronegative. This is especially important for health care workers and day care workers. It is also true that over 70% of adults with a negative history for varicella infection have serologic evidence of past infection.[7] A study published in July 1998 in the *Journal of the American Board of Family Practice* convincingly demonstrated that serologic testing should be performed on any individual who does not have a positive varicella history. The positive predictive value of a history of varicella is .985 (or, more simply, the history accurately predicts a past infection more than 98% of the time). However, the negative predictive value of a negative history is only .23. Therefore, we cannot reliably depend upon the patient's negative history to be the determining factor for administering or not administering the vaccine.[13] If a patient does not relate a history of varicella infection, the patient should have a serologic test for varicella antibodies and, if the result is negative, be administered the vaccine. This is the most cost-effective and evidence-based approach.

ROTAVIRUS

Rotavirus is the most common cause of severe gastroenteritis in preschool children. Annual hospitalization rates for rotavirus in the U.S. range from 2300 to 110,000, with data published in 1999 suggesting that the rate is closer to 50,000.[16–18] Since the virus is transmitted by the fecal-oral route, transmission among family members and within day care and preschool settings is very common. Other burdens of this illness include approximately 410,000 physician visits per year, $264 million spent for medical costs (66% of which was related to hospitalizations), and $1.001 billion in costs related to lost work time for parents.[16] It is also estimated that administration of the vaccine could result in a 73% reduction in physician office visits per year.[16] Armed with these statistics, many argued *initially* for the universal administration of this vaccine, including the AAP and the ACIP.

However, four counter concerns should be taken into consideration when discussing the need for universal rotavirus vaccination.[16] First, the patient-centered and evidence-based approach should be honored in the case of this vaccine. The rotavirus vaccine confers no herd immunity because a significant number of children will not benefit from immunization of a large portion of the child population. Second, there appears to be a real potential for decreased acceptance of vaccines in general on the part of parents. At this time, 28 vaccinations are recommended in the first 18 months of life. Adding three more injections may be the proverbial last straw for some parents. This is particularly important in the case of parents who already have a low compliance rate for obtaining immunizations for their children and for those who are at highest risk for rotavirus infection. Third, there is the important factor of cost. The cost of the vaccine from the manufacturer is $38.75 per dose, or $116.25 for the three doses at 2, 4, and 6 months of age.[18] To date, managed care organizations have not yet had enough experience with this vaccine to know the impact of this cost on capitation rates for primary care physicians. Fourth, and most importantly, data are inadequate to support a universal recommendation. The CDC staff has reminded the ACIP group that the CDC's initial findings are pilot data and argued that more documentation and a further observation period of 1 to 2 years is needed.[16] This is especially prophetic in light of the CDC's actions in 1999 that first postponed and later removed this vaccine from the market because of a cluster of intussusception reports among 15 infants who received the rotavirus vaccine. Although this vaccine may offer substantial benefits to children in underdeveloped countries, it currently seems to have been removed from general use within the U.S.

MENINGOCOCCUS

Neisseria meningitidis is an important cause of bacterial meningitis and sepsis in children and young adults in the U.S. The meningococcal vaccine effective against serotypes C and Y (but not B) has been available for many years and has been used with approximately 70% success in foreign travelers and the American military. "At its October 20, 1999 meeting, the ACIP, citing results of two CDC studies done in 1998 which identified a slightly higher risk among [college] freshman dormitory residents, recommended that those who provide medical care to this group give information to students and their parents about meningococcal disease and benefits of vaccination. . . . Approximately 300 cases . . . occur each year in the U.S., and 10–13% . . . die despite [early treatment]."[9] Although less than 30 of these cases occurred in freshman college students during 1998, the American College Health Association (ACHA) has recommended a proactive education campaign about this disease and vaccination option pending more definitive studies by the CDC.

HEPATITIS

The hepatitis A vaccine is currently recommended for residence in or travel to endemic areas and to those who engage in anal or anal-oral sexual relations. The hepatitis B vaccine confers protection from hepatitis D, since hepatitis B is required for the D virus to replicate. Hepatitis C is responsible for more than 50% of all cases of chronic liver disease. Within the next 10 or more years, it is hoped that a vaccine may become available to prevent hepatitis C, which is prone to mutation, much as the HIV virus.

VACCINATION AND DISEASE

Periodically local activists or the media explore allegations regarding sensational associations between vaccination and disease. On November 12, 2000, CBS's "60 Minutes" aired a segment investigating allegations of an association between the MMR vaccine and autism. Similar concerns have been voiced regarding an association between this same vaccine and inflammatory bowel disease. While there is plentiful credible evidence in the literature that may satisfy the health care provider that no such association exists, the clinician engaged in patient education is most successful combating parental concerns when armed with information sources about such concerns. The CDC offers resources, links, and patient education materials on its web page at http://www.cdc.gov/nip/vacsafe/concerns.

CONCLUSION

This chapter summarizes the current immunization schedule for children (see Fig. 11–1), adolescents, and adults, discusses the current rationale for these immunizations, and also briefly discusses the current controversies in immunization recommendations. Immunizations are an important element in the health care and health counseling offered to patients. In fact, in the CDC's list of Top Ten Prevention Interventions, childhood immunizations and the pneumococcal vaccine are listed as numbers one and three, respectively. It is hoped that the reader will be able to use this information to guide discussions with patients and/or parents in the office setting. For a more in-depth discussion of the topics raised in this chapter, the reader is referred to the resources and references at the end of this chapter and additional CDC resources in the Resources Appendix at the end of this book.

REFERENCES

1. Cogswell B, Eggert M. People want doctors to give more preventive care. Arch Fam Med 1993;2:611–619.
2. Kamerow D. Prioritizing prevention [editorial]. J Fam Pract 1994;38:229–230.
3. United States Preventive Services Task Force. Guide to Clinical Preventive Services: An Assessment of the Effectiveness of 169 Interventions, 2nd ed. Baltimore, Williams & Wilkins, 1996.
4. Stoto MA, Behrens R, Rosemont C (eds). Healthy People 2000: Citizens Chart the Course. Washington, DC, National Academy Press, 1990.
5. Stange KC, Fedirko T, Zyzanski SJ, et al. How do family physicians prioritize delivery of multiple preventive services? J Fam Pract 1994;38:231–237.
6. What Would Happen if We Stopped Vaccinations? CDC web site, 1999.
7. Zimmerman RK, Spann SJ. Poliovirus vaccine options. Am Fam Physician 1999;59:113–118.
8. Physician Peer Education Project on Immunization. Michigan Department of Community Health, 1998.
9. Vaccine-preventable childhood diseases. CDC web site, 2000.
10. AAP Committee on Infectious Diseases. Acellular pertussis vaccine: Recommendations for use as the initial series in infants and children. Pediatrics 1997;99:282–288.
11. Atkinson W, Furphy L, Gannt J, et al. Epidemiology and prevention of vaccine-preventable diseases, 3rd ed. Department of Health and Human Services, Centers for Disease Control and Prevention, 1996.
12. Michigan Immunization Update. Michigan Department of Community Health, 6:1–20, 1999.
13. Jerant AF, DeGaetano JS, Epperly TD, et al. Varicella susceptibility and vaccination strategies in young adults. J Am Board Fam Pract 1998;11:296–306.
14. Michigan Department of Community Health, Fact Sheet on Immunizations, 1999.
15. Michigan Department of Community Health Immunizations in Michigan: Fact Sheet. 8/20/97.
16. Zimmerman RK, Ganiats TG. Controversies in family medicine: Universal

rotavirus immunizations. Should rotavirus vaccine be recommended for universal use? J Fam Pract 1999;48:146–148.

17. Reeg MP. Rotavirus vaccine for prevention of rotaviral gastroenteritis. AAFP Home Study Self-Assessment, Therapeutic Update #239. April 1999.

18. A vaccine for rotavirus. The Medical Letter 1999;41:50.

RESOURCES

The National Immunization Program (NIP) of the CDC, web site: http://www.cdc.gov/nip. (See also Boxes 11–1, 11–2, and 11–3 of this chapter for three excellent promotional flyers produced by the CDC for patient/parent education.)

All Kids Count (AKC) has compiled a directory of vendors offering immunization registry software and support. http://www.allkidscount.org

Vaccine information for Spanish speakers. The Michigan State University Extension's Physician Peer Education Project on Immunization has developed a videotape set of vaccine information statements (VISs) in Spanish. The six videos cover polio, Hib, varicella, DTP, hepatitis B, and MMR. Call 517-353-2596 for ordering information. Cost: ~$25.

Vaccine information in foreign languages. Foreign language VISs translated by California's DHS and Minnesota's DH can be downloaded from the Immunization Access Coalition (IAC) web site at: http://www.immunize.org/vis/.

IAC Express. To subscribe to the IAC listserv, send an e-mail to express@immunize.org. Then place the keyword "subscribe" in the subject field and send.

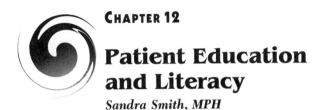

CHAPTER 12

Patient Education and Literacy

Sandra Smith, MPH

INTRODUCTION

This chapter describes two literacy problems plaguing the health care system at the turn of the millennium: hypoliteracy and hyperliteracy. *Hypoliteracy* (low literacy) refers to undeveloped or atrophied literacy skills. Hypoliteracy negatively affects health through lack of knowledge, resources, and empowerment. Hypoliteracy leaves patients unable to make sense of clinicians' instructions and unprepared to marshal the resources of an increasingly complex and technological health care system. *Hyperliteracy* refers to extremely high literacy, which can leave clinicians unable to communicate effectively with most patients. This chapter focuses on information necessary to clinicians to assist patients with low literacy levels while improving communication to all patients. After reading this chapter, providers will have

* Explored communication gaps resulting from mismatches in logic, language, and experience, that is, differences in the ways clinicians and patients think and talk about health and illness, and differences in their experience of the health care system
* Considered universal precautions to bridge communication gaps and help all patients understand, recall, and act on information about their conditions, treatments, self-care, and self-management
* Reviewed their legal responsibility and considered methods to communicate effectively with all patients in a language the patients can understand
* Identified resources for managing education for patients of all literacy levels

LITERACY AND HEALTH

WHAT IS LITERACY?

The definition of literacy has evolved over the last two centuries from the ability to write one's name, to the ability to recite prose, to the ability to read, and now to a new, broader concept. About 1950, literacy was defined as the ability to read; a person was said to be literate or illiterate based on various standards related to comprehension. The United States Army was among the first to realize that illiteracy could be hazardous to health and designated fifth grade reading ability as the threshold for recruits' literacy. The U.S. Census Bureau recorded as literate persons who could read at a sixth grade level, while the Department of Education said literate students read at the eighth grade level.[1]

Literacy took on a new definition under the 1991 National Literacy Act. Congress defined literacy as the ability to:

* Read, write and speak *in English*
* Compute and solve problems
* Function on the job and in society
* Achieve one's goals
* Develop one's knowledge and potential[2]

The National Literacy Act both broadened and narrowed the concept of literacy in the U.S. Its new definition of literacy recognizes that life in the Information Age requires higher levels of basic skills (word recognition, comprehension) and expands the concept of literacy to include problem solving and higher level reasoning skills (synthesis, analysis).

In this broadened view, a person is no longer said to be literate or illiterate, but rather more or less *functionally literate*. An individual's skills may be adequate to function day to day at a satisfactory level in one environment, e.g., a rural farming community, but inadequate in another environment, such as a university medical center. This line of thinking led to the concept of *health literacy*, described by Baker[3] as *ability to read and understand health-related materials*. Health literacy is discussed later in this chapter.

The 1991 National Literacy Act also narrowed the concept of literacy in the U.S. to English language proficiency. Following suit, at least 18 states have enacted "English-only" laws making English the official state language. For example, the Arizona constitution requires state employees to "act in English and no other language." The U.S. House of Representatives considered similar legislation in 1996. The proliferation of English-only statutes threatens the ability of persons with limited English proficiency (LEP) to access health care services and contradicts other laws requiring health care providers to bridge communications barriers. The constitutionality of these English-only laws has been challenged, and their future remains clouded.[4]

WHO IS LITERATE?

Little was known about the literacy skills of American adults until 1993, when the U.S. Department of Education published results of the National Adult Literacy Survey (NALS). This monumental study interviewed 26,000 adults and tested their literacy skills in three areas, each reflecting a different type of literacy task. Reading tasks, such as finding information in a newspaper story, reflect *prose literacy.* Document *literacy* is demonstrated, for example, by completing forms. *Quantitative literacy,* also called *numeracy,* is reflected in tasks requiring computing or interpretation of charts or tables.

NALS makes clear that literacy is not something someone has or does not have. NALS measured literacy on a continuum divided into five *Functional Competency Levels.* Level 1 reflects the lowest skill level and Level 5 the highest. An individual may perform at different levels on different skills and under different conditions (Fig. 12–1).

NALS found about one in five American adults at Functional Competency Level 1. Although NALS levels are not designed to be comparable to school grades, Level 1 prose literacy is roughly equivalent to a fifth grade or lower reading level.[2] This means that about 40 to 44 million of the 191 million Americans over age 16 are hypoliterate—they have low functional literacy. Of these, about 4%, or 1.6 million, cannot complete the most basic literacy tasks, such as finding one piece of information in a sports article. It is also notable that the vast majority of adults in Level 1 describe themselves as reading well or very well.

Hypoliteracy may result from lack of education or poor quality education; 62% of adults in NALS Level 1 did not graduate from high school. Hypoliteracy may also be attributable to atrophied skills among those unaccustomed to learning by reading and many years out of school; 71% of Level 1 adults are over age 60. Low functional literacy also may be the result of LEP, common among immigrant and refugee populations; 25% of those in Level 1 are immigrants who have just begun to learn English.

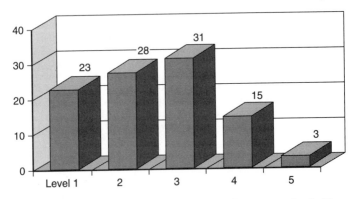

Figure 12–1. Percentage of U.S. adults in functional competency levels. (From U.S. National Adult Literacy Survey 1993, U.S. Department of Education, 1993.)

Most Americans in Level 1 are white and U.S.-born. Disproportionately represented are people with low incomes, minorities, and inner city and rural populations. Since persons of low income, low education, and advanced age carry the largest disease burden and have the highest need for health and medical information, literacy is a critical issue for the health care system, particularly for clinicians.

Although hypoliteracy crosses all social, economic, educational, and political boundaries, it carries a significant stigma and is a source of shame, feelings of inadequacy, fear, and vulnerability. Most hypoliterate persons are adept at hiding their difficulty from their spouses, children, friends, coworkers, and doctors.[5] Clinicians encounter hypoliterate patients daily without recognizing them.

NALS data have been variously interpreted and misinterpreted in the medical literature, sometimes confounding common sense. Recent journal articles have reported that adults in Level 1 "cannot read and write well enough to meet the needs of everyday living and working,"[3] and that "they are unable to assimilate the information that could improve their health."[6] Katz[7] describes illiteracy as a "permanent barrier to learning." Titles of several journal articles refer to "patients who cannot read" or to "illiterate patients."[8, 9]

NALS data show that hypoliterate persons are at a disadvantage in society. They do not have the full range of economic, social, and personal options that are available to Americans with higher levels of literacy skills. However, researchers who developed NALS emphasize that patients in Level 1 are not "illiterate." They are able to perform a variety of literacy and other tasks that life may require of them. They may be highly functional in familiar surroundings.[10]

Most people with hypoliteracy have average intelligence and function quite well by compensating in other ways for lack of literacy skills. They can learn what they need to know to maintain their health or manage disease. They can learn from nearly any health instruction that is designed and presented in ways suitable for them[11] (see Box 12–1).

THE HEALTH-LITERACY CONNECTION

However health is defined or measured, it is negatively affected by low literacy, both directly and indirectly. It is hardly surprising that failure to understand information about medications, health practices, and safety risks can result in health problems.

Three themes emerge from consideration of variables through which literacy affects health.

1. Lack of knowledge—about health and health services, about how to get information and assistance
2. Lack of resources—safe living conditions, food, medical care and supplies, health services

---

Box 12-1–SKILL LEVELS OF ADULTS AT FUNCTIONAL COMPETENCY LEVEL I

Usually Can

- Sign one's name
- Identify a country in a short article
- Locate one piece of information in a sports article
- Locate expiration date on a driver's license
- Total a bank deposit

Usually Cannot

- Locate an intersection on a street map
- Locate two pieces of information in a sports article
- Fill out a social security application
- Total costs on an order form

From Reader S. The State of Literacy in America. Washington, DC, National Institute for Literacy, 1998.

3. Lack of empowerment and control—patients' limited self-advocacy and self-efficacy, unemployment and low income, limited control over their own health.[12]

Direct impacts of hypoliteracy on health include not following medical instructions and incorrect use of medication, such as mixing up bottles. Similarly, infant health is directly impacted by parents' hypoliteracy when parents improperly administer infant formula. These occurrences are frequently mistaken for noncompliance.

Safety risks are another direct impact of hypoliteracy. Low-literacy workers often are limited to dangerous work environments and have higher than average rates of accidents, often owing to inability to read or understand warnings.[12]

The major impact of low literacy on health status occurs indirectly and has significant implications for preventive services.

Literacy and Poverty

Documentation of links between poverty and ill health is extensive.[13] In turn, education and literacy are the primary factors in poverty.[14] Literacy is a critical determinant of employability. It is closely related to employment and income. According to the U.S. Department of Labor, about 40% of existing jobs can be done by unskilled workers, but only 27% of newly created jobs will be in that category.[1] Because hypoliteracy severely limits employment opportunities, it can "cause" poverty. Without literacy skills, chances of escaping poverty are slim.

In addition, people with low literacy are likely to live in low-quality housing and in unsafe areas with higher rates of pollution, traffic, and crime. They are less likely to be in a position to install smoke detectors and other safety devices. For these reasons, accidents are more common among hypoliterate persons.[12]

Lifestyle Practices and Literacy

Hypoliteracy limits one's options to make lifestyle choices by limiting opportunities, knowledge, resources, and control. People with low literacy are more likely than others to engage in unhealthy behaviors such as smoking, poor nutrition, inactivity, not using seatbelts and bicycle helmets, not breastfeeding, and not obtaining blood pressure checks and Pap smears. Hypoliterate persons are less likely to be aware of the importance of healthy lifestyle practices.[15]

Stress, Lack of Control, and Literacy

For someone who lacks literacy skills, coping with the literacy demands of a technologically advanced society is stressful by itself. In addition, hypoliteracy may introduce stress from unemployment, poverty, unsafe living and working conditions, uncertainty, or lack of control of one's own life. At the same time, low literacy severely limits resources available to cope with these stressors.

Stress is recognized as a health problem in itself. For example, stress is a major factor in depression and other mental illnesses and can lead to other diseases. Change is a source of stress for everyone but a severe disadvantage for persons with limited literacy who rely on routines, landmarks, and set processes. In a stable environment, they may function very well, but they are likely to suffer increased stress when environments change.

The stigma attached to low literacy leads to stress, shame, and low self-esteem. Many persons with low literacy have invested a lifetime in hiding their disability.[15] Stress and shame related to low literacy have significant implications for preventive services. The stress involved in the process of obtaining care can discourage hypoliterate patients from seeking care, especially preventive services. Shame and low self-esteem interfere with efforts to change health-related behavior. According to Bandura,[16] a feeling of confidence that one can do what is asked of him or her is the most important prerequisite for successful behavior change.

Health Affects Literacy

Clinicians need only observe themselves to notice that stress, hunger, fatigue, pain, illness, and medication reduce ability to apply literacy skills. Newcomer[17] showed that hormones secreted when an individual is under stress affect cognitive ability and memory. Greater stress corresponds to greater impairment. Therefore, even persons with well-developed reading, reasoning, and numeracy skills are likely to become less functionally literate when their condition warrants medical treatment, particularly hospitalization. Feeling stressed and lacking medical vocabulary, the patient may be unable to clearly describe his or her complaint, to answer or articulate questions, or to understand answers.

However health is measured, it is negatively impacted by hypoliteracy, both directly and indirectly. Conversely, poor health reduces literacy skills, even among the most proficient. Hypoliteracy limits opportunities, knowledge, resources, and control over one's own life. Persons with limited literacy are likely to have a high need for health care and to experience significant barriers to obtaining health information, locating health services, and accessing care.

◼◼◼◼LITERACY AND HEALTH CARE

Communication gaps between hyperliterate clinicians and hypoliterate patients have been described as mismatches in logic, language, and experience, that is, differences in the ways clinicians and patients think and talk about health and illness, and differences in their experience of the health care system.[11] The National Adult Literacy Survey found that about 20% of American adults are at Level 1 functional literacy, roughly equated to a fifth grade reading level or lower. Only 3% function at Level 5, the highest level of competence, roughly equivalent to a college graduate level of ability.

Because of their training and daily practice of advanced literacy skills, most, but not all, clinicians have Level 5 literacy skills and can be said to be hyperliterate. Although hyperliteracy—very high literacy—is generally considered an advantage, in health care delivery it leads to communication problems. Whereas hypoliteracy leaves patients unable to make sense of clinicians' instructions and unprepared to marshal the resources of an increasingly complex and technological health care system, hyperliteracy can leave clinicians unable to communicate effectively with most patients.

DIFFERENCES IN HOW PERSONS PROCESS INFORMATION

Although most people think of literacy in terms of reading comprehension, literacy skills also affect listening comprehension, the ability to understand verbal instruction.[3] There are significant differences in the ways that hypoliterate and hyperliterate persons obtain information and learn. Clinicians typically are highly successful, life-long learners with a gourmet's taste for knowledge. In contrast, patients with low literacy skills typically have had negative learning experiences associated with failure and embarrassment. For them, learning leaves a bitter taste, so they approach it with apprehension.

Even when highly motivated to learn, a hypoliterate patient may read or hear all or most words in an instruction and still obtain little or no meaning. While most clinicians, as skilled learners, are adept at interpreting meaning, patients with low literacy skills take words literally without interpreting them for new situations.[11] Therefore, as the cartoon illustrates, a patient who appears noncompliant in fact may be highly motivated to follow instructions to the letter, even if the instructions make no sense (Fig. 12–2).

Where hyperliterate persons read and listen with fluency and draw on broad vocabulary, hypoliterate persons often read or listen to one word at a time. When listening to verbal instruction, they may not hear the second half of a sentence because they are still digesting the first part, especially if the terms are unfamiliar. This may cause them to appear uninterested or distracted. Similarly, when people read one

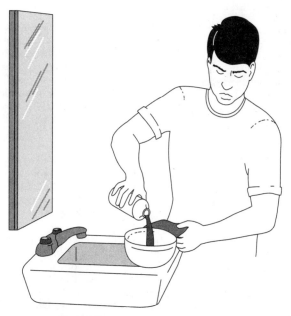

Figure 12–2. One capful every 4 hours.

word at a time, they may easily forget the beginning of a sentence by the time they get to the end, particularly if the sentence is long. Even when they can read and understand all the words, unskilled readers can miss the meaning of a sentence or paragraph.[11]

Although skilled readers are accustomed to deciphering the meaning of uncommon words, looking them up in a dictionary, or asking clarifying questions, unskilled readers typically skip over unfamiliar terms and avoid asking questions out of fear of revealing their low literacy or of appearing ignorant.

Unskilled readers may miss the context. For example, a person with low literacy skills may not infer from a brochure or discussion that the facts about a particular disease and how it affects other people also relate to his or her own life, unless the connection is specifically explained.

Although most people with hypoliteracy have adequate intelligence, their skills in decoding words and meaning, and in analyzing and synthesizing information tend to be inadequate to understand unfamiliar terms or complex presentations of facts.

THE ROLE OF LLE—LOGIC, LANGUAGE, EXPERIENCE

Additional communication problems arise in health care settings out of mismatches in clinicians' and patients' logic, language, and experience (LLE).[11] Humans learn by adding new information to what they already know, their logic, language, and experience. The cartoon illustrates what can happen when new information does not fit into the patient's LLE. In the cartoon, the patient adds new information—instruction to "take one capful" of medicine—to his existing LLE, which tells him that "cap" is his hat, and that he can drink from it in a pinch. So, being motivated to follow instructions, he pours the elixir into his cap.

Because of their training, clinicians think about illness and treatment in ways foreign to persons outside the medical professions. For example, most patients take medication to feel better. In this manner of thinking, it is logical to stop taking medication when symptoms abate; it does not make sense to continue taking antibiotics when feeling fine.

This mismatch in logic is particularly problematic in preventive services and with patients from certain cultural backgrounds. For example, Hispanic women view pregnancy as a normal, healthy condition, and view the health care system as a place to seek treatment for serious injury or disease. Another characteristic of Hispanic culture is fatalism, a sense that health and disease—including fetal and infant health—are divinely ordained and unlikely to be changed by human efforts. Further, in some Hispanic cultures, only a woman's husband can properly touch or examine her.[18] From this cultural background, seeking early prenatal care is illogical. It should not be surprising, then, that utilization of prenatal care services is low among Hispanic women.

Consider also the mismatch in experience of health care settings between clinicians and patients with low literacy levels. Whereas clinicians have daily experience in the medical office or hospital and so feel at home and in control in that setting, for patients, a visit to the doctor is by definition a stressful event. For many immigrants, a trip to the hospital may represent their first encounter with an institution of any kind.

The medical encounter can be particularly difficult for hypoliterate and LEP patients, who may experience significant difficulties just locating the facility. The usual signage, forms, questions, and instructions that are daily routine for health care professionals can be overwhelming to persons with low literacy. They may hesitate to ask for help, either because they do not speak English well, or out of fear of discovery of their low literacy and the attendant shame and potential discriminatory treatment. By the time the clinician sees the patient, the patient's stress level can be high enough to prevent effective application of whatever literacy skills he or she may possess. Newcomer[17] showed that hormones secreted when an individual is under stress affect cognitive ability and memory. Greater stress corresponds to greater impairment. Feeling stressed and lacking medical vocabulary, the patient may be unable to clearly describe his or her complaint and answer or articulate questions. Such a situation is ripe for missed or delayed diagnosis and inappropriate or unnecessary testing and treatment.

Perhaps the most apparent mismatches in health care settings are mismatches in language. Medicine has its own terminology, which is rarely heard outside the profession. Few English-speaking Americans understand even basic medical words, such as *void, laceration*, or *tumor*. Communicating risk information is particularly challenging, since hypoliterate persons have difficulty with fractions and statistics and may not connect facts about risks to others with risk to themselves.[11]

UNIVERSAL PRECAUTIONS FOR HYPOLITERACY

Goals of Patient Education: Enable patients to

* Make informed decisions
* Engage in self-care to survive and recover
* Recognize problems

* Seek timely, appropriate assistance
* Get information and find resources[19]

"Half the adult population needs easy-to-read materials, and the other half who do not need them wants them anyway."[20] People at all literacy levels can better understand simply written materials.[21, 22] College-educated readers report increased recall of key messages and express extreme satisfaction with fifth grade level health information materials.[23] A study comparing a simplified sixth grade level brochure to a tenth grade level brochure on the same topic demonstrated that patients of all reading levels and socioeconomic levels preferred the shorter, simpler material.[24]

Hypoliteracy affects more than just reading. Information that is incomprehensible in writing is still incomprehensible presented in person or on audio- or videotape. Whether reading, viewing, or listening, and regardless of their literacy skills, people under stress have limited ability to understand, and otherwise able learners prefer their information brief, clear, picturesque, and accurate.

Therefore, it makes sense to approach low literacy in health care settings with universal precautions. Universal precautions are principles and practices applied to all patients to prevent or mitigate the effects of literacy mismatches in health care settings.

A universal precautions approach recognizes that all patients' literacy skills are reduced by the physical and mental effects of illness and the stress associated with needing and obtaining medical care. In addition, since low literacy is associated with factors that increase need for health services, such as poverty, advanced age, and lack of education, it is likely that the majority of patients have low functional literacy.

A universal precautions approach further recognizes that most people outside the health and medical professions have low "health literacy," since medical topics are increasingly complex, technological, anxiety-producing, and unrelated to people's lives until they become patients—an occurrence most seek to avoid. Medical terms are rarely used in everyday conversations and are unfamiliar, even to the highly literate. Since a universal precautions approach anticipates that all patients will have difficulty understanding the language of medicine, it begins to position clinicians for a multicultural future and for treating increasing numbers of patients with LEP.

Because the same strategies that help patients with low literacy also help highly literate patients,[25, 26] there is no need to identify individuals with low literacy. There is no need to rate patients' "health literacy," and no need to provide printed information at various reading levels. Successful clinicians and health care systems are those who develop skills for communicating orally and in writing with persons with low functional literacy and lower health literacy, and who practice those skills with all patients.

Clinicians cannot change some factors in the effectiveness of health communications, such as cultural beliefs and values, formal education, socioeconomic status, language differences, and intellectual ability. However, research on patient education, patient satisfaction, adult learning, memory, and compliance indicates that clinicians can improve patients' comprehension of health messages. With the universal precautions described hereafter, clinicians can expect to achieve gains in patients' recall (knowledge), satisfaction, compliance, and outcomes.[23, 27–29]

Joseph Pulitzer's formula for prize-winning writing serves as a succinct and memorable statement of principles that can mitigate mismatches in literacy in health care settings:

> *Put it before them briefly so they will read it, clearly so they will appreciate it, picturesquely so they will remember it, and above all, accurately so they will be guided by its light.*
>
> —Joseph Pulitzer

Pulitzer offers an elegant guide to preparing or selecting materials for patients and planning educational interventions. The formula is applicable to all types of materials—printed, audio, video—as well as face-to-face communications.

At least 22 factors are known to affect suitability and effectiveness of materials. Detailed assessment instruments are available, notably the Suitability Assessment of Materials (SAM).[11] Clinicians who rigorously apply Pulitzer's formula will address most factors covered in more complex instruments.

Now, consider each element of Pulitzer's advice and its implications for practice.

Put it before them briefly so they will read it, . . .

Brief means short. Here it refers not only to the length of materials, but also to all aspects of the information package.

* Short words—one- or two-syllable common words
  Quick test: Hold your chin as you say the word. It should move once per syllable.
* Short sentences in writing and speaking—less than 15 words, one idea
* Short paragraphs—two to five sentences, one topic
* Short lines—30 to 50 characters and spaces
* Short lists—not more than 5 items

Put it before them . . . clearly so they will appreciate it, . . .

Clearly means clear to the reader, not open to interpretation. *Appreciate* does not mean grateful, although patients will be grateful for clear information and instruction. *Appreciate* means to understand and value the information so they can act on it. To speak or write *clearly*:

* Focus on behavior, not facts.

In other words, do not describe a condition the way clinicians are taught in medical school. Patients do not need to know the etiology, incidence, and prevalence of a disease. They need practical how-to information to make informed decisions, engage in self-care, recognize problems, seek timely and appropriate assistance, and get information or resources.

* Use the learners' LLE—logic, language, and experience—not yours.

When planning an educational intervention, start by inviting a group representative of the learners to tell you about their condition, what they think caused it, what it means in their lives, how they cope, and their experience of seeking treatment. This will allow you to think about the condition as the patients do, and to recognize their concerns and questions. It will give you specific words and phrases to use when discussing the condition that will make sense to them.

When administering a formal education intervention or initiating an informal teaching conversation, start with a learning needs assessment.[19] This can be a quick step that saves time and frustration for both patient and clinician. Informal conversation is an effective and unintimidating method of assessment.

- Set the stage by reminding patients that learning is part of treatment and recovery, that they should expect teaching from clinicians, and that their job is to understand and to ask questions when they do not.
- Find out what the learner knows already. Reinforce desired behaviors and correct misperceptions. Listen carefully to the patient's words and use them in your response.
- Determine the patient's readiness to learn. Ask directly what the patient wants to know and why it is important to him or her. Whatever that is, address it first. The patient is ready to learn about that topic.
- Find out what the patient believes. Tailor instruction for this patient by framing the conversation around his or her beliefs. Keep the focus on the critical minimum that the patient needs to know (despite your urge to teach something else).
- Recognize when you are not getting through. Any resistance is a

"red flag" that tells you to stop teaching and check for mismatches between your LLE and the patient's. Are you lecturing? Are you talking to the right person—should you be addressing the caregiver instead of the patient? Does the information conflict with something the patient already knows or believes? Does the advice seem irrelevant, impractical, or impossible in the patient's situation? In each case, stop and ask a question to refocus on what the patient needs to know to make an informed decision, engage in self-care, recognize problems, seek assistance, or get information and resources.

- In each sentence, start with what the patient already knows and believes. To get information into memory where it can become knowledge, the brain needs a place to put it. By starting with what the patient/learner already knows, you put the information on an established pathway into memory. Construct sentences with the known information first, followed by new information. For example, say *When you have a stomachache* (the part the patient knows), *call the doctor* (the new information). This construction is especially important to unskilled readers who may forget the first part of the sentence by the time they work through to the end.
- Replace or explain value judgment terms. Instructions that require patients to make a judgment are unclear. Rephrase to be specific and not open to interpretation. For example, instead of *heavy bleeding*, say *bleeding that soaks a pad in 2 hours*. Instead of *large clots*, say *clots the size of a golf ball or larger*—unless your learners do not play golf. Then you might say *the size of a walnut*. Instead of *fever* say *a temperature higher than 100 degrees*.
- Review, repeat, summarize. Adults learn by repetition. Say the most important thing three times. Do not be concerned about repeating yourself. Ask the patient to summarize the discussion about one topic before going on to the next.
- Test readability. *Readability*, the relative difficulty of decoding the words, typically is expressed as a school grade reading level required to recognize most of the words in a text. For example, materials with an eighth grade readability rating require reading skills equal to those of the average middle school student. Formulas that rate readability are based on syllables (or characters) per word and words per sentence. Some include a vocabulary list. A too-high readability rating readily identifies materials that exceed most patients' literacy skills.[30]

Readability is only one of many factors that make materials more or less useful for patients. Readability rating has well-known shortcomings.[31] Since it is quite possible to recognize all the words and still miss the meaning, a good (low) readability score cannot stand alone as a predictor of easy reading and understanding.

Clinicians who apply Pulitzer's formula as described in this section will likely achieve an appropriate readability level. Still, the importance of this factor warrants a policy requiring readability testing of all materials for patients. Several software programs, including Microsoft Word, apply one or more of the more than 40 readability formulas in existence, and, when properly applied, these formulas produce a rating that is accurate within a grade or two.[11]

For most patient populations, a fifth to sixth grade reading level is a reasonable standard. Materials at this level that are otherwise well designed can be independently understood by about 80% of the U.S. adult population. Patients with low literacy skills may stretch their capacity in order to understand information that is immediately applicable to a problem they have now.

Put it before them . . . picturesquely so they will remember it, . . .

Picturesque means attractive.

❋ We *do* judge books by their covers. Patients/learners will decide whether or not to read your instructions in a few seconds. The appearance of materials communicates loudly and clearly the importance the clinician places on the information. If it's only worth a quick and dirty photocopy, maybe it's not worth reading and following.

Picturesque also means the words paint a picture in the learner's mind. This returns to the issue of clarity and LLE. Familiar words make meaningful mental pictures. Technical terms, acronyms, and other jargon make static.

Replace this:	*With this:*
limbs	arms and legs
ambulate	walk
bacteria	germs

Put it before them . . . accurately so they will be guided by its light.

A rigorous expert review process is appropriate for all information on which patients rely. Clinicians typically are content experts. Content must be current, evidence-based, and independently reviewed for adherence to national guidelines as well as to local conventions.

Clinicians rarely are experts on materials development or specialists in health education, so presentation (format, design, graphics, typography) must be reviewed for adherence to health education theory separately from evaluation of design and graphics factors that affect readability, comprehension, and persuasiveness.

Patients themselves are the only reliable experts on the suitability and effectiveness of particular content and presentation. Information can be accurately stated and inaccurately interpreted. Misinterpretation may be due to the patients' low literacy skills, but more likely it is a problem of the writers'/teachers' failure to adequately consider the patients' LLE. Only patients/learners can tell you if information is attractive, understandable, and persuasive to them.

Brief interviews with 10 representative patients will be sufficient to reveal weaknesses in materials and suggest remedies. (Doak, Doak, and Root[11] offer details on how to involve patients in review and revision of materials.) Only when materials and planned oral presentations are pretested with patients and revised according to their suggestions are materials ready to be put before them as Pulitzer suggests.

Put it before them . . .

Briefly reviewing materials with each patient increases the proportion of patients for whom the materials are useful. This practice improves understanding and reinforces the key messages for readers at all literacy levels. Reviewing materials adds the motivating power of the clinician's endorsement. In the process, the materials cue the clinician to reinforce key messages.[29]

Give the patient a pen to write his or her name on the materials to demonstrate the importance of the information and of the patient's role. Refer to the materials to answer questions. Use a highlighter to point out areas of particular importance to the patient, such as warning signs to report and how to report them. This makes materials more useful when patients refer to them later or share them with a caregiver.

Reviewing printed information with the patient also gives the clinician opportunities to assess understanding by asking a question such as *What will you do if you have trouble breathing?* Do not ask *Do you understand?* No one wants to appear ignorant, so almost everyone will respond positively. Instead, take responsibility for the communication by asking *Is there something you'd like to go over again?*

▬ ASSURING LINGUISTIC ACCESS TO CARE

CLINICIANS' LEGAL RESPONSIBILITIES

Before 1975 only a few languages could be heard in the U.S. Since then, immigration patterns have changed dramatically. Now, U.S. residents speak at least 328 languages in addition to English. About 32 million U.S. residents, in both urban and rural areas, speak a language other than English at home.[32]

Increasingly, clinicians encounter patients who are immigrants or refugees unfamiliar with English. While these patients may be well educated and proficient in another language, by U.S. standards and for practical purposes they are hypoliterate owing to LEP—limited English proficiency. Many may have limited literacy skills in their primary language, or no literacy skills. According to the U.S. Department of Health and Human Services, non-English speakers face substantial communication barriers at almost every level of the health care system.[33]

When communication barriers prevent health care professionals from understanding their patients' symptoms, proper medical care and informed consent can be nearly impossible. Lack of appropriate linguistic services to facilitate communication between clinicians and patients with LEP is associated with failure to use preventive care.[36] In addition, cost of care may be increased by unnecessary testing,[35] extended treatment times,[36] delayed diagnosis, and increased chances of patients' inability to follow instructions.[37]

In most cases, providers have the means to overcome language barriers. Still, according to a report from the National Health Law Program,[4] current practice in most communities reflects an assumption that providers have no obligation to bridge language barriers, or that it is the patients' obligation to make themselves understood. In most instances, this assumption is wrong as a matter of law. Federal and state laws and accreditation standards require access to linguistically appropriate care.

Federal Law

> *No person in the United States shall, on the grounds of race, color or national origin, be excluded from participation in, be denied benefits of, or assistance, or be subjected to discrimination under any program or activity receiving Federal financial aid.*
>
> Title VI of the 1964 Civil Rights Act

Nondiscrimination language similar to that of Title VI in the Hill Burton Act and in Medicaid laws provides an additional base for requiring clinicians to overcome language barriers. In addition, the Health Care Financing Administration (HCFA), the agency in charge of Medicaid at the federal level, specifically requires states to communicate orally and in writing *in a language understood by the beneficiary.*[38]

The Office for Civil Rights has consistently taken the position that these federal laws place the burden of ensuring effective communication with LEP patients on the recipient of federal funds.[4] The obligations of Title VI and its implementing regulations apply to all recipients of federal funding, without regard to the amount of funding or the number of non-English speakers in a program. Since federal funding of medical care is so pervasive, nearly every health care provider is bound by Title VI.[4]

Liability for Negligence

Clinicians who fail to overcome language barriers run the risk of malpractice claims arising from injuries suffered as a result of miscommunication.[39] Providers also face potential claims that failure to ensure their understanding of the patient's complaints is a breach of professional standards of care.[4] Failure to ensure that the patient understands treatment options, risks, and benefits is a breach of informed consent requirements.

Accreditation Standards

Additional requirements to overcome language barriers are imposed by accrediting organizations. The Joint Commission on Accreditation of Healthcare Organizations (JCAHO) standards require hospitals to offer education to patients and families to enable them to meet patients' ongoing health care needs. Explanations and instructions must be presented in ways that are understandable to patients and their families, taking into account their culture and language.[40]

The National Committee for Quality Assurance (NCQA) accredits managed care organizations (MCOs) and produces the Health Plan Data and Information Set (HEDIS) to enable health care purchasers to evaluate the performance of MCOs. HEDIS asks MCOs to report how many doctors and staff serving Medicaid patients speak a language other than English, and the availability of out-of-plan interpreters for all members. HEDIS also asks for an inventory of all materials in languages other than English.

Many of the federal and state laws requiring health care providers to take steps to understand and be understood by LEP patients are relatively unknown and infrequently enforced. However, MCOs are dealing with language problems because of government regulation and to compete for market share. In an attempt to assure that MCOs prepare adequately for multicultural populations, states are including requirements for culturally sensitive services, translated written materials, use of interpreters, and multilingual staff in managed care contracts and requests for grant proposals.[4] Clinicians can anticipate growing pressure to comply with federal, state, and private mandates to ensure linguistic access to services and information for immigrant and refugee populations.

STEPS TO BRIDGE THE COMMUNICATION GAP WITH LEP PATIENTS

❋ Increase data collection.

Lack of data on the language and health needs of LEP patients makes it difficult to determine what specific steps clinicians should take to overcome language barriers, determine costs of linguistic services, and monitor provision of services. A logical first step for clinicians is to advocate for data collection in their service areas. At the same time, clinicians should consider involving consumers and their advocates in designing and implementing solutions.

❋ Translate patient education materials.

For cost-conscious clinicians and organizations, translating printed materials is a particularly attractive method of communicating with LEP patients. Materials can be reproduced and reused easily. Member service information and informed consent forms are now translated with some frequency. However, patient care instructions, satisfaction surveys, grievance forms, and bills are rarely available in any language other than English.

Availability of translated materials of any kind is limited. The quality of available materials varies widely. Straight translations that do not take into account differences within cultures and subtleties in language are likely to confuse and alienate readers. Since most English language materials exceed the literacy skills of most Americans,[11] translations of these materials are likely to be unsuitable for LEP patients. Certified professional translators should translate materials. Before use with patients, translated materials must be tested with representatives of the target audience, revised according to their recommendations, and retested. Clinicians can bridge language barriers, increase understanding and compliance, and reduce liability exposure by using quality materials to guide discussions and reinforce key messages.

❋ Hire bilingual staff and qualified interpreters.

Recruitment and hiring of bilingual and bicultural physicians, nurses, and health aides may be vital to delivering language-appropriate services to LEP patients. Professionally trained staff interpreters or a shared pool of contract interpreters can also improve services. Experts emphasize the need for interpreters to demonstrate skill in medical interpretation.

Clinicians should not rely on family, friends, or health care workers untrained for interpretation. Children should never be asked to translate. Untrained interpreters are prone to omissions, additions, substitutions, volunteered opinions, and semantic errors that can distort care.[41] Patients may speak less freely when family members, especially children, interpret.[42] Family interpreters might not translate accurately out of fear of the impact on the patient.[41] They rarely know medical terminology and may be uncomfortable discussing sensitive conditions (see Box 12–2).

How to Locate Qualified Interpreters

To locate medical interpreter services in your area, consult the telephone directory under Translators and Interpreters. Also, professional organizations specifically for medical interpreters are emerging around the country and can help clinicians locate services. These include the National Council on Interpretation in Health Care, the Massachusetts Medical Interpreter Association, the California Healthcare Interpreters Association, and the American Translators Association. For more information on these and other interpreters' organizations, visit the DiversityRX website at http://www.diversityrx.org/HTML/MOASSO.htm.

Clinicians who do not have ready access to qualified interpreters can obtain telephone interpretation services from English into 140

Box 12-2–The Use of Family and Friends as Interpreters

- Results in omissions, substitutions, and semantic errors that distort care
- Breaches confidentiality
- Creates barriers to the provider/patient relationship
- Upsets family relationships and hierarchies that are deeply rooted in culture
- Is particularly problematic in areas of gynecology, reproductive health, and sexually transmitted diseases
- Inhibits mental health treatment

From Perkins J, Simon M, Cheng F, et al. Ensuring Linguistic Access in Health Care Settings: Legal Rights and Responsibilities. Menlo Park, CA, The Henry J. Kaiser Family Foundation, 1998, p 11, reprinted with permission from the Henry J. Kaiser Family Foundation of Menlo Park, CA. The Kaiser Family Foundation is an independent health care philanthropy and is not associated with Kaiser Permanente or Kaiser Industries.

languages through AT&T Language Line Services. Call 1–800–752–0093, Ext. 196, or see http://www.languageline.com.

■ CONCLUSION

According to the 1990 census, U.S. residents speak more than 300 languages. Approximately 32 million persons, both in urban and rural areas, speak a language other than English at home. One in five U.S. adults are hypoliterate, medical conditions reduce functional literacy for all learners, and, since virtually all patients have low "health literacy"—little understanding of health and medical concepts and terminology—universal precautions are appropriate to mitigate communication problems in health care settings. Universal precautions for low health literacy recognize that strategies to assist low literacy patients help all patients, and, consequently, there is no need to identify patients with low literacy or to design educational interventions geared to particular literacy levels. Joseph Pulitzer's formula for prize-winning writing serves as an elegant guide to developing materials, planning education interventions, and engaging in informal teaching conversations with patients.

References

1. Ohio Literacy Network. Adult Literacy: Foundation for Progress. Online at wysiwyg://710http://archon.educ.kent.edu/Oasis/Resc/Educ/fb2.html.
2. Kirsch IS, Jungblut A, Lenkins L, et al: Adult Literacy in America: A First Look at the Results of the National Adult Literacy Survey. Washington, DC, U.S. Department of Education, 1993.
3. Baker DW, Parker RM, Williams MV, Clark, WS. Health Literacy and the Risk of Hospital Admission. J Gen Intern Med 1998;13:791–798.
4. Perkins J, Simon H, Cheng F, et al. Ensuring Linguistic Access in Health Care Settings: Legal Rights and Responsibilities. Menlo Park, CA, The Henry J. Kaiser Family Foundation, 1998, p 1.
5. Parikh NS, Parker RM, Nurss JR, et al. Shame and health literacy: The unspoken connection. Patient Educ Couns 1996;27:33–39.
6. Marwick C. Patients' lack of literacy may contribute to billions of dollars in higher hospital costs. JAMA 1997;278:971–972.
7. Katz, JR. Back to basics: Providing effective patient teaching. Am J Nurs 1997;97:33–36.
8. Medical Practice Communicator 1998;5:6. Online at medscape.com/HMI/MPCommunicator/1998/v05.n05/mpc0505.11.html.
9. Weiss BD, Coyne C. Communicating with patients who cannot read. N Engl J Med 1997;337:272–276.
10. Reader S. The State of Literacy in America. Washington, DC, National Institute for Literacy, 1998.

11. Doak L, Doak C, Root J. Teaching Patients with Low Literacy Skills, 2nd ed. Philadelphia, JB Lippincott, 1996.

12. Perrin B. Literacy & Health Project, Phase I Research Report. Ontario Public Health Association, 1989.

13. O'Campo P, Rojas-Smith L. Welfare reform and women's health: Review of the literature and implications for state policy. J Public Health Policy 1998; 19:420–446.

14. Calman KC. Equity, poverty and health for all. BMJ 1997;314:1187–1191.

15. Weiss BD, Hart G, McGee DL, D'Estelle S. Health status of illiterate adults: Relation between literacy and health status among persons with low literacy skills. J Am Board Fam Pract 1992;5:257–264.

16. Bandura A. Social Foundations of Thought and Action: A Social Cognitive Theory. Englewood Cliffs, NJ, Prentice-Hall, 1986.

17. Newcomer JW, Selke G, Melson AK, et al. Decreased memory performance in healthy humans induced by stress-level cortisol treatment. Arch Gen Psychiatry 1999;56:527–533.

18. Acalay R, Ghee A, Scrimshaw S. Designing prenatal care messages for low-income Mexican women. Public Health Rep 1993;108:354–362.

19. London F. No Time to Teach? A Nurses Guide to Patient & Family Education. Philadelphia, JB Lippincott, 1999, p 16.

20. Plimpton S, Root J. Materials and strategies that work in low literacy health communication. Public Health Rep 1994;109:86–92.

21. Ley P, Jain VK, Skilbeck CE. A method for decreasing patients' medication errors. Psychol Med 1976;6:599–691.

22. Mareaux EJ, Murphy PW, Arnold C, et al. Improving patient education for patients with low literacy skills. Am Fam Physician 1996;53:205–211.

23. Smith SA. Information giving: Effects on birth outcomes and patient satisfaction. Int Electronic J Health Educ 1998;3:135–145. Online at http://www.prenataled.com/newsv2n7.htm

24. Davis TC, Jackson RH, Bocchini JA, et al. Comprehension is greater using a short vaccine information pamphlet with graphics and simple language. J Gen Intern Med 1994;9(suppl 2):103.

25. Davis TC, Bocchini JA Jr, Fredrickson D, et al. Parent comprehension of polio vaccine information pamphlets. Pediatrics 1996;97:804–810.

26. Meade CD, Byrd JC, Lee M. Improving patient comprehension of literature on smoking. Am J Public Health 1989;79:1411–1412.

27. Arthur V. Written patient information: A review of the literature. J Adv Nurs 1995;21:1081–1086.

28. McCann S, Weinman J. Empowering the patient in the consultation: A pilot study. Patient Educ Couns 1996;27:227–234.

29. Doak C, Doak L, Friedell GM, Meade CD. Improving comprehension for cancer patients with low literacy skills: Strategies for clinicians. CA Cancer J Clin 1998;48:151–162.

30. Meade CD, Smith CF. Readability formulas: Cautions and criteria. Patient Education and Counseling 1991;17:153–158.

31. Foltz A, Sullivan J. Get real: Clinical testing of patients' reading abilities. Cancer Nurs 1998;21:162–166.

32. U.S. Department of Health and Human Services, Office for Civil Rights. Limited English Proficiency as a Barrier to Health & Social Services. Washington, DC, Macro International, 1995.

33. U.S. Department of Health and Human Services. Draft LEP Regulation,

45 C.F.R. Part 80 (on file with National Health Law Program). August 1993.

34. Woloshin S, Schwartz LM, Katz SJ, Welch HG. Is language a barrier to the use of preventive services? J Gen Intern Med 1997;12:472.

35. Donovan S. Language barriers hinder health care. USA Today, April 15, 1991.

36. Hagland MM, Sabatino F, Sherer JL. Crossing cultures: Hospitals begin breaking down the barriers to care. Hospitals (United States) 1993;67:22–25, 28–31.

37. Woloshin S. Language barriers in medicine in the United States. JAMA 1999;274:724–725.

38. Health Care Financing Administration. State Medicaid Manual. Washington, DC, March 1990.

39. Health Literacy Project (Brandes W, ed.). Literacy, Health and the Law. Philadelphia, Health Promotion Council of Southeastern PA, 1996.

40. Joint Commission on Accreditation of Healthcare Organizations. Comprehensive Accreditation Manual for Hospitals, 1996:PF-9-10, 1997.

41. Baker DW, Parker RM, Williams MV, et al. Use and effectiveness of interpreters in an emergency department. JAMA 1996;275:783–788.

42. Hafner L. Translation is not enough: Interpreting in a medical setting, West J Med 1992;197:255–259.

RESOURCES

PRACTICE GUIDELINES FOR CONTENT EVALUATION OR DEVELOPMENT

National Guideline Clearinghouse (NGC)

http://www.guidelines.gov

A public resource for evidence-based clinical practice guidelines. NGC is sponsored by the Agency for Health Care Policy and Research in partnership with the American Medical Association and the American Association of Health Plans.

http://www.PrenatalEd.com

PrenatalEd is a resource for health and medical professionals in their role as patient educators. It is an electronic handbook of scientific and practical information on developing and evaluating health related content and materials. The site editor is the author of this chapter. The site is sponsored by the award-winning prenatal patient education series, Beginnings: A Practical Guide Through Your Pregnancy.

PRIMARY CARE PRACTICE GUIDELINES

http://medicine.ucsf.edu/resources/guidelines/guide11.htm

This site is for primary care providers. Clinical or practice guidelines are "quality-improving strategies." Sackett DL, et al, in Evidence-based Medicine, define them as "user-friendly statements that bring together the best external evidence and other knowledge necessary for decision-making about a specific health problem."

PRENATAL EDUCATION GUIDELINES

http://www.PrenatalEd.com/hpbib.html

TOOLS TO EVALUATE AND IMPROVE PATIENT EDUCATION MATERIALS

Reviewers Guide and Checklist for Health Information Materials

http://www.prenataled.com/story7.html

University of Utah Substitute Word List

http://www.med.utah.edu/pated/authors/substitute2.html
Use this list to find simpler, more common words to replace medical terms.

REFERENCE BOOKS TO GUIDE PATIENT TEACHING

Doak L, Doak C, Root J. Teaching Patients with Low Literacy Skills, 2nd ed. Philadelphia, JB Lippincott, 1996.
London F. No Time to Teach? A Nurses Guide to Patient & Family Education. Philadelphia, JB Lippincott, 1999.
Lorig K. Patient Education: A Practical Approach. St. Louis, Mosby–Year Book, 1992.

RESOURCES EMPHASIZING COMMUNICATION SKILLS

http://hub1.worlded.org/health/comp/index.html
An annotated bibliography of print and web-based health materials for use with limited literacy adults.

RESOURCES FOR INTERPRETATION AND TRANSCULTURAL HEALTH SERVICES

Diversity RX
http://www.DiversityRx.org

Includes demographics and statistics on cultural and linguistic diversity in the U.S. models and strategies for overcoming linguistic barriers in health care, model policies and protocols, legal issues, networking opportunities, and links to interpreter services and additional cross cultural health care resources.

Ten Core Competencies for Interpreters in Community and Health Care Settings

http://wwwl.umn.edu/ccch/comp%26standard.html

Coughlan J. Bibliography for Medical Interpreting, 1998.

Online at CultureMed, State University of New York Institute of Technology

http://wwwl.sunyit.edu/library/culturemed/bib/medical/index.html

Also find here additional bibliographies on transcultural nursing; Bosnian, Russian, and Asian cultures and medicine; and links to culture and health web sites, refugee/immigrant health databases, and statistics.

CHAPTER 13

Nutrition Education in the Clinical Setting

Mark Abramson, MD,
Linda L. Summers, FNP, MA, MSN
and Sunnie Bell, RN, CDE

INTRODUCTION

Obesity, eating disorders, and other nutrition problems have been recognized as common health concerns affecting millions of Americans. The combined efforts of both patients and providers have had little impact on the problem of achieving successful weight loss in the majority of patients who are put on food management programs. Many disciplines have tackled this difficult problem, including primary care and internal medicine practitioners, midlevel providers, diabetic educators, dietitians, exercise physiologists, behavioral and psychological counselors, and clergy. All lend their particular areas of expertise and personal perspectives to the task. The real challenge for health care providers remains to identify those patients who would benefit from information and treatment and to determine at what point they should be provided with sound advice and skills for long-term lifestyle change and support.

On a daily basis health care providers find themselves telling, encouraging, threatening, and cajoling patients to stop smoking, lose weight, eat right, take medication as directed, exercise more, and implement stress-reducing measures. Health care providers are convinced that in order to improve health, the patient needs to assume new responsibilities and initiate change. Information overload can be costly and detrimental to motivating patients to change. During an office visit new information should be provided in blocks, remembering that retention of large amounts of material is not likely to occur once the patient steps out of the office. Important issues to include as time and patient interest warrant are dietary information (with visual aid), exercise information (with a reasonable exercise prescription), stress management (individualized to the patient), and behavioral changes (have a list of these in mind and offer them a few at a time). Other topics that can be covered include self-esteem, rituals involving food, depression and anxiety (and their impact on eating), food as an addiction, and identifying and intervening in stressful thinking patterns.[1] The health care provider needs a sound and up-to-date basis for information provided to the patient and a variety of food programs, exercise ideas, and interventions in order to ensure individualization.

An assessment of the patient should include an interview, as assessment of readiness to change (what stage of readiness rather than "ready-or-not"), and a functional analysis of the eating problem. The health care provider should explore what situations and feelings trigger eating behaviors, and what are the risks and benefits to both changing and not changing. Finally, the health care provider should avoid focusing entirely on the weight-related problem, and should explore how the patient is managing other areas of life, including health, work, family, social, and recreational needs.

There are no "magic bullets" in weight management. Recognizing this is an important start for both patients and health care providers. Clearly some behavioral techniques (planning and record keeping, specific reward systems, group work) have been shown to be helpful in the challenging but medically important task of weight loss. Most patients who are motivated to lose or gain weight, or to follow a specific eating plan for other health reasons, or who desire to improve the nutritional status of their meal plan, will benefit from close provider support and follow-up, information about specific eating plans, behavior modification, and social support.

PRINCIPLES AND PURPOSES

There is no mystery to a healthy diet. Except for a relatively small group of conditions (such as end stage renal failure, tropical sprue, or congenital metabolic deficiencies such as phenylketonuria, or maple syrup urine disease), the principles of good nutrition are similar for the vast majority of patients. In Western society, by far the most common reasons to offer nutrition education are obesity, hypercholesterolemia, hypertension, diabetes, and health maintenance (including counseling for adequate growth in children). For these common conditions encountered every day by primary care providers, the goal is a low-fat diet with the proper proportions of carbohydrate, fat, and protein, including appropriate amounts of calories as well as essential vitamins and minerals. The specifics of such a healthy diet follow in this chapter.

For most people, knowing the principles of what and how much to eat is only part of the "battle." Often the challenge is to change eating behaviors. Will patients put the education to use? The success rate of diet therapy alone or in combination with other treatment modalities varies by condition, use of exercise, patients' own perceived motivation, and other factors. Most reports show that long-term weight loss, for example, is quite low. At most, about 20% of patients achieve success, and those odds drop considerably in the morbidly obese. Your patients' past experiences in trying to lose weight and/or eat right for medical conditions may well reflect this low success rate. They and you may well be skeptical of succeeding at weight loss. When faced with these discouraging odds, should we as health care providers give up? The answer is to be analytical, not skeptical. Once you and your patients address these conflicts and concerns, any nutrition program can be evaluated as to whether it adheres to principles of sound nutrition.

The limiting factor in most nutritional treatment is compliance. The adverse consequences of obesity, hypertension, dyslipidemia, and diabetes are very prevalent. Even if noncompliance limits successful treatment to a small percentage of patients, that small percentage of successful patients still significantly reduces population morbidity and mortality. Hyperlipidemia has been proved to increase risk of heart attack and stroke. Obesity has been strongly linked to cardiovascular disease, type II diabetes, obstructive sleep apnea, and adverse social and psychological effects. Improving glycemic control in type II diabetes decreases the risk and severity of retinopathy, neuropathy, and renal disease.

Someone who has a genetic tendency for obesity may need to work harder to lose weight than someone who does not, but he or she still can lose weight. For the morbidly obese, the goal need not be, and probably should not be, achieving "ideal" body weight. The right nutritional behaviors will lead to some weight loss and decreased associated health risks.

Although obesity is not entirely inherited, congenital factors play a substantial role. Studies, including studies of identical twins separated at birth, have demonstrated the heritability of body fat distribution to be 65–75%.[2] The other side of the coin, however, is that there is still a significant part of anyone's weight over which he or she has more control. The prevalence of obesity has been shown to be increasing over the past several decades. A higher proportion of the population is overweight. Genetics does not explain this phenomenon. The gene pool of the human race cannot change that rapidly. Environment, namely less physical activity and increased fat intake, is the most likely cause of the trend. High-fat "fast foods" are more readily available, and sedentary activities such as watching television are more prevalent, than in the past. Many people "eat on the run," consuming high-fat, low-fiber foods. Also, more people own automobiles than in past years.

How much nutrition counseling primary care practitioners do themselves, and how many patients they refer to nutritionists or diabetes educators, usually depends on how comfortable a practitioner is in reviewing these issues, on economic factors, and on the resources that are available in the community. Whether or not the patient is seeing a nutrition educator, it is important for the primary care provider to be familiar with the issues and to discuss them with the patient during an office visit. As with most behavior modifications, the frequency of reinforcement is important, as is a consistent message from the nutritionist and the primary care provider.

Do all patients need nutrition education? Probably not, but they all should be evaluated. We routinely screen for diabetes and hypercholesterolemia, but we should also screen for obesity and discuss it with our patients. Several tools for obesity screening are included later in this chapter. If an obese patient is identified and the subject of obesity is not discussed, an understandable and probably common reaction by the patient will be to think, "Well, he didn't say anything, so it must not be that important." The interpretation is that tacit approval has been given. A few words from a health care provider identifying obesity as a problem may make a significant difference in how motivated patients may be to take behavioral steps to lower their health risks. The prevalence of obesity in children has been increasing since the 1970s. Education for good nutrition habits and exercise is certainly just as appropriate for children as for adults. Ideally, and almost necessarily, the whole family should have the same healthy eating habits.

The need for nutrition assessment and treatment may not always be obvious. Malnutrition may be overlooked as a cause or contributor to symptoms such as weakness, anemia, or jaundice. In addition, malnutrition must also be considered in the elderly, or on initial evaluation of the syndrome of failure to thrive in children. Difficulty chewing and ingesting food may go unnoticed in an elderly person with poorly fitting dentures and mild dementia. Someone may have an eating disorder, such as anorexia nervosa, bulimia, or binge eating. Infant powdered formula that is being mixed with too much water, either to save money or by mistake, will lead to malnutrition. A vegetarian may lack sufficient vitamin B_{12} and folate, leading to anemia and neurologic manifestations. Someone getting a large portion of calories from alcohol or other carbohydrates may have subclinical protein malnutrition. It is important to remember that the obese may also have underlying malnutrition related to essential nutrients. Clearly, education has a role in improving nutrition. Before education, other treatment, and improvement can start, however, nutrition must first be considered as an issue before it can be identified as one requiring attention.

■■■ MICRONUTRIENTS

Most nutrition counseling revolves around the three macronutrient, calorie-providing categories of carbohydrate, protein, and fat. Dietary fiber and the micronutrient vitamins and minerals also have important roles in primary and secondary disease prevention related to nutrition. Micronutrient deficiencies may lead to well-defined syndromes, for example, vitamin C deficiency and scurvy. "Fast foods" often have plenty of carbohydrate and protein, as well as too much fat, but are often lacking in vitamins and minerals found in fresh vegetables. An all-around healthy diet as detailed in this chapter should automatically incorporate adequate amounts of all essential vitamins and minerals.

Multivitamin supplements are generally safe; however, one must avoid amounts that are far above recommended daily amounts for the fat-soluble vitamins A, D, E, and K. Overdoses of these vitamins can be toxic and life-threatening.

The beneficial effects of the "antioxidant" vitamins A, E, and C have only been widely accepted in the traditional medical establishment relatively recently. Vitamin E has been shown to decrease risk of coronary artery disease. Folic acid deficiency in pregnant women has been shown to increase the risk of neural tube birth defects, and its supplementation, especially prior to and during pregnancy, will decrease this risk.[3] It may take a month or two of daily oral doses of folic acid to replenish depleted body stores. Thus, as part of the screening of any woman of reproductive age, if there is even a remote possibility she may become pregnant, she should be educated about folic acid and its benefits. Folic acid supplementation may help lower homocysteine levels, thus possibly lowering risk of vascular and heart disease.[4, 5]

Calcium is important for women of any age, and sufficient amounts lower risks for osteoporosis and hip fracture as well as for spinal compression fractures and their sequelae. Sufficient calcium intake is especially important in preadolescent and adolescent girls as well, with even greater amounts required for those who are participating in athletics or dance. Phosphate in carbonated beverages interferes with calcium absorption. Calcium is best absorbed with food.

Sodium chloride, while necessary for human life, is abundant and perhaps overly abundant in many foods. Some but not all people with hypertension are "salt (sodium) sensitive," and will have higher blood pressure if too much sodium is ingested. Excess sodium may also worsen pulmonary and peripheral edema.

When ingested in sufficient volume, dietary fiber is believed to decrease risk of colon cancer and diverticulosis.

GENERAL GUIDELINES FOR THE HOSPITALIZED PATIENT

Sometimes nutrition may be overlooked as an issue in the hospitalized patient. Most hospitals have nutritionists and diabetes educators. A serum prealbumin level is a useful test to help assess nutritional status and is often used in the hospital setting. When a patient is in the hospital for a condition that has a primary nutritional component to it, such as diabetes or diverticulitis, it makes sense to have the nutritionist educate the patient further, or simply to review dietary issues with him or her.[6] Obesity frequently contributes to patients' conditions or increases the risk of complications, such as degenerative joint disease and deep vein thrombosis. As the primary care provider, remember to read what the nutritionist has written in the chart. This will better help you to continue and reinforce the education on follow-up. Good nutrition is important for any type of healing. A variety of factors may necessitate enteral or parenteral nutrition, and your nutritionist or pharmacist will be able to guide you in these matters.

GUIDELINES AND TOOLS FOR INTEGRATION OF NUTRITION INTO A CLINICAL PRACTICE

Many components of a balanced, healthy diet can be adapted for use in healthy individuals for disease prevention as well as for disease management in people with chronic conditions requiring dietary interventions. General principles of meals based on high fiber, low fat, low cholesterol, lessened sodium and sugar, and higher complex carbohydrate food choices can be applied to many disease states. Since a good meal plan also considers overall improvements in thermogenic increases in metabolic rate as well as promotion of release of stored excess fat, consistency and regularity in meal timing and quantity are also important. A variety of foods with an abundance of low-calorie vegetables, sufficient fruits, grain products, and lean choices of dairy and meat products helps to ensure that nutrient needs are met while still controlling caloric intake.

Integrating principles of a balanced, healthy diet into a provider's practice can be easily accomplished with use of the food guide pyramid as long as the pyramid is specifically adapted to individual patient need based on states of health and disease. In the simple and practical program presented in this chapter, serving size aspects of the American Diabetes Association and the American Dietetic Association Exchange System have been joined to the food guide pyramid distribution of foods and numbers of servings. Total caloric intake and general principles of good nutrition as previously discussed are also included. This combination of systems makes the plan fully functional for a wide group of people who can benefit from improved nutrition. The succeeding sections of this chapter explain the combined system as well as provide simple-to-use tools for establishing a need for nutrition prescriptions, guidelines for determining caloric requirements for weight loss, weight gain, and weight maintenance, and calorie-specific plans utilizing guides included in this chapter.

TOOLS TO DETERMINE NEED FOR NUTRITIONAL WEIGHT CHANGE INTERVENTION

Waist Measurement

Men: Should be 40 inches or less for ages under 40.
       Should be 35 inches or less for ages 40 and above.

Women: Should be 35 inches or less for all ages.

Measure waist at the midpoint between the lower frontal rib and the iliac crest. Supine measurement is recommended to avoid inaccurate representation. Particularly in older people and/or the extremely obese, waist measurement may be altered by gravity shift of body mass.

Body Mass Index

Body Mass Index (BMI) =
      Weight in kilograms divided by squared height in meters

Conversions: Kilograms = pounds divided by 2.2
            Meters = inches multiplied by .0254

See Figure 13–1, a BMI chart.[7] The chart lists findings only for BMIs from 22 to 46. Underweight individuals are not represented on this chart. Therefore, calculation will be necessary (Fig. 13–2).[8]

* BMI between 19 and 24 is recommended.
* BMI less than 19 is underweight.
* BMI 25–29 is overweight.
* BMI 30 and above is obese.

Note: Consider muscle mass while computing BMI. Bodybuilders or heavily muscled individuals may have a relatively higher BMI that does not require intervention. Normal BMI calculations are based on average individuals who are not involved in bodybuilding exercise.

Weight Measurement

See the at-risk weight chart (Table 13–1) or calculate recommended weight based on height.

Male: First 60 in = 100 lb. Then add 6 lb for each additional inch of height over 5 ft.

Example: 6'2" male: 100 + (6 × 14) = 184 lb.

Female: First 60 in = 100 lb. Add 5 lb. for each additional inch of height over 5 ft.

Example: 5'5" female: 100 + (5 × 5) = 125 lb

  • Weight measurement up to 19% above recommended weight = Overweight
  • Weight measurement 20% or more above recommended weight = Obesity

Figure 13–1. Body Mass Index (BMI) Chart. The Body Mass Index does not consider gender. The chart is for both men and women. To use, find the height at the left and move right to find the weight. The number at the top of the column is the BMI. BMIs of 25 to 29 are considered overweight. Obesity is defined as 30 and above. Adapted from National Heart, Lung, and Blood Institute Body Mass Index Charts.

BMI	22	23	24	25	26	27	28	29	30	31	32	33	34	35	36	37	38	39	40	41	42	43	44	45	46
Height	Healthy			Overweight					Obese																
4'10"	105	110	115	119	124	129	134	138	143	148	153	158	162	167	172	177	181	186	191	196	201	205	210	215	220
4'11"	109	114	119	124	128	133	138	143	148	153	158	163	168	173	178	183	188	193	198	203	208	212	217	222	227
5'0"	112	118	123	128	133	138	143	148	153	158	163	168	174	179	184	189	194	199	204	209	215	220	225	230	235
5'1"	116	122	127	132	137	143	148	153	158	164	169	174	180	185	190	195	201	206	211	217	222	227	232	238	243
5'2"	120	126	131	136	142	147	153	158	164	169	175	180	186	191	196	202	207	213	218	224	229	235	240	246	251
5'3"	124	130	135	141	146	152	158	163	169	175	180	186	191	197	203	208	214	220	225	231	237	242	248	254	259
5'4"	128	134	140	145	151	157	163	169	174	180	186	192	197	204	209	215	221	227	232	238	244	250	256	262	267
5'5"	132	138	144	150	156	162	168	174	180	186	192	198	204	210	216	222	228	234	240	246	252	258	264	270	276
5'6"	136	142	148	155	161	167	173	179	186	192	198	204	210	216	223	229	235	241	247	253	260	266	272	278	284
5'7"	140	146	153	159	166	172	178	185	191	198	204	211	217	223	230	236	242	249	255	261	268	274	280	287	293
5'8"	144	151	158	164	171	177	184	190	197	203	210	216	223	230	236	243	249	256	262	269	276	282	289	295	302
5'9"	149	155	162	169	176	182	189	196	203	209	216	223	230	236	243	250	257	263	270	277	284	291	297	304	311
5'10"	153	160	167	174	181	188	195	202	209	216	222	229	236	243	250	257	264	271	278	285	292	299	306	313	320
5'11"	157	165	172	179	186	193	200	208	215	222	229	236	243	250	257	265	272	279	286	293	301	308	315	322	329
6'0"	162	169	177	184	191	199	206	213	221	228	235	242	250	258	265	272	279	287	294	302	309	316	324	331	338
6'1"	166	174	182	189	197	204	212	219	227	235	242	250	257	265	272	280	288	295	302	310	318	325	333	340	348
6'2"	171	179	186	194	202	210	218	225	233	241	249	256	264	272	280	287	295	303	311	319	326	334	342	350	358
6'3"	176	184	192	200	208	216	224	232	240	248	256	264	272	279	287	295	303	311	319	327	335	343	351	359	367
6'4"	180	189	197	205	213	221	230	238	246	254	263	271	279	287	295	304	312	320	328	336	344	353	361	369	377

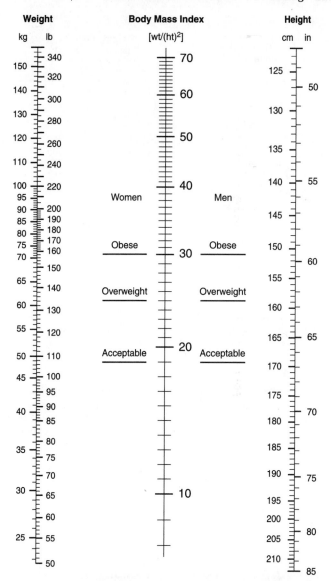

Figure 13–2. Nomogram for body mass index. (From Bray GA. Definitions, measurement, and classification of obesity. Int J Obes Relat Metab Disord 1978; 2:99–112, with permission.)

Table 13–1. At-Risk Weight Chart

Height (Feet/ Inches, Without Shoes)	Weight (Pounds, Without Clothing)	
	Women	*Men*
4' 9"	134	
4' 10"	137	
4' 11"	140	
5' 0"	143	
5' 1"	146	157
5' 2"	150	160
5' 3"	154	162
5' 4"	157	165
5' 5"	161	168
5' 6"	164	172
5' 7"	168	175
5' 8"	172	179
5' 9"	175	182
5' 10"	178	186
5' 11"	182	190
6' 0"		194
6' 1"		199
6' 2"		203
6' 3"		209

Waist-Hip Ratio

While any of the above methods may be used independently to document medical need for weight loss, waist-hip ratio (Fig. 13–3)[9] indicates relationship of high-risk upper body fat to lower risk peripheral fat. However, simple supine waist measurement is recommended as an adequate indicator of visceral (upper body) fat.

Generally, individual conditions or diseases define dietary need. When it is necessary to convince patients without obvious problems of the need for dietary modifications, the preceding measurements may prove helpful. Other indicators that may assist in creating patient awareness include the presence of acanthosis nigricans as a sign of compensatory hyperinsulinemia and pendulous abdominal fat.

RECOMMENDED TOOLS FOR DETERMINING CALORIC PRESCRIPTIONS

Methods of determining caloric prescriptions vary from simple to complex. Collaboration with registered dietitians and certified diabetes

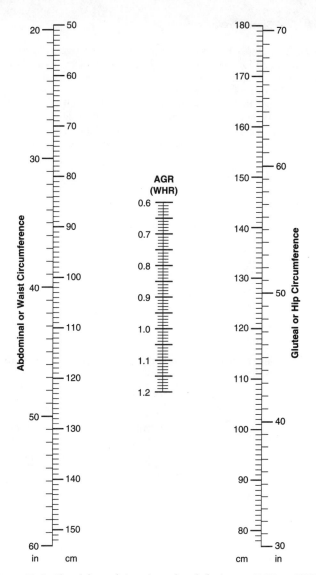

Figure 13–3. The abdominal (waist) to gluteal (hip) ratio (AGR or WHR) can be determined by placing a straightedge on the measurement for waist circumference and the measurement for hip circumference and reading the ratio from the point where this straightedge crosses the AGR or WHR line. The waist or abdominal circumference is the smallest circumference below the rib cage and above the umbilicus, and the hip or gluteal circumference is taken as the largest circumference at the posterior extension of the buttocks. (From Bray GA, Gray DS. Obesity, Part 1—Pathogenesis. West J Med 1988; 149:429–441, with permission.)

educators may be necessary in many cases. For basic prescriptions involving need for weight loss, weight gain, and uncomplicated diabetes management, the following methods may be helpful. They are arranged in order from simplest to complex.[10, 11]

Remember that, in general, women should consume at least 1200 calories, and men should consume at least 1800 calories per day to meet essential nutritional needs. Vitamin and mineral supplementation should be considered if caloric needs for weight loss fall below this range.

General Estimation

For weight loss, prescribe 10 calories per day for every pound of desirable weight.

> Examples: Female adult with desirable weight of 120 lb: 10 × 120 = 1200 calories/day
>
> Male adult with desirable weight of 180 lb: 10 × 180 = 1800 calories/day

For weight gain, prescribe 15 calories per day for every pound of desirable weight.

> Examples: Female adult with desirable weight of 120 lb: 15 × 120 = 1800 calories/day
>
> Male adult with desirable weight of 180 lb: 15 × 180 = 2700 calories/day

For weight maintenance, prescribe 12 calories per day for every pound of current weight.

> Examples: Female adult with current weight of 120 lb: 12 × 120 = 1400 calories/day
>
> Male adult with current weight of 180 lb: 12 × 180 = 2200 calories/day

General Formula A

(Assumes under age 55 unless otherwise specified, includes weight maintenance and weight reduction prescriptions)

10 × present weight in pounds = calories for obese, inactive, chronic dieters

13 × present weight in pounds = calories for active women, sedentary men, and most persons over age 55

15 × present weight in pounds = calories for active men, very active women

20 × present weight in pounds = calories for very thin persons or very active men

General Formula B

(For weight maintenance only)

Active men: 14 calories per pound or 30 calories per kilogram

Sedentary men <55, active women all ages, active men >55: 13 calories per pound or 28 calories per kilogram

Sedentary women all ages, sedentary men >55: 9 calories per pound or 20 calories per kilogram

General Formula C

(For weight loss only)

Active or sedentary, male or female, overweight or obese: 9 calories per pound or 20 calories per kilogram

Calorie Adjustment

(For slow, sustained weight loss or weight gain of about 1 lb per week in adult men or women)

Determine number of daily calories for weight maintenance using any recommended formula.

Add 500 calories per day for weight gain.

Subtract 500 calories per day for weight loss.

Harris-Benedict Equation for Adult Caloric Requirements

Measure of basal energy expenditures (BEE)

❋ Step 1. Determine BEE

Female: BEE = 655 + (9.6 × [weight in kg]) + (1.8 × [height in cm] − (4.7 × [age in years]))

Male: BEE = 66 + (13.7 × [weight in kg]) + (5 × [height in cm]) − (6.8 × [age in years])

Obese female or male: ([actual weight − ideal weight] × .25) + ideal weight

* Step 2. Determine Activity Factor as follows:

    Restricted: 1.1

    Sedentary: 1.2

    Aerobic: 3×/week, 1.3; 5×/week, 1.5; 7×/week, 1.6

    True athlete: 1.7

* Step 3. Multiply BEE by Activity Factor to find calories per day.

    Example. Obese 45-year-old female weighs 195 lb (with desirable body weight of 135 lb), 65″ in height, doing aerobic activity three times per week.

* Step 1. Make special obese weight calculation:

    ([195 − 135]) × .25) + 135 = 60 × .25 + 135 = 15 + 135 = 150

    Convert weight to kg: 150 ÷ 2.2 = 68

    Convert height to cm: 65 × 2.54 = 165

    Calculate BEE formula:

$$655 + ([9.6 \times 68] + [1.8 \times 165]) - (4.7 \times 45)$$
$$= 655 + (653 + 297) - 212 = 655 + 950 - 212 = 1393$$

* Step 2. Activity Factor is 1.3
* Step 3. 1393 × 1.3 = 1811 ~ 1800 calories per day

For Infants, Toddlers, Children, and Teens

Infants

A healthy term infant usually requires 100 calories per kilogram per day. Formula is usually 20 calories per ounce. If there are no apparent growth or nutritional problems noted and the infant is following its growth curve, it is not usually necessary to measure nutritional intake. The amount of time breast feeding on each breast and how frequently the baby breast-feeds may be useful as indirect measures of intake in the initial evaluation.

Toddlers

Whole milk, rather than low-fat milk, is recommended from ages 1 to 2 years. Because the neurologic system continues to rapidly develop during this age period, and because fat is a vital building block for the myelin sheath of the neurons in the central and peripheral nervous systems, it is wise not to strictly restrict fat intake during this age period.

Children and Teens

(Weight maintenance and normal growth)

Record height and weight on National Center for Health Statistics growth charts every 6 months

* 1–11 years
  1000 calories for first year of life + 100 calories for each additional year
  Example: 8-year-old girl = 1000 + 700 = 1700 calories

* 12–15 years
  1000 calories for first year of life + 100 calories for each additional year up to age 11, then add 100 additional calories per year for girls or 200 additional calories per year for boys

  Example: 14-year-old boy = 1000 + 1000 (for next 10 years to age 11) + 600 (for years to age 14) = 2600 calories

Older Teens

Girls > 15 years: Same as adults
Boys > 15 years: Very active: 23 calories × weight in pounds
Moderately active: 18 calories × weight in pounds
Sedentary: 16 calories × weight in pounds plus encourage at least moderate activity, which may require additional lifestyle intervention
Boys > 19 years: Same as adults
For weight reduction in children, use weight maintenance calories first. If adequate weight loss is not achieved, reduce calories by 100–300 calories per day, depending on the child's age. Consider referral to a nutrition specialist owing to the high probability of overriding issues (e.g., athletic participation, incipient onset of eating disorders, family conflict).[12, 13]

Tips

* At the start of treatment many people are consuming more calories per day than they realize. They may state that they have already been eating fewer calories than what is now the recommended prescription. Consider the possibility of their underestimation of actual intake.

* Patients and providers often err in judgment about appropriate serving sizes. Initially, instruct patients to make size decisions based on exact measurements. After a period of time, it may be possible to judge serving sizes based on experience, but a periodic time of re-measuring may be advisable.

* Caloric need may decrease with progressing weight loss. Re-evaluate at regular intervals. Generally, do not prescribe weight loss plans less than 1200 calories per day for moderately active women and less than 1800 calories per day for moderately active men.

* Progressive weight loss in diabetic patients requires frequent re-evaluation of medication needs. Anticipate reduction in the need for insulin and/or oral diabetes medications with successful weight loss.

* Consider the risks and management of hypoglycemia in diabetic patients on insulin and/or sulfa-based oral medications.

* In all meal plans, consider the need for sufficient overall macronutrients and micronutrients. Vitamin and mineral supplementation may be advisable in some cases, especially the lower calorie meal plans.

* Since a great number of patients in any family practice need to lose weight, those who need to gain weight may be less frequently identified. A BMI under 19 requires weight-gain intervention.

CALORIE-SPECIFIC PRESENTATION TOOLS[14]

This section includes tools to use for teaching calorie-specific prescriptions. Patients will need two items:

1. A serving guide plan that lists foods and serving sizes based on the six groups (starches, vegetables, fruits, dairy, meat/meat substitutes, and extras such as salad dressings, spreads, sweets, and oils). A serving guide such as the one found in Figure 13–4 can be used in conjunction with the circle-pyramid exchange guides pictured in Figure 13–5. Or a more detailed serving guide can be ordered from the American Dietetic Association (ADA) at a minimal cost (www.eatright.org).

2. The calorie-specific, circle-pyramid guides (seen in Fig. 13–5) demonstrate examples of an exchange plan based on the popular food pyramid. Each diagram demonstrates the number and type of food exchanges (represented by circles) allowed each day for a given calorie-count diet. One circle-pyramid guide sheet (for the chosen calorie count) will be needed each day. The diagram may be

SERVING CHOICES AND SIZES
PYRAMID GUIDE

Look for low calorie versions that equal 35 calories for a larger serving.

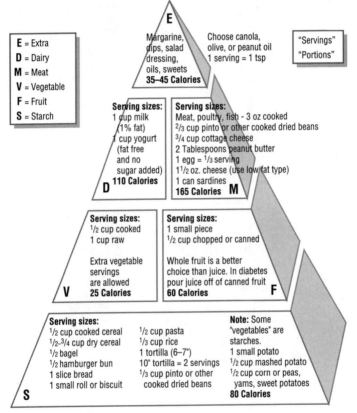

E = Extra
D = Dairy
M = Meat
V = Vegetable
F = Fruit
S = Starch

E

Margarine, dips, salad dressing, oils, sweets
35–45 Calories

Choose canola, olive, or peanut oil
1 serving = 1 tsp

"Servings"
"Portions"

D Serving sizes:
1 cup milk (1% fat)
1 cup yogurt (fat free and no sugar added)
110 Calories

Serving sizes:
Meat, poultry, fish - 3 oz cooked
2/3 cup pinto or other cooked dried beans
3/4 cup cottage cheese
2 Tablespoons peanut butter
1 egg = 1/3 serving
1 1/2 oz. cheese (use low fat type)
1 can sardines
165 Calories **M**

V Serving sizes:
1/2 cup cooked
1 cup raw

Extra vegetable servings are allowed
25 Calories

Serving sizes:
1 small piece
1/2 cup chopped or canned

Whole fruit is a better choice than juice. In diabetes pour juice off of canned fruit
60 Calories **F**

S Serving sizes:
1/2 cup cooked cereal
1/2–3/4 cup dry cereal
1/2 bagel
1/2 hamburger bun
1 slice bread
1 small roll or biscuit

1/2 cup pasta
1/3 cup rice
1 tortilla (6–7")
10" tortilla = 2 servings
1/3 cup pinto or other cooked dried beans

Note: Some "vegetables" are starches.
1 small potato
1/2 cup mashed potato
1/2 cup corn or peas, yams, sweet potatoes
80 Calories

Use these serving sizes as general guidelines.
Other sources such as the ADA Exchange Book may be used for additional ideas.
Remember! Your portion may be more or less than one serving. Count correct number of serving circles when combining for one portion or count a partial serving.

Figure 13–4.

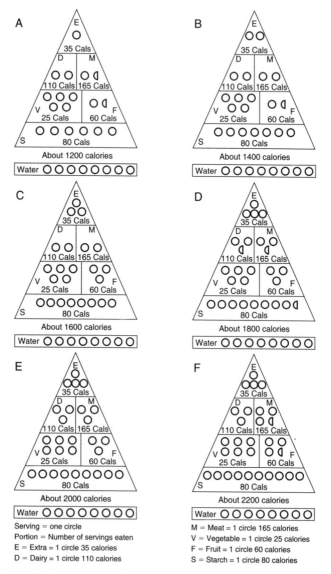

Figure 13–5. Circle-pyramid guides. *A*, 1200 calorie plan. *B*, 1400 calorie plan. *C*, 1600 calorie plan. *D*, 1800 calorie plan. *E*, 2000 calorie plan. *F*, 2200 calorie plan.

enlarged as needed using an ordinary copier. The provider or patient may then reproduce them as necessary. Another option is to laminate a copy of the sheet and have the patient use an erasable marker to indicate servings as consumed each day, thus allowing reuse of the sheet each new day.[15]

Sample meal plans may be included as patient handouts or may be used simply as an instructional tool. The sample should not be interpreted as a singular guideline for food choices (see Table 13–2). For example, patients need to understand that a breakfast starch choice may be based on any of the several items included in the detailed list rather than the example of cold cereal given in the sample meal plan.

Patients will need definitions of a few terms.

* *Serving*—One item and amount as described on the detailed guide. One circle on the meal plan sheet equals one serving. More than one serving of any group may be used at one meal if sufficient circles are remaining.
* *Portion*—The number of servings (circles) used at any meal. One circle, more than one circle, or less than one circle may constitute a portion in any given meal.

  Example: A *small* fast-food hamburger dressed with mayonnaise, lettuce, tomato, and onion.

The patient would therefore mark through two starch, one meat, one or two vegetable, and one extra (fat) circle.

* *Serving Guide*—This lists typical foods and their serving sizes for each group. This guide can be ordered from the ADA or supplied by a nutritionist.
* *Circle-Pyramid Guide*—This indicates the numbers of servings allowed for each calorie plan. They are provided in 1200, 1400, 1600, 1800, and 2200 calorie plans.

Remember, the goal is to put an X through all serving circles by the end of each day. There is no advantage to consuming fewer than the recommended servings. Also, ask the patient to accurately show his or her true food intake by adding additional circles when necessary. Adjustments may be made based on this realistic reporting.

The patient should be instructed to space selections from the six different groups throughout the day, choosing the majority of circles during daylight hours rather than at night. In other words, avoid eating all starches or all dairy products at one or two meals, but instead spread them throughout as many meals and snacks as possible.

Special Cautions

* Eight water serving circles, each representing one eight-ounce glass of water, are included on the Circle-Pyramid Guide. Adjustments may be needed for special diets requiring fluid restriction.

Table 13–2. 1200 Calorie Sample Meal Plan*

Foods	Serving Count (Number of circles to X out at each meal and snack)
Breakfast	
¾ cup cold cereal flakes	1 Starch circle
½ cup milk (1% fat)	½ Dairy circle
Small banana	1 Fruit circle
Midmorning Snack	
1 fat-free, no sugar added fruit yogurt (6 oz)	¾ Dairy circle
Lunch	
Hamburger with 1 cup of raw vegetables (such as lettuce, tomato slices, onion, sprouts)	2 Starch circles 1 Meat circle 1 Vegetable circle
(No cheese, no mayonnaise or creamy spread; mustard is permissible.)	
4 oz milk (1% fat)	½ Dairy circle
Afternoon Snack	
1 cup raw cauliflower and broccoli	1 Vegetable circle
1 tablespoon low calorie salad dressing (about 35 calories)	1 "Extra" circle
Dinner	
1 cup spaghetti noodles	2 Starch circles
½ cup spaghetti sauce	1 Vegetable circle
1½ ounces chicken strips	½ Meat circle
1 cup green beans	2 Vegetable circles
1 small roll	1 Starch circle
Evening Snack	
¼ cup chopped fruit	½ Fruit circle
2 oz milk (1% fat)	¼ Dairy circle
Sprinkle with plain cinnamon	
Suggestion: If additional snack is needed, use diet gelatin or raw vegetables.	

*Explain to patients that these are merely sample suggestions. Meal planning should be based on a wider variety of choices selected from the pyramid guide. Remind patients to drink eight circles worth of water, herbal tea, or other noncaffeinated sugar-free beverages to complete the bottom part of the circle-pyramid plan.

● Servings allowed on the 1200 calorie plan provide less than the minimum number of servings recommended by the ADA. For those patients requiring 1200 calories (or less), consider the addition of vitamin and mineral food supplements and/or two or three additional 25-calorie vegetable servings each day. Any meal plan should allow two to four extra vegetable servings per day if necessary for appetite satiation.

* Using the basic food guide pyramid plan can be problematic without an explanation of recommended numbers of servings. The food guide pyramid shows recommended numbers of servings in general terms, such as 6–11 servings of starches. This is not adequate information.

* DASH (Dietary Approach to Stop Hypertension) should also be considered as part of the treatment plan when indicated and is perfectly adaptable to the pyramid plan. In the DASH diet, six vegetable servings, three fruit servings, and three dairy servings are included each day. A 2000 calorie plan will accommodate the DASH diet. Adjusting starch servings downward will reduce calories as needed to achieve weight loss. Each starch serving is worth 80 calories. Salty foods and salt used at the table are to be avoided. Flavor enhancers that are salt-free can be substituted.

* Free foods, such as no-calorie sodas, unsweetened or artificially sweetened coffee and tea, and diet gelatin may be added to the meal plan without having to add any additional circles.

The pyramid-based meal planning method included in this chapter is intended for broad use in many case situations not requiring more complex intervention. For instruction on carbohydrate counting for intensive diabetes therapy and for detailed use of the ADA Exchange System, and in cases involving significant co-morbid conditions, the services of a registered dietitian should be employed. Morbid obesity, severe anorexia or bulimia, severe malnutrition, and diabetes with presence of renal complications are examples of conditions that require more complex dietary assessment and intervention.

It should also be noted that the ADA Exchange System was recently revised to combine the various carbohydrate sources into more integrated groups. In addition, dietary information about many combination foods has been included in this revision. Other combination foods, such as casseroles and soups, can also be adapted to the pyramid plan by considering their basic components and applying them to the appropriate serving circles. Some general patient education tips for the diabetic are included in Box 13–1.[16]

Patients need defined numbers of servings per day rather than ranges. Teach patients that when they can find lower calorie versions of foods, for larger quantity serving sizes, they may substitute. But remind them that "there is no such thing as a free lunch," and that many "fat-free" foods contain calories equal to or higher than the original fat-containing foods. Patients must understand that portions (how many servings are eaten at one meal or snack) may be part of a serving or more than one serving, depending on how many circles are available and desired. Instruct patients that on days when they have exceeded their meal plan circles, they should add circles and half circles as needed to honestly reflect what was eaten. It may be necessary to adjust the plan to a higher calorie level and gradually

Box 13-1–DIABETES PATIENT EDUCATION HANDOUT[15]

In diabetes, a lack of insulin (type I) or a problem with use of insulin (type II) causes problems with using food for energy, growth, and healing. Levels of sugar and insulin in the blood stream that are out of balance can cause serious problems, both short term and long term. Long-term complications are caused by damage to blood vessels and nerves. They may result in disability or early death. Complications can be delayed or prevented by good diabetes management.

- The three parts of food, carbohydrates, proteins, and fats, are all important. The simplest form of carbohydrate is glucose, a one-molecule sugar. Glucose is used by cells as the main source of energy. Insulin allows this sugar to enter cells and be used for energy. If sugar is not used well, it builds up in the blood. High levels of sugar in the blood are not healthy at any time. Over a long period, a high level of sugar can cause damage to blood vessels in all parts of the body. This explains why the complications of diabetes include blindness, kidney failure, nerve disease, heart disease, strokes, and circulation problems in the feet. Diabetes affects all parts of the body. The long-term complications often result from several combined problems that may include high blood sugar, high blood pressure, abnormal blood fats, and tobacco use of any kind.
- There are two main types of diabetes, type I and type II. They have different origins, but the outcomes and risks for complications are similar. Both types of diabetes should be treated very seriously.

Type I	Type II
5% of cases	95% of cases
Lack of insulin	Insulin made by pancreas but does not work well
Immune reaction	
Must take insulin shots	Liver produces too much sugar
	May be helped by oral medication, but some take insulin

*Box 13-1–*DIABETES MELLITUS[15] *Continued*

- Common symptoms of diabetes include

Lack of energy	Blurry vision	Dry skin
Too much urine	Headaches	Problems with healing
Too much thirst	Weight loss, mostly in Type I	
Too much hunger	Weight gain, in many cases of Type II, but sometimes weight stays the same and sometimes there is weight loss	

- Risks for diabetes include

Type I:
Family background and immune reaction, possibly to viral infections or even to a person's own insulin-producing cells.
Type II:
Family background, lack of exercise, being overweight, especially in the upper part of the body, too much stress, aging, ethnicity (Hispanics, Native Americans, and African Americans are at higher risk), and a history of high blood sugar during a stressful time, during a pregnancy, or at any other time.

- Good treatment for diabetes should include
  Medical Management
    Medications
    Monitoring—including self testing of blood glucose and foot examination and care
    Prevention of complications—control of blood sugar, blood pressure, blood fats, and stopping all tobacco use
  Lifestyle Adjustments
    Nutrition
    Physical Activity
  Social and Cultural Adjustments
    Stress Management
    Motivation
    Education
- Excellent control of diabetes is possible. Success depends on the person with diabetes working with a good health care team for lifelong shared management.

decrease the calorie intake as patients learn and adjust to the system. Set calorie intakes sufficiently high and reasonable early goals to encourage success.

■ CONCLUSION

The system of pyramid-guided food choices based on generally accepted serving sizes and categories is scientifically sound, easy to use, and offers patients both a visual and a practical way to accomplish their meal planning goals. Frequent performance and caloric-need re-evaluations should be included in the normal process of clinical management. Once a patient has mastered the pyramid system, only minimal re-education will be needed to adapt to a different calorie prescription. Patients should be positively assured and encouraged to view this program as long term and preferably lifelong. They need to guard against the temptations of "fad diets" and other misconceptions that frequently are reported by the general media. Encourage patients to ask questions of their medical support team regarding popular ideas or trends in nutrition management. Given simple instructions, regular feedback, and patient empowerment for control of one's own nutritional choices and meal planning, the majority of patients' nutritional and weight goals can be accomplished in the clinical office setting.

REFERENCES

1. Poor Success Weight Loss: Methods for voluntary weight loss and control. NIH Technology Assessment Conference Panel. Consensus Development Conference, 30 March to 1 April 1992 [Review]. Ann Intern Med 1993;119:764–770.
2. Stunkard AJ, Sorenson TI, Hanis C, et al. An adoption study of human obesity. N Engl J Med 1986;314:193–198.
3. Czeizel AE, Dudas I. Folic acid may prevent or decrease the incidence of neural tube defects. N Engl J Med 1992; 327:1832.
4. Graham IM, Daly LE, Refsum HM, et al. Plasma homocysteine as a risk factor for vascular disease. The European Concerted Action Project. JAMA 1997;277:1775–1781.
5. Diaz MN, Frei B, Vita JA, Keaney JF Jr. Antioxidants and atherosclerotic heart disease. N Engl J Med 1997;337:408–416.
6. ASPEN Board of Directors Guidelines for the use of parenteral and enteral nutrition in adult and pediatric patients. JPEN J Parenter Enteral Nutr 1993;17:1SA–26SA.
7. Adapted from the National Heart, Lung, and Blood Institute Body Mass Index Charts.
8. Bray GA. Definitions, measurement, and classification of obesity. Int J Obes Relat Metab Disord 1978;2:99–112.

9. Bray GA, Gray DS. Obesity, Part I—Pathogenesis. West J Med 1988;149:429–441.
10. The American Dietetic Association. Manual of Clinical Dietetics, 5th ed. Chicago, 1996.
11. Hunt SM. Advanced Nutrition and Human Metabolism. St. Paul, MN, West Publishing Company, 1990.
12. Christian JL, Greger J. Nutrition for Living. The Benjamin/Cummings Publishing Co., Inc, Redwood City, CA, 1993.
13. Zeeman FJ. Clinical Nutrition and Dietetics, 2nd ed. New York, MacMillan Publishing Company, 1991.
14. American Dietetic Association publications, 1998. (See Resources section of this chapter.)
15. Bell S. Memorial Medical Center, Las Cruces, NM, 1998.

RESOURCES

American Dietetic Association. www.eatright.org

American Dietetic Association. American Diabetes Association Complete Guide to Diabetes. American Diabetes Association, 1997.

American Diabetes Association. The New Family Cookbook for People with Diabetes. American Dietetic Association. Simon & Schuster, 1999.

American Diabetes Association, American Dietetic Association. The Official Pocket Guide to Diabetic Exchanges. 1998.

Colorado Dietetic Association. Simply Colorado Too: More Nutritious Recipes for Busy People. 1999.

CHAPTER 14

Trauma

*James W. Gordon, PA-C, EMT-P, BSM, BBA,
and Tomas B. Garcia, MD, FACEP*

INTRODUCTION

To a degree, society has accepted trauma as an inevitable part of life (and death). However, trauma can be prevented with an awareness of and respect for the mechanisms that are involved. When trauma does occur, improved understanding of posttrauma care improves outcomes.

Injury prevention occurs at both the societal and the individual level. Society prevents injury through regulations and mandatory safety measures. Clinicians identify individuals at risk and attempt to prevent high-risk behaviors leading to trauma. Accidents would not be so named if one could anticipate their occurrence. Rationalizing not wearing seat belts or helmets because of the length of the trip, discomfort, or heat can result in significant injuries, disabilities, and death simply because traumatic events cannot be foreseen. Protective gear and risk-reduction practices must be maintained at all times in order to reduce the rate and sequelae of both accidental and intentionally violent trauma.

EPIDEMIOLOGY

While uncommon traumatic events are frequently sensationalized in the media, approximately 400 people die every day because of acute traumatic injury.[1] Trauma is the leading cause of death in the first 44 years of life (Table 14–1).[2, 3]

Within the next 10 min approximately 350 people will have a disabling injury requiring at least 24 h off work, and approximately $7.8 million will be spent on unintentionally injured patients in the United States.[1] The leading cause of death for all ages is the motor vehicle accident (MVA), including motorcyclists, bicycle riders, and pedestrians injured by motor vehicles. MVAs are followed closely by firearm deaths, the vast majority being suicide or homicide. In descending order, the next most frequent causes of traumatic deaths are falls, drowning, thermal injuries by fire or hot objects, cutting or piercing injuries, and machinery-related trauma. The complete breakdown, by age, is listed in Table 14–2.[4]

Text continued on page 325

Table 14–1. Deaths and Death Rates for the 10 Leading Causes of Death in Specific Age Groups for All Races and Both Sexes: United States, 1997

Cause of Death (Based on the 9th Revision, International Classification of Diseases, 1975)

Rank[1]	Age	Number[2]	Rate[2]
	All Ages[3]		
	All causes	2,314,245	864.7
1.	Diseases of heart (390–398, 402, 404–429)	726,974	271.6
2.	Malignant neoplasms, including neoplasms of lymphatic and hematopoietic tissue (140–208)	539,577	201.6
3.	Cerebrovascular diseases (430–438)	159,791	59.7
4.	Chronic obstructive pulmonary diseases and allied conditions (490–496)	109,029	40.7
5.	Accidents and adverse effects (E800–E949)	95,644	35.7
	Motor vehicle accidents (E810–E825)	43,458	16.2
	All other accidents and adverse effects (E800–E807, E826, E949)	52,186	19.5
6.	Pneumonia and influenza (480–487)	86,449	32.3
7.	Diabetes mellitus (250)	62,636	23.4
8.	Suicide (E950–E959)	30,535	11.4
9.	Nephritis, nephrotic syndrome, and nephrosis (580–589)	25,331	9.5
10.	Chronic liver disease and cirrhosis (571)	25,175	9.4
	All other causes (Residual)	453,104	159.3
	Ages 1–4		
	All causes	5501	35.8
1.	Accidents and adverse effects (E800–E948)	2005	13.1
	Motor vehicle accidents (E810–E825)	768	5.0
	All other accidents and adverse effects (E800–E807–E826–E949)	1237	8.1
2.	Congenital anomalies (740–759)	589	3.8
3.	Malignant neoplasms, including neoplasms of lymphatic and hematopoietic tissue (140–208)	438	2.9
4.	Homicide and legal intervention (E960–E978)	375	2.4
5.	Diseases of the heart (390–398, 402, 404–429)	212	1.4
6.	Pneumonia and influenza (480–487)	180	1.2
7.	Certain conditions originating in the perinatal period (760–779)	75	0.5
8.	Septicemia (038)	73	0.5
9.	Benign neoplasms, carcinoma in situ, and neoplasms of uncertain behavior and of unspecified nature (210–239)	65	0.4
10.	Cerebrovascular diseases (430–438)	56	0.4
	All other causes (Residual)	1433	9.3

Table 14–1. Deaths and Death Rates for the 10 Leading Causes of
Death in Specific Age Groups for All Races and Both
Sexes: United States, 1997 *Continued*

Cause of Death (Based on the 9th Revision, International Classification of Diseases, 1975)

Rank[1]	Age	Number[2]	Rate[2]
	Ages 5–14		
	All causes	8061	20.8
1.	Accidents and adverse effects (E800–E949)	3371	8.7
	Motor vehicle accidents (E810–825)	1967	5.1
	All other accidents and adverse effects (E800–E807, E828, E949)	1404	3.6
2.	Malignant neoplasms, including neoplasms of lymphatic and hematopoietic tissues (140–208)	1030	2.7
3.	Homicide and legal intervention (E960–E978)	457	1.2
4.	Congenital anomalies (740–759)	447	1.2
5.	Diseases of heart (390–398–402–404–420)	313	0.8
6.	Suicide (E950–E959)	307	0.8
7.	Pneumonia and influenza (480–487)	141	0.4
8.	Chronic obstructive pulmonary diseases and allied conditions (490–496)	129	0.3
9.	Human immunodeficiency virus infection (°042–°044)	102	0.3
10.	Cerebrovascular diseases (430–438)	75	0.2
10.	Benign neoplasms, carcinoma in situ, and neoplasms of uncertain behavior and of unspecified nature (210–239)	76	0.2
	All other causes (Residual)	1612	4.2
	Ages 15–25		
	All causes	31,544	86.2
1.	Accidents and adverse effects (E900–E949)	13,367	36.5
	Motor vehicle accidents (E810–E825)	10,208	27.9
	All other accidents and adverse effects (E800–E807, E826, E949)	3159	8.6
2.	Homicide and legal intervention (E960–E978)	6146	16.8
3.	Suicide (E950–E959)	4186	11.4
4.	Malignant neoplasms, including neoplasms of lymphatic and hematopoietic tissue (140–208)	1645	4.5
5.	Diseases of the heart (390–398, 402, 404, 429)	1098	3.0
6.	Congenital anomalies (740–759)	420	1.1
7.	Human immunodeficiency virus infection (°042–°044)	276	0.8

Table continued on following page

Table 14–1. Deaths and Death Rates for the 10 Leading Causes of Death in Specific Age Groups for All Races and Both Sexes: United States, 1997 *Continued*

Cause of Death (Based on the 9th Revision, International Classification of Diseases, 1975)

Rank[1]	Age	Number[2]	Rate[2]
	Ages 15–25 continued		
8.	Pneumonia and influenza (480–487)	220	0.6
9.	Chronic obstructive pulmonary diseases and allied conditions (400–496)	201	0.5
10.	Cerebrovascular diseases (430–438)	188	0.5
	All other causes (Residual)	3797	10.4
	Ages 25–44		
	All causes	134,946	161.4
1.	Accidents and adverse effects (E800–E949)	27,129	32.4
	Motor vehicle accidents (E810–E825)	14,167	16.9
	All other accidents and adverse effects (E800–E807–E826–E949)	12,962	15.5
2.	Malignant neoplasms, including neoplasms of lymphatic and hematopoietic tissue (140–208)	21,706	26.0
3.	Disease of heart (390–398, 402, 404, 429)	16,513	19.8
4.	Suicide (E950–E959)	12,402	14.8
5.	Human immunodeficiency virus infection (°042–°044)	11,066	13.2
6.	Homicide and legal intervention (E960–E978)	8752	10.5
7.	Chronic liver disease and cirrhosis (571)	4024	4.8
8.	Cerebrovascular diseases (430–438)	3465	4.1
9.	Diabetes mellitus (250)	2478	3.0
10.	Pneumonia and influenza (480–487)	1928	2.3
	All other causes (Residual)	25,483	30.5
	Ages 45–64		
	All causes	376,875	679.7
1.	Malignant neoplasms, including neoplasms of lymphatic and hematopoietic tissue (140–208)	131,743	237.8
2.	Diseases of the heart (390–398, 402, 404–429)	101,235	182.6
3.	Accidents and adverse effects (E800–E949)	17,521	31.8
	Motor vehicle accidents (E810–E825)	8134	14.7
	All other accidents and adverse effects (E800–E807–E826–E949)	9387	16.9

Table 14–1. Deaths and Death Rates for the 10 Leading Causes of
Death in Specific Age Groups for All Races and Both
Sexes: United States, 1997 *Continued*

Cause of Death (Based on the 9th Revision, International Classification of Diseases, 1975)

Rank[1]	Age	Number[2]	Rate[2]
	Ages 45–64 continued		
4.	Cerebrovascular diseases (430–438)	15,371	27.7
5.	Chronic obstructive pulmonary diseases and allied conditions (490–496)	12,947	23.4
6.	Diabetes mellitus (250)	12,705	22.9
7.	Chronic liver disease and cirrhosis (571)	10,875	19.6
8.	Suicide (E950–E959)	7894	14.2
9.	Pneumonia and influenza (480–487)	5992	10.8
10.	Human immunodeficiency virus infection (°042–°044)	4578	8.3
	All other causes (Residual)	56,014	101
	Ages 65 and Over		
	All causes	1,728,872	5073.6
1.	Diseases of the heart (390–398, 402, 404–429)	606,915	1781.1
2.	Malignant neoplasms, including neoplasms of lymphatic and hematopoietic tissue (140–208)	382,913	1123.7
3.	Cerebrovascular diseases (430–438)	140,366	411.9
4.	Chronic obstructive pulmonary diseases and allied conditions (490–496)	94,411	277.1
5.	Pneumonia and influenza (480–487)	77,561	227.6
6.	Diabetes mellitus (250)	47,289	138.8
7.	Accidents and adverse effects (E800–E949)	31,386	92.1
	Motor vehicle accidents (E810–E825)	8027	23.6
	All other accidents and adverse effects (E800–E807, E826–E949)	23,359	68.6
8.	Alzheimer's disease (331.0)	22,154	65.0
9.	Nephritis, nephrotic syndrome, and nephrosis (580–589)	21,787	63.9
10.	Septicemia (038)	18,079	53.1
	All other causes (Residual)	286,013	839.3

[1]Rank based on number of deaths.

[2]Figures for age not stated are included in "All ages" but not distributed among age groups. Rates per 1,000,000 population in specified group.

[3]Includes deaths for "Under 1 year."

°Figure does not meet standards of reliability or precision.

Source: Centers for Disease Control and Prevention (CDC), National Vital Statistics Report, Vol. 47, No. 19, June 30, 1999. The numbers in parentheses following each cause of death are ICD9 diagnostic codes.

Table 14–2. Deaths, Death Rates, and Age-Adjusted Death Rates for Injury Deaths According to Mechanism and Intent of Death: United States, 1997

Mechanism and Intent of Death (Based on the 9th Revision, International Classification of Diseases, 1975)	All Ages	Under 1	1–4	5–14	15–24	25–34	35–44	45–54	55–64	65–74	75–84	85 and Over	Age Not Stated
							Age (Years)						
All injury deaths (E800–E869, E880–E929, E960–E999)	148,400	1110	2383	4150	24,010	23,982	26,048	17,567	10,749	11,202	13,866	11,148	185
Unintentional (E800–869) E880–E929	92,353	736	1968	3338	13,318	12,519	14,343	10,117	6726	7870	11,180	10,138	100
Suicide (E950–E959)	30,535	—	—	307	4186	5672	6730	4948	2946	2663	2260	805	18
Homicide (E960–E969)	19,491	317	375	456	6083	4961	3569	1829	834	539	332	149	47
Undetermined (E960–E969)	3657	57	40	48	360	716	1297	632	224	120	88	56	19
Other (E970–E978, E990–E999)	364	—	1	1	63	114	109	41	19	10	6	—	1
Cut/pierce (E920, E956, E966, E974, E986)	2864	3	10	44	499	666	733	394	193	154	109	51	8
Unintentional (E920)	104	—	3	7	12	13	20	18	7	9	10	7	—
Suicide (E956)	499	—	—	1	18	75	131	110	54	45	43	22	—
Homicide (E966)	2246	2	7	36	467	575	577	266	132	99	55	22	8
Undetermined (E966)	14	1	—	—	2	3	5	2	—	—	1	—	—
Other (E974)	1	—	—	—	—	—	—	—	—	1	—	—	—
Drowning (E830, E832, E910, E954, E964, E984)	4724	78	474	458	731	744	745	526	337	271	232	95	33
Unintentional (E830, E832, E910)	4051	60	456	449	665	631	602	422	265	218	188	70	25
Suicide (E954)	384	—	—	—	35	59	85	71	47	33	32	22	—
Homicide (E964)	58	14	11	5	9	7	6	2	2	2	—	—	—
Undetermined (E964)	231	4	7	4	22	47	52	31	23	18	12	3	8

Cause													
Fall (E880, E888, E957, E968.1, E967)	12,555	17	50	57	349	502	798	783	834	1638	3433	4088	6
Unintentional (E880, E886, E888)	11,858	11	48	53	249	353	637	701	779	1580	3382	4061	4
Suicide (E957)	600	—	—	3	79	130	138	73	46	56	48	25	2
Homicide (E968.1)	28	3	1	—	6	3	7	3	3	—	2	—	—
Undetermined (E967)	69	3	1	1	15	16	16	6	6	2	1	2	—
Fire/hot objects/substance (E890–E899, E924, E958 [.1,.2,.7], E961, E968 [.0,.3], E988 [.1,.2,.7])	4083	58	381	311	248	374	510	458	424	458	537	313	11
Unintentional (E890–E899, E924)	3601	53	354	277	200	292	423	381	366	423	519	303	10
Suicide (E958 [.1,.2,.7])	203	—	—	1	24	38	45	43	33	13	3	3	—
Homicide (E961, E968 [.03])	192	4	20	28	22	30	27	19	14	14	9	4	1
Undetermined (E988 [.1,.2,.7])	87	1	7	5	2	14	15	15	11	8	6	3	—
Firearm (E922, E955 [.0–.4], E965 [.0–.4], E970, E985 [.0–.4])	32,436	9	75	546	8173	7045	5802	3872	2390	2202	1740	555	27
Unintentional (E922)	961	—	20	122	300	165	130	96	58	51	24	15	—
Suicide (E955 [.0–.4])	17,566	—	—	127	2587	3010	3321	2647	1859	1906	1608	494	7
Homicide (E965 [.0–.4])	13,252	9	53	284	5110	3706	2217	1068	437	224	88	39	17
Undetermined (E985 [.0–.4])	367	—	2	12	115	76	63	33	23	17	17	7	2
Other (E970)	270	—	—	1	61	88	71	28	13	4	3	—	1
Machinery (E919)	1,055	—	17	32	82	137	181	171	162	155	96	22	—
Motor vehicle traffic, all (E810–E819, E958.5, E988.5)	42,473	160	657	1866	10,056	7389	6513	4704	3252	3308	3309	1237	22
Unintentional (E810, E191)[1]	42,340	160	657	1864	10,027	7351	6487	4689	3245	3304	3302	1232	22
Occupant (E810–E819 [.0,.1])	25,089	123	360	909	6559	4307	3592	2621	1876	1965	2020	753	4
Motorcyclist (E810–E819 [.2,.3])	1645	—	—	16	380	483	396	235	98	24	12	7	—
Pedal cyclist (E810–E819 [.6])	757	—	4	197	123	96	137	84	45	36	28	7	—

Table continued on following page

Table 14-2. Deaths, Death Rates, and Age-Adjusted Death Rates for Injury Deaths According to Mechanism and Intent of Death: United States, 1997 Continued

Mechanism and Intent of Death (Based on the 9th Revision, International Classification of Diseases, 1975)	All Ages	Age (Years)												
		Under 1	1-4	5-14	15-24	25-34	35-44	45-54	55-64	65-74	75-84	85 and Over	Age Not Stated
Pedestrian (E810–E819 [.7])	5497	5	200	470	605	757	951	724	518	521	506	224	16
Unspecified (E810–E819 [.9])	9302	31	93	263	2349	1697	1405	1022	707	756	731	246	2
Suicide (E958.5)	124	—	—	1	24	36	26	15	7	4	7	4	—
Undetermined (E988.5)	9	—	—	1	5	2	—	—	—	—	—	1	—
Pedal cyclist, other (E800–E807 [.3], E820–E825 [.6], E826 [.1,.9], E827–E829 [.1])	141	—	3	21	10	23	30	20	12	13	7	2	—
Pedestrian, other (E800–E807 [.2], E820–E825 [.7], E826–E829 [.0])	878	3	103	45	111	139	177	102	64	54	53	21	6

Totals for selected causes of death differ from those shown in other tables that utilize standard mortality tabulation lists. Rates per 100,000 in specified group; age-adjusted rates per 100,000 U.S. standard population. The numbers in parentheses following each Mechanism are ICD9 diagnostic codes.

DEFINITION AND MECHANISMS OF TRAUMA

Acute trauma can be prevented or its incidence reduced in much the same way as chronic conditions or diseases can be prevented or reduced in incidence. By understanding mechanisms that lead to injury, acute harm frequently can be avoided. Trauma occurs as a result of too much energy applied to the body (e.g., falls resulting in fractures) or from insufficient energy exerted by the body (e.g., asphyxiation). Intervention anywhere along the continuum of events leading to trauma can result in prevention of the traumatic outcome.[1] Theoretical models of injury have been developed, such as this epidemiologic model applied to trauma:

* Reservoir: Refers to where the agent is found in the environment
* Agent: Energy supplied via mechanical, electrical, chemical, radiation, or thermal means
* Vector (vehicle): The vector conveys energy from the reservoir. This energy may result in injury to the host if the amount of energy exceeds the tolerance level of the host. Examples of vectors include bullets, a human fist, and an automobile.
* Host response: How the body reacts to the force applied.[1]

For example: The reservoir is the roadway, and the agent (mechanical energy) is supplied by a motor vehicle. If the vehicle strikes a person, then the resulting injury is a factor of the speed of the vehicle and the host response (diving out of the way). Efforts to prevent pedestrian versus motor vehicle accidents can involve the reservoir, the agent, the vehicle and/or the host response. For vectors conveying much smaller amounts of energy, host response can be modified to accommodate the energy. A football player conditioning himself to withstand the blows of an opposing player and wearing protective gear is such an example.

The ten basic strategies for injury prevention, as developed by Dr. William Haddon, Jr., have been assembled to combine historical constructs of the mechanisms of trauma into potential preventive interventions. They are intended as an aid to considering countermeasures in a logical and systematic fashion.[1]

1. Prevent the creation of the hazard (stop producing poisons).
2. Reduce the amount of the hazards (package toxic drugs in smaller amounts).
3. Prevent the release of a hazard that already exists (make bathtubs less slippery).
4. Modify the rate or spatial distribution of a hazard (require automobile air bags).
5. Separate, in time or space, the hazard from that which is to be protected (use sidewalks to separate pedestrians from automobiles).

6. Separate the hazard from that which is to be protected by material barriers (insulate electric cords).
7. Modify relevant basic qualities of the hazard (make crib slats too narrow for a child to insert his or her head and strangle).
8. Make what is to be protected more resistant to damage from the hazard (improve the host's physical condition through appropriate nutrition and exercise programs).
9. Begin to counter the damage already done by the hazard (provide emergency care).
10. Stabilize, repair, and rehabilitate the object of the damage (provide acute care and rehabilitation facilities).

However, theories need to be put into a realistic framework in order to address problems that confront society and the clinician every day. Health care providers need to be involved on both the individual and the societal levels to reduce injuries. In order to address some specific public health issues, it is necessary for government agencies to become involved with regulatory assistance. Trauma can be reduced through persuasion, requirements of law, alterations of vehicles or environments, and improving postinjury emergency care and rehabilitation programs.

* Persuasion: Persuasion is targeted at changing individual behavior through education at the personal or at the societal level. Identifying at-risk individuals is paramount in preventing trauma to individuals or groups. One of the strongest correlates to high-risk behavior is the early age of onset of cigarette smoking and substance abuse.[5] Schools, pediatrician offices, and family practices are the ideal settings for trauma prevention at the individual level.

    Counseling seems to have some benefit when given to parents of small children. Counseling provided at 3 months postpartum has been shown to reduce children's injuries at age 1 year. Parents tend to institute household safety measures when asked to do so by the health care provider. Free devices such as cabinet locks and smoke detectors (often provided as part of a safety promotion campaign) also seem to increase compliance. Counseling is more beneficial when provided by the patient's primary care provider, suggesting that continuity of care and trust play a significant role in compliance. Counseling along with community efforts also have a positive influence on injury reduction.[6, 7]

* Requirements of law: Behaviors such as the use of seat belts, child restraints, and motorcycle and bicycle helmets can be mandated by law. The desired behavioral change may be accomplished both indirectly, by media attention, and directly, by enforcement of the law. For example, a mandatory drinking age requires storeowners not to sell to underage drinkers, which may affect targeted advertising or media attention from groups such as Mothers Against Drunk Driving (MADD).

* Alterations of vehicles or environments to increase automatic, pas-

sive, or involuntary protection: Changes in the design of, for example, automobiles, streets, architecture, work sites, and clothing to improve safety do not require individual behavior changes. Safety features can be inherent in the product design. Changes can be motivated by government action, response to litigation, economic pressure, or because of consumer demands.

* Improve postinjury emergency care and rehabilitation programs: Improving the response time and training of emergency medical personnel improves survival rates of trauma victims. Rehabilitation strategies improve functional outcomes for survivors of trauma.

▬ TRAUMA PREVENTION COUNSELING

Many traumatic situations have similar origins. These similarities include risk-taking behaviors, such as speed, alcohol and/or substance abuse, improper use of available safety features, and denial of and/or minimizing risks. Patients need to be aware that trauma is not just a choice between living and dying. Injury or even passive suicide attempts can result in significant morbidity, such as permanent disability, pain, disfigurement, and/or a vegetative state. It should also be pointed out that the individual engaging in the risk-taking behaviors is often not the only victim. Other members of the community may be injured or killed and their family/families significantly affected. Parents and peers should be included to support and enforce adolescent counseling beyond the clinical setting.[1]

Specific causes of trauma form a framework in which to outline specific preventive counseling strategies. The distribution and type of injuries are listed in Tables 14–3 and 14–4.[8]

FACTS AND TIPS USEFUL IN COUNSELING

Motor Vehicle Accidents[1, 2]

* General
  * Eighty percent of all accidents take place near the home or workplace at speeds less than 35 miles per hour.
  * The majority of fatal motor vehicle crashes contain one or more of the following contributing factors: speed, alcohol, and failure to use the restraint system.
  * The majority of fatal vehicle crashes occur on dry, straight, rural roadways! Environmental and highway design factors are rarely the cause.
* Seat belts
  * There is a decrease of death and nonfatal injuries by 50% with seat belt use.

Table 14-3. Number and Percent Distribution of Emergency Department Visits by Selected Characteristics of the Injury, According to Patient's Age: United States, 1998

Selected Characteristic of the Injury	All Ages		Under 18		18-64 Years		65 Years and Over	
	Visits in Thousands	Percent Distribution	Visits in Thousands	Percent Distribution	Visits in Thousands	Percent Distribution	Visits in Thousands	Percent Distribution
All injury-related visits	37,111	100	10,458	100	22,560	100	4093	100
Place of occurrence								
Residence	10,679	28.8	3602	34.4	5042	22.4	2034	49.7
Street or highway	5195	14.0	1063	10.2	3814	16.9	317	7.7
Recreation/sports area	2290	6.2	1151	11.0	1083	4.8	*	*
Industrial places	2263	6.1	*	*	2166	9.6	*	*
Other public building	1185	3.2	155	1.5	886	3.9	*	*
Schools	785	2.1	697	6.7	86	0.4	*	*
Other	1226	3.3	211	2.0	806	3.6	208	5.1
Unknown	13,488	36.3	3498	33.4	6676	38.5	1314	32.1
Intentionally								
Yes (self-inflicted)	671	1.8	105	1.0	549	2.4	*	*
Yes (assault)	1824	4.9	363	3.5	1403	6.2	*	*
No, unintentional	30,046	81.0	8980	85.9	17,534	77.7	3528	86.2
Unknown/blank	4569	12.3	1009	9.6	3071	13.6	489	12.0
Work-related								
Yes	4444	12.0	223	2.1	4159	18.4	*	*
No	21,844	58.9	7782	74.4	11,211	49.7	2,851	69.6
Unknown/blank	10,822	29.2	2453	23.5	7189	31.9	1,180	28.8

*Figure does not meet standard of reliability or precision.

Note: Numbers may not add to totals because of rounding.

Source: Advance Data, No. 313, May 10, 2000, National Hospital Ambulatory Medical Care Survey, 1998 Emergency Department Summary, from Vital and Health Statistics of the Centers for Disease Control and Prevention/National Center for Health Statistics (Tables 8 and 9, page 17).

Table 14-4. Number and Percent Distribution of Injury-Related Emergency Department Visits by Intent and Mechanism of External Cause: United States, 1998

Intent and Mechanism[1]	Number of Visits in Thousands	Percent Distribution
All injury-related visits	37,111	100.0
Unintentional injuries	28,636	77.2
Falls	7712	20.8
Struck against or struck accidentally by	4717	12.7
objects or persons	4259	11.5
Motor vehicle traffic	3142	8.5
Cutting or piercing instruments or	1456	3.9
objects	1238	3.3
Overexertion and strenuous movements		
Natural and environmental factors		
Poisoning by drugs, medical substances, biological, other solid and liquid substances, gases, and vapors	754	2.0
Fire and flames, hot substances or objects, caustic or corrosive material, and steam	531	1.4
Pedal cycle, nontraffic and other	496	1.3
Machinery	411	1.1
Motor vehicle, nontraffic	391	1.1
Other transportation	174	0.5
Other mechanism[2]	2171	5.9
Mechanism unspecified	1183	3.2
Intentional injuries	2168	5.8
Assault	1618	4.4
Unarmed fight or brawl, striking by blunt or thrown object	873	2.4
Cutting or piercing instrument	160	0.4
Other and unspecified mechanism[3]	585	1.6
Self-inflicted	443	1.2
Poisoning by solid or liquid substances, gases, and vapors	298	0.8
Other and unspecified mechanism[4]	145	0.4
Other causes of violence	107	0.3
Injuries of undetermined intent	323	0.9
Adverse effects of medical treatment	1197	3.2
Blank cause[5]	4778	12.9

[1]Based on the Supplementary Classification of External Cause of Injury and Poisoning, International Classification of Diseases, 9th Revision, Clinical Modification.

[2]Includes drowning, suffocation, firearm, and other mechanisms.

[3]Includes assault by firearms and explosives, and other mechanisms.

[4]Includes injury by cutting and piercing instruments, and other and unspecified mechanisms.

[5]Includes illegible entries and blanks.

Note: Numbers may not add to totals because of rounding.

- Wearing a seat belt offers a 75% efficiency rate in preventing fatal injury and a 30% chance of preventing injury altogether.
- Lap and shoulder belts reduce the risk of fatal injury to front seat passenger car occupants by 45% and the risk of serious injury by 55%. In light trucks, these risks are reduced by 60–65%.
- There is a 20–30% higher risk of fatality with an increase in speed from 55 to 65 miles per hour, even with seat belt use and air bags.
- Nearly 50% of all serious head injuries could be avoided through the use of seat belts.
- People who consistently wear seat belts are less likely to be involved in an accident.
- An unrestrained occupant of a 35-mile-per-hour vehicular crash must be able to bench press approximately 17,000 pounds to "brace" himself or herself.
- A vehicle occupant who is thrown from a car is 25 times more likely to be injured than one who is belted in place. The forces in a crash can be great enough to throw an occupant as far as 150 ft (about 15 car lengths).
- In a 30-mile-per-hour collision, a driver or passenger who is not wearing a seat belt slams into the windshield or other interior surface of the vehicle with the same impact as a fall from a three-story building.
- Alcohol/Drugs
  - Forty percent of fatal automobile accidents involve drivers with blood alcohol levels greater than or equal to 0.10.
  - Driving after as little as 1 or 2 drinks can be dangerous.
  - An individual whose blood alcohol content is 0.15 is 300–600 times more likely to have an accident.
  - A designated driver should be appointed whenever a combination of alcohol and driving is a possibility.
  - Screen patients for problem drinking, as alcoholics have an 8 times greater risk of dying in an MVA than a nondrinker.
  - Patients should also be screened for use of other drugs in addition to alcohol, as 10–32% of people injured in MVAs have other drugs (marijuana, cocaine, alcohol) present in their blood, with or without alcohol.
  - Other drugs in addition to alcohol may be a cause of an accident or may be present in those more likely to take risks.
  - Alcohol is involved in approximately 40% of all deaths resulting from MVAs.
  - Almost 30% of drivers ages 15–20 who were killed in MVAs during 1996 had been drinking.
- Child safety seats
  - Child safety seats in motor vehicles should be installed correctly and used in accordance with the manufacturer's instructions.
  - Child safety seats save approximately 160 lives each year.

- As many as 52,600 pediatric injuries can be avoided with their proper use.
- When used correctly, child safety seats are 71% effective in preventing fatalities, 67% effective in reducing serious injuries, and 50% effective in preventing minor injuries.
- Over the period from 1982 through 1994, an estimated 2655 lives were saved by child restraints.
- In a crash at highway speeds of 30 miles per hour, a 15-lb child can generate a sudden force of greater than 300 lb.
- Make sure all children are secured in safety seats no matter where they sit in a vehicle. Child safety seats are best used in the back seat away from air bags.
- An adult not wearing a seat belt and holding a child in his or her lap in a 30-mile-per-hour crash is thrown forward with the force of 1.5 tons.
- Drivers are less likely to be involved in MVAs if all children are properly secured in safety seats.

* Motorcycles and all terrain vehicles (ATVs)
  - Helmet use by motorcyclists resulted in a 30% reduction in mortality and 75% reduction in head injuries.
  - Eighty percent of motorcyclists killed in MVAs are intoxicated at the time of the accident.
  - Helmet use with ATVs reduces the risk of death by 42%.

* Age
  - Trauma is primarily a disease of younger people, with more than half of all persons killed in MVAs less than 25 years of age.
  - Young drivers between 15 and 20 years old account for only 6.7% of the total number of drivers, but are involved in the majority of fatal crashes.
  - Almost one third of the 15-to-20-year-old drivers involved in fatal crashes who had an invalid operator's license at the time of the crash also had a previous license suspension or revocation.
  - The elderly or infirm are also at greater risk of MVAs. Therefore, functional aids (hearing amplification or corrective lens), and/or avoidance of certain medications should be considered when operating a motor vehicle.

Firearms[1, 6, 7, 9]

* Three basic rules of firearm safety should be followed at all times:
1. Every gun should be treated as loaded and ready to fire.
2. Never point a gun at any object that is not an intended target.
3. Unload and secure all firearms after use.
* Firearms should be kept out of reach of children and others who are not intended to use the firearm.

* Trigger locks prevent firing of the weapon but should not substitute for keeping the weapon unloaded and out of the reach of children.
* An absolutely childproof safety device does not exist!
* If the firearm is to be used for recreational purposes or hunting, appropriate use, carrying, handling, and safety should be taught.
* The shooter should be aware of the target and anything along the trajectory to prevent unintended injury.
* Children and others may encounter firearms outside the home or a controlled setting. It is best to counsel the individual or the child to remove himself or herself from the setting, not to touch the weapon, and to immediately inform a responsible adult to prevent potential injury (e.g., in the situation of another child playing with a gun or finding a firearm).
* Firearm deaths have been steadily reduced through individual and community safety education, hunter safety classes, requiring hunters to wear blaze orange apparel, and improved equipment (e.g., rifle scopes and appropriate recognition of the target). See Figure 14–1.[9]
* See also Chapter 10, Safety Precautions In and Around the Home.

Falls[1, 6, 7]

* Appropriate barriers should be used to prevent children from falling down stairs, off tables, and out of windows.
* Falls in the elderly are caused by medical conditions, gait dysfunction, medications (e.g., sedative), visual difficulty, and/or cognitive impairment.

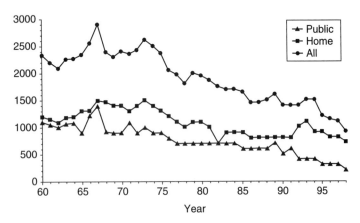

Figure 14–1. Accidental Firearms-Related Fatalities, 1960–1998. (From National Shooting Sports Federation, nssf.org, with permission.)

* Stairs, walking surface irregularity, slippery surfaces, inadequate lighting, unexpected objects, and improper footwear increase the risk of falls.
* Preventive efforts in the elderly include exercise, balance therapy, external protective devices (handrails, carpeting), medication adjustments, measures to increase bone density, improved lighting, risk-proofing the living area, appropriate footwear, and corrective lenses.
* Fifty percent of serious fall injuries in the elderly result in nursing home admissions.
* With a hip fracture, there is a 10–20% decrease in expected survival within the first year following the injury.
* Normal function is not regained in approximately 50% of older people following hip fractures.
* See also Chapters 9 and 10, Geriatrics and Safety Precautions In and Around the Home.

Poisoning[1, 6, 7]

* A poison control telephone number should be immediately available.
* Have ipecac available and accessible, but do not use it unless instructed to do so by poison control personnel.
* Keep poisons out of the reach and access of children.
* Childproof caps should be used on all medication bottles (if an older person who is unable to use childproof caps is present, store and secure the medications out of a child's reach).
* Poison warning labels, including those targeted at children, do not seem to prevent poisonings.
* Cabinets and doors containing and concealing potentially toxic substances should be secured with childproof latches.
* Young adult men account for approximately 40% of unintentional poisoning deaths, usually due to alcohol, heroin, and cocaine use.

Burns[6, 7]

* To prevent scald injuries, water heaters should be set at a temperature of <120–130°F.
* Death in fires is 2–3 times more likely in homes without smoke detectors.
* Smoke detectors require proper installation, testing, and maintenance.
* A fire escape plan should be formulated and understood by all family members and visitors to the home.
* A sign in the window (available at many fire departments) should identify children's rooms.
* Fire-retardant clothing (especially pajamas) should be worn. If clothing ignites, "drop and roll" anticipatory guidance reduces extent of burn injuries.

* Alcohol is involved in about 40% of deaths in residential fires.
* Fires are prevalent in winter, with the use of portable heaters and fireplaces, or the presence of Christmas trees.
* Common causes of fires set by children include playing with matches or lighters and smoking.
* Preventive measures include keeping matches and lighters out of a child's reach and counseling those who smoke not to smoke in bed or when intoxicated.
* "Learn Not To Burn" education programs should be encouraged through mass media and/or schools.
* The elderly suffer a higher mortality if burned.
* Seventy-five percent of clothing ignition occurs in the elderly (over age 65) and is thought to be caused by a combination of impaired coordination and smoking.

Drowning[6, 7]

* Death rates from drowning are greatest for children younger than age 5 and for men from 15 to 24 years of age.
* The majority of infant drownings occur in bathtubs, usually due to inadequate supervision
* In children, 40–90% of drownings occur in swimming pools, with about 75% of cases occurring despite the child's being supervised.
* Adolescent and adult drownings occur more often in lakes, rivers, and ponds and are associated with recreational activity.
* Alcohol is associated with 25–50% of drownings (other drugs are associated with 10% of drownings).
* Life preservers or personal flotation devices (PFDs) were not used in 75% of drownings associated with boating.
* Preventive efforts include
  * Discouraging alcohol use when participating in water activities
  * Encouraging water safety and boating classes
  * Swimming lessons
  * PFDs on nonswimmers around or in pools or other bodies of water
  * Childproof fencing around pools
  * PFD use for all persons regardless of age or skill levels when on the water. Special suits to prevent hypothermia should be worn by all persons on the water when low water temperatures exist or delay in rescue is a possibility.
  * Basic cardiac life support (BCLS) training should be encouraged

Elderly at Risk for Asphyxiation Deaths Caused by Choking

* Preventive efforts include proper denture fit, reduction in use of sedatives, appropriate dietary changes, and BCLS training.

Sports[1, 6, 7, 10]

* Appropriate protective gear should be worn when participating or practicing any athletic activity.
* Certain sports should be discouraged (e.g., boxing, trampolines).
* Proper training, conditioning, and warm-ups should be advocated before any athletic activity.
* Recreational activities and sports should not be performed when intoxicated.
* Injury rates for all sports are included in Table 14–5.[10]

Bicycle[1, 2, 6, 7, 10]

* Mandatory helmet laws and community-based education have increased helmet use and decreased head injuries, hospitalizations and fatalities (by 80%).
* Ninety percent of bicycle-related deaths are the result of collisions with motor vehicles, with 80% of the deaths related to head injury.
* Bicycle helmets reduce the risk of head injury by 85%.
* Only about 18% of bicyclists wear helmets.
* Bicyclists treated for head injury are anywhere between 4.5 and 19.6 times more likely to be unhelmeted than those without head injury.
* Bicycle-related deaths are highest in children 10 to 14 years of age.
* Bicycles are associated with more childhood injury than any other consumer product directly operated by children.
* Nearly half of all bicycle fatalities occur between 4 PM and 8 PM Friday through Sunday.[11]
* About six times as many males experience bicycle-related deaths compared with females. At every age, more male than female bicyclists are killed.
* Alcohol use—either by the driver or by the bicyclist—was reported in more than one third of the traffic accidents that resulted in bicyclist fatalities in 1995.[12]

Farm/Agricultural Accidents[6, 7, 13]

* Tractors should be equipped with rollover protective structures (ROPS) and seat belts.
* Tractors should be shut off every time the operator leaves the seat and certainly before machines are serviced, adjusted, or unclogged.
* Permit NO RIDERS on tractors or machinery, or on the outside of vehicles.
* All guards and shields on machinery should be in place.
* All vehicles should be properly maintained and equipped with safety belts. Operators and passengers must wear safety belts.

Table 14-5. Sports Injuries: Sports Participation and Injuries, United States, 1997

Sports	Participants	Injuries	Percent of Injuries by Age				65 and Over
			0-4	5-14	15-24	25-44	
Archery	4,800,000	3,213	4.9	27.8	17.8	47.4	2.1
Baseball and softball	30,400,000	326,714	0.0	36.0	26.0	36.0	0.0
Basketball[a]	33,300,000	644,921	0.3	30.5	47.7	21.4	0.1
Bicycle riding[a, b]	45,100,000	544,561	7.0	56.8	14.1	19.8	2.2
Billiards, pool	36,000,000	3685	7.9	27.2	28.5	29.1	7.3
Bowling	44,800,000	23,317	7.1	17.7	17.8	46.7	10.6
Boxing	(*)	7257	1.3	10.8	55.8	32.2	0.0
Exercising with equipment[c]	47,900,000	86,024	10.0	16.2	24.7	45.1	4.0
Fishing	44,700,000	72,598	4.0	25.8	13.6	49.3	7.2
Football[d]	20,100,000	334,420	0.3	44.9	43.3	11.3	0.2
Golf	26,200,000	39,473[e]	6.1	26.4	10.6	39.9	17.0
Gymnastics	(*)	33,373[f]	2.4	76.3	19.9	1.4	0.5
Handball	(*)	2517	0.0	31.5	38.9	29.5	0.0
Horseback riding	(*)	58,709	2.1	20.6	17.7	57.0	2.5
Ice hockey	1,900,000	77,491[g]	0.0	26.8	43.3	28.8	0.6
Ice skating	7,900,000	25,379[h]	2.1	49.3	18.3	28.4	1.7
Racquetball[i]	4,500,000	10,438	0.2	5.5	24.1	67.9	2.3

Roller skating	37,500,000	153,023[h,i]	1.3	60.2	16.9	21.4	0.2
Skateboarding	6,300,000	48,186	1.6	50.8	41.3	6.0	0.3
Snowboarding	2,800,000	37,638	0.0	24.0	54.0	21.9	0.2
Snowmobiling	(°)	12,676	0.5	10.0	27.1	62.4	0.0
Soccer	13,700,000	148,913	0.2	48.0	35.5	16.2	0.1
Swimming	59,500,000	83,772	10.4	43.4	20.3	24.5	1.5
Tennis	11,100,000	22,794	1.2	14.6	18.0	49.8	16.4
Volleyball	17,800,000	67,340	0.1	23.2	41.0	35.4	0.2
Water skiing	6,500,000	10,657	0.0	2.8	27.9	68.2	1.0
Wrestling	(°)	39,829	0.3	31.8	57.9	9.9	0.0

Source: Participant—National Sporting Goods Association (NSGA); figures include those 7 years of age or older who participated more than once per year except for bicycle riding and swimming, which include those who participated six or more times per year. Injuries—Consumer Products Safety Commission (CPSC); figures include only injuries treated in hospital emergency departments.

a Basketball and bicycle riding each accounted for more than half a million emergency department visits in 1997.
b Excludes mountain biking.
c Includes weight lifting.
d Includes touch and tackle football.
e Excludes golf carts (8304 injuries).
f Excludes trampolines (82,722 injuries).
g There were 4444 injuries in street hockey, 5584 in roller hockey, 4830 in field hockey, and 45,306 in hockey (unspecified).
h There were 22,748 injuries in skating, unspecified.
i Includes squash and paddle ball.
j Includes 2 × 2 (54,609 injuries) and in-line (98,414 injuries).
° Numbers not available.
(From Sports Participation and Injuries, United States, 1997. Injury Facts, National Safety Council, Itasca, IL, 1999, with permission.)

* When repairing electrical systems or equipment, the electrical power must be locked out.
* Working surfaces should be dry, free of objects and conditions that could cause falls, and well lighted.
* Mechanical devices should be used to lift heavy objects, and repetitive lifting, carrying, or handling of materials should be mechanized. Forklifts, loaders, and conveyors should be used in place of "back power" whenever possible.
* Jobs and workstations should be redesigned to eliminate repetitive reaching, pulling, pushing, and lifting activities.
* Workers must be instructed in the proper way to get on and off a tractor or bed of a truck, and how to go up and down ramps, ladders, and stairs.
* Workers must be forced to wear safe footwear and other protective clothing and gear (e.g., goggles and respirators) needed for the job.

ADVANCED TRAUMA LIFE SUPPORT

When clinician or community education efforts are not initiated or not heeded, the next encounter with the health care provider is following the traumatic event. It is at this time that secondary preventive efforts must predominate to reduce the effect of the damage that has already occurred.

Immediately after the injury occurs the *golden hour* begins. The *golden hour* refers to intervention for shock and restoration of functional circulation and blood pressure within 1 h after the traumatic event. This term was initially coined by R. Adams Cowley of the Maryland Institute for Emergency Medical Services.

For all health care providers who treat trauma, especially those who handle it infrequently, the Advanced Trauma Life Support (ATLS) course (as taught by the American College of Surgeons) provides a systematic, easily remembered method for diagnosing and treating the victims of trauma. The following is a brief overview of ATLS basic concepts. Participation in a provider course cannot be overemphasized, as didactic concepts, simulated drills, and practical procedure skill workshops are included in the program.

Trauma patients encountered may have very minor, moderately serious, or very serious and life-threatening injuries. Trauma patients are initially evaluated by a system called triage. The word *triage* is derived from the French *trier,* which means "to sort out."[14] Initially, trauma patients can be categorized as Category I (e.g., multiple system trauma, severely bleeding open fractures, severe head injury, pelvic fractures), Category II (e.g., nonbleeding open fractures, minor bleeding soft tissue wounds), or Category III (e.g., uncomplicated fractures, no hypotension or hypovolemia, no neurologic injury).[14]

The assessment of a trauma patient begins with the first encounter with a health care professional, usually an emergency medical technician. All trauma patients are initially evaluated by the AVPU method to evaluate the level of consciousness of a patient:

A: Alert

V: Responds to Vocal stimuli

P: Responds only to Painful stimuli

U: Unresponsive to all stimuli[2]

The next step is the Primary and Secondary Survey that each trauma patient must undergo so that the appropriate treatment plan can be developed.

The process by which the Primary Survey is made constitutes the A-B-C-D-Es of trauma care and identifies life-threatening conditions.[2]

A. **Airway** with Cervical Spine Protection
   1. Assessment
      a. Ascertain patency.
      b. Rapidly assess for airway obstruction.
   2. Management—Establish a patent airway
      a. Perform a chin lift or jaw thrust maneuver.
      b. Clear the airway of foreign bodies.
      c. Insert an oropharyngeal or nasopharyngeal airway.
      d. Establish a definitive airway.
         i. Orotracheal or nasotracheal intubation
         ii. Surgical cricothyroidotomy
   3. Maintain the cervical spine in a neutral position with manual immobilization as necessary when establishing an airway.
   4. Reinstate immobilization of the cervical spine with appropriate devices after establishing an airway.

B. **Breathing:** Ventilation and Oxygenation
   1. Assessment
      a. Expose the neck and chest; ensure immobilization of the head and neck.
      b. Determine the rate and depth of respirations.
      c. Inspect and palpate neck, chest for tracheal deviation, unilateral and bilateral chest movement, use of assessory muscles, and any signs of injury.
      d. Percuss the chest for presence of dullness or hyperresonance.
      e. Ascultate the chest bilaterally.
   2. Management
      a. Administer high concentrations of oxygen.
      b. Ventilate with a bag valve mask device.
      c. Alleviate tension pneumothorax.
      d. Seal open pneumothorax.
      e. Intubate if indicated; attach a CO_2 monitoring device to the endotracheal tube (as soon as available).
      f. Attach the patient to a pulse oximeter.

C. **Circulation** with Hemorrhage Control
  1. Assessment
     a. Identify source of external, exsanguinating hemorrhage.
     b. Identify potential source(s) of internal hemorrhage.
     c. Determine pulse: quality, rate, regularity, paradox.
     d. Assess skin color.
     e. Determine blood pressure, time permitting.
  2. Management
     a. Apply direct pressure to external bleeding site.
     b. Consider presence of internal hemorrhage and potential need for operative intervention, and obtain surgical consultation.
     c. Insert two large-caliber intravenous catheters.
     d. Simultaneously obtain blood for hematologic and chemical analyses, pregnancy test, type and crossmatch, and arterial blood gas analysis.
     e. Initiate IV fluid therapy with warmed Ringer's lactate solution and blood replacement.
     f. Apply the pneumatic antishock garment (e.g., military antishock [MAST] trousers) or pneumatic splints as indicated to control hemorrhage.
     g. Prevent hypothermia.
D. **Disability:** Brief Neurologic Examination
  1. Determine the level of consciousness using the AVPU method or the Glasgow coma score.
  2. Assess the pupils for size, quality, and reaction.
E. **Exposure/Environment:** Completely undress the patient but prevent hypothermia.

The Secondary Survey is a more detailed, comprehensive examination after all life-threatening conditions have been addressed. A history is taken using the AMPLE method:

  A: Allergies
  M: Medications currently used
  P: Past illnesses/Pregnancy
  L: Last meal
  E: Events/Environment related to the injury

A special "trauma series" of radiographs is made as indicated during the primary and secondary survey.

All trauma patients should be questioned concerning their tetanus immunization status and treated according to the Centers for Disease Control guidelines (DT boosters preferred to TT; see Chapter 11, Immunizations).

All those who encounter a trauma patient should use personal protective devices (PPDs). These items include goggles, gloves, head covers, shoe covers, and gowns that are fluid resistant. The risk of infection (AIDS, hepatitis, tuberculosis, and other communicable diseases) from contact with body fluids is a very serious concern during contact with a trauma patient. Because of these risks, universal protection against body fluids is absolutely necessary.[2]

CONCLUSION

Trauma is the leading cause of death in persons under the age of 45 and continues to be a significant source of mortality and morbidity throughout life. Prevention focused upon a knowledge of the mechanisms of injury and potential methods of prevention and counseling can make a significant impact upon patients of the primary care provider. Successful interaction between the provider and the community can reinforce preventive efforts. When primary prevention fails, careful attention to the concepts and skills contained in the ATLS provider program and the maximal use of the *golden hour* reduce mortality and morbidity. Rehabilitation of the patient and renewed educational efforts form the cornerstone of tertiary prevention of traumatic injuries.

REFERENCES

1. Last JM, Wallace RB. Public Health and Preventive Medicine, 13th ed. Appleton & Lange, 1992.
2. American College of Surgeons, Committee on Trauma. Advanced Trauma Life Support for Doctors, Instructor Course Manual, 6th ed. American College of Surgeons, 1997.
3. Centers for Disease Control and Prevention (CDC), Deaths and death rates for the 10 leading causes of death in specified age groups, by race and sex: United States, 1997. National Vital Statistics Reports 1999; 47, 19, June 30, 1999 (Table 8).
4. Centers for Disease Control and Prevention (CDC), Deaths, death rates, and age-adjusted death rates for injury deaths according to mechanism and intent of death: United States, 1997. National Vital Statistics Reports 1999; 67, no. 19, June 30, 1999 (Table 19).
5. DuRant RH, Smith JA, Kreiter SA, Krowchuk DP. The relationship between early age of onset of initial substance use and engaging in multiple health risk behaviors among young adolescents. Arch Pediatr Adolesc Med 1999; 153:286–291.
6. Guide to Clinical Preventive Services, 2nd ed. Report of the U.S. Preventive Services Task Force. Williams & Wilkins, 1996.
7. Woolf SH, Jonas S, Lawrence RS. Health Promotion and Disease Prevention in Clinical Practice. Williams & Wilkins, 1995.
8. Advance Data, No. 313, May 10, 2000, National Hospital Ambulatory Medical Care Survey. 1998 Emergency Department Summary, from Vital and Health Statistics of the Centers for Disease Control and Prevention/ National Center for Health Statistics (Tables 8 and 9, page 17).
9. Accidental Firearms-Related Fatalities, 1960–1998. National Shooting Sports Federation. nssf.org.
10. Sports Participation and Injuries, United States, 1997. Injury Facts, National Safety Council, 1999. National Safety Council, Itasca, IL, 1999.
11. American College of Surgeons, Committee or Trauma Advanced Trauma Life Support for Doctors, Instructor Course Manuals, 6th ed. American College of Surgeons, 1997, pp 436–437.
12. National Center for Injury Prevention and Control, Fact Sheet: Bicycle-Related Head Injury, 04-29-97

13. University of Florida, Fact Sheet AE-92, Florida Cooperative Extension Service, 11/91.
14. Wilkins EW Jr., Emergency Medicine: Scientific Foundations and Current Practice, 3rd ed. Baltimore, Williams & Wilkins, 1989, pp 6–7, 42–58, 977.

RESOURCES

FURTHER READINGS

Barker LR., Principles of Ambulatory Medicine, 4th ed., Baltimore, Williams & Wilkins, 1995.

Flaherty L, Maclean S, Jagim M, et al. A Crash Course in Motor Vehicle Injury Prevention. Park Ridge, IL. Emergency Nurses Association, 1996.

Harwood-Nuss AL. The Clinical Practice of Emergency Medicine, 2nd ed. Philadelphia, Lippincott-Raven, 1996.

Mortiere MD. Principles of Primary Wound Management, A Guide to the Fundamentals. Gaithersburg, MD, PFP Printing Inc., 1996.

National Committee for Injury Prevention and Control. Injury Prevention: Meeting the Challenge. New York, Oxford University Press, 1989.

National Highway Traffic Safety Administration. Campaign Safe & Sober Planner 21, National Highway Traffic Safety Administration, Washington, DC. February 2000.

Salyer SW. The Physician Assistant Emergency Medicine Handbook. Philadelphia, WB Saunders, 1997.

Tintinalli JE. Emergency Medicine: A Comprehensive Study Guide. New York, McGraw-Hill, 1996.

Wilkins Jr. EW, Emergency Medicine: Scientific Foundations and Current Practice. 3rd ed. Baltimore, Williams & Wilkins, 1989.

INTERNET RESOURCES

www.projecthomesafe.org
Project HomeSafe partners distribute, free of charge, safety kits that include a gun locking device. The site also provides links for safety information and education.

http://www.nrahq.org/safety/eddie/info.shtml
The Eddie Eagle GunSafe Program
Regardless of one's stance on the political perspective of firearms or whether or not a particular family owns firearms, chances are that neighbors and relatives do, making it likely that children will encounter a firearm at some point.
Just as Smokey Bear teaches children not to play with matchbooks, Eddie Eagle teaches them not to play with firearms with a simple, memorable, four-part plan.

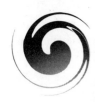

CHAPTER 15

Health Planning and Illness Prevention for International Travel

Christopher A. Ohl, MD, FACP,
and Charles C. Lewis, MPH, PA-C

INTRODUCTION

Travel medicine, or "emporiatrics," has emerged since the 1970s as a medical subspecialty concerned with the health of the international traveler. Each year over 500 million travelers cross international borders with itineraries that vary from a short business trip in a modern city to an adventure tourism trek in a deep tropical rainforest. Although most patients inquire initially about "required shots" and treatment or prevention of "Montezuma's revenge," the spectrum of preventable disease and injury for overseas travelers is quite broad and ranges from trivial to life-threatening. Thus, medical providers who consult with international travelers should consider a wide range of health issues to prevent illness and injury in these special-circumstance patients.

The incidence of travel-related illness increases as exposure time and intensity increase. Some studies report that 50–75% of United States citizens who travel abroad will experience illness that may be directly attributable to their travel. Fortunately, serious morbidity or mortality is rare, with the death rate for Americans traveling overseas less than five per 100,000. At the same time, the cost of prevention can be extremely high. It is common for many travelers to spend $100–$400 for advice, medications, and vaccinations.[1] Moreover, the cost-effectiveness of pretravel vaccination is controversial. Nevertheless, travelers and businesses must individually weigh these uninsured expenses against the potential financial loss of an expensive business trip or vacation that was ruined by illness or mishap. Thus, the prudent traveler and travel medicine practitioner will individualize preventive advice and interventions based on the ultimate risk for illness determined by the traveler's health, itinerary, activities, and behaviors.

The association between a traveler and a travel medicine provider involves three aspects.

* Pretravel preparation
* Medical assistance while traveling
* Post-travel evaluation of illness

This chapter is predominantly concerned with illness and injury prevention, which, ideally, should be provided months prior to the traveler's embarking on a trip.

PRETRAVEL ASSESSMENT

A pre-overseas travel visit to a travel clinic or medical provider ideally should be scheduled several months prior to the expected departure date in order to allow adequate time for consultation and recommended sequential immunizations. Patients who have medical or dental problems may need additional time to consult with their primary care provider in order to adjust medications or stabilize chronic illnesses. Unfortunately, many wait until the last minute for consultation, leaving little time for proper vaccination and procurement of medications.

Preparation

Travel and living arrangements should be made far enough in advance to allow the traveler to determine what special needs may occur. For example:

* Will mosquito netting be needed; if so, where will it be obtained?
* How will safe food and water be obtained?
* What access to modern health care will be available and how far away from the traveler's destination will it be?
* Aside from routine items, what else will the traveler need to bring, and will it fit properly in the luggage allowed for the trip.
* Does the country being visited require specific immunizations?
* Would the patient benefit from any routine boosters?
* How long will the patient be away from home? The answer to this question may influence how prescriptions are written and how much empowerment for self-treatment should be considered.

PATIENT INTERVIEW AND HISTORY

The travel medicine provider should ascertain and record a brief history of the traveler's medical and psychiatric illnesses. A complete list of medications and allergies (including past vaccination reactions) should be documented. The vaccination status of the traveler should be obtained, if possible, from available medical records and vaccination certificates. The travel itinerary must be explored, with attention to details such as destination(s), length of stay, accommodations, voca-

Box 15-1–TRAVELERS WITH SPECIAL NEEDS

1. Patients with current medical problems
2. Pregnant women
3. Children
4. Immunocompromised patients (e.g., patients with HIV/AIDS, transplant recipients, patients receiving steroids)
5. Returning expatriates
6. High altitude travelers
7. Travelers planning expeditions involving diving or other risky activities

tional and recreational activities, and access to medical care and medications. Elucidating the patient's knowledge of his or her destination and past overseas travel experience will provide the clinician with insight into the amount of information that must be provided to the patient during the visit.[2] Special attention may be required for travelers with special needs (Box 15–1). The traveler should be informed that most health insurance policies do not provide coverage while overseas. Health insurance can often be purchased for overseas destinations from insurance companies specializing in travel coverage. Putting together a travel medical kit to be included in the carry-on luggage is often advised (Box 15–2).

Box 15-2–TRAVEL MEDICAL KIT

1. Bottled water for use in areas where safe beverages cannot be purchased, e.g., at airports, at customs stations, on bus trips
2. First aid items, e.g., bandages, mole skin for blister prevention
3. Medications, including prescription and nonprescription items, e.g., pain relievers, cold remedies, antacids, over-the-counter topical steroids, medication for vaginitis
4. Medications specific to the travel destination, e.g., antimotility agents, antibiotics, antimalarials
5. Materials for water purification such as bleach or iodine
6. Insect repellents
7. Sun block
8. Mosquito bed netting for use in malarious areas (should be treated with permethrin and allowed to dry prior to departure)
9. Immunization certificates (should be kept with passport)

TRAVEL RISK ASSESSMENT

The risk for specific illness or injury in an individual traveler can often be estimated from the patient's initial interview and history (see Table 15–1). Assessing the level of risk to the traveler's health is important in order to adapt specific preventive education, medications, and vaccinations to the individual journey. For example, consider two travelers visiting Thailand. One is a healthy person visiting Bangkok for 2 days of business meetings, staying in a quality hotel and eating in established tourist restaurants. The other traveler is a college student visiting the country for a few months to study Southeast Asian temple artistry, who plans to stay in student hostels and explore the culture of Thailand through its food. The business traveler needs only education about safe drink and food, and minimal vaccinations, whereas the student requires extensive education about safe drink and food, insect avoidance, and how to seek medical care in the country of destination. In addition, the student will need antibiotics for self-treatment of diarrhea, antimalarial medication, and vaccination against hepatitis A, typhoid fever, and Japanese encephalitis. Both should be advised on the risk of sexually transmitted diseases and avoidance of sex with strangers and professional sex workers. If sexual relations are anticipated, the hepatitis B vaccination and safe sex education should be discussed.

In general, those who prefer adventure or a more intense and prolonged cultural experience will assume greater risk and require greater preventive measures.

Table 15–1. Assessment of Travel Risk for Injury or Illness

	Higher Risk	**Lower Risk**
Destination climate	Tropical	Temperate
Destination	Developing nation, rural region	Industrialized nation, urban regions
Number of destinations	Several nations or localities	One nation or locality
Travel activity	Adventure tourism, outdoor vocations, religious or medical missions	Common tourism destinations, business travel
Travel accommodations	Low quality hotels, hostels, homes of friends or relatives; dormitories	High quality hotels
Exposure to local citizens	Frequent and intimate	Limited
Health of traveler	Chronic illness, impaired immunity	Good health and fitness

Other considerations include the sequence order of border-crossings when visiting multiple countries, which may impact on required vaccinations such as yellow fever, and the climatic season of the visit. Many endemic infectious diseases such as meningococcal meningitis and several arthropod-borne diseases have a seasonal predilection. Conversely, diseases considered seasonal in North America are transmitted year-round in tropical climates. Cruise ships, although generally equated with high-quality hotels, have been implicated in extraseasonal outbreaks of influenza.[3]

PREVENTION OF TRAVELER'S DIARRHEA AND OTHER ENTERIC DISEASES

Enteric diseases, in particular traveler's diarrhea, pose the greatest risk of illness to travelers journeying to the developing world. Several studies have shown that approximately 40% of such travelers will develop traveler's diarrhea, with considerable impact on the individual traveler's health and finances. Although mortality caused by traveler's diarrhea is very uncommon, one third of those who suffer from this ailment are confined to bed, and up to 40% are forced to change their travel plans. Although the term traveler's diarrhea is commonly applied, the health care provider should attempt to distinguish watery diarrhea from true dysentery by the absence or presence of fecal red blood cells and leukocytes. Some examples are included in Table 15–2.

Fortunately, the more severe enteric diseases such as dysentery, hepatitis A, typhoid fever, cholera, and polio are rare in routine travelers. However, the potential mortality and morbidity of these latter illnesses necessitate that many overseas travelers take preventive

Table 15–2. Causes of Infectious Diarrhea in Travelers, According to Common Clinical Presentation

Watery Diarrhea	Dysentery
Aeromonas spp.	*Campylobacter jejuni*
Plesiomonas shigelloides	*E. histolytica*
Entamoeba histolytica	Invasive *E. coli*
Giardia lamblia	*Salmonella* spp.
Noncholera vibrios	*Shigella* spp.
Norwalk agent	*Yersinia enterocolitica*
Rotavirus	
Salmonella spp.	
Toxigenic *E. coli*	
Vibrio cholerae	
Vibrio parahaemolyticus	

measures when visiting regions where these diseases are endemic. As enteric pathogens are almost always acquired through contaminated food and water, the prevention of these diseases can partly be accomplished by motivating the traveler to seek safe cuisine and beverages. Additional protection for selected enteric diseases can be obtained through pretravel immunization. Other measures for the prevention and therapy of traveler's diarrhea can lessen the frequency and severity of this common scourge.[4]

DIETARY ADVICE FOR AVOIDING ENTERIC DISEASES

Most authorities recommend strict adherence to standard dietary advice while traveling in the developing world. Unfortunately, it is difficult for even the most motivated of travelers to adhere to a safe diet. This difficulty most likely explains the fact that many studies have failed to show the efficacy of diet modification for the prevention of traveler's diarrhea. Nevertheless, acquisition of safe food and beverages most likely has a favorable effect on the risk of traveler's diarrhea. Table 15–3 and Box 15–3 outline standard dietary precautions for food and beverages acquired overseas. Travelers should be informed that

Table 15–3. Dietary Advice for the Avoidance of Enteric Disease

	Safe	Unsafe
Beverages	Bottled water (sealed and labeled)	Tap water
	Bottled carbonated soft drinks	Ice—particularly chipped
	Beer	Mixed alcoholic drinks
	Boiled water	Unpasteurized milk and juices
	Self-chlorinated or iodinated water	Teeth brushing with tap water
	Self-filtered water (commercial kits)	
	Pasteurized milk and juices	
	Teeth brushing with bottled water	
Food	Cooked and served hot	Raw or uncooked
	Peeled fruit	Food served cold
	Cracked nuts	Soft cheeses and pastries
	Processed and packaged	Salads and vegetables
	Food from established restaurants	Food from street vendors

Box 15-3–COOKING IN THE HOME

1. Obtain food from known safe sources whenever possible.
2. "Raw" or unpasteurized dairy products and fresh fruit juices are of higher risk.
3. Meat, fish, and poultry should be fresh and clean in appearance.
4. Frozen foods in Third World countries may not have been maintained and stored at proper temperatures.
5. Thoroughly cook all foods and dispose of leftovers (unless adequate and reliable refrigeration exists). Do not allow foods to sit out for periods of time between preparation, cooking, and serving. Serve hot foods hot and keep cold foods cold.
6. Wash and sanitize pots, pans, counter surfaces, and utensils before using them in another level of preparation. This will minimize cross-contamination.
7. When hot water is not available, use a strong chlorine solution to clean surfaces and utensils.
8. Do not allow cooked foods to come in contact with any surface on which raw foods were cut or combined.

---

food and beverage safety should be questioned even in luxury hotels overseas, as most produce used in hotel meals is bought in local markets, and water is often obtained from the municipal water supply. Diseases transmitted by food handlers, such as hepatitis A, can be just as likely to occur in luxury settings as in less luxurious hotels.

Travelers well off the beaten path may have difficulty finding a safe source of food and water.[5] When a heat source is available, it is a simple mater to boil water 3–5 min, which is sufficient to kill most enteric pathogens.

Alternatively, if no heat source is available:

* Water can be filtered with a commercial grade filter.
* Water can be halogenated with iodine (tablets or tincture).
* Two to four drops of household bleach (4–6% sodium hypochlorite) may be added to each liter of water, which is then allowed to stand for 30 min prior to drinking.

Fruits and vegetables can be washed in halogenated water as prepared above and allowed to air dry.

Other factors influencing a traveler's risk for enteric disease include

* Alcoholic beverages, as the alcohol concentration found in most mixed drinks usually fails to kill pathogenic bacteria, and imbibing may well lessen inhibitions and impair dietary discretion.

* Travelers with achlorhydria, either intrinsic owing to disease or surgery or extrinsic owing to use of antacids or medications that raise gastric pH, are at increased risk for enteric disease because of the loss of this important host defense mechanism.

PREVENTION AND THERAPY OF TRAVELER'S DIARRHEA

Traveler's diarrhea is a self-limited diarrheal illness characterized by four or more loose stools occurring in a 24-h period (or three or more stools in an 8-h period). The loose stools are generally accompanied by nausea, crampy abdominal pain, fecal urgency, and, less often, by vomiting and fever. Traveler's diarrhea should be distinguished from dysentery, which is usually accompanied by fever and stool containing red and white blood cells. Traveler's diarrhea is usually caused by bacterial pathogens (see Table 15–2), with enterotoxigenic *Escherichia coli* being the most commonly isolated pathogen. Some bacterial organisms that can be responsible both for this syndrome and for a dysentery form of illness include nontoxogenic *E. coli*, *Campylobacter jejuni*, *Salmonella* spp., and *Shigella* spp. Viruses and protozoa are isolated less commonly in routine travelers. Among the parasitic causes of traveler's diarrhea, *Giardia lamblia* predominates and can be treated empirically with metronidazole (Flagyl) if diarrhea does not respond to antibacterial therapy as outlined below. Risk for traveler's diarrhea is highest in tropical developing nations and lowest in temperate developed countries.[6]

Therapy for traveler's diarrhea can generally be classified as either preventive or abortive. The mainstay of preventive therapy is dietary discretion but may include other modalities as listed in Table 15–4. While there is little question that preventive therapy with bismuth subsalicylate (BSS) or antibiotics is effective in preventing traveler's diarrhea, most clinicians with expertise in travel medicine prefer abortive self-therapy, with the traveler taking steps to stop the illness at its first appearance. The arguments *against* routine antibiotic use for prevention of traveler's diarrhea include

* Frequent adverse reactions (rash, photosensitivity, diarrhea)
* Selection of resistant bacteria in the traveler
* Encouragement of a cavalier attitude toward safe food and drink
* Potential for antibiotic resistance in the destination country

Bismuth subsalicylate is safer and without major concerns for resistance, but many travelers find inconvenient the black coloration of tongue and stools, frequent dosing schedule, and loss of precious luggage space that is required for this volume of medication (liquid or tablets). Although the consensus is against antibiotic prophylaxis for traveler's diarrhea, selected travelers may benefit from it. These travel-

Table 15–4. Agents Used to Prevent Traveler's Diarrhea in Adults

Agent	Dose	Comments
Bismuth subsalicyate (BSS)	Two 262-mg tablets chewed 4 times per day	Less effective than antimicrobials; safe; produces dark stools
Trimethoprim/ sulfamethoxazole	One double-strength tablet once per day	Resistance now common; occasional adverse reaction such as rash
Fluoroquinolones Ciprofloxacin Ofloxacin Levofloxacin	500 mg once daily 300 mg once daily 250 mg once daily	Most effective antibiotic; occasional rash or photosensitivity reaction; usually reserved for self-treatment

ers include those with severe underlying health problems, those with abnormal secretion of gastric acid, and those on extremely important trips where a diarrheal illness would cause severe economic or personal hardship (for example, salvage divers, diplomats, or physicians to medical missions).

The recommended approach to traveler's diarrhea is early self-treatment with replacement fluids, antimotility agents, and BSS or antimicrobial agents. Several studies have shown the efficacy of such an approach.

Loperamide (Imodium) is the antimotility agent of choice for traveler's diarrhea and can be purchased over the counter by the traveler prior to the voyage. Loperamide decreases the frequency of watery bowel movements, relieves abdominal cramping, and shortens the duration of illness. Loperamide should be avoided in very young children and if diarrhea is accompanied by high fever or severe abdominal pain, or if blood or pus is noted in the stool.

Antibiotic therapy is more effective than BSS. Fluoroquinolone antibiotics are more effective than trimethoprim/sulfamethoxazole (TMP/SMZ) because of antimicrobial resistance to the latter. Doxycycline is no longer considered an ideal treatment for diarrhea owing to widespread antimicrobial resistance and photosensitivity reactions. Self-treatment with fluoroquinolone antibiotics decreases the number of diarrheal stools per day and reduces the duration of diarrhea by approximately 50%. Because fluoroquinolones are not indicated in children and pregnant women, TMP/SMZ is still recommended for these patients. Table 15–5 outlines the approach to therapy of traveler's diarrhea using these agents. Rehydration for severe diarrhea may require administration of oral electrolyte solutions.

DISEASES TRANSMITTED BY INSECT AND OTHER ARTHROPOD VECTORS

Those who travel to a tropical or subtropical country potentially risk exposure to insects and/or arthropod-borne disease. Table 15–6 gives a partial list of such diseases and their vectors. Fortunately, with the exception of malaria and dengue fever, most of these afflictions are extremely rare and seen only in long-term travelers. Many arthropod-borne diseases can be prevented through insect and tick bite avoidance, while chemoprophylaxis further decreases the odds of acquiring malaria. Highly protective vaccines are available for yellow

Table 15–5. Treatment of Traveler's Diarrhea

Severity of Diarrhea	Agent	Dose
Occasional loose stool	None	
Mild diarrhea	Loperamide° OR	One tablet every 3–8 h
	Bismuth subsalicylate (BSS)	Adult dose: 2 tablets every 2 h Pediatric dose: 5–10 mL every 2 h
Moderate or severe diarrhea (interferes with social or occupational functions)	Loperamide PLUS	One tablet every 3–8 h
	Fluoroquinolone (preferred)† Ciprofloxacin OR Ofloxacin OR Levofloxacin	500 mg twice daily 300 mg twice daily 500 mg twice daily
	Alternate Antibiotic Trimethoprim/ sulfamethoxazole (TMP/ SMZ)‡	Adult dose: 1 double strength tablet twice daily Pediatric dose: 5 mL liquid per 10 kg per dose twice daily

°Most pediatricians do not recommend loperamide for small children and infants.
†Fluoroquinolone antibiotics are not approved for use in ages less than 18 years old.
‡In most regions TMP/SMZ is not as effective as a fluoroquinolone antibiotic.

Table 15–6. Diseases Associated with Arthropods

Arthropod Vector	Transmitted Disease
Mosquitoes	Malaria
	Dengue fever
	Yellow fever
	Japanese encephalitis
	Arboviral encephalitis
	Filariasis
	Myiasis
Flies	Dysentery
	Leishmaniasis
	Onchocerciasis
	African trypanosomiasis (sleeping sickness)
Bugs *(Hemiptera)*	American trypanosomiasis (Chagas disease)
Fleas	Plague
Ticks	Rickettsial disease (e.g., Rocky Mountain spotted fever, boutonneuse fever)
	Lyme disease
	Tick-borne encephalitis
	Congo-Crimean hemorrhagic fever
	Relapsing fever
Lice	Typhus
	Relapsing fever

Allergy, skin irritation, and cellulitis may result from contact with hairs, scales, stings, and bites from both disease- and non-disease–causing arthropods.

fever, Japanese encephalitis, plague, and tick-borne encephalitis (the vaccine for the latter is not available in the United States).

MALARIA

Clearly malaria is the most important insect-borne disease that threatens both short- and long-term travelers. About seven million Americans visit regions endemic for malaria each year, with approximately 1000 cases of malaria reported annually within the U.S. An additional 10,000–30,000 cases of malaria are diagnosed in travelers from other industrialized countries. The majority of cases of malaria due to *Plasmodium falciparum*, the most dangerous malaria species, are acquired in sub-Saharan Africa. Rates of malaria due to *Plasmodium vivax* appear to be increasing in travelers to the increasingly popular tourist destinations in Central and South America. Malaria, particularly *falciparum*, is a serious disease for nonimmune travelers and can progress from asymptomatic infection to severe malaria within 48 h. Thus, a considerable amount of time should be spent educating the traveler about the prevention of this disease when visiting a malaria-endemic region.[6] Unfortunately, drug-resistant malaria is now found over much of the world and should be taken into account when prescribing chemoprophylaxis or treatment for malaria.

Prevention of malaria starts with mosquito avoidance. By avoiding the bite of the pre–dusk-to-dawn feeding *Anopheles* mosquito, patients can reduce the hazard of malaria considerably. Personal protection measures to avoid insect bites include the use of window screens, bed netting, protective clothing, and insect repellents and insecticides. Travelers visiting malaria-endemic regions who are not staying in screened or air-conditioned quarters should use bed nets. Lightweight nets and frames can be purchased from most outfitters or outdoor adventure supply stores and should be framed or hung so that they are not in contact with the skin of the sleeping person. Impregnating the net with a pyrethroid insecticide such as permethrin (Permanone) will increase its effectiveness. Individuals who are outdoors during evening or nighttime hours should wear clothing that minimizes the amount of exposed skin (long sleeves, long pants, socks). They should also regularly apply an insect repellent that contains at least 30–35% diethyltoluamide (DEET) to all exposed skin. DEET-containing lotions or creams are preferred over spray aerosols. The percentage concentration of DEET is often indicated on the label of most commercially available repellents. For children, DEET concentrations of 12–15% should be used to minimize the potential for encephalopathy or seizures. Non-DEET or "natural" repellents have limited efficacy and are not recommended. Impregnating outdoor clothing with permethrin can increase protection against insect bites. Permethrin-soaked clothing should be allowed to air dry for at least 30 min before wearing.[5, 8]

In addition to taking measures to avoid mosquito bites, chemoprophylaxis is recommended for many travelers to malaria-endemic regions. As all antimalarials have potential adverse effects, the benefit versus risk of prescribing these medications should be weighed when counseling the traveler. Factors to consider include

* Risk of exposure to mosquitoes
* Rate of malaria in the region of the country to be visited
* Odds of being infected with *P. falciparum* or drug-resistant malaria
* Traveler's access to medical care
* Potential contraindications, such as pregnancy
* Adverse effects of medication, for example, hemolysis due to G-6-PD deficiency

For patients traveling from the U.S., the regimens listed in Table 15–7 are usually employed. Patients must be cautioned that strict compliance with instructions is essential and that malaria can still occur even with adherence to chemoprophylaxis. Medication with chloroquine should be started 1 week prior to entering the malarious region, and mefloquine should be started 2 weeks before entering the

Table 15-7. Chemoprophylaxis of Malaria

Geographic Region	Drug	Adult Dose	Pediatric Dose	Adverse Effects
Chloroquine Sensitive				
Central America (west of Panama Canal), Hispaniola, Egypt, Middle East (most areas)	**Primary** Chloroquine (Aralen)	500 mg (salt) weekly	8.3 mg/kg (salt) weekly **Maximum Dose**	Occasional: Nausea, pruritus, headache
	Alternative Doxycycline (Vibramycin, Doryx, Monodox)	100 mg daily	2 mg/kg/day up to 100 mg but relatively contraindicated in children less than age 7.	
Chloroquine Resistant				
Sub-Saharan Africa (except much of South Africa), Panama, Amazonia, Indian subcontinent, Southeast Asia, Oceania	**Primary** Mefloquine (Lariam)	250 mg (salt) weekly	5 mg/kg (salt) weekly; maximum dose: 250 mg	Frequent: Dizziness, nausea, diarrhea, headache, strange dreams, insomnia Rare: Seizures, psychosis
	Alternative Doxycycline	100 mg daily	2 mg/kg/day up to 100 mg but relatively contraindicated in children less than age 7.	
Chloroquine and Mefloquine Resistant				
Borders of Thailand, Cambodia, and Myanmar (Burma)	**Primary** Doxycycline	100 mg daily	2 mg/kg/day up to 100 mg but relatively contraindicated in children less than age 7.	Occasional: Nausea, vaginal candidiasis, photosensitivity rash

Notes:
1. Current, specific information on malaria within the destination country, region, and city should be solicited (see text) in order to choose the most appropriate chemoprophylaxis.
2. Medication may not be appropriate for low-risk activities (e.g., no nocturnal exposure) in low-risk areas.
3. Chloroquine and mefloquine should be started 1–2 weeks prior to entering a malarious region. Doxycycline should be started 1–2 days before entering. All drugs should be continued for 4 weeks after departure.

region. Doxycycline can be initiated 2 days prior to malaria exposure. Chemoprophylactic medication should be continued for 4 weeks after leaving the malaria-endemic region. Postexposure prophylaxis with primaquine (15 mg base daily for 14 days) is appropriate for travelers with prolonged exposure to regions with endemic *P. vivax* or *P. ovale*.

Because of widespread chloroquine resistance, mefloquine is now the mainstay recommended antimalarial for chemoprophylaxis. It is of high efficacy and is generally well tolerated. However, recently, the media, the Internet, and some vocal travelers have focused attention on the safety of mefloquine. Many of these reports focus on possible adverse central nervous system (CNS) effects, including seizures and neuropsychiatric reactions. It should be emphasized that severe CNS reactions are rare with prophylactic doses (less than one occurrence per 10,000 individuals) and that less than 1% of travelers discontinue the drug because of reactions such as anxiety, depression, or nightmares. The risk of serious CNS effects due to mefloquine is higher in patients with a history of depression or anxiety, and the medication is relatively contraindicated in these individuals. Overall, only 1–6% of individuals taking this drug for chemoprophylaxis discontinue the medication because of any side effect (usually nausea, headache or dizziness)—a rate not significantly different from other chemoprophylactic agents. Certainly for those at risk for chloroquine-resistant *falciparum* malaria, the benefit from mefloquine greatly outweighs the risk of these self-limited adverse effects.

In September 2000, Malarone, a new combination antimalarial consisting of atovaquone and proguanil, was made available in the U.S. This drug appears to be as effective as mefloquine for the prevention and treatment of acute *falciparum* malaria with less adverse reactions. The dose for a prophylactic course in adults is one tablet (250 mg atovaquone and 100 mg proguanil) per day to begin 2 days before travel to a malarious area and continued daily through 7 days after return. For children, pediatric tablets are available, with the dose based on weight.

Travelers who have visited any malaria-endemic region should be cautioned that any significant fever (higher than 101°F for 24 h) that occurs within 3–6 months after returning from a malarious region may be a symptom of malaria. Travelers returning from travel to malarious regions should inform their health care provider that evaluation for malaria should be included as part of their evaluation for a febrile illness.

■■■ VACCINE-PREVENTABLE DISEASES[9]

A real or perceived need for pretravel vaccination may well be the traveler's primary reason for contacting a travel clinic or medical care provider. The question, "What shots do I need to go to . . . ?" often begins a traveler's call to the clinic. As outlined in this chapter, however, a capable travel medicine provider will consider many preventive interventions other than vaccines. Nevertheless, immunizations are an important component of the pretravel visit and should be carefully selected—based on destination, degree of disease exposure, length of stay, and potential legal requirements. Table 15–8 lists vaccines that might be considered prior to overseas travel.

The medical care provider and traveler should thoughtfully weigh the benefits and risks of pretravel vaccination. In doing so they must consider that no vaccine is 100% effective or safe and that pretravel immunization can be quite expensive. Travelers will differ in the amount of risk that they are willing to assume for illness. Some individuals may not wish to receive certain vaccines, despite an expected benefit, while others, who are more risk-averse, may request multiple vaccinations—regardless of the chance of disease exposure. The decision on whether or not to vaccinate ultimately rests with the traveler who has been provided with appropriate information on the benefits, risks, and alternatives to each specific immunization. Informed consent should be obtained for all vaccinations. While some travel visas may still require certain immunizations, re-entry into the home country may require others. Patients (via their travel agents) should be aware of any special requirements and so advise the provider. Unfortunately, patients may be completely unaware of special visa requirements, and the provider may need to consult the database of the United States Centers for Disease Control and Prevention (CDC), whose contact information is provided at the end of this chapter.

Very few absolute contraindications exist for vaccine administration

Table 15–8. Immunizations and Screens Used in International Travelers

Vaccines Considered for Short- and Long-Term Travelers	Vaccines and Screens Considered for Long-Term Travelers
Enteric Diseases	Japanese encephalitis
Hepatitis A	Hepatitis B
Typhoid	Rabies (pre-exposure)
Polio	PPD (pre- and post-travel)
Cholera (seldom indicated)	
Arboviral Diseases	
Yellow fever	
Communicable Diseases	
Meningococcal	
Influenza	
Pneumococcal	
Diphtheria/tetanus	

(e.g., severe allergy to a vaccine component). Some relative contraindications, however, may be encountered. These include administration of some live attenuated vaccines to pregnant women, immunosuppressed hosts, and those with severe concurrent illness. Specific recommendations of the Advisory Committee on Immunization Practices (ACIP) can be found on the CDC's web site, cdc.gov. The following invalid reasons have been cited in the past for withholding vaccines:

* Concurrent minor illness or antibiotic therapy
* Disease exposure or convalescence
* Pregnancy in the household
* Need for tuberculosis testing or multiple vaccines

None of these constitutes a valid contraindication. The provider must, however, take into account potential interactions that may exist between vaccines or between vaccines and other pharmaceuticals. Vaccine interactions are occasionally encountered with live attenuated viral vaccines or when coadministering immunoglobulin.

Although a comprehensive discussion of the various vaccines listed in Table 15–8 is beyond the scope of this chapter, an overview of the more commonly administered vaccines follows. The reader is referred to the CDC web site, to the vaccine manufacturer's product insert, or to a vaccine administration handbook for specific information.

HEPATITIS A

This enteric viral infection, once highly endemic to the U.S. and other regions of the developed world, has become less common in these regions in recent times. Thus, a growing segment of the population from these areas is not immune to hepatitis A and risks infection when visiting the developing world. Many countries in Eastern Europe, Latin America, Africa, and South and Southeast Asia are highly endemic for hepatitis A, and travelers who consume contaminated food and water in these areas are at considerable risk for infection. Two vaccines are now available and highly protective for hepatitis A, Havrix and Vaqta. Both should be administered in a series of two vaccinations given 6–12 months apart. These vaccines are long lasting, and current available information indicates that further boosters are not required. A full serologic response requires 4 weeks, but vaccination up to 2 weeks before travel may still be effective. Adverse effects of hepatitis A vaccine include mild pain and occasional redness at the injection site. Systemic side effects are extremely rare. If there is less than 2 weeks available prior to travel, passive immunization with immune globulin (IG) provides immediate but temporary protection from hepatitis A infection. Immune globulin can be administered intramuscularly simultaneously with vaccine for both immediate and long-term protection. Unfortunately, passive immunization is often not practical in the U.S. because of periodic lack of availability of this pooled human serum product.

TYPHOID FEVER

The incidence of typhoid fever has steadily declined in the U.S. and most cases are now attributed to travelers returning from the underdeveloped world. Even so, typhoid fever is a rare illness among travelers, with an overall case rate of 1 in 30,000. In selected countries such as Haiti, Peru, India, Pakistan, and Indonesia the rate is higher. Exposure to typhoid fever may be avoided by insisting on well-cooked foods and safe beverages. Adventuresome eaters, travelers off the beaten path, long-term travelers, or those visiting highly endemic areas may wish to be immunized for further protection. Three vaccines currently exist: an inactivated whole cell parenteral vaccine with an unacceptably high incidence of injection site and systemic febrile reactions and two newer, less reactive vaccines. Vivotif Berna is a live attenuated, oral vaccine produced from typhoid strain Ty21a. It is given as four capsules (U.S. and Canada) or three capsules (outside North America), one every other day, to adults and children over the age of 6. The period of protective immunity from this vaccine is up to 5 years. Refrigeration of the capsules is required during the series, and compliance with the full dosing schedule must be stressed. Typhim Vi is a capsular polysaccharide vaccine for intramuscular injection. One dose is effective for 2 years and can be given to children as young as 2 years. The oral and capsular polysaccharide vaccines have a protective efficacy of 43–96% and 60–72%, respectively.

CHOLERA

This severe diarrheal illness is transmitted through food and water contaminated with *Vibrio cholerae* and is endemic or epidemic in selected regions of the developing world. Fortunately, cholera is rarely seen in travelers, and the disease is rarely fatal if medical attention is promptly sought. It is best prevented by careful attention to acquiring safe food and drink. The current inactivated whole cell parenteral vaccine for cholera is marginally protective at best and is associated with local and systemic adverse reactions. It is currently not recommended by the World Health Organization (WHO) or the CDC for travel to any region. Occasionally, however, some travelers may encounter local governments, usually in Africa, that will require proof of cholera vaccination for border crossings. If so advised by U.S. or a local authority, the vaccine can be given as one dose and entered on the official WHO International Certificate of Immunization. A more efficacious oral vaccine has been licensed in some countries (but not the U.S.) and offers greater protection with fewer side effects. For this reason, some persons at high risk for exposure may choose to break their journey in Europe for this immunization.

POLIO

This disease, which is nearing global eradication, is still occasionally seen in sub-Saharan Africa and South Asia, including the Indian subcontinent. Infection in American travelers is extremely rare because of universal childhood immunization. Adult travelers who never received the primary vaccination series should immediately start the polio vaccination series with inactivated parenteral vaccine (IPV) and be advised to exercise strict food and water precautions. Previously immunized adults traveling to a known endemic area should receive a one-time booster of IPV or oral polio vaccine.

YELLOW FEVER

Yellow fever is a potentially severe mosquito-borne viral infection that is best prevented by vaccination. The CDC recommends this vaccine for travelers entering yellow fever epidemic or rural endemic regions in equatorial South America and Africa. Most countries within this zone require proof of yellow fever vaccination for border entry. In addition, many countries that lie outside endemic regions but have susceptible mosquito populations require vaccination for travelers arriving from countries infected with yellow fever. A list of countries that require yellow fever vaccine for entry can be found on the CDC's web site or in the publication *Health Information for International Travel*. Yellow fever vaccine is highly protective, well tolerated, and requires boosting every 10 years. Redness and pain at the vaccination site are occasionally noted, but systemic reactions are rare. It is a live virus vaccine that is contraindicated in pregnant and lactating women, immunocompromised hosts, and children younger than 6 months of age (many recommend against vaccination for children younger than 12 months of age). This vaccine is valid 10 days after administration and must be recorded on an official WHO International Certificate of Immunization with a uniform stamp that is issued by federal and state immunization programs to official yellow fever immunization centers. A letter from a physician on letterhead stationery stating that yellow fever vaccine is contraindicated on the basis of a medical condition is acceptable in place of a validated vaccination certificate.

JAPANESE ENCEPHALITIS

Japanese encephalitis virus is a cause of sporadic and epidemic encephalitis in rural Southeast Asia, China, and the Indian subcontinent. Symptomatic infection is rare in routine short-term travelers. The mosquito vector breeds in the rice paddies of these regions. An effective vaccine exists for Japanese encephalitis that is given in a three-dose series over 3-4 weeks. This vaccine is associated with local reactions, fever, headache, and malaise in approximately 20% of vaccine recipients and is uncommonly associated with allergic reactions such as urticaria (1 in 100), angioedema (1 in 1000), and anaphylaxis. These allergic responses may occur up to 10 days after vaccination. This vaccine should be reserved for short-term travelers with intense mosquito exposure and for those who will be spending 1 month or more in a known endemic region. Travelers should be cautioned to use personal protection measures against mosquito bites.

RABIES

Pre-exposure vaccination may be recommended for travelers making extended trips to the developing world. Persons such as missionaries (including medical missionaries), teachers, adventure travelers, and others who will be in contact with domestic and wild animals should be considered for this vaccine. Children are at higher risk than adults because of their tendency to play with unknown animals. Patients receiving chloroquine or mefloquine may not mount a sufficient antibody response to this vaccine.

HEPATITIS B

Hepatitis B is a major health problem throughout the world affecting both developed and developing countries. The U.S. has reportedly more than one million chronically infected individuals. A very safe, effective vaccine is currently available in the U.S. and is now routinely given in infancy. Long-term travelers visiting the developing world and short-term travelers who will be involved in health care or intimate contact with local inhabitants should be immunized. The standard dosing schedule requires vaccination at 0, 1, and 6–12 months. An accelerated schedule for Engerix-B (Smithkline Beecham) utilizes doses at 0, 1, and 2 months, with a booster at 12 months.

OTHER VACCINE-PREVENTABLE DISEASES

Other vaccines that should be considered for selected travelers include

* Tetanus-diphtheria boosters if one has not been received within 5–10 years (The shorter interval is used if access to care is limited after receiving a wound.)
* Influenza vaccine for travelers boarding cruise ships or visiting regions with influenza activity
* Pneumococcal vaccine for individuals with chronic medical conditions or anyone over the age of 65
* Tetravalent meningococcal vaccine for travelers to sub-Saharan Africa during the dry season, when epidemic meningococcal disease occurs, for military personnel or students confined in close barrack-style housing. (In addition, pilgrims visiting Saudi Arabia for the haj pilgrimage are required to show proof of vaccination for entry into the country.)

■■■MISCELLANEOUS PREVENTIVE MEASURES

International travelers who plan extended stays, partake in adventure activities, or venture well off the beaten path should make contingency plans prior to departure for emergency medical care in case they become sick or injured. This might include researching competent medical providers in the destination country and purchasing special travel insurance that includes arrangements for medical evacuation by airlift.

Persons planning visits to high altitude regions (above 2500 m/8200 ft) are at risk for altitude sickness (AS). About 25% of adults experience symptoms of AS with ascent from sea level to 2000 m, 30% with ascent to 3000 m, and 75% with exposure to 4500 m (14,800 feet). The risk increases as acclimatization time decreases. Headache, malaise, fatigue, nausea, vomiting, and insomnia characterize mild AS. More severe illness can result in life-threatening cerebral or pulmonary edema. AS is best prevented by maintaining hydration, obtaining adequate rest, and gradually ascending in altitude with occasional overnight stays prior to reaching maximal elevations. For those who are unable to acclimate, acetazolamide (Diamox) at a dose of 125–250 mg twice daily may be initiated 1–2 days prior to ascent and continued for 2–3 days at altitude. High altitude travelers should be instructed to descend to lower altitudes should AS occur and to seek medical care for signs and symptoms of the more severe form of illness.

Sexually transmitted diseases (STDs), including HIV, are endemic throughout much of the world. Travelers may acquire an STD from

Box 15-4–PREVENTIVE MEASURES FOR PERSONAL SAFETY

1. Use only government-approved public conveyances such as taxis and buses (inquire at your hotel or with local authorities).
2. Determine fees and tipping in advance (it is considered impolite in some countries to offer a tip; inquire as to local customs and amounts).
3. Avoid crowds and large public gatherings (pickpockets and vandals may be present in crowds, or anti-American groups may be operating).
4. Do not carry large sums of cash, and do not use a bag with a shoulder strap.
5. Avoid confrontations with local citizens; this is sometimes a ruse used to extort cash.
6. Do not move about alone in unfamiliar surroundings.
7. Do not show interest in items at markets or from street vendors that you do not wish to purchase; know local customs on bartering.
8. Use safety devices such as seat belts when driving or helmets when bicycling.
9. Avoid swimming in fresh water, which may be heavily contaminated or harbor the parasite that causes schistosomiasis.
10. Wear foot gear when walking on beaches.

the local populace or from fellow travelers. Individuals should be advised against high-risk sexual activity and to use latex or polyurethane condoms for any sexual contact. Furthermore, tattoos, intravenous needle use, and elective dental work while traveling, should be discouraged.

Lastly, international travelers should be advised on measures to increase personal safety. Box 15–4 lists common recommendations. The State Department routinely posts advisories on personal safety for selected countries, and the local U.S. embassy can provide further information on crime and safety.

CONCLUSION

With over 500 million travelers crossing international borders each year and medical missions or adventure travel increasing in frequency, the number of primary care patients seeking travel medicine advice is escalating exponentially. A variety of resources are available to the travel medicine provider regarding country-specific information on endemic disease activity, required and recommended vaccinations, malaria chemoprophylaxis, and other issues pertinent to the traveler's health.

* The CDC publishes the "Yellow Book" *Health Information for International Travel* and the CDC world wide web page on International Travelers' Health.
* Computer programs (e.g., Travex) that compile and frequently update health and safety information from official and unofficial sources can be purchased. Many of these programs will generate itinerary-specific documents for the traveler and health care provider.
* The International Association for Medical Assistance to Travelers (IAMAT) publishes a comprehensive list of English-speaking medical care providers overseas who have agreed to a set fee for IAMAT members. Membership can be arranged through the home page listed in the Resources section of this chapter.

Whether the provider chooses to handle these issues personally or to refer patients to a specific travel clinic or health department, a basic knowledge of travel medicine and the advanced planning required is necessary to every clinician.

REFERENCES

1. Centers for Disease Control and Prevention. Epidemiology & Prevention of Vaccine Preventable Diseases: The Pink Book. 1999.
2. Blair DC. A week in the life of a travel clinic. Clin Microbiol Rev 1997; 10:650–673.
3. Centers for Disease Control and Prevention. Health Information for the International Traveler: The Yellow Book. 1999.
4. Jong E, McMullen R. The Travel and Tropical Medicine Manual, 2nd ed. Philadelphia, W. B. Saunders, 1995.
5. Auerbach PS. Wilderness Medicine, Management of Wilderness and Environmental Emergencies. 3rd ed. St. Louis, Mosby, 1995.
6. Dupont HL, Steffan R. Textbook of Travel Medicine and Health. St. Louis, BC Decker, 1997.
7. Freedman DO, ed. Travel medicine. Infect Dis Clin North Am 1998;12.
8. Wallace RB, ed. Maxcy-Rosenau-Last Public Health and Preventive Medicine, 14th ed. Stamford, CT, Appleton & Lange, 1998.
9. Thompson RF. Travel and Routine Immunizations: A Practical Guide for the Medical Office. Milwaukee, WI, Shoreland, Inc., 1999.

RESOURCES

Centers for Disease Control and Prevention (toll free number 877–394–8747 or 877–FYI–TRIP; http://www.cdc.gov/travel)

International Association for Assistance to Travelers (IAMAT) (http://www.sentex.net/~iamat/)

Pan-American Health Organization (www.paho.org/english/media/htm)

Promed Emerging Diseases web page (www.healthnet.org/programs/promed.html)

U.S. Department of State Consular Information and Travel Advisories (http://www.travel.state.gov/travel_warnings.html)

Shoreland's Travel Health On-line (www.trippprep.com)

University of Alabama-Birmingham Core Travel Medicine Resources (http://www.medinfo.dom.uab.edu/geomed/links.html)

World Health Organization (www.who.ch)

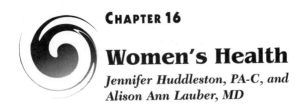

CHAPTER 16

Women's Health

Jennifer Huddleston, PA-C, and
Alison Ann Lauber, MD

INTRODUCTION

For more than half of the women in the United States, access to primary care revolves around the annual gynecologic examination. Whether the health care provider is a gynecologic specialist or a primary care provider, this patient encounter should be viewed as an opportunity for a comprehensive periodic health examination. The annual gynecologic examination can bridge gaps in primary preventive health care by providing education and counseling to promote healthy lifestyles. The health care provider can use this encounter to coordinate often underutilized health maintenance screening and disease prevention strategies, facilitating patient referrals to specialty care as needed. In addition to offering an opportunity to address the holistic health needs of the female patient, this visit should also include preconception counseling to those with reproductive potential. This chapter is an overview of selected patient education topics and high-priority routine health screening recommendations that providers should consider in the care of the female patient.

FERTILITY

PRECONCEPTION COUNSELING

By age 45 more than 80% of women have given birth. While the average woman living in the U.S. has 2.2 children, surveys report that up to 50% of all pregnancies are unintended.[1] A significant number of women, using an effective method of reversible contraception, become pregnant each year. Therefore all women of reproductive age should be considered capable of conception. Because substantial reductions in perinatal morbidity can be accomplished by even brief patient encounters, preconception counseling, when appropriate, should become a routine feature of the woman's health visit.

An individual risk assessment can be done simply and quickly for most patients. Important topics to address are high-risk lifestyle practices that include

* Alcohol, tobacco, and drug use
* Multiple sexual partners

* Workplace hazards and exposures to infectious diseases (such as cytomegalovirus and toxoplasmosis), toxins, and/or radiation

For women residing in the U.S. vaccination status can erroneously be assumed to be adequate. Many women lack immunity and/or vaccination to rubella, while other women may have inadequate acquired immunity. The goal of rubella vaccination in women is to prevent disease transmission to the fetus. Women born before 1957 are considered immune to rubella; however, immunity ideally should be documented by an antibody titer. The National Immunization Program of the Centers for Disease Control and Prevention recommends that reproductive-capable women who lack vaccination documentation, were born between 1963 and 1967 (during a time when only inactivated measles vaccines were available), or who were immunized before their first birthdays should receive one additional dose of live attenuated vaccine. Because of outbreaks of measles on college campuses in the early and mid-1990s, many health care employers and universities now require documentation of two doses of the measles, mumps, and rubella (MMR) vaccine, or documented immunity before work or enrollment may begin. In addition to MMR vaccination, immunization prophylaxis for varicella and hepatitis A and B in susceptible individuals may be recommended. Diphtheria-tetanus (DT) boosters are indicated every 7 to 10 years (see also Chapter 11, Immunizations).

A quick nutritional screening evaluation can be obtained by using a simple 24-h diet recall. This activity can serve as an educational tool to teach women about the importance of sensible nutritional habits and of preconception folic acid supplementation in the prevention of birth defects. Patients who are planning a pregnancy should initiate folic acid supplementation at least 3 months before conception. Adequate daily folic acid intake is associated with a decreased incidence of neural tube birth defects.[2] Although exact amounts of folic acid supplementation for the general population have been debated, all authorities agree that, given that 50% of pregnancies are unplanned, dietary intake without supplementation is unlikely to provide amounts adequate to significantly reduce birth defect rates. Increasing efforts have been made to supplement foodstuffs with folic acid to ensure adequate intake; however, most providers still advocate a minimum 400 μg to 1 mg folic acid supplement daily for all women of potential fertility. Women with an impoverished nutritional status, eating disorders, or a previous history of birth defects should have an opportunity to access formal counseling and treatment before planning conception. In counseling multiparous women, child spacing and identifying factors that may have led to previously poor perinatal outcomes should be discussed. Finally, a basic psychosocial evaluation exploring readiness for motherhood will benefit most women. Providers should be equipped to offer information on how to access economic and social support services in the community.

INFERTILITY

Patients often express concerns regarding fertility. Pregnancy probability in healthy heterosexual couples engaging in frequent intercourse is estimated at approximately 30% per month. When no contraceptive method is used, approximately 80% of these couples will conceive within 12 months, and an additional 10% will conceive within the second year.[1] Infertility is therefore defined as an inability to conceive after 12 months of unprotected intercourse. Approximately 1 in 6 heterosexual couples in the U.S. experience difficulty in achieving pregnancy during a 1-year period.[2] Some "infertile" couples may simply have an inadequate understanding of the events of the reproductive cycle and timing of coitus. General information and education regarding the reproductive cycle is necessary for all couples who report difficulty conceiving.

Infertility affects approximately 10–15% of heterosexual couples in the U.S.[1,2]; however, it is a mistake to assume that conception inquiries will be restricted to traditional married couples. Women seeking conception advice may be in stable lesbian relationships, interested in single parenthood, or investigating the possibility of becoming a surrogate for a friend or family member. Initiating an infertility evaluation depends largely on desire to conceive, opportunity and/or access to fertile sperm or ovum, and age of the mother. In addition to a complete history and physical examination of both partners, a sexual history, including previous conceptions, frequency and/or timing of coitus, and use of any type of lubricants, should be obtained. Partners should be screened for asymptomatic infection. Causes of infertility are generally classified in three basic categories: (1) female factors and (2) male factors, with each accounting for 40% of infertility, and (3) mixed male and female factors, accounting for 20% of infertility.[2] In up to 20% of cases, no identifiable cause of infertility can be found with standard investigation.

The initial infertility investigation usually begins with a noninvasive and inexpensive semen analysis. Male partners or donors should be instructed to abstain from ejaculation for 2 to 3 days prior to the analysis. Specimens can be collected at home in a clean container if the patient can bring the specimen to the laboratory within 30 mins. Smaller labs may request a "reservation" for this test to ensure that adequate personnel are available when the specimen is received. The first milliliter of ejaculate contains the most spermatozoa. Since ejaculate can vary in quality, at least two specimens over a period of a few weeks should be obtained. While parameters of normal analysis are variable, minimum normal values have been established. Other specialized tests are available when indicated.[2]

Although most women who complain of infertility report regular menstrual cycles, practitioners are often compelled to verify normal ovulatory function. Presumptive ovulation can be determined inexpensively by evaluating basal body temperature (BBT). The patient is instructed to take her temperature each morning before getting out of bed. Owing to the influence of progesterone, the BBT normally rises during the luteal phase by approximately 0.5°F to 0.8°F (or 0.3°C) over the proliferative phase BBT.[2] In addition to suggesting ovulation, the BBT allows assessment of the length of the luteal phase. If the luteal phase is normal, the patient should experience at least 11 days between the rise of BBT and the onset of menses. Conception may be suspected when the luteal elevation persists more than 15 days. Patients with irregular menses may require more complex or expensive evaluations and/or treatments to determine whether or when ovulation may occur.

Laboratory documentation of ovulation can be obtained by examining serum progesterone levels between days 19 and 23 of the "normal" 28-day menstrual cycle. Serum progesterone levels above 4 mg/mL indicates ovulation. Luteinizing hormone (LH) and follicle stimulating hormone (FSH) can be measured to screen for polycystic ovary syndrome or ovarian failure. Urine LH detection kits are available over the counter and are useful in determining the time of ovulation more precisely. If a luteal defect is suspected, an endometrial biopsy or aspirate may be obtained within 3 to 5 days of the anticipated menses.

Women may require imaging studies to rule out tubal pathology. While simple pelvic ultrasonography may reveal cystic ovaries, a hysterosalpingogram, a radiographic study with instillation of radiopaque dye into the uterine cavity, can reveal tubal obstruction or congenital abnormalities of the upper reproductive organs. Postcoital evaluations may reveal abnormalities in cervical mucus and sperm transport caused by previous cryotherapy, conization, or "hostile mucus" due to infection, allergy, or congenital exposure to diethylstilbestrol (DES).

CONTRACEPTION

Nearly 65% of reproductive-aged women use some method of contraception.[1] Because of the increased use and improved efficacy of contraceptives, the unplanned pregnancy rate has dipped by more than 15% since the late 1980s.[1, 3, 4] While this decline is encouraging, nearly half of all pregnancies occurring in 1994 were undesired, and almost 50% of women with unintended pregnancies reported using some form of birth control. Failure rates of this magnitude support what women have known for years: There is no perfect method of contraception. Successful contraception depends largely on patient education and the patient's ability to comply with the form of contraception she has chosen. With the numerous options now available, deciding which contraceptive method is best for a patient can be a daunting task. Each patient must be approached individually to determine which contraceptive choices may be best for her. Methods vary greatly in cost, convenience, potential side effects, reversibility, and, most importantly, effectiveness. Additional concerns for some women may center around religious beliefs and/or the desire to keep her contraceptive method concealed.

ORAL CONTRACEPTIVES

The oral contraceptive pill (OCP) debuted on the American market in 1960, and within the span of a decade the original high-dose pill had become the cause of considerable alarm among women and their health care providers. OCPs manufactured today are formulated with significantly lower levels of estrogen and progestin, making them safe, effective, and well tolerated by nearly all users. With an estimated 10.4 million users, the OCP is the most commonly used reversible birth control method.[1, 4]

Most women are candidates for OCPs. Relative and absolute contraindications are, however, important considerations that should be discussed with each patient before prescribing them (Table 16–1). Long-term use has been determined to be safe, and many noncontraceptive benefits accompany OCP administration. Still, women continue to worry about the potential side effects and dangers mostly associated with older formulations. Common concerns among women include risks of cancer, heart disease, and subsequently infertility. Thorough patient education regarding individual risk factors, danger signs (Table 16–2), and overall benefits of OCP use greatly improves compliance and reduces the number of patients who discontinue OCPs because of minor side effects such as breakthrough bleeding, amenorrhea, and misconceptions about weight gain.

Table 16–1. Relative and Absolute Contraindications to OCP Use

Relative	Absolute
Migraine headaches	Thrombotic event
Hypertension	Cerebrovascular accident
Uterine leiomyomas	Liver dysfunction
Use of anticonvulsant drugs	Hepatic tumor
Sickle cell disease	Coronary artery disease
Diabetes mellitus	Estrogen-dependent malignancy (breast, endometrial or other estrogen receptor-positive cancer)
Gallbladder disease	Undiagnosed vaginal bleeding
Recent or planned surgery	Smoker over age 35
Obstructive jaundice	Pregnancy

Table 16–2. Warning Signs for OCP Users
A: Abdominal pain
C: Chest pain and acute shortness of breath
H: Headaches, dizziness, or weakness
E: Eye or vision changes
S: Severe leg pain or speech problems

Noncontraceptive Benefits

Studies have shown up to a 50% reduction in the incidence of endometrial cancer and a 40% reduction in the incidence of ovarian cancer and cysts in patients using OCPs.[4] Oral contraceptive users also experience fewer episodes of benign breast disease, irregular bleeding, and pelvic inflammatory disease, and have fewer menstrual complaints and ectopic pregnancies compared with non-users. Other noncontraceptive benefits include treatment of acne, hirsutism, and endometriosis, and possible protection against atherosclerosis.

Choosing an OCP

Many OCP preparations are available. Current formulations differ in type and dose of estrogen or progestin used. OCPs can contain combined estrogen and progestin in a 21- or 28-day monophasic, biphasic, or triphasic regimen, or as a progestin-only "mini-pill."

Choosing the best OCP for a patient depends on her unique risk factors, whether she is lactating, and/or whether specific noncontraceptive benefits such as treatment of acne are desired. Generally, all new users are best offered the lowest-dose estrogen-progestin combination pill with the least androgenic effects. Triphasic regimens have an overall lower progestin content with efficacy equal to their monophasic counterparts. Low-dose pills containing third generation progestins such as norgestimate and desogestrel have been shown to reduce acne and have fewer potential cardiovascular effects.[3] Desogestrel, however, has been linked to a slight increase in thrombotic events, and some experts recommend against beginning new users with desogestrel-containing OCPs.[3, 4] Further research is needed to validate this practice. In addition to newer progestin OCPs, studies have conclusively proved the safety of older, low-dose formulations containing norethindrone, norethindrone acetate, and levonorgestrel. Because combined OCPs have been shown to reduce milk volume, lactating women may be better served by a progestin-only containing OCP. It is important to note, though, that the efficacy of progestin-only pills in nonlactating women depends on the patient's ability to take the pill regularly at the same time each day. If a breast-feeding mother chooses to use a combination pill, the pill should be started only after the milk supply is established (a minimum of 6 weeks and better after 6 months). Combined OCPs are a better choice for adolescents and adults who may forget to take pills (Box 16–1).

Injectable and Implantable Forms of Hormonal Contraception

Surveys performed in 1995 reported only 2% of women as using injectable forms of contraceptives (medroxyprogesterone acetate), and less than 1% reported using implanted levonorgestrel contraception.[1, 5, 6] Many women find the convenience of injectable and im-

---

Box 16-1–What Happens If I Forget a Pill?

Taking your pill every day is important in successfully avoiding pregnancy. Plan to take your pill at the same time every day. Choose a time that is convenient and that might help you remember. You should always have a back-up method of birth control, like condoms, available in case you forget to take your pills. If you do forget to take a pill, follow these instructions carefully and contact your health care provider for more advice:

One missed pill:

- As soon as you notice that you forgot to take a pill, take the missed pill.
- Take your regularly scheduled pill for that day as well—you will take two pills in one day.
- Then resume your pill schedule as usual the next day.

Two consecutive missed pills:

- If you miss two pills in a row, take two pills one day and then two pills the next day.
- Then resume your pill schedule as before.
- You should use a back-up method for 7 days.

If you missed two pills in the 3rd week of your cycle:

- Start a new pack of pills. You may become pregnant, so you must use a back-up method of contraception for at least 7 days.
- If you think that you might already be pregnant, speak with your health care provider right away about what you should do next.

planted contraception attractive. Failure rates with these methods are extremely low. Since progestins do not affect clotting or thromboembolic phenomena, nearly all women are candidates for progestin-only contraceptives. Despite the convenience and benefits of these methods, the undesirable side effects that many women experience have mitigated their popularity.

Depo-Provera (medroxyprogesterone acetate) is a sustained-release suspension that is injected intramuscularly every 12 weeks. Failure rate is approximately 1.2 in 100 woman years.[5] Several noncontraceptive benefits of Depo-Provera have been documented. Depo-Provera has been shown to increase milk volume in lactating mothers and to improve seizure control, and has it been approved by the U.S. Food and Drug Administration for the treatment of endometriosis.[5]

Many women who discontinue Depo-Provera report unpredictable or persistent breakthrough bleeding. However, by the end of the first year of use, most women experience amenorrhea. While cessation of menses would be considered a benefit by many women, some users are disturbed by a lack of menstruation, feel chronically anxious about an unwanted pregnancy, and/or express cultural beliefs that failure to have regular menses is unhealthy. Other possible side effects are weight gain, depression, and decreased bone density with prolonged use (defined in most studies as 5 or more continuous years of use).[6, 7] Because of questions regarding the risk of decreased bone mineralization, some experts recommend prescribing calcium supplementation for users. Considering the risk of decreased bone density, it may be advisable to avoid prescribing Depo-Provera during the first 2 years following menarche.[7] Nevertheless, given that the average teen misses two or more OCPs per cycle, Depo-Provera's advantage in teen compliance makes it an attractive option.

Return of fertility in Depo-Provera users is variable. Some women experience continued ovarian suppression for more than a year after discontinuing injections, with a return to normal ovulatory cycles generally by 18 months.[6, 7] Counseling regarding the expected side effects and ways to minimize breakthrough bleeding, and reassurance of the efficacy of injectable contraceptives can greatly improve satisfaction and continuance of a very effective and safe method of birth control.[6, 7]

Norplant is a long-term, reversible method of contraception that consists of six subdermal Silastic tube implants each containing 36 mg of levonorgestrel. The implants provide 5 years of effective contraception. Insertion requires a small incision on the medial area of the upper arm distal to the axilla. The implants are inserted below the skin using a small trocar. Usually the small scar and the implants are barely noticeable. They may be slightly more prominent in thin women, and darker-skinned women report an increase in pigmentation over the implants. Complications are uncommon when insertion is performed by an experienced practitioner. Both injections or implants may be initiated immediately post-partum. Unlike Depo-Provera, return to fertility occurs within 2 days of implant removal.[8]

Similar to Depo-Provera, many women experience irregular bleeding during the first year of Norplant use. However, even with increased episodes of vaginal bleeding, concentrations of hemoglobin rise because overall blood loss is reduced. Amenorrhea occurs less frequently. Approximately 10% of women report cessation of menses or oligomenorrhea. After irregular bleeding, headache is the most common side effect reported by Norplant users and represents the leading nonmenstrual cause for removal of implants.[6, 8] While there are few contraindications to Norplant use, women who are taking certain medications such as anticonvulsants and rifampin may well experience reduced efficacy.

BARRIER METHODS

These methods include condoms (male and female), spermicidals (gels, foam, suppositories, and VCF, an impregnated film), diaphragms (disposable sponge and fitted, reusable), and cervical caps. Latex barriers and nonoxynol-9 spermicidal products have been shown to reduce transmission of many sexually transmitted diseases (STDs) but do not offer the same degree of contraceptive protection as their hormonal counterparts, largely owing to compliance issues.

INTRAUTERINE DEVICES

The intrauterine device (IUD) is a simple, cost-effective contraceptive choice assuming correct patient selection and a desire for at least 2 years of continuous contraception. The Cu T 380A (Paragard) has a 2.6% probability of failure over a 10-year period and currently enjoys the largest market share in the U.S. with its only competition the 1-year Progestasert. By 2002 it is hoped that the levonorgestrel 5-year IUD will be released on the American market. All currently available IUDs are thought to work by interfering with fertilization. The risk of pelvic inflammatory disease associated with IUD use is a result of insertion and subsequent exposure to a sexually transmitted disease (STD). The greatest risk is within the first few weeks following insertion. The progestin IUD actually lowers the associated risk of pelvic inflammatory disease. Expulsion rates range from 2% to 10% (higher expulsion rates are usually postpartum) within the first year following insertion, and expulsion can occur without the patient's notice. For this reason careful education should include:

P: Period late (pregnancy) or abnormal bleeding
A: Abdominal pain or dyspareunia
I: Infection exposure or symptoms
N: Not feeling well (systemic symptoms of fever or chills)
S: String missing, longer, or shorter

FERTILITY AWARENESS, WITHDRAWAL, AND ABSTINENCE

Rhythm and other more scientific forms of periodic abstinence based on fertility awareness can be an acceptable method of family planning (spacing) for a stable monogamous couple. Coitus interruptus, traditionally viewed as ineffective, is actually as successful as most barrier methods under typical conditions. However, withdrawal does not eliminate the risk of infectious exposures. Celibacy certainly is a reasonable option to avoid the risk of deadly sexually transmitted infections and does not exclude the possibility of alternative means of sexual intimacy.

STERILIZATION

Sterilization still remains one of the safest and effective means of reliable contraception. However, reversal is expensive and requires major surgery, its results cannot be guaranteed, and it is not readily available on an equitable basis. For these reasons careful counseling over time should precede the selection of this contraceptive option.

EMERGENCY CONTRACEPTION

Emergency contraception (EC) should be available to all women at risk for an unintended pregnancy. Reports from abortion clinics suggest that up to 60% of women would have been candidates and would have used postcoital contraception had it been available to them.[9, 10] Adolescents and women who use barrier methods are at particular risk for coital accidents, as are any women who experience a lapse in contraceptive method. It is not uncommon for adolescents to be sexually active for months before seeking contraceptive advice. An obvious need for emergency contraception also exists in cases of sexual assault. Discussion regarding access to emergency contraception should become part of routine education counseling for all women of reproductive potential who desire pregnancy prevention. Ideally patients would have access to these methods before an accident occurs; practitioners should consider offering emergency contraception kits to all patients who are at increased risk for coital accidents (Table 16–3). When patients can appropriately self-administer emergency contraception pills (ECPs), efficacy rates increase and thereby potentially reduce the large numbers of unwanted pregnancies and subsequent abortions performed each year.[9, 10]

While the exact mechanism of action is not known, it is believed that high doses of estrogen, progesterone, or both interfere with

Table 16-3. Post-Coital Emergency Contraception			
Brands	Formulations	Pills per Dose	Dosing Instructions
Plan B	Levonorgestrel, 75 μg	1	First dose within 72 h of unprotected coitus; second dose in 12 h
Preven	Ethinyl estradiol, 50 μg, levonorgestrel, 25 μg	2	First dose within 72 h of unprotected coitus; second dose in 12 h
Ovral	Ethinyl estradiol, 50 μg, norgestrel, 0.50 mg	2	First dose within 72 h of unprotected coitus; second dose in 12 h
Lo/Ovral	Ethinyl estradiol, 30 μg, norgestrel, 0.30 mg	4	First dose within 72 h of unprotected coitus; second dose in 12 h
Levlen, Nordette	Ethinyl estradiol, 30 μg, levonorgestrel, 0.15 mg	4 (peach)°	First dose within 72 h of unprotected coitus; second dose in 12 h
Triphasil, Tri-Levlen	Ethinyl estradiol, 30 μg levonorgestrel, 0.125 mg	4 (yellow)°	First dose within 72 h of unprotected coitus; second dose in 12 h
Ovrette	Norgestrel, 0.075 mg (progestin only)	20	First dose within 48 h of unprotected coitus; second dose in 12 h
Copper T (Paragard)	Intrauterine contraceptive device		Placement within 5 days of unprotected coitus

°Some OCP packages include pills of different dose combinations, identified by different colors; colors indicated are the mid-cycle pills.

fallopian tube transport and/or implantation. Efficacy rates of combined OCPs used for emergency contraception administered within 72 h of an isolated exposure approach 98%.[9] Treatment must be initiated as soon as possible within the 72-h window; efficacy increases with earlier administration.

Practitioners must rule out an existing pregnancy prior to prescribing hormones. Commercially available kits containing a home pregnancy test in addition to ECPs are useful in cases where women may not be able to obtain a clinical evaluation. Usual contraindications to OCP use also apply in decisions to use emergency contraception. Since ECPs are used on a short-term basis, clinicians can carefully consider each patient's potential risk factors and determine whether the risks of hormonal ECPs outweigh the benefits of avoiding pregnancy. Common side effects of ECPs include nausea, vomiting, headaches, and dizziness. Women who vomit pills within 1 h of administration require another dose as soon as possible. Prescribing an antiemetic may be advisable. Though the failure rate of ECPs is only 2%, women should be counseled about the unlikely but potential teratogenic effects of high-dose hormonal administration and should be offered information about elective termination in the event of emergency contraception failure.[10]

In women who are not candidates for hormonal emergency contraception, insertion of a copper intrauterine contraceptive device within 5 days of a coital accident can prevent implantation in more than 99% of cases.[9, 10] Though the failure rate is remarkably low, women who have identifiable risk factors for IUD use (such as multiple partners, uncertainty of STDs, or sexual assault) should be offered other alternatives. With either approach, the patient should be advised to schedule a follow-up examination and pregnancy test within 3 weeks of administration of emergency contraception.

VOLUNTARY INTERRUPTION OF PREGNANCY (VIP)

Ideally every conception would be planned and desired; unfortunately this is not the case. Since the 1973 Supreme Court decisions (Roe v. Wade and Doe v. Bolton), therapeutic abortions have been legalized through a trimester framework.

1. During first trimester, the decision is left to the privacy of the patient and her health care provider, with little opportunity for the state to interfere.
2. During the second trimester, each state may regulate or restrict procedures as reasonably related to a woman's health.
3. During the third trimester, fetal viability is assumed, and the state may prohibit abortion as long as the restriction does not interfere with the life of the mother.

Each provider and patient will have personal feelings about abortion. It is the primary care provider's responsibility to provide the patient with relatively unbiased options, counseling, and/or referrals as needed. Methods of first trimester VIPs include RU-486 and/or suction D&C. Methods of second trimester terminations should be discussed in detail with an experienced provider of this service, as publicity in the late 1990s has clouded public perceptions surrounding these procedures.

▬▬ SEXUALLY TRANSMITTED DISEASES

Sexually transmitted diseases (STDs) account for significant morbidity in women worldwide. Although not all patients are at an increased risk for STDs, hundreds of thousands of new cases of STDs are reported each year.[1, 11] Preventive approaches and screening strategies that can be adapted to all women's needs are crucial in efforts to control disease transmission and complications.

Chlamydia and Gonorrhea. *Chlamydia trachomatis* and *Neisseria gonorrhoeae* represent the most common sexually transmitted pathogens in women.[1, 11] Over 500,000 new cases of chlamydia and nearly 180,000 new cases of gonorrhea were reported in 1998.[1, 11] Sexually active women younger than age 20 have three times the rate of infection of older women.[1, 12] Lower socioeconomic status and multiple sexual partners also increase risk. The greatest incidence of infection occurs in the 15–19-year-old age group, and 25% of adolescent females contract at least one STD each year.[1, 11, 12]

Pelvic Inflammatory Disease. Each year an estimated one million women are treated for pelvic inflammatory disease (PID), an infection of the upper reproductive organs.[1] The usual pathogens implicated in PID include chlamydia, gonorrhea, and polymicrobial vaginal flora. The groups most commonly affected are sexually active adolescents and IUD users.[1, 11, 12] Adolescents are particularly susceptible, due, in part, to their developing anatomy and less mature natural immunity. Ectopic pregnancy related to PID complications is one and a half times more likely in African American women compared with any other group. Women with a previous history of PID have a 25% recurrence rate.[11]

Syphilis. During the 1980s cases of syphilis in reproductive-aged women were the highest since the 1940s. With increased attention given to screening and treatment by the late 1980s, rates of infection in all ethnic groups had once again declined by 1997.[11] Approximately 18,000 new cases of syphilis were reported in 1998.[1, 11] Despite substantial reduction in the incidence of syphilis in all racial groups, this STD continues to disproportionately affect African American women.[1, 11]

Genital Herpes. More than 45 million individuals in the U.S. are reported to have recurrent genital herpes simplex virus (HSV-2).[11, 12] An estimated one in four women are infected with genital herpes but many remain undiagnosed. Persons infected with HSV-2 may be only mildly symptomatic and unaware of infection. Such persons may unknowingly shed virus and transmit disease to others, making infection control difficult. Suppressive treatment only becomes possible in symptomatic and diagnosed patients. The use of acyclovir anytime during pregnancy is generally considered safe, its benefits far outweighing its risks, when treating a case of primary HSV. Suppressive therapy for patients at risk for recurrence during the third trimester of pregnancy should be strongly considered, as acyclovir has been shown to be safe and effective.

Human Papillomavirus. Over 100 types of human papillomavirus (HPV) have been identified. Twenty types of HPV are associated with genital tract disease, making HPV the most common sexually transmitted viral disease. HPV types 6 and 11 often cause visible genital warts. Other types, such as 16, 18, and 31 reportedly possess oncogenic potential and have been linked to cervical dysplasia and cancer.[11-13] Women can be infected with multiple types of HPV and may demonstrate severe cervical dysplasia in the absence of visible genital warts. Although barrier methods are effective at preventing transmission of other STDs, they are of little help in the prevention of HPV exposure.[11-13]

Hepatitis. Hepatitis B virus (HBV) is a common sexually transmitted disease. Although the majority of children in the U.S. are vaccinated against hepatitis B virus, large numbers of older teens and adults are at risk. Screening for HBV "catch-up" immunization programs should be strongly encouraged even if not covered by some insurance programs. An estimated 240,000 new cases of HBV and 6000 HBV-related deaths occur each year in the U.S.[11] Up to 6% of persons infected with HBV will become chronic carriers capable of infecting others. Infants infected with HBV at birth are at substantially increased risk for being a chronic carrier and for chronic liver disease. Hepatitis A is not generally thought of as a potentially sexually transmitted disease. However, for women engaging in anal or oral-anal sexual stimulation, this vaccine series should be strongly encouraged. Hepatitis C is perhaps an even greater problem for the future, and screening should be considered for all patients at risk for STDs. (For further details see Chapter 21, Infectious Diseases.)

STD Education

STD education and risk reduction center on identifying and eliminating behaviors that increase the likelihood of sexual disease transmission. Health care providers should discuss the following topics at the initial encounter with each patient at risk for an STD:

* Risk assessment, STD identification, and prevention measures (including the correct application and use of condoms and dental dams)

* HIV, syphilis, hepatitis, and cervical cancer screening
* Importance of periodic chlamydia and gonorrhea screening and complications such as pelvic inflammatory disease, cervical dysplasia, increased risk for HIV transmission
* Need for partner notification and treatment
* Sexual abstinence or use of barrier methods during treatment
* Access to preexposure hepatitis vaccination
* Psychosocial and substance abuse issues that may contribute to high risk behavior

When discussing issues of sexuality, a health care provider must take a nonjudgmental approach. It is vital that health care providers feel comfortable and competent when asking direct, specific questions about sexual history and individual risk factors. In response to a nonjudgmental approach, most patients will feel secure and reveal an accurate history. Once high risk behaviors are identified, the health care provider can discuss prevention measures with the patient and adapt these strategies to fit her individual needs. Examples of preventive strategies involve the proper and consistent use of barrier methods, such as condoms and dental dams, abstaining from sexual contact with partners who have an unclear STD status or history of injection drug use, and pre-exposure vaccination for vaccine-preventable diseases such as hepatitis A and B. All patients should be encouraged to require HIV and STD screening of partners before initiating sexual encounters.

DETECTION AND COUNSELING

Many women infected with an STD lack remarkable symptoms for weeks to months. Detection of asymptomatic disease is crucial in the control of STD transmission and complications associated with prolonged disease. Papanicolaou (Pap) smears are an inadequate method of STD detection. Annual screening for STDs in all sexually active women is recommended even if they do not complain of symptoms. Diagnosis of chlamydia and gonorrhea may be obtained by the use of DNA probes.[11] While vaginal/cervical probes done at the time of a woman's annual examination screen for asymptomatic disease, newer technology may soon allow for more frequent screening through random urine specimens. In most cases, syphilis, HIV, and hepatitis must be screened for by blood serology.[11] Pretest and post-test counseling are important when screening for HIV infection. A risk assessment of behaviors that contribute to HIV infection must be realistically discussed with the patient. Explanations of the significance of results are often deferred to the post-test encounter, but ideally these issues should be discussed before the test is performed. When appropriate pretest counseling is provided, informed consent for HIV testing can be ensured. Post-test counseling focuses on the meaning of the result, reinforcement of risk-reducing behaviors, and understanding the need for follow-up testing in the event of a negative test. Women who test positive for HIV should be referred for comprehensive medical care and psychosocial support services as soon as possible. All pregnant women should be encouraged to be tested for HIV, even if they are in a low-risk population, as the benefits to the fetus are great if an HIV+ mother is diagnosed and treated throughout her pregnancy.

Advising women on partner notification and treatment may be the most delicate of all issues in dealing with sexually transmitted disease. Women who reveal an STD diagnosis may be in danger of physical abuse, homelessness, or separation from their families. Though confidential STD reporting requirements vary by states, infections with syphilis and gonorrhea, and the active disease, AIDS (although not simply the HIV infection) are reportable in all states. Chlamydial infections are reportable in many areas. In most states local agencies can provide anonymous notification in cases of selected disease. It is essential that all women understand the risks of reinfection from an untreated partner. While sexual abstinence from an infected partner is optimal, barrier methods and careful instructions for use should be offered to all women unwilling or unable to inform partners.

VAGINITIS AND VAGINOSIS

Most commonly these terms refer to candidal or trichomonal vaginitis and bacterial vaginosis (BV). Diagnosis usually is based on clinical presentation, vaginal pH, and/or wet prep microscopic examination. While any of these infections may be sexually transmitted, frequently they are not. Patients with frequent recurrences should be evaluated for underlying disease (diabetes, HIV), noncompliance with treatment, and reinfection by a partner (frequently asymptomatic), and/or fomite transmission (infected toys, diaphragms). Generally symptoms prompt treatment, and these infections are rarely associated with complications or sequelae. However, there has been evidence that treatment of BV in pregnancy reduces the risk of premature labor.

BREAST EXAMINATIONS AND MAMMOGRAMS

The United States Preventive Services Task Force (USPSTF) has determined that there is no conclusive evidence to recommend for or against regular self-examination of the breasts. Though the value of self-examination may be unclear, it is reported that 90% of breast masses are discovered by the patient. A painless breast lump is the presenting complaint in approximately 70% of patients diagnosed with breast cancer. Even so, most women do not regularly examine their breasts, and even fewer women are familiar with the characteristics of a suspicious breast mass. Many women report that they feel discouraged from performing monthly breast self-examinations because they are not aware of the signs of breast cancer. Perhaps the best approach to encouraging patients to perform regular breast self-examinations includes a combination of general education about breast cancer, proper self-examination techniques, and specific information about the characteristics of malignant breast masses (Box 16–2). Currently recommendations regarding provider breast examinations and mammography frequency have been debated among many groups, including the USPTF, the American College of Obstetricians and Gynecologists, and the American Cancer Society. Generally provider breast examinations should be included as part of the annual well-woman encounter, and annual mammography should begin by age 40. Mammograms in young women are poor screens owing to technical difficulties in penetration and imaging. Therefore all new masses should be carefully considered for needle aspiration and/or excisional biopsy.

OTHER HEALTH RISKS

CARDIOVASCULAR DISEASE

Heart disease kills more American women than any other condition. More than 20% of women living in the U.S. have a serious form

---

Box 16-2–EASY STEPS TO A CONFIDENT BREAST SELF-EXAMINATION

Breast cancer strikes one in eight women. Early detection is the key to full recovery from breast cancer. Women over the age of 20 should examine their breasts monthly. Self-breast examinations are best performed approximately 1 week after your menstrual period. During your menses, hormones may affect your breasts and cause tenderness and inflammation. Waiting to examine your breasts until after your menstrual period ends allows the hormonal effects of the menstrual cycle to subside. If you do not have a menstrual period, you can choose an easy date to remember, such as the first day of each month, to perform your regular examination. The most convenient time to examine your breasts may be while you are preparing to shower or bathe. Here are a few simple steps that will help you thoroughly and confidently examine your breasts:

First inspect your breasts in front of a mirror. Observe your breasts and nipples carefully for lumps, asymmetry, dimpling of the skin, or any new changes while holding your hands over your head and then at your sides. Now, place your hands on your hips and press down. This will cause your pectoral muscles in your chest to contract and may reveal changes like skin dimpling or retraction of the nipple that you could not see before.

The next part of your breast examination may be performed in the shower or bath. Sensitivity to touch can be increased by examining your breasts with warm, soapy water. Begin the second part of your exam by placing your left hand on the back of your neck.

- Take your right hand and place it at the tip of your left collar bone just below your neck.
- Using the flat portion of your middle three finger tips, press in small circular motions, inching your way down toward the bottom of your ribs.
- Once you have checked downward to the area below the breast, slide your fingers slightly to the left and inch your way back up toward your collar bone.
- Repeat this thin "strip pattern" until you have checked your entire breast and your underarm.
- Once you have completely examined your breast tissue, take a minute to check for lumps on all sides of your underarm area and along the flaps of muscle between your underarm and chest.
- Now repeat these steps to exam your right breast.

Many women are unaware of how breast cancer might feel. Breast masses that are suspicious for cancer may be painless, feel very firm, feel attached to the skin, or feel stuck to the surrounding tissue. They may also have an irregular or lumpy shape and may result in changes of skin color or texture on the breast. Bloody discharge from the breast should also be reported to your health care provider. If you detect any changes in your breasts, report these findings to your health care provider. Ask your provider if a mammogram and/or biopsy is right for you.

of cardiovascular disease.[1] Each year strokes claim twice the number of women's lives compared with breast cancer, making strokes the third leading cause of death among women. African American and Hispanic women are especially susceptible to stroke.[1] While heart disease more commonly affects young men, equal numbers of men and women over age 50 die each year from cardiovascular disease. Though general mortality from cardiovascular disease had begun to decline, the increase in female obesity has soared to as much as 36% in the general population, with estimates of approximately 50% in certain ethnic groups.[1] Obesity, high blood pressure, tobacco use, and family history are major risk factors for cardiovascular disease in women. Morbidity increases with compounding numbers of risk factors.

Counseling and support of lifestyle habits that reduce cardiovascular disease risks are imperative in the treatment and prevention of heart disease. Women may have symptoms that are less "classic" than symptoms in men, and/or they are less likely to be as intensively evaluated as their male counterparts. Only recently has significant research begun to target disease in women. The use of the high-sensitivity C-reactive protein test as an early screen for coronary artery disease in women has shown some early promise, but has yet to be validated for both efficacy and/or cost as a worthwhile screening test. Patient education should be focused on a healthy diet, weight reduction, exercise, smoking cessation, and the identification of early signs of disease (see also Chapter 18, Cardiology.)

TOBACCO AND CANCER

During the 1990s mortality from lung cancer decreased in men, while this form of cancer has continued to claim the lives of more and more women each year. Lung cancer is now the leading cause of cancer deaths among women, accounting for 25% of all cancer-related deaths.[1] Between 1960 and 1990, the death rate from lung cancer among women increased by more than 400%, and the rate continues to increase.[14] Despite these facts, few women would identify lung cancer as their biggest cancer risk. A woman who has smoked the equivalent of one pack of cigarettes per day for 40 years has a cancer risk three times higher than a man with a similar smoking history.[14]

When tobacco companies introduced a "feminine" cigarette along with accompanying advertisements, the number of women smoking increased by over 110%. Eighty percent of women report that they began smoking while they were adolescents.[1] Female smokers are not only at risk for lung cancer. Tobacco use is a major risk factor for cancers of the oropharynx, esophagus, kidney, pancreas, bladder, and cervix.[14]

SUPPORTING WOMEN THROUGH MENOPAUSE

One third of the average woman's life remains after the cessation of her monthly menses. Menopause, or the time when menstrual bleeding ceases, usually occurs between ages 48 and 55. By age 55, 95% of women have completed menopause.[1, 15] The climacteric, the transitional years before menopause, can be characterized by irregular menses, vasomotor symptoms, sleep disturbances, and affective disorders. In addition, decreased estrogen secretion may lead to urogenital dryness, along with associated dyspareunia, cystitis, or urinary incontinence.[15, 16] The elevation of vaginal pH permits increased colonization of the vagina and urethra by bacteria and an increased likelihood of urinary tract infections and vaginitis. Lower estrogen levels permit increased osteoclastic activity, osteoporosis, and an increased risk of fracture and fracture-related morbidity. Menopausal estrogen

Table 16–4. Contraindications to Hormone Replacement Therapy

Unexplained vaginal bleeding
Active liver disease or impaired hepatic function
Breast cancer
Endometrial cancer (untreated or advanced)
Recent or past thrombotic event associated with hormonal therapy

declines also permit increases in low-density serum lipoproteins and reductions in high-density lipoproteins that contribute to the increased rates of cardiovascular disease.[17]

A health care provider's approach to caring for women throughout the climacteric and menopause is twofold: providing emotional support and relieving the physical symptoms. Although many women complain of both emotional and cognitive disturbances during this time, it is unclear exactly what role menopause actually plays in mood alteration. Menopause is viewed as a significant life event in most cultures and tends to occur within the same time period as many other personal or social changes. Therefore this time of transition can represent a real emotional and psychological challenge on many levels and may result in depression and irritability. Individual counseling, support groups, and education are generally beneficial in assisting women in coping with the emotional experience of menopause.

RISKS AND BENEFITS OF POSTMENOPAUSAL HORMONE REPLACEMENT THERAPY

Relief of the physiologic changes of menopause can be achieved within 4 to 6 weeks of the start of estrogen replacement therapy (ERT). Most women can benefit from ERT or combined hormone replacement therapy (HRT); however, it is important to consider each patient's individual risk factors before beginning replacement therapy (Tables 16–4, 16–5, and 16–6). Absolute contraindications to HRT include undiagnosed vaginal bleeding, active deep vein thrombosis, and current endometrial or breast cancers. Other disease processes that require special consideration but do not necessarily preclude HRT are cured Stage I endometrial or breast cancers, hepatobiliary disease, and hypertriglyceridemia. Estrogen may be used with caution

Table 16–5. Benefits Associated with Hormone Replacement Therapy

Relief of vasomotor symptoms such as night sweats and hot flashes
Improvement in vaginal dryness and urinary incontinence
Increased libido
Decrease in severity of osteoporosis
Possible cardioprotective effect in some women
May delay or prevent the development of Alzheimer's disease

Table 16–6. Relative Risks Associated with Hormone Replacement Therapy

Endometrial hyperplasia (unopposed estrogen replacement therapy only)
Hypertension (reversible)
Thromboembolism (more common with use of oral contraceptive pills)
Progestins may adversely affect lipid balance
Breast cancer (studies conflict)

in women with identifiable risk factors; however, its use in these populations remains controversial. Thus far, treated Stage I endometrial cancers have not been linked to adverse effects with subsequent HRT administration.[18] Conclusive evidence is currently unavailable regarding either the safety or oncogenicity of ERT in breast cancer survivors.[19] Oral estrogen can pose complications in women with active liver disease, as oral estrogen involves first pass hepatic metabolism. Non-oral estrogen, such as estrogen creams or transdermal estrogen patches, avoids the first pass metabolism in the liver and may provide a reasonable alternative for such patients.

INITIATING HRT

The goals of hormone replacement differ with each patient. Some patients prefer therapy to target symptomatic relief, while others desire long-term prevention of chronic disease. Doses, routes of administration, and types of hormones used vary depending on the needs of each patient. Vasomotor instability may require short-term treatment with higher-dose systemic estrogen that may be administered orally or transdermally. Vaginal topical estrogen, commonly used to relieve symptoms of atrophic vaginitis, has a local effect on the vaginal epithelium theoretically without stimulating other estrogen-sensitive tissues. Systemic absorption from vaginal application is erratic but may be significant. Therefore, as with any other form of estrogen administration, it is always important to consider each patient's potential benefits versus contraindications to therapy. In the postmenopausal woman with an intact uterus, concurrent progesterone replacement prevents endometrial hyperplasia and reduces the risks of endometrial cancer associated with past unopposed ERT.

Hormone regimens vary. Continuous administration is the least confusing and most convenient, and it reduces symptom breakthrough. Progesterone, when indicated, may be given continuously or cyclically on days 1–12 of each month. Continuous progesterone administration often causes irregular breakthrough bleeding for up to 1 year after initiation. Higher doses of progesterone (5 mg vs. 2.5 mg of medroxyprogesterone acetate) are associated with a shorter duration of vaginal spotting. Women who adhere to the cyclical HRT regimen usually experience regular bleeding beginning after the ninth day of progesterone administration. Suspicious bleeding patterns in any postmeno-pausal woman requires investigation. A symptom journal and bleeding calendar are helpful in determining possible etiologies of bleeding in women who are new initiates to HRT. However, a transvaginal sono-graphic measurement of the endometrial stripe width and/or an endo-metrial aspirate should be considered whenever there is any question about postmenopausal bleeding.

HRT AND OSTEOPOROSIS

Many women express concern regarding potential complications of HRT, possibly because much of the information that patients receive from the media and popular literature is often inaccurate or incom-plete. While it is true that estrogen replacement is not without risk, many more women benefit from HRT than experience serious side effects from it. For example, osteoporosis causes more than 1.5 million fractures each year.[1] Women aged 65 and over have a 50% incidence of osteoporosis.[1, 20] By age 75 nearly 90% of women are affected.[20] Greatest bone loss occurs during the fifth and sixth decades of life, the years following menopause. Ideally osteoporosis prevention should begin in adolescence. Women benefit from additional calcium supple-mentation as early as their menarche. All women should consume a diet with a minimum of 800 mg of daily calcium.[20] By menopause women should be advised to supplement their diets with an additional 1000 mg of elemental calcium and 400 units of vitamin D per day, preferably consumed with meals for improved absorption.[20] If women prefer to take supplements between meals, calcium citrate may be preferable. Women over age 70 may have significantly decreased absorption of vitamin D and thus may require doses of 800 units per day. Women can also minimize loss of bone mass with a regular routine of weight-bearing exercises and walking.

Particular risks for osteoporosis include:

* Smoking
* A history of hyperthyroidism
* Use of certain medications (Table 16–7)
* A sedentary lifestyle
* A strong family history of osteoporosis

Most women and especially those with any risk factors for osteopo-rosis should be counseled to abstain from tobacco and alcohol use, to engage in exercise programs, and to consider ERT at the onset of natural or surgical menopause. ERT is currently the gold standard of osteoporosis prevention treatments. The minimum recommended daily dose is 0.625 mg of oral conjugated estrogens. Other forms of estrogen, such as estradiol, are equally effective in controlling symp-toms, but may have fewer longitudinal studies to prove long-term

Table 16–7. Medications Associated with Worsening of Osteoporosis

Thyroid replacement hormone (inappropriate use)
Benzodiazepines (long acting)
Steroids (prolonged use)
Anticonvulsants
Antipsychotics
Tricyclic antidepressants
Heparin

equal efficacy.[20] Higher risk patients unsuitable for traditional ERT may benefit from alternative and/or adjunctive therapies, including biphosphonates, calcitonin, or selective estrogen receptor modulators (SERMs) such as raloxifene.[18, 20]

▬CARING FOR THE PEDIATRIC AND YOUNG ADOLESCENT PATIENT

The American College of Obstetricians and Gynecologists suggests that adolescents should receive their first exposure to gynecologic care as early as age 13.[21] While young women do not require a pelvic examination in the absence of gynecologic complaints or sexual activity, they do benefit from the opportunity to access information about their developing bodies, from anticipatory guidance regarding menstrual changes and comfort measures, and from clarification of misinformation. In addition, age-appropriate sex education and strategies to cope with peer pressure discussed in early adolescence may help to build self-esteem, avert early coitus, and prevent unintended pregnancy or infection.

Issues of confidentiality need to be discussed in advance with both the young patient and the parent. Parents need to be informed of the importance of creating a secure and confidential environment that will help the adolescent to take responsibility for her health care and decision-making. In addition to ensuring patient confidentiality, health care practitioners also need to reassure parents that communication is encouraged so that healthy parent-child relationships will be facilitated. History taking may initially involve both the parent and the adolescent. A menstrual history noting age at menarche, frequency and duration of menses, and presence of dysmenorrhea should also be elicited. Reasons prompting the current visit should be clarified. Once the initial history is obtained, the teen must be allowed the opportunity to discuss issues of concern privately. Obtaining a sexual history is uncomfortable for many practitioners. Questions should be presented in the same phrasing and tone as other questions asked during the health history. Practitioners should avoid using clinical or sophisticated terms obscure to teenagers. Of importance are the number and gender of sexual partners, frequency of coitus, use of contraceptives, and whether sexual encounters are consensual.[22] Many young women are not familiar with what constitutes normal vaginal secretions versus an abnormal discharge. Educating the patient about changes in normal vaginal secretions in relation to the menstrual cycle and the signs of infection (such as color, odor, pain, lesions, dysuria, and adenopathy), exemplifies one topic worthy of discussion during an encounter.[23] Finally, it is important to directly ask the teen if there are any concerns not addressed during the initial conversation. Adults frequently may presume to know what is most important, while the teen may be struggling with issues not immediately apparent or simply dismissed by others as unimportant.

Most young women approach their first pelvic examination with a sense of dread or at least apprehension, often basing these fears on misinformation obtained from peers or family members. Addressing the patient's concerns and giving a detailed explanation of the pelvic examination beforehand greatly relieves many of these feelings. In addition to receiving a verbal explanation, all patients should have an opportunity to see and touch any instruments that will be used during the examination. The use of illustrations or models further enhances the patient's understanding and purpose of the pelvic examination. Patients should be reassured that the examination does not imply a loss of virginity. Perhaps most important is explaining to the patient that she will control the examination. While she may experience a sensation of pressure or discomfort, she should not experience significant pain and may at any time ask the examiner to stop. Relaxation techniques and comfort measures can be explored before the pelvic examination begins. Many patients prefer not have their parent present; therefore, parents should be in attendance only at the teen's request. Most adolescents find the presence of a supportive female assistant reassuring.

THE ADOLESCENT GYNECOLOGIC EXAMINATION

The examination should begin with the assessment of secondary sex characteristics. With puberty, secondary characteristics should become apparent. Breast buds appear and pubic hair begins to take on the typical triangular distribution pattern in early adolescence (Table 16–8). A demonstration of breast self-examination techniques should be given during the clinical breast examination. Once the inspection and breast examination is completed, the patient can be positioned for the pelvic examination. Many patients prefer a semisitting rather than the traditional lithotomy position more frequently offered. In a semisitting position, patients can maintain eye contact with the health care pro-

Table 16–8. Tanner Classification—Sexual Maturity Rating in Females

Stage	Breast	Pubic Hair
I	No breast buds	None
II	Areolar diameter increased, breast buds present, papillae elevated	Sparse, straight, slightly pigmented medial borders of labia
III	Breast and areola enlarged, confluent	Coarser, darker, curly
IV	Areola and papillae project, forming mound	Adult distribution, lesser quantity
V	Mature breast contour, nipple projects	Adult distribution, spread to lateral thigh

Adapted from Nelson WG, Behrman RE, Kliegman RM, Arvin AM. Nelson Textbook of Pediatrics, 15th ed. Philadelphia, WB Saunders, 1996, p 60, with permission.

vider and feel like an active participant in the examination. The increased sense of control serves to enhance the teen's sense of comfort and aids in relaxation. Providing the patient with a hand-held mirror to use during the examination offers the teen an opportunity to view the anatomy of the external genitalia, and practitioners should reassure the patient, when appropriate, that the genitals appear normal and healthy.

The external genitals should be inspected for lesions, discharge, inflammation, or signs of trauma. Clitoral size is normally 2–4 mm in width. A clitoris larger than 10 mm may indicate virilization.[21] If infection is suspected, the Skene's glands should be gently milked and cultures taken if any discharge is noted. The hymen and vagina can be visually inspected by downward traction on the labia minora. Any hymenal abnormalities such as an imperforate hymen should be noted and recommendations for correction offered. By early adolescence the vagina grows to its adult size.[23] However, the hymenal opening may still be too small to admit a speculum or finger without significant discomfort. In the absence of gynecologic complaints, one may consider deferring a speculum examination to a later date. Vaginal cultures and wet mounts can be easily obtained without discomfort by using small damp swabs, or secretions can be aspirated with a soft plastic catheter and syringe.

Choosing the appropriate size and style of speculum reduces a significant amount of discomfort. The Huffman-Graves speculum is specially designed for use with the adolescent patient. The long, narrow speculum blades are more easily inserted in a small hymenal opening and allow for easier visualization of the cervix. If this style of speculum is not available, a small Pederson speculum can be substituted. A small or medium Graves' traditional style speculum may be suitable for sexually active teens. Pediatric specula are inappropriate because the blades are too short to allow adequate visualization. A good general rule is to use a narrow speculum in the younger patient, but to remember that a longer length may be necessary to comfortably view the cervix if the patient is obese. Before insertion, the speculum should be lubricated with warm water. The practitioner can help the patient relax by identifying the pelvic floor muscles and encouraging the patient to relax. This can be done by inserting one or two fingers into the introitus and applying downward pressure. Once the patient relaxes, the speculum can be gently inserted. An adolescent cervix is usually pale pink and may exhibit ectopia, which can at times be confused with cervicitis.[23] A Papanicolaou (Pap) smear and cultures should be obtained from all sexually active teens or teens with a gynecologic complaint. The bimanual examination may be done by inserting only one or two fingers into the vagina. The ratio of uterus to cervix size varies with the age of the patient.[23] Any mass, irregularity, or tenderness requires further evaluation. After the examination is completed, the teen should have an opportunity to dress and then privately discuss any findings or plans with the health care practitioner. Patient and practitioner should decide what information will be revealed to or withheld from the parent or guardian. Any limitations in confidentiality must be discussed with the patient, and she must be advised in advance of any information that will be disclosed to parents or legal entities.[22]

EXAMINING THE PREPUBERTAL CHILD

Examining the prepubertal child is an especially sensitive task. Often young children have been specifically instructed not to allow others to see or touch their genitals. Even in the presence of a parent, a gynecologic examination can be particularly distressful to a young patient. Performing a nontraumatic pediatric gynecologic examination requires experience, patience, kindness, and time. Young children may be distracted by the use of toys or puppets, whereas older children may be engaged in conversation about school or sports. As with adolescents, all children should be allowed to see and touch any instruments that will be used during the examination, and they should be told that at any time they may ask that the examination stop. The presence of the child's parent is usually reassuring, but in select cases, when privacy or abuse issues arise, it may be advisable that parents be escorted to the waiting area. Before the examination begins, the practitioner should explain in understandable terms that the genitals are a special, private area of the body, and the purpose of the examination is to evaluate her health or address a specific gynecologic complaint. Reinforcing beliefs that the genitals are a special part of the body and explaining the importance of informing parents if any one attempts to touch the child can be discussed at this time.

Selecting a position for examination depends on the child's age and level of comfort with the examination. Older children are usually comfortable in the supine froglike position. The patient is asked to recline in a semisitting position with the legs flexed, the knees abducted, and the soles of the feet together. Younger children can sit in the parent's lap in a modified froglike position with the parent supporting the child's legs. Another comfortable position for younger children is a knee-chest position. The child may start on all four arms and legs, "like a puppy"; then she may lower her head and chest down toward the table and raise the hips upward. This position allows close inspection of the perineum and hymen. If a full gynecologic speculum examination is indicated, the parent may lie on the table with feet in the stirrups and the child lying on the parent's abdomen. The child's legs may then be draped over the parent's legs. Alternatively, the parent may assume the supine froglike position behind the child and support the child's legs with his or her own legs. In either position the child is cradled and comforted in her parent's arms. Restraints are never indicated in a nonemergency gynecologic examination. In emergency cases, children who have been traumatized by abuse or are extremely frightened by the examination may require sedation. In some cases examination under anesthesia is necessary.

In the absence of gynecologic complaints or abnormalities, a modified pediatric gynecologic examination (omitting the speculum examination) usually suffices. Unlike the adolescent female, the ovaries in a young female are situated in the upper pelvis. Ovarian neoplasms may be mistaken for abdominal masses. Prepubescent females exhibit thinner, flatter labia majora and minora. Pubic hair is absent. Nevertheless, the child may exhibit physical findings influenced by ovarian activity. The labia and mucosa begin to thicken, and leukorrhea may be present.[24] The vulvovaginal area and introitus can be examined by asking the child to preform the Valsalva maneuver. The lower third of the vagina can also be inspected by applying gentle upward and outward traction on the labia. If the child is fearful, she should be allowed to hold the labia open herself. Inspection of the vestibule will reveal any discharge. Culture and wet mounts can be painlessly obtained with small dampened swabs or aspirated via catheter. A light source and some source of magnification to examine genital tissues are useful. A simple otoscope is often adequate for this purpose.

A complete bimanual pelvic examination is indicated in the presence of complaints such as pain, bleeding, discharge, or suspected retained foreign body. Abdominal or pelvic masses, precocious puberty, or evidence of sexual abuse should also prompt a complete gynecologic examination.[24]

Gentleness and patience are absolutely required when attempting to insert any instruments into the vagina of a young child. The practitioner's approach and the child's experience of the examination if traumatic, could potentially cause long-term psychological consequences. The child should have a chance to see and hold the instrument. It is important to point out that the instrument is smooth and may feel cold but should not cause pain. This point should be reiterated throughout the examination. Before insertion, the instrument should be placed on the child's thigh near the perineum, then on the labia, and finally inserted. Insertion is facilitated with gentle, downward pressure on the perineum. The Cameron-Myers and Mueller vaginoscopes are commonly used instruments when such an examination is required in the younger child.[24] In younger patients, a 0.5 cm diameter scope is usually required, while older pediatric patients can usually tolerate the 0.8 cm size.[23] The bimanual examination may be accomplished by inserting a lubricated small finger into the hymenal orifice of older children. However, this commonly is too uncomfortable for many young patients. A rectal examination is usually better tolerated, as the rectum is more easily distended.[24]

CHILD SEXUAL ABUSE

Sadly, current statistics suggest that 25% of women in the U.S. will experience sexual abuse by the age of 18.[25] More than a quarter of a million cases of sexual abuse per year are suspected. Many young victims do not report abuse out of shame or fear. Health care practitioners are often the first point of discovery in these unreported cases. It is crucial that all health care practitioners be astute at recognizing the signs of sexual abuse. Physical signs include the more obvious ones such as vaginal discharge, bleeding, or vulvar irritation, as well as less specific signs, including abdominal pain, anorexia, enuresis, urethritis, and dyschezia. Emotional signs of sexual abuse may manifest as aggression, fearfulness, nightmares, phobias, or displays of precocious sexual or other high risk behaviors.

Careful documentation is paramount in managing suspected sexual abuse cases. Often the medical examination is the substantiating evidence. The practitioner should remain nonjudgmental and interested in the child's report of events. Open-ended questions are often useful for older children, while younger children may require general questions with yes or no answers. During the interview it is helpful to allow the child some distraction with coloring books or puzzles. Play-talk often allows the child an opportunity to reveal painful information more comfortably. Audio and photographic documentation, when available, should be utilized and social services involved immediately if abuse is suspected. The determination of abuse and the need for intervention are best managed by legal authorities and their specialized consultants.

In cases of abuse a modified pelvic examination is usually sufficient unless a retained foreign body or a vaginal trauma requiring surgical repair is present. Children requiring a complete pelvic examination usually require sedation. The physical examination should be brief and focus on documenting signs of abuse, such as bruising patterns consistent with restraint, bites, and trauma to the pharynx. The anogenital area must be carefully inspected. Specific signs of child sexual abuse include the presence of semen, an STD, an unusually enlarged hymenal opening, suspicious trauma, and pregnancy. True culture techniques, rather than "gen-probes," should be used so there will be less chance of dispute should a case go to court. However, physical examinations are often unremarkable, and not all forms of sexual abuse leave behind detectable evidence. If suspected sexual penetration occurred within 72 h, it may be possible to identify sperm. A rape kit, modified for children, should be used to collect semen and hair samples. Cultures for STDs must also be obtained. All specimens should be handled with great care and considered forensic evidence.

Once all documentation is collected, the practitioner must discuss the findings with the parents and explain the legal obligations of reporting the findings to authorities and/or Child Protective Services. Parents may also benefit from referral to support services to assist in coping with such a difficult situation.

CONCLUSION

Women's health care encompasses not only health care issues traditionally limited to obstetric/gynecology specialists, but also conditions relevant to all phases of a woman's life. It is vitally important that providers of women's health care recognize this spectrum as not limited to reproductive functions or age. As with their more mature counterparts, young women's needs benefit from equal attention. Regardless of age, it should be the goal of health care providers to encourage positive lifelong behaviors and to educate patients throughout their various physical and emotional challenges. It is important to view the woman as a whole person and not simply as a sum of her reproductive parts.

REFERENCES

1. Statistical Information on Women and Women's Health. http://4women. gov.media.statistics.htm
2. DeCherney AH, Pernoll ML. Current Obstetric and Gynecologic Diagnosis and Treatment, 8th ed. Norwalk, CT, Appleton & Lange, 1994, pp 1996–1006.
3. Darney P. Safety and efficacy of a triphasic oral contraceptive containing desogestrell: Results of three multicenter trials. Contraception 1993;48:323.

4. Cerel-Suhl S, Yearger B. Update on oral contraceptive pills. Am Fam Physician 1999;60:2073–2084.
5. Westhoff C, Wieland D, Tiezzi L. Depression in the users of depomedroxyprogesterone acetate. Contraception 1995;51:351.
6. Cromer B, Smith R, Blair J, et al. A prospective study of adolescents who choose among levonorgestrel implant (Norplant), medroxyprogesterone acetate (Depo-Provera), or the combined oral contraceptive pill. Pediatrics 1994;94:687.
7. Cromer B, Blair JM, Maham JD, et al. A prospective comparison of bone density in adolescent girls receiving depot medroxyprogesterone acetate (Depo-Provera), levonorgestrell (Norplant), or oral contraceptives. J Pediatrics 1996;129:671–676.
8. Salah M, Ahmed A, Abo-Eloyoun M, Shaaban MM. Five-year experience with Norplant implants in Assiut, Egypt. Contraception 1987;35:543.
9. Young L, McCowan LM, Roberts HE, Farquhar CM. Emergency contraception—Why women don't use it. N Z Med J 1995;108:145.
10. Haspels AA. Emergency contraception: A review. Contraception 1994;39:459.
11. 1998 Guidelines for treatment of sexually transmitted diseases. MMWR Morb Mortal Wkly Rep 1998;47:1.
12. Woodward C, Fisher MA. Drug treatment of common STDs: Part II. Vaginal infections. Pelvic inflammatory disease, and genital warts. Am Fam Physician 1999;60:1716–1722.
13. Pelvic Inflammatory Disease and Genital Warts. Am Fam Physician 1999;60:1387–1399.
14. National Cancer Institute: Physician's Data Query—Screening and Prevention recommendations: http://cancernet.nci.nih.gov.clinpdq/screening_h.html
15. Greendale GA, Lee NP, Arriola ER. The menopause. The Lancet 1999;353:571.
16. Canavan T, Doshi N. Endometrial cancer. Am Fam Physician 1999;59:3069–3074.
17. The Writing Group for the PEPI Trial: Effects of estrogen or estrogen/progesterone regimens on heart disease risk factors in postmenopausal women. JAMA 1995;273:199–208.
18. Mack TM, Pike MC, Henderson BE, et al. Estrogen and endometrial cancer in a retirement community. N Engl J Med 1976;294:1267–1267.
19. Steinberg KK, Thaker SB, Smith J, et al. Meta-analysis of the effect of estrogen replacement therapy on the risk of breast cancer. JAMA 1991;265:1985–1990.
20. Ullom-Minnich P. Prevention of osteoporosis and fractures, Am Fam Physician 1999;60:194–202.
21. DeCherney AH, Pernoll ML. Current Obstetric and Gynecologic Diagnosis and Treatment, 8th ed. Norwalk, CT, Appleton & Lange, 1994, pp 633–661.
22. Confidentiality in Adolescent Health Care. ACOG Educational Bulletin No. 249. August 1998.
23. Emans SJ, Laufer MR, Goldstein DP. Pediatric and Adolescent Gynecology, 4th ed. Philadelphia, Lippincott-Raven, 1998, pp 1–48.
24. Nelson WE, Behrman RE, Kliegman RN, Arvin AM. Nelson Textbook of Pediatrics, 15th ed. Philadelphia, WB Saunders, 1996, pp 1554–1566.
25. Giardino AP, Finkel MA, Giardino ER, et al. A Practical Guide to the

Evaluation of Sexual Abuse in the Prepubertal Child. Newbury Park, CA, Sage Publications, Inc., 1992, pp 1–7.

RESOURCES

Fertilityplus.org
Hatcher RA, Trussell J, Stewart F. Contraceptive Technology, 17th rev. ed. New York, Ardent Media, 1998. (Includes special sections on emergency contraception and STD treatment guidelines.)

CHAPTER 17

Men's Health

Donna Gamero, PA-C,
O. Michael Obiekwe, MD,
and Fred Shessel, MD

INTRODUCTION

Despite the increased publicity and attention currently focused on many of the problems unique to men's health, including erectile dysfunction, prostate cancer, and sexual orientation, men still are overall more reluctant to seek medical attention.[1] This statement does not simply apply to prostate-related clinical complaints or sexual dysfunction, but to all other medical problems as well. Whether this is due to intrinsic stoicism, worries about appearing weak or inadequate, fears of potential disability, or concerns about loss of household "breadwinner" status remains to be fully understood.

The focus of this chapter includes

* The use of prostate-specific antigen (PSA) testing
* Prostatitis and benign prostatic hypertrophy (BPH)
* Sexual dysfunction
* Mid-life crisis and depression

Other topics to be briefly touched on include

* Tobacco and alcohol use
* Accidents and violence
* Coronary artery disease
* Cancer
* Infertility
* Contraception and safe sex
* Men who have sex with men

Many of these topics are dealt with in greater depth in other chapters of this text.

The fear of developing prostate cancer and dying as a result is a palpable concern for most men. The odds of an American man developing prostate cancer are one in three after age 50. The odds are significantly increased for African American men and for those with a positive family history.[2] Prostate cancer is the leading type of cancer in men.[2] Although an increase in public awareness and improved public health education efforts have prompted more men to present for routine screening and evaluation, many may not be inclined to seek screening or evaluation unless someone they know has been recently diagnosed.

Health care practitioners need to develop rapport with their male patients, often based on fewer contacts compared with female patients. When a practitioner makes it a habit to inquire about sexual and psychosocial questions as a regular part of encounters, patients develop a comfort level that allows them to feel less inhibited in discussing concerns such as erectile dysfuction (ED). In fact, all patients become more comfortable and honest in answering "private" questions when their health care providers routinely incorporate those types of assessments into their medical practice. Some of the topics most difficult for men to discuss are urinary excretion (often due to BPH), sexual performance, and/or sexual orientation. Although many women commonly discuss both individual and family health problems with their peers, men are less inclined (whether due to nature or nurture).

Still other patients may not bring up such problems because they assume that these difficulties are an inevitable result of aging. Men may also be unaware that their complaints could be caused by other conditions and medications, or that successful treatment options exist.[3]

Another factor to consider when dealing with men's health concerns is the rapidly expanding use of the Internet and the availability of "alternative" over-the-counter medications and therapies. Many American consumers are using these alternative therapies in place of or to augment ongoing treatment by their health care providers for complaints including lower urinary tract problems and symptomatic BPH.[4] It is estimated that 30–90% of patients under a urologist's care are using additional homeopathic or herbal agents that are marketed for "men's health" and "prostate health."[4] Men who are reluctant or too self-conscious to seek out traditional medical care may turn to Internet resources or seek out alternative therapies. Many of these therapies may have value, such as the use of saw palmetto berry extract. However, these complaints still warrant the appropriate initial medical evaluation to avoid misdiagnoses and counsel patients about available options for care.

▬▬ PROSTATE-SPECIFIC ANTIGEN

The issue of PSA screening is addressed in Chapter 24, Neoplastic Conditions, in the section on prostate cancer, but it deserves further mention and elaboration in the setting of men's preventive health and its role in BPH evaluation. Prostate-specific antigen is a 33-kD protein that is almost exclusively produced by the epithelium of the prostate. It functions to prevent coagulation of seminal fluid. Increases in PSA occur with both benign and malignant prostatic abnormalities (and sometimes following lower genitourinary instrumentation or manipulation). A PSA value of up to 4.0 ng/dL is considered by most laboratories to be the upper limit of normal.[2] Alternatively, a "normal" PSA value is relative, and should be evaluated in the context of the clinical condition. Serial PSA values in a particular patient are a more accurate means of assessing the significance of any given elevated PSA level. Perusal of PSA values should also be interpreted in regard to racial and age differences seen within the general population by using reference PSA ranges. The ratio between free and bound PSA may help differentiate between cancer and BPH with levels between 4 and 10.

Age-specific PSA has been recommended as a more specific reference standard when determining whether a patient should be referred and/or considered for further evaluation. These values reduce unnecessary biopsies in the elderly and improve cancer detection in the younger man who is more likely to benefit from earlier detection (Table 17–1).[5]

The use of PSA as a prostate cancer–screening tool continues to be controversial. PSA levels increase as the size of the prostate increases. The PSA level will also be elevated with prostatitis. This hypertrophy of the prostate is nearly always due to BPH. This factor complicates the evaluation of an abnormally elevated PSA. The question then arises of when biopsy is indicated, and what is a truly "normal" PSA value. Current recommendations for biopsy in the setting of an elevated PSA are based on the patient's risk factors, life expectancy, comorbid conditions, and the patient's own motivation and wishes. However, PSA elevation due to BPH can be distinguished from that caused by cancer by calculating the PSA density (PSAD).[6] A transrectal ultrasound is used to measure prostatic volume and related to the total PSA to produce the PSAD. A PSAD of 0.15 or greater in men with PSAs between 4–10 ng/dL has been recommended as a threshold for prostatic biopsy.[7, 8]

$$PSAD = PSA/prostate \text{ volume or mass}$$

The one incontrovertible fact regarding this issue is that PSA testing has led to an increased rate of detection of prostate cancer. Between

Table 17–1. Age-Adjusted PSA Reference Values

Age in Years	Normal PSA (ng/dL)
40–49	0–2.5
50–59	0–3.5
60–69	0–4.5
70–79	0–6.4

From Osterling JE, Jacobson SJ, Chute CG, et al. PSA in a community-based population of healthy men: Establishment of age-specific reference ranges. JAMA 1993;270:860–864, with permission.

1990 and 1995, the death rate from prostate cancer for white U.S. males under the age of 75 fell by > 14% and was attributed to PSA screenings.[9] There are currently several large trials taking place in the United States and Europe. These studies are designed to specifically determine whether PSA-based screening cost-effectively reduces mortality due to prostate cancer and/or leads to an improved quality of life.[2]

Because of these unanswered questions, the International Union against Cancer, the U.S. Preventive Services Task Force, and the Canadian Task Force have not yet endorsed routine PSA screening.[2] Conversely, the American Urological Association and American Cancer Society currently recommend that all men undergo PSA screening along with a digital rectal examination (DRE) beginning at age 50. If the man belongs to a high-risk group, as do African American males and men with first-degree relatives with prostate cancer, screening is recommended to begin at age 40.[2, 10, 11]

When the asymptomatic patient with no risk factors requests a PSA, it is advisable to counsel him regarding

* The controversy over PSA determination
* The pros and cons of early detection of prostate cancer
* The differential diagnosis of an elevated PSA
* The types of further diagnostic testing that may be triggered by an elevated PSA level

In the patient who has symptoms that may be attributable to a prostate problem or risk factors, discussion regarding the need and benefits of early detection and/or screening should begin before age 50, and as young as age 40. The clinical consensus, pending further evidence, is that when a man is

* Between the ages of 50 and 75, and
* Has at least a 10-year life expectancy,
* He should receive both a PSA and DRE screening.

If either test is abnormal, referral to a urologist is recommended.[2]

■■■PROSTATITIS AND BENIGN PROSTATIC HYPERTROPHY

Traditionally, prostatitis has been divided into four categories: acute bacterial, chronic bacterial, chronic nonbacterial, and prostadynia. Perhaps the most surprising fact is that <10% of prostatitis is of bacterial etiology. This acute febrile illness is usually associated with low back, perineal, or rectal pain as well as myalgias, urinary symptoms, and/or dysuria. Treatment with antibiotics for 4–6 weeks generally is required to prevent chronic prostatitis or abscess. Eighty percent of these infections are due to *Escherichia coli*, whereas the remainder are caused by *Pseudomonas, Neisseria gonorrhoeae, Mycobacterium tuberculosis, Serratia, Klebsiella, Proteus*, or other enteric organisms. Chronic prostatitis is caused by the same organisms, but it is more common in older men. Antibiotics poorly penetrate the uninflamed prostate; therefore, treatment usually requires 3 months.

Nonbacterial prostatitis and prostadynia are much more common than bacterial prostatitis, in fact, almost eight times more common. Pain and inflammation are present and secretions expressed after prostate massage reveal leukocytes, but routine cultures remain negative. Prostadynia simply refers to pain and localized symptoms without signs of inflammation of the prostate. Associated symptoms can include weakened urinary stream, hesitancy, nocturia, painful ejaculation, and hematospermia. Although bacterial etiologies are unproved, empirical antibiotics, alpha-blockers, and nonsteroidal anti-inflammatory drugs (NSAIDs) can ameliorate symptoms >50% of the time.[12]

After the age of 70, 90% of men have detectable BPH. Fortunately, only 15% have clinically significant symptoms and sequelae. BPH is the underlying etiology in 90% of urinary retention in men.[10] Prostate gland size is not necessarily proportional to degree of symptoms, but is important in determining the most appropriate treatment. The etiology of BPH is relatively unclear, although hormonal changes are believed to be involved in the alterations that occur within the prostate gland. It has been noted that, as men age, multiple fibroadenomatous nodules begin to develop within the gland, displacing the more normal prostate tissue. This displacement of prostate tissue can occur either medially or laterally. Medial displacement, which is often the initial event, leads to constriction of the urethra as it passes through the prostate gland. This causes the obstructive urinary symptoms that are the most common complaints in BPH.

The symptoms of BPH include

* A slow urine stream
* Intermittent stream
* A change in voiding characteristics, such as double voiding

BPH can lead to detrusor instability, urinary infections, formation of genitourinary (GU) calculi, bladder diverticula, and upper GU tract dilatation, often associated with renal insufficiency.[10] Evaluation of these complaints should include a thorough history and focused physical examination. The International Prostate Screening Questionnaire can be a useful tool in screening for potential BPH-related problems (Box 17–1).[13] The physical examination should focus on the abdominal and GU examinations and should include the DRE. A urinalysis including microscopic analysis and/or a urine culture aids in ruling out urinary tract infections (UTI), hematuria, and proteinuria. The question of whether or not to do a PSA test should be based on the clinical picture and the patient's risk factors.

Box 17-1—INTERNATIONAL PROSTATE SCREENING QUESTIONNAIRE*

Questions pertain to symptomatology over the previous 1–2 months

How many times do you most typically get up to urinate from the time you go to bed at night to the time you get up in the morning?

How often do you have a sensation of not emptying your bladder completely after you finish urinating?

How often do you have to urinate again in <2 hours after you finished urinating previously?

How often do you find that you stopped and started again several times while urinating?

How often do you find it difficult to postpone urination?

How often do you experience a weak urinary stream?

How often do you have to push or strain in order to begin urination?

Add scores of all questions: A score of >10 is considered clinical.

---

*Each question is scored from 0 to 5, with 0 being no symptoms ranging to 5 as experiencing symptoms almost all the time.

Adapted from Barry MJ, Fowler FR Jr, O'Leary M. The American Urological Association Symptom Index for Benign Prostatic Hypertrophy. J Urol 1992;148(5):1549–1557.

The goals of treating symptomatic BPH are to improve the patient's quality of life. The health care provider should keep in mind any other chronic medical problems the patient may have and other medications he may be taking. Current medical treatment involves the use of alpha-blockers. Patients on certain antihypertensives, such as terazosin (Hytrin) and doxazosin (Cardura), were observed to have an added benefit beyond blood pressure control, specifically, improvement in prostatism or urinary retention symptoms. These medications were found to be equally effective in nonhypertensive patients, although peripheral vasodilatory side effects can be problematic. Another alpha blocker, tamsulosin hydrochloride (Flomax), is a fairly new medication developed specifically for BPH. It has been found to produce less systemic vasodilatory side effects, although it does cause delayed or absent ejaculation and commonly an aggravating rhinitis. Finasteride (Proscar), another relative newcomer to the market, is a 5-alpha-reductase inhibitor. It is a selective inhibitor of alpha$_1$-receptors in the prostate, although it too can cause some peripheral vasodilatory effects. Finasteride is the only medication that results in a reduction in the size of the prostate gland. Unfortunately, it takes 6–12 months to obtain results, and it is successful in only approximately 50% of men.

Surgical treatment usually is reserved for medication failures and those with exceptionally large prostate glands. Traditionally, either transurethral prostatectomy (TURP) or suprapubic prostatectomy was the treatment of choice. Currently, there are other, less invasive options to choose from, including laser prostatectomy, transurethral prostate vaporization, microwave thermotherapy, and transurethral needle ablation.[10] For acute-onset urinary retention, urethral or suprapubic catheterization may be necessary on a short-term basis.

SEXUAL DYSFUNCTION

Erectile dysfunction (ED) is one aspect of the overall syndrome of impaired sexual function, which affects both men and women. Men more commonly present to their health care provider with a complaint of sexual impairment in the form of ED, whereas women are more likely to present with pain or libido issues. In women this is frequently termed "lack of interest" and often has physiologic causes including early pregnancy, lactation, fear of an unintended pregnancy, stress and/or fatigue, medications such as selective serotonin reuptake inhibitor (SSRI) antidepressants, and hormonal imbalances, particularly in the perimenopausal period.[14]

The definition of erectile dysfunction is "the inability to achieve and/or maintain a penile erection sufficient to permit satisfactory vaginal intromission."[15, 16] Twenty to 30 million American men between the ages of 40 and 70 suffer from some degree of ED. This translates to 52% of men in this age group.[3, 15] As men age, frequency increases so that by the age of 70, 67% of men have some manifestations of ED.[3] In addition to countless outpatient visits, ED accounts for up to 30,000 hospital admissions every year.[17]

ED is frequently a difficult issue for men to broach with their health care providers. Men may use Internet or other electronic resources to self-diagnose and even seek treatment which, as discussed earlier in this chapter, can be inappropriate or even dangerous. When evaluating a patient who presents with complaints of ED, it is advisable to inquire about what, if any, therapies or medications the patient may have already tried. It is also enlightening to ask what type of research he may have already done on this subject, particularly using the Internet.

Not only do men experience difficulty or reticence in talking about sexual dysfunction, health care practitioners often are reluctant or uncomfortable in obtaining a good sexual history or even broaching the subject of sexuality. As has been reiterated several times previously, the health care provider must make the psychosocial and sexual parts of the history and physical examination routine and objective. There are many ways of approaching the subject if the patient does not voluntarily bring it up. For example, one method is to make a statement. To a diabetic patient, one might state, "Many men who have diabetes often experience some sexual difficulties as a result of their disease. Have you had any concerns or complaints regarding your sexual activity?" During a checkup when doing a review of symptoms, simply ask, "Assessing a patient's sexual health is an important part of the routine physical. Do you have any particular concerns or questions regarding your sexual activity?"

During the workup of ED, the man should be strongly encouraged to include his partner in evaluation and treatment decisions. Treatment decisions can be better made if the expectations of the man and his partner are discussed openly. This also aids in patient education, including treatment side effects and mechanisms of action.

When evaluating ED, one must always be suspicious of concomitant medical problems as an etiology. The three main categories of ED etiologies are organic, psychogenic, or mixed.[15] The most common, chronic medical conditions that can cause organic ED are

* Hypertension
* Diabetes mellitus
* Hyperlipidemia
* Medication side effects

Other conditions that can also result in ED are

* Low testosterone
* Renal failure
* Hepatic disease
* Neurologic conditions, especially post-trauma or cerebrovascular accident (CVA)
* A history of GU surgery

Factors such as smoking, anemia, pituitary adenoma, thyroid disorders, depression, and chronic alcoholism also can predispose a man to ED.[3, 18] If a patient is on antihypertensive medication, the health care provider must routinely inquire specifically about sexual difficulties. Fifteen percent of patients on this broad class of drugs develop ED within the first year of therapy.[3] The patient may not be aware that his medication is causing the problem, and simply assumes that this is part of the aging process. Other medications such as diuretics, digoxin, cimetidine, and many antidepressants are also notorious for causing sexual dysfunction. The most difficult aspect of evaluating ED is differentiating between the organic and psychogenic causes.

Often, ED that is psychogenic in origin tends to be abrupt in onset and the symptom course may be intermittent. Additionally, the patient usually is able to obtain an erection with masturbation or erotic stimuli. Nocturnal or morning erections are generally present in psychogenic or mixed etiology ED, whereas they are absent if there is a purely organic etiology.[3, 19] Many psychogenic causes result from problems in one's relationship. Problems with stress, anxiety, anger, fears about previous sexual performance or even sexual inhibition can also lead to problems with ED. Another reason frequently advanced for developing ED is that the man's partner is no longer sexually appealing.[14]

In addition to the clinical symptoms of ED, the patient can also experience feelings of depression, decreased self-esteem, and a decrease in relationship satisfaction. As was stated by Dr. Althof, "Health care providers must remember that ED does not just affect the penis" (Box 17–2).[1] The man (and sometimes his partner) perceives the ED as an inadequacy. He may be reluctant to discuss it with his partner and/or may elect to avoid intimacy and love-making situations. Feelings of failure and being "unmanly" are also common thoughts. Relationship concerns may then arise in regard to questions of infidelity, and loss of love and desire in both partners.[1] An effective screening tool is the Sexual Health Inventory for Men.[1, 20] If an untreated depressed patient has developed ED in temporal association with the depression, medical treatment of the dysthmia may resolve the issue. However, if problems of decreased libido or ED develop on antidepressant therapy, especially SSRI medications, consider changing to another such as nefazodone, bupropion or mirtazapine. If the offending medication must be continued, a trial of sildenafil or buspirone can be used to counter these unwanted side effects.[21, 22]

The history should include a full evaluation of the chief complaint, the past medical history, a comprehensive sexual history, and psychosocial assessment.[23] The physical examination should be fairly comprehensive with particular focus on the GU system, evaluation of the secondary sexual characteristics, a cardiovascular examination including assessment of the peripheral pulses, and a focused neurologic examination. The rectal examination should always be included.

Laboratory evaluation should consist of a serum glucose, lipid profile, and basic metabolic panel, if none of these have been done recently. The use of testosterone testing is controversial. It has been found that even if testosterone levels are low, treatment with testosterone supplementation may not significantly improve sexual function.[3] A free testosterone is best drawn as two morning specimens (pooling the sera) and submitted as one test. If the value is less than 250–350 ng/dL, this level may be considered relatively deficient and a trial of supplementation could be considered.[24] There is agreement that some type of assessment of the hypothalamic-pituitary-gonadal axis should be done, by measurement of prolactin or testosterone levels.[18, 23] Other diseases should be screened for as the clinical picture dictates. A 12-lead electrocardiogram and a serum PSA may also be included as part of the evaluation.[14] Consider potential reversibility of the problem. Always keep available the option for referral if

* This is a younger patient with a history of GU or spinal trauma
* The patient is diagnosed with Peyronie's disase

Box 17-2–PATIENT GUIDE TO ERECTILE DYSFUNCTION

What is erectile dysfunction?

Erectile dysfunction (ED) is the inability to achieve or maintain an erection satisfactory for sexual intercourse over a period of time.

Do many men experience ED?

You are not alone; 20 to 30 million men in the U.S. suffer from ED. This condition affects men of all ages: 39% of 40-year-olds and up to 67% of 70-year-olds.

What causes ED?

Some 80% of ED has an organic cause, which means it is caused by a physical condition such as diabetes, high blood pressure, high cholesterol, or other physical problems. Some 20% of cases are caused by psychological factors such as stress, depression, or anxiety. ED can also be caused by a combination of both. When the blood vessels and muscles do not relax enough to allow blood to enter the penis, an erection cannot happen.

What else affects ED?

Other things can decrease blood flow to the penis and reduce the possibility of having an erection. Smoking tobacco or taking certain medications (such as some medicines to lower high blood pressure or to combat depression) can decrease your chance of having an erection. Also, how much stress you have in your life is a big factor that can affect sexual function.

How is ED diagnosed?

Your health care provider may ask you questions about your sexual health such as if you have an erection when sleeping or when you wake up. He may also ask if you have any history of sexual problems or if you have any problems staying erect during sex or when you masturbate.

Your health care provider may also ask about your relationship with your partner. Stress between partners can be a cause of ED. He will then perform a complete physical examination.

How is ED treated?

ED can usually be easily treated in several different ways. First, your health care provider will need to determine if the ED is caused by an underlying illness that needs to be treated. If the ED is caused by a particular kind of medication, your health care provider may choose to change your prescription. Remember, too, that lifestyle can affect ED. If you smoke, you should stop; you should also decrease alcohol intake.

Box 17-2–PATIENT GUIDE TO ERECTILE DYSFUNCTION (Continued)

Whatever the cause, ED is best resolved when you and your partner are involved in the treatment decision together. If you and your partner are experiencing stresses in your relationship, your health care provider can help you find ways of dealing with your problems. If you are under a considerable amount of stress, doing things to decrease your stress, such as exercising, can help.

Your health care provider might prescribe an oral medication such as sildenafil (Viagra) to help you achieve an erection. This medication works by allowing the muscles and blood vessels of the penis to relax so that blood can fill the penis, giving you an erection. You usually take it about 1 hour before having sex. Avoid a fatty meal if faster action is preferred.

Viagra is not for everyone; it cannot be taken by patients on certain heart medicines (called nitrates) because they dilate your blood vessels. The combination may cause your blood pressure to drop too quickly, which could cause you to become dizzy or have other medical problems.

Another treatment is using a vacuum device, which, when placed on the penis, pulls blood into it and keeps it there until intercourse is finished. Some patients may need other treatments, such as injections into the penis or medication inserted into the penis. A penile implant is available for patients when the other methods do not work.

What else should I know about ED?

You should never be afraid to bring up any sexual problems that you are having to your health care provider. An important thing to remember is that you are never too old to have sex, and sex is an important part of your overall health. You may feel embarrassed talking to your health care provider about these kinds of problems, but remember that he or she is there to help you. Also remember that your health care provider will always keep whatever you say and any treatments you decide on confidential and private.

Adapted from Patient guide: Erectile dysfunction; a teaching aid. PA Journal 2000;24(Supplement):21.

* An abnormality within the hypothalamic-pituitary-gonadal axis has been diagnosed
* The patient fails to respond to initial therapy

Treatment options are varied. In part, due to the intensified re-search on ED and the development of newer oral medications, such as sildenafil (Viagra), patients have seen better treatment outcomes and have more options to choose from since the mid-1990s. Viagra has become a household word, and the number of prescriptions written for it over the past few years is staggering. Although the indications for prescribing sildenafil are for significantly severe ED, off-label use is very prevalent. If a patient elects to use sildenafil, its proper use, side effects, and contraindications need to be clearly explained to the patient and his partner. The patient must be warned that the medication may not be very effective the first time it is used due to the anxiety engendered by ED. If the man hasn't recently engaged in intercourse or other physical activity, the health care provider should consider the possibility of vascular disease and the advisability of stress cardiac testing and/or Doppler studies before considering a trial of Viagra. Adverse effects include headache, flush-ing, nasal congestion, and dyspepsia. Its use is contraindicated in those taking nitroglycerin in any form, or those using other organic nitrates or nitric oxide drugs (e.g., nitroprusside).[19, 23, 25] If a patient has been advised not to engage in sexual activity for medical reasons, that patient should also not be prescribed sildenafil.[25]

The use of other oral medications remains controversial. Yohimbine (which blocks the presynaptic alpha-2 adrenergic receptors and is derived from the bark of the tree *Corynanthe yohimbi*) has fallen in and out of favor for many years as treatment for ED. One article stated that, under the 1996 American Urological Association guide-lines, yohimbine was not considered an effective treatment of ED.[26] Subsequently, in an article published 1 year later, yohimbine was again mentioned as possibly being beneficial in patients with ED who had minimal organic dysfunction, but had a significant functional compo-nent to their ED.[19] Newer medications such as sublingual apomor-phine (Uprima) may benefit some men who fail on Viagra.

Adolescents frequently search for medications to enhance duration and hardness of their erections in the belief that their partners will admire their prowess. Use of yohimbine, amyl nitrate "poppers," and rubbing cocaine powder topically on their erections are examples of the self-experimentation that goes on among young men.

Other primary ED treatment options consist of vacuum constrictive devices and psychological evaluation and treatment, based on the diagnostic findings. Second-line management options involve the use of intracavernosal self-injection of papaverine or the synthetic form of prostaglandin E_1, alprostadil (Caverject), or the intraurethral adminis-tration of alprostadil (Muse). Third-line therapy, which is reserved for refractory cases of ED, involves surgical implantation of a semirigid or inflatable penile prosthesis.[19, 23, 25, 26]

Naturally, any organic problems that have exacerbated or caused the ED need full evaluation and appropriate management. Lifestyle changes include tobacco cessation, moderation of alcohol use, and dietary management along with exercise to lower cholesterol. These changes should be recommended and the appropriate education provided to the patient. Unfortunately, although lifestyle modifications may often be the most effective long-term management, they can be difficult to enforce, and the long-term compliance rate is often very poor.

In the past, urologists almost exclusively treated ED. With the ongoing changes under managed care, primary care providers are being called on to manage these problems with greater frequency. Education of both health care providers and patients can only serve to enhance the quality of health care provided for all patients, especially those with ED. This enhanced health care is brought about by emphasis on patient education during the evaluation, and by allowing both the patient and his partner to clarify their expectations and needs to the health care practitioner (Box 17–3). Continued follow-up after treatment is initiated is important and is usually carried out at 6–12-month intervals or as needed by the patient.[23]

Persistent or recurrent ejaculation with only minimal stimulation, upon penetration or before the partner desires it, is considered premature ejaculation (PE). The treatment cornerstone is relationship counseling, behavioral modification, and less commonly pharmacologic interventions. Behavioral modification has had reported success rates of upward to 95%; however, long-term outcomes are less favorable and depend on ongoing involvement of a committed sexual partner. Clomipramine and sertraline modify the ejaculatory response by lengthening the latency period by 4–6 min.[27, 28]

There are many ways to approach patients about sexual concerns. The health care practitioner who approaches the sexual history just as one might handle a chest pain workup provides the patient a comfort

---

Box 17-3–PATIENT AND PARTNER EDUCATION IN ED

Basic review of the anatomy and physiology of the sexual response

Discussion of the pertinent etiologies and associated risk factors such as lifestyle and/or medication side effects

Description of the initial results of the evaluation

Review of treatment options

level that permits him to discuss issues of sexuality or sexual dysfunction in the future. It also gives the patient a sense of validation that his sexual problems and concerns are genuine and in need of proper evaluation.

MID-LIFE CRISIS AND DEPRESSION

Despite the fact that evidence-based medicine is strongly biased toward studies of male patients, there is a paucity of research or evidence to support the notion of a "male menopause." However, there is a transitional period, between ages 40–60, when men become aware of their own mortality and must begin to adjust to the aging process. Many other changes occur during this same interval, including the "empty nest," divorce, disenchantment with one's life's work, retirement, bereavement due to the loss of parents, friends, family, or spouse, and/or physical decline. Mid-life is a natural period of changes and should be viewed as such. Nevertheless, different personalities handle the stresses of social change quite differently. Men who have low self-esteem, high anxiety, and resentment may note an exacerbation of symptoms during this developmental period of their life.[29]

Although depression is two to three times more common in women, men are more likely to commit suicide. Risk factors for depression in men include

* Medical illness and/or physical disability
* Medications, for example, barbituates, benzodiazepines, reserpine, methyldopa, and beta-blockers or H_2 blockers
* Alcohol or drug abuse
* Single status and/or lack of social supports
* New life stressors
* Previous depression episode
* Family history of depression and suicide

Although advancing age is not by itself a risk factor for depression, suicide rates in depressed men do increase with increased age. Studies have revealed that 75% of elderly suicide victims had visited their primary care provider within 1 month of their attempt, and nearly 40% had visited their health care provider in the preceding week![30, 31] Classic presentations of depression are less common in the elder patient, although a new complaint of insomnia may hint at a deeper problem. Consider the Beck Depression Inventory or the Geriatric Depression Scale when the diagnosis is unclear. While SSRIs continue to be the first line for medical therapy, many alternatives exist if side effects are noted or the patient fails to respond. If a tricyclic antidepressant is considered remember to obtain a baseline ECG to rule out the possibility of an underlying block that could be worsened by the cholinergic effects of these medications. Prompt diagnosis, medication, psychiatric consultation or, in extreme cases, hospitalization form the basis for successful intervention.

OTHER PERTINENT ISSUES IN MEN'S HEALTH

Women live, on the average, 8 years longer than their male counterparts. Therefore, there are more elderly women than elderly men. This is postulated to be the result of genetic, biologic, and environmental factors. Survival differences have remained unchanged at the beginning of the 21st century, despite women smoking more and moving into the more traditional male job markets. Therefore, risk factors in men that can be changed need to be especially emphasized during patient education and preventive health encounters.

TOBACCO AND ALCOHOL USE

Smoking in the U.S. is still more common in men than in women—28% versus 23%—according to statistics from the Centers for Disease Control's (CDC) Tobacco Information and Prevention Source Page for 1999.[32] If men quit smoking by the age of 35, they can add 2 years to their life expectancy, whereas a woman will add 3 years to her life expectancy. Initially, smoking was a male prerogative until the 1960s, when the percentage of women smokers increased dramatically due to social acceptability and as a feminist social statement. Because men have a higher prevalence of developing coronary artery disease up to 60 years of age, smoking cessation, especially in younger men, cannot be overstressed. Patient education for men needs more focus on these specifics.

Statistics show that male adolescents are still more likely than females to start using tobacco products, particularly smokeless tobacco. A component of an adolescent's well-care physical examination should include questions about tobacco use, including smokeless tobacco use in young men (its use by females is still rare outside of isolated regional and cultural groups). If a patient acknowledges the use of smokeless tobacco products, the physical examination should include a thorough oral, head, and neck examination. He should also be counseled on the risks of smokeless tobacco use, and changes to look for that could signal the development of leukoplakia or oral cancer.

Alcoholism also continues to be more common in men, although the rates of alcoholism in both sexes are converging. Denial of alcohol abuse is common in both men and women. However, men tend to be more reluctant to seek medical care or even to be able to acknowledge that they have a problem. Denial, an important but dangerous coping mechanism in both sexes, may be raised to an even higher form by the younger, active man.

ACCIDENTS AND VIOLENCE

Men aged 16–35 are at especially high risk of serious injury and death from accidents and acts of violence. These risks appear to be even greater for African American and Latino males; however, this may be due to cultural machismo or simply skewed representation in poverty zones. In all racial groups, more young men die in motor vehicle accidents and are more likely to be the victims of injury or death from gunshot wounds. A recent study completed in California showed that 88% of handguns were purchased by men. It also revealed that 62% of suicides in men are secondary to gunshot wounds.[33] Men of all ages are also more likely to be perpetrators of violence.[34]

CANCER

Cancer is the second most common cause of death in the U.S. As this topic is covered in more depth in Chapter 24, highlights regarding neoplastic diseases in men's health promotion and patient education are noted here. The ten most common cancers in the U.S. in men (in decreasing order of occurrence) include[35]

* Prostate
* Lung
* Colorectal
* Bladder
* Lymphoma
* Melanoma
* Oropharyngeal
* Kidney
* Leukemia
* Pancreas

Of particular note is the finding that until the age of 50, the incidence of cancer is higher among women. However, after age 60, the cancer frequency rises remarkably among men.

Testicular cancer is a relatively rare cancer, accounting for <7000 new cases each year. The 5-year survival rate has increased to 95% in the last 15 years. Public awareness and celebrity advocacy for testicular self-examination (TSE) and prompt treatment of this cancer of young men (teens–35) are largely responsible for this success. Box 17–4 provides details regarding TSE.[36]

Box 17-4–TESTICULAR SELF-EXAMINATION

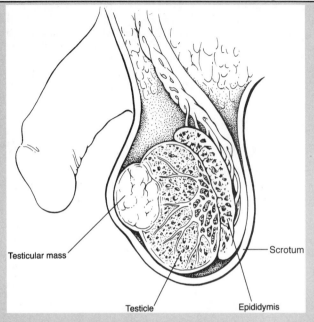

Testicular mass

Testicle

Scrotum

Epididymis

- Should be taught and learned between ages 13 and 18
- Perform monthly after a warm bath or shower. Warm temperature makes the scrotal skin relax and easier to examine
- Stand naked in front of a mirror:
  - Look for any swelling on the skin of the scrotum
  - It is normal for one testicle to be slightly larger than the other
  - A normal testicle feels smooth, rubbery, and is egg-shaped
- Examine each testicle with both hands:
  - The index and middle finger should be placed on top
  - Roll your testicle gently between thumbs and fingers
  - Feel for a lump about the size of a pea on the front or side of the testicle
  - These lumps are usually painless
- Find the epididymis (a cord-like structure on top and back of the testicle that stores and transports sperm)
- Feel for any lumps or masses. These may be as small as a pea, but are generally painless and firm. If you find a lump, mass, or have symptoms such as swelling, pain, or heaviness, this does not necessarily mean that you have cancer. It simply means that it needs to be promptly checked by your health care provider. If cancer is detected and treated early, >90% of testicular cancer patients are cured by surgery and radiotherapy.

(Illustration from Strauss RH. Sports Medicine, 2nd ed. Philadelphia, WB Saunders, 1991, p 524, with permission.)

Breast cancer, which is of such concern in women, is relatively uncommon in men. However, it has been established that the risk of male, like female, breast cancer increases with advancing age. Breast cancer in men accounts for 1% of all new breast cancer cases. The breast examination should not be omitted from the routine male physical examination, as this cancer in men tends to progress more rapidly compared to its female counterpart (see also Chapter 24, Neoplastic Conditions).[37]

CORONARY ARTERY DISEASE

The incidence of coronary artery disease (CAD) in men is cumulatively higher than in women by a lifetime ratio of 4:1. Alarmingly, the odds ratio in men, up to 40 years of age, is eight times greater than that of women. Conversely, after age 70, the ratio is 1:1.[35] Risk factors for developing CAD include being male, with particular risk if the man is ≥35 years of age. If a man has at least one additional risk factor for CAD, daily aspirin prophylaxis is recommended (unless specifically contraindicated). In the patient who has had a myocardial infarction one needs to address treatment expectations and any concerns about the resumption of sexual relations or performance anxieties of the patient or his partner. Men generally tend to have better treatment outcomes and better survival rates following myocardial infarctions. Given greater risk factors and frequency of CAD in the general male population, it is not clearly understood why men's survival rates are better than women's. Theories suggest this may be due to underdiagnosis and delay in the treatment of women presenting for care with the chief complaint of chest pain, although others suggest that less is known about female CAD due to skewed research studies in the past.

INFERTILITY

The incidence of infertility has increased due to a variety of factors. There has also been an increased awareness about the plethora of therapeutic options available to the infertile couple. Male-only infertility occurs in approximately 22% of couples who are unable to conceive.[38] For a male to be able to reproduce without the assistance of contraceptive technology, he must have:

1. A normal semen analysis including sperm count, motility, and morphology.
2. The ability or access to convey sperm successfully into the female reproductive tract. The ability to obtain and maintain an erection, achieve ejaculation, and the capacity to place the ejaculate into the

vaginal vault all must occur with sufficient frequency to achieve fertilization.

Although the most common cause of male-only infertility is unknown, the other established causes are listed in Box 17–5. The age of a man may not affect sperm function, but does increase the possibility of sexual dysfunction, such as ED. Because of a prolonged refractory period as they age, men tend to have fewer coital episodes. Medications, including monoamine oxidase inhibitors, narcotics, most antihypertensives, and cimetidine, can directly affect male fertility by causing ED, retrogade ejaculation, or temporary impairment of spermatogenesis. Smoking, alcohol, sickle cell disease, cocaine or marijuana use, tight-fitting clothing, and prolonged heat exposures can affect many aspects of sperm function, numbers, and morphology. The treatment for male infertility is to address the factors that can be controlled, that is, stop smoking, decrease alcohol intake, avoid tight-fitting clothing, and repair any varicoceles. If the problem cannot be resolved, then artificial insemination via donor sperm or in vitro fertilization are options.

The infertile couple, whether heterosexual or same-sex, has special emotional needs that must be met during the workup and treatment process. Feelings of inadequacy abound, and the primary care provider needs to be sensitive to signs of depression that may develop in otherwise well and "unstressed" couples.

CONTRACEPTION AND SAFE SEX

Preventing pregnancy and sexually transmitted disease (STD) is a responsibility that should be shared by both partners. Taking the initiative of initiating contraception use has traditionally been the woman's role, but is now much more equally shared by men because of safe-sex issues. As men have become more involved in the parenting and household aspects of family life, they have started taking a more proactive part in preventing unintended pregnancies.

Condom use is the most common form of birth control used by men. Although there is a female condom available, the frequency of

---

Box 17-5–COMMON CAUSES OF MALE INFERTILITY

Varicocele
Primary testicular failure
Accessory gland infection
Idiopathic low sperm motility/count

its use remains sporadic. Latex condoms are the most common type of condom used and are most effective at preventing transmission of STDs. Natural membrane condoms are also effective in avoiding pregnancy, but do not protect against STDs. Currently, in the U.S., there are only a few brands of polyurethane condoms (synthetic and latex-free). Both the polyurethrane and latex condoms seem to provide an adequate barrier to both STDs and pregnancy. The failure rate of appropriate condom use is 3% in the first year of use, although condom effectiveness is further enhanced if spermicidal creams or vaginal contraceptive films are used concurrently.[38] The disadvantages of condom use for men include complaints of reduced sensitivity, interference with erection, embarrassment, feelings of losing control over one's partner, and latex allergy. Most men are unaware of the large variety of condoms available internationally, which may solve most of these common concerns. Although most condoms are purchased by women, a man can be educated in comparison shopping and proper application using several Internet sites:

* condommania.com
* wearyourrubbers.com
* gaycondoms.com

Emergency contraception is a well-kept secret, but fertile men need to know what to do when the "rubber" breaks (for details see Chapter 16, Women's Health).

The withdrawal method (coitus interruptus) can be as effective as other vaginal barrier methods. However, it is not a contraceptive method recommended by most practitioners since it provides no protection from STDs. It also requires a great degree of control by the male partner to be able to withdraw prior to ejaculation. In addition, the preejaculate fluid may contain a small number of spermatozoa that may still persevere against all odds.

Vasectomy is considered a permanent form of contraception or sterilization. Prior to a man electing to have a vasectomy procedure, he should be fully informed of the procedure, risks, and the fact that it is considered permanent sterilization. Vasectomies are considered safe procedures that are convenient and can be done in an office setting. Complications such as bleeding, hematoma, and infection are relatively rare. If reversal is desired, the success rate is fair (as measured by a resultant pregnancy), ranging from 16–79% depending primarily on the length of time since the vasectomy was performed.[38]

MEN WHO HAVE SEX WITH MEN

Not all men who have sex with other men describe themselves as gay or bisexual. Because of methodologic problems and legitimate concerns about prejudices, studies report wide variations in the number of persons who have had sex with their same gender or have been attracted by their own gender at some point in their life. Although >9% of all men admit to having had sex with another man, <3% of the general population identify themselves as gay.[39, 40] One must also consider the transgender patient, who may be at any point in the reassignment process when he or she presents for routine care. Regardless of expressed sexual preferences or orientation, such men have additional health concerns that often remain unmet by the insensitive or judgmental health care provider.

Before 1973, homosexuality was categorized as a mental illness. Following years of advocacy, sexual orientation has finally achieved "equality" within health care planning circles. It has been recently targeted as one of six specific patient populations with acknowledged health disparities that will be addressed in the upcoming report *Healthy People 2010*. Nevertheless, studies continue to confirm that 31–89% of health care providers respond negatively to patients "coming out," and 40% of health care providers describe themselves as uncomfortable or threatened by same-sex orientation.[41, 42]

Important health issues include:

1. General

   * Smoking
   * Alcohol
   * Depression/suicide
     * Especially as youth, 30–40% attempt or seriously consider suicide
     * Teens more prone to suffer poor school performance, substance abuse, avoidance of health care, and violence
     * Elders may depend on support systems outside of biologic family and may become isolated if they have no children
   * Noninfectious sexual problems
   * Gastrointestinal problems
   * STDs, including HIV and hepatitis
     * Strongly advise both hepatitis A and B vaccination
     * Screen for STDs, including hepatitis A, B, and C
   * Cancer: Colon, anal, hepatocellular, and lung
     * Nontraditional families emphasize need for advanced directives
   * Eating disorders and/or anabolic steroids
     * The Adonis complex
   * Recreational drugs
     * 3,4-Methylenedioxymethamphetamine (MDMA; also known as Ecstasy, XTC, X, or Adam)
     * Amyl nitrate ("poppers")
     * Cocaine and marijuana

2. Transgender

   * Female to male

- Hormone evaluation
- Lipid and liver function monitoring
- CAD risk issues
- Breast, mammograms, and Pap smears, if sex not yet surgically reassigned
- Male to female
  - Hormone evaluation
  - Risk of thrombosis in smokers
  - Blood pressure elevations
  - Kidney stones
  - Mammograms and breast examinations

To improve health in these patient populations, the health care provider should

- Maintain a nonjudgmental attitude
- Avoid assumptions
- Ask about sexual function
- Use gender-neutral terms (such as partner rather than wife)
- Differentiate risk groups from high-risk behaviors[43]

Good communication and sensitive primary care go a long way toward improving existing health disparities within these groups of persons. However, one must also be prepared to provide specific useful information, resources, or referrals:

- Gay and Lesbian Medical Association www.glma.org
- National Gay Lesbian Task Force www.ngltf.org
- Parents, Families and Friends of Lesbians and Gays www.pflag.org

CONCLUSION

Men's reticence and reluctance to seek medical care requires focus through public health initiatives and the efforts of individual health care providers. Attention to gender-specific concerns such as BPH, sexuality, and use of screening and self-examination techniques to detect cancers are all issues that should be addressed with men as important to both their health and well-being. The health care provider's interest in and openness to discussing these topics lends them more importance. This, along with careful attention to routine primary care, can serve to enhance provider-patient relationships and overall medical compliance.

Adolescent males need an approach to their routine physicals that focuses on issues relevant to all teenagers—sexuality, safe sex concepts, contraceptive use, and alcohol, tobacco or illicit drug use. However, special attention should also focus on the issues of safe driving, violence, guns, and substance abuse. Medical issues and diseases in men, such as cardiovascular conditions, cancer, sexual dysfunction (including ED and premature ejaculation), gender preference, and infertility, all need to be approached with a perspective sensitive to men's health concerns.

In general, the health care provider must remain open, nonjudgmental, and empathetic. Always keep options open by providing opportunities for the male patient to bring up uncomfortable subjects and offer referral when a patient seems to be unable to discuss certain personal issues with you.

REFERENCES

1. Althof S. The patient with erectile dysfunction: Psychological issues. PA Journal 2000;(Suppl):17–19.
2. Cookson MS, Smith JA. PSA testing: Update on a diagnostic tool. Consultant 2000;40:670–676.
3. Moskowitz MA. The challenges of diagnosing erectile dysfunction in the primary care setting. PA Journal 2000;24(Suppl):1–4.
4. Lowe FC, Fagelman E. Using complementary medications to treat BPH. Patient Care 2000;34:191–203.
5. Oesterling JE, Jacobson SJ, Chute CG, et al. Serum prostate-specific antigen in a community-based population of healthy men. Establishment of age-specific reference ranges. JAMA 1993;270:860–864.
6. Benson MCS, Whang IS, Olsson CA, et al. Specific antigen density to enhance predictive value of intermediate levels of serum PSA. J Urol 1992;147:817–821.
7. Seamen E, Whang M, Olsson CA, et al. Prostatic specific antigen density (PSAD): Role in patient evaluation and management. Urol Clin North Am 1993;20:653–663.
8. Rommel FM, Augusta VE, Breslin JA, et al. Use of PSA and PSAD in diagnosis of community-based urology practice. J Urol 1994;151:88–93.
9. Smith RA, Mettlin CJ, Jarvis KJ, Eyr H. Guidelines for early detection of cancer. CA Cancer J Clin 2000;50:34–49.
10. Reznicek SB. Common urologic problems in the elderly. Postgraduate Medicine 2000;107:163–178.
11. Von Eschenbach A, Ho R, Murphy GP, et al. American Cancer Society guidelines for early detection of prostate cancer. Update, June 10, 1997. Cancer 1997;80:1805–1807.
12. Roberts RO, Lieber MM, Bostwick DG, Jacobsen SJ. A review of clinical and pathological prostatitis syndromes. Urology 1997;49:809–821.
13. Barry MJ, Fowler FR Jr, O'Leary MP, et al. The American Urological Association Symptom Index for Benign Prostatic Hypertrophy. J Urol 1992;148:1549–1557.
14. Ringel M. Patients with sexual dysfunction: Your guidance makes a difference. Patient Care 1999;33(7):99–123.
15. Vetrosky D. Erectile dysfunction: The role of concomitant diseases. PA Journal 2000;24(6)(Suppl):12–16.

16. Tabor CW. Tabor's Cyclopedic Medical Dictionary. Philadelphia, FA Davis Co, 1997.

17. Kochar MS, Mazur LI, Patel A. What is causing your patient's sexual dysfunction? Postgrad Med 1999;106:149–157.

18. Miller TA. Diagnostic evaluation of erectile dysfunction. Am Family Physician 2000;61:95–104.

19. Jordan GH. Erectile function and dysfunction. Postgrad Med 1999;105:131–147.

20. Vroege JA. The Sexual Health Inventory for Men. Int J Impot Res 1999;11:177.

21. Landen M, Eriksson E, Agren H, et al. Effect of buspirone on sexual dysfunction in depressed patients treated with SSRIs. J Clin Psychopharmacol 1999;19:268–271.

22. Hargreave T. Sildenafil in SSRI induced sexual dysfunction. Poster presentation. Congress International Neuropsychiatry, Glasgow, Scotland, 1997.

23. Padma-Nathan H, Forrest C. Diagnosis and treatment of erectile dysfunction: The process of care model. PA Journal 2000;24(Suppl):5–11.

24. Winters SJ. Current status of testosterone replacement therapy in men. Arch Fam Med 1999;8:257–263.

25. Viera AJ, Clenney TL, Schenenberger DW, Green GF. Newer pharmacologic alternatives for erectile dysfunction. Am Fam Physician 1999;60:1159–1166.

26. Guay AT, Levine SB, Montague DK. New treatments for erectile dysfunction. Patient Care 1998;32:30–52.

27. Balon R. Antidepressants in the treatment of premature ejaculation. J Sex Marital Ther 1996;22:85–96.

28. Kim SC, Seo KK. Efficacy and safety of fluoxetine, sertraline and clomipramine in patients with premature ejaculation: A double-blind, placebo controlled study. J Urol 1998;159:425–427.

29. Kruger A. The mid-life transition: Crisis or chimera. Psychol Rep 1994;75:1229–1305.

30. Lebowitz BD, Pearson JL, Schneider LS, et al. Diagnosis and treatment of depression in late life. Consensus statement update. JAMA 1997;278:1186–1190.

31. Sharma HS, Mouton CP, Behl JR. Selected Diseases in Elderly Persons: Depression. AAFP Home Study Self-assessment. Monograph 233. Kansas City, MO, American Academy of Family Physicians, 1998, pp 24–31.

32. CDC's Tobacco Information and Prevention Sourcepage. http://www.cdc.gov/nccd/osh/tobacco.htm

33. Wintemute GJ, Parham CA, Beaumont JJ, et al. Mortality among recent purchasers of handguns. N Engl J Med 1999;341:1583–1589.

34. National Center for Injury Prevention and Control. http://www.cdc.gov/ncipc/ncipchm.htm

35. Tierney LM Jr, McPhee SJ, Papadakis MA. Current Medical Diagnosis and Treatment, 39th ed. New York, Lange Medical Books/McGraw Hill, 2000.

36. American Cancer Society. Cancer Facts and Figures 2000. Atlanta, ACS, 2000.

37. The Merck Medical Manual. 17th ed. PDR Electronic Library. Ramsey, NJ, Medical Economics Co, 1999.

38. Hatcher RA, Trussell J, Stewart F, et al. Contraceptive Technology, 17th ed. New York, Irving Publishers, 1998.

39. Herdt GM (ed). Third Sex, Third Gender: Beyond Sexual Dimorphism in Culture and History. New York, Zone Books, 1994.
40. Millman M. Access to Health Care in America. Washington, DC, National Academy Press, 1993.
41. Schatz B, O'Hanlan K. Anti-Gay Discrimination in Medicine: Results of a National Survey of Lesbian, Gay and Bisexual Physicians. San Francisco, American Association of Physicians for Human Rights-Gay-Lesbian Medical Association, 1994.
42. Wolfe A. One Nation After All: What Americans Really Think About God, Country, Family, Racism, Welfare, Immigration, Homosexuality, Work, the Right, the Left and Each Other. New York, Viking Press, 1988.
43. Laumann O, Gagnon JI I, Michael RT, Michael S. The Social Organization of Sexuality: Sexual Practices in the United States Chicago, University of Chicago Press, 1994.

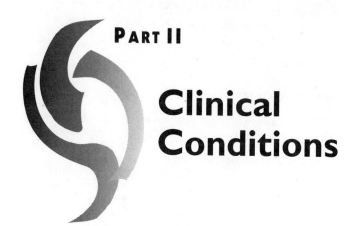

PART II

Clinical
Conditions

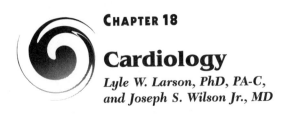

CHAPTER 18

Cardiology

*Lyle W. Larson, PhD, PA-C,
and Joseph S. Wilson Jr., MD*

▬ INTRODUCTION

The heart is a complex organ with a conical structure consisting of two atria and two ventricles separated by a fibrous annulus containing four valves. The fibrous annulus functions as the skeleton of the heart. The heart is a sequence of four pumps arranged in series, each separated by a one-way valve. The right atrium and ventricle are separated by the tricuspid valve. The pulmonic valve, a semilunar valve with three leaflets, separates the right ventricle from the pulmonary artery. The mitral valve separates the left atrium from the left ventricle and consists of two scalloped leaflets. The left ventricle is isolated from the systemic circulation by the aortic valve, a three-leaflet valve with each cusp named for the origin of the coronary arteries.

Coronary arteries supply oxygen and nutrients to the myocardium during diastole. The coronary arteries and capillaries are unable to receive blood flow during systole because the capillary pressure cannot equal the systolic pressure. The heart is the only organ capable of receiving blood during diastole. The left main coronary artery originates from the left cusp of the aortic valve and immediately separates into the left anterior descending artery (LAD) and circumflex artery. The LAD and its diagonal branches supply blood to the anterior surface of the left ventricle as well as to the intraventricular septum. The circumflex artery and its obtuse marginal branches supply the lateral and sometimes the posterior aspects of the heart. The right coronary artery originates from the right cusp of the aortic valve and courses down the interventricular groove to supply the right ventricle and the inferior surface of the heart. If the posterior descending artery (PDA) originates from the right coronary artery, the coronary artery blood supply is said to be "right dominant."[1] The PDA is supplied by the LAD or by the circumflex artery in "left dominant" systems. Venous return from the myocardium drains into the right atrium via the coronary sinus.

The conduction system of the heart consists of the sinus node, the atrioventricular (AV) node, the bundle of His, the Purkinje system, the right and left bundles, and the myocardium. In a normal heart, an automatic electrical stimulus proceeds from the sinus node down the atrium to the AV node, through the bundle of His, through the Purkinje system, and into the right and left bundle branches to initiate myocardial contraction. Cardiac muscle possesses three properties, contractility, conductivity, and automaticity. These functions ensure the normal progression of blood through the various chambers and valves of the heart.

Both sympathetic and parasympathetic, afferent and efferent nerves innervate the heart. Sympathetic neurons originate from the upper T5–T6 thoracic levels of the spinal cord, while parasympathetic neurons originate from the dorsal efferent nucleolus of the medulla.[2]

The principal purpose of the heart is to assure adequate blood supply for oxygenation and metabolic needs. Stroke volume is the amount of blood expelled from the heart with each cardiac contraction. Cardiac output increases proportionally to heart rate as long as stroke volume remains constant. Cardiac output (CO) is a product of heart rate (HR) and stroke volume (SV): CO = HR × SV. With acceleration of heart rate, the duration of systole slightly decreases. At the same time, the diastolic filling period is significantly diminished. This decreases ventricular filling time, limiting the maximum effective heart rate to 180 to 200 beats per minute in the normal heart. As demand increases, the heart increases its work by increasing its rate and force of contraction.

The normal, healthy heart without vagal or sympathetic tone (denervated or transplanted) has a rate of 100 beats per minute. The heart rate at rest is relatively slow. As activity increases, heart rate increases as a byproduct of reduced vagal impulse rate, augmentation of sympathetic discharge, and increased circulation of catecholamines. Catecholamines, vasodilatation, and sympathetic activation also augment myocardial contraction.

Neural regulation plays a pivotal role in cardiac physiology. Increased force of contraction (inotropy) is augmented by humoral and neural mechanisms. The sympathetic nervous system provides both a positive chronotropic (increase in rate) and positive inotropic (increase in contraction) response to stimulation. The parasympathetic innervation, on the other hand, produces a negative chronotropic and a slightly negative inotropic response to stimulation. Vagal stimulation slows heart rate and slows conduction through the AV node.

For additional resources, see the Resources Appendix at the end of this book.

CARDIAC ARRHYTHMIAS

Pathophysiology

Alterations of cardiac rhythm are a common clinical problem. Although arrhythmias have been classified in many different (and often confusing) ways, they can be divided into two major categories, abnormal impulse formation and abnormal conduction. Complex arrhythmias may incorporate both mechanisms.[1, 2]

Disturbances of impulse formation modify or alter the normal conduction sequence and may be either active or passive. Sinus rhythm disturbances include sinus bradycardia and tachycardia, sinus arrhythmia, and sinus arrest. Passive impulse formation manifests as escape beats within the atrium, AV node, or ventricle, and includes ectopic or premature atrial, nodal, or ventricular beats. Active impulse formation includes such arrhythmias as atrial tachycardia (paroxysmal or nonparoxysmal), atrial flutter or fibrillation, AV nodal tachycardia, and ventricular tachycardia and fibrillation.

Conduction disturbances may occur anywhere within the conduction system and include the entire spectrum of heart block from first degree AV block to complete heart block.

Mixed disturbances incorporate both mechanisms. This complex group of conduction disturbances includes complete or incomplete AV dissociation, reciprocating tachycardia from Wolff-Parkinson-White syndrome, electrical alternans, and parasystole.

Pediatric Issues

Infrequent premature atrial contractions (PACs) and premature ventricular contractions (PVCs) are normal and usually benign. Sinus node dysfunction, tachycardias, and bradycardias are usually due to underlying heart disease but are uncommon in the absence of underlying pathology. Re-entrant tachycardias (e.g., Wolff-Parkinson-White syndrome) represent approximately 80% of pediatric arrhythmias.[3]

Obstetric Issues

If a patient with significant arrhythmia becomes pregnant, a cardiologist should be consulted to assess the benefits and risks of administering pharmacologic therapy, owing to the potential for teratogenesis. Some drugs, such as beta blockers, are relatively safe in pregnancy. Palpitations increase during pregnancy as the blood volume increases; however, most ectopic beats are not hemodynamically significant. Women with pre-existing arrhythmias may experience either improvement or worsening of their symptoms during pregnancy. The major consideration with arrhythmia during pregnancy is perfusion of the fetus. In general, if the mother's brain is well perfused, the fetus is sufficiently perfused.

Geriatric Issues

In this population, there tend to be more arrhythmias related to underlying cardiac pathology. It is very important to conduct complete evaluations to determine the cause of new-onset arrhythmias. Sick sinus syndrome and bradycardia in this population are underdiagnosed and undertreated, leading to premature loss of memory and mental deteriorations.[2, 4, 5]

Epidemiology

The incidence of arrhythmias is very difficult to deduce, as it varies among locations and types of institution, patient population, and clinician interest in making the diagnosis. Arrhythmias may be benign and self-limiting, or they may represent the first evidence of underlying heart disease. The most common arrhythmias are extrasystoles (premature beats), occurring in the atria and in the ventricle, almost all of which are benign. Atrial fibrillation is the most commonly encountered sustained arrhythmia, affecting roughly 4% of the population. Approximately 90–95% of patients with acute myocardial infarction have some arrhythmia associated with their infarction. Digoxin toxicity, which is much less common now than in the past, is a well-recognized cause of arrhythmias, as are congenital conditions such as congenital heart block and Wolff-Parkinson-White syndrome.[2, 6]

Treatment Options

Most benign arrhythmias need no treatment. If necessary, treatment is directed first to control rate, followed by management of the underlying etiology. Simply stated, if the rate is too slow, causing failure to maintain adequate perfusion (depending on symptoms), it must be increased. This may be achieved either pharmaceutically or mechanically (pacing). If the rate is too fast (depending on symptoms), it must be decreased, either pharmaceutically or mechanically (cardioversion, defibrillation, or ablation). Once the rate is controlled, attention can then be directed toward management of the underlying etiology. This is not always possible (e.g., complete, permanent third-degree heart block). In determining etiology, the first step is to determine whether the arrhythmias are occurring in an otherwise normal heart, or in one with structural or functional defects. In general, those occurring in a heart without disease are benign.[7]

Bradycardia caused by enhanced vagal tone is best treated with atropine to facilitate AV nodal conduction. Vasovagal episodes, which may be frequent, abrupt, and unpredictable, are managed by blockade of left ventricular baroreceptor stimulation. This may be accomplished with drugs, including beta blockers and calcium channel blockers, to prevent reflex peripheral vasodilatation. Drugs that enhance vagal tone or act directly upon the sinoatrial or AV node should be discontinued if in use. Temporary or permanent pacing is required in any instance where bradycardia causes symptoms of cerebral hypoperfusion or hemodynamic compromise. High-grade or complete AV block usually requires permanent pacemaker insertion.

The approach to treatment of tachycardia depends on the rhythm strip and 12-lead electrocardiogram (ECG) to differentiate between narrow (<0.12 sec) and wide (≥0.12 sec) complexes. If a narrow complex is encountered, the ventricle may be excluded as the source of the arrhythmia. On the other hand, wide complexes may arise from the ventricle or from the atrium, with aberrant conduction to the ventricle. In cases of wide complex tachycardia, ventricular tachycardia is three times more prevalent than supraventricular tachycardia. Modification of the AV node is successful in treating AV nodal reciprocating tachycardia (PAT) from dual AV nodes. Modification of the AV node or ablation of the node and pacemaker insertion are rarely needed but can be successful in treating atrial fibrillation refractory to rate control. Focal tachycardias, such as ectopic atrial tachycardia and monomorphic ventricular tachycardia, may also be eliminated successfully by catheter ablation. Congenital tachycardias, such as reciprocating tachycardia from Wolff-Parkinson-White syndrome, can be cured with ablation of the accessory pathway.

Atrial fibrillation is the most commonly encountered atrial tachycardia. The two options for treating this disorder include correcting by restoring sinus rhythm (if possible), or by controlling rate and reducing the risk of cerebral vascular accident with anticoagulation. Advantages of maintaining sinus rhythm include more physiologic rate control, better atrial contribution to cardiac output (atrial "kick"), better exercise tolerance, and avoidance of rate-related atrial dilation. Advantages of rate control and anticoagulation include avoiding proarrhythmic complications from antiarrhythmic drugs and reducing compliance issues and cost of management.[2, 5, 6]

Polymorphic ventricular tachycardia and ventricular fibrillation, both potentially fatal arrhythmias, have been shown to respond favorably to treatment with an implantable defibrillation system. Future generations of defibrillators will possess the ability to control rhythms in both chambers. Advances in intracardiac mapping and ablation catheter construction will most certainly expand the range of arrhythmias treatable by ablation.

Patient Education

Most simple symptomatic arrhythmias are benign, and reassuring the patient of this fact is important. An explanation of the etiology, degree of severity, and treatment options (if required) of diagnosed arrhythmias is crucial to alleviating anxiety and enhancing compliance in patients. Although premature atrial and ventricular contractions are usually benign, palpitations may be a significant source of anxiety to certain patients. Accurate assessment of pulse, to determine rate, regularity, and strength of pulse, should be taught to any patient with suspected arrhythmias. Patients with implanted devices (pacemaker, defibrillator) require counseling and education regarding the purpose of the device, management, follow-up, changes in lifestyle, and recognition of potential complications before they become life-threatening.

A "gas and brake" analogy can be used for arrhythmias. Acceleration is caused by sympathetic input, and vagus input is the brake. An imbalance in this gas/brake cycle leads to arrhythmia.

With atrial fibrillation, an association with systemic embolism is well established, and anticoagulation with Coumadin (warfarin) is usually recommended.[1, 5]

Prevention

Although many arrhythmias are transient and unavoidable, several measures can be implemented to reduce the incidence and severity. Drugs with known proarrhythmic potential, including those with sino-atrial or AV nodal blocking properties, should be avoided if possible. Myocardial ischemia and volume overload require early intervention and control. Valvular dysfunction should be treated. Prevention is directed at the underlying cardiac pathology and avoidance of drugs that can enhance cardiac excitability, such as caffeine, alcohol, cocaine, and sympathomimetics (e.g., pseudoephedrine).

The AFFIRM (Atrial Fibrillation Follow-up Investigation of Rhythm Management) trial currently underway addresses the long-term treatment of either paroxysmal or persistent atrial fibrillation in patients at risk for systemic embolism or stroke. Its primary endpoint is to control total mortality in rate control versus rhythm control, with secondary endpoints including total mortality, disabling stroke, and anoxic encephalopathy.[6]

Screening Recommendations

Arrhythmias are very common and range from benign to fatal. Successful treatment depends on an accurate diagnosis. Arrhythmias may be primary, caused by an inherent conduction anomaly, or secondary, such as ischemia-induced tachycardia following myocardial infarction. Once a diagnosis is made, a search for the underlying etiology is imperative.

▄▄CORONARY ARTERY DISEASE

Pathophysiology

Coronary arteries (that fill during diastole) provide the primary blood supply to the myocardium. Coronary artery disease (CAD) results when this blood supply cannot meet the oxygen demands of the myocardium, as a result of atherosclerotic changes due to plaque and/or thrombus within the lumen, or as a result of nonatherosclerotic changes from conditions such as collagen vascular disease, aortic or coronary dissection, or congenital anomalies. The major determining factor of total blood flow through the normal coronary artery is coronary vascular resistance. Arterial dilatation is a normal response to exercise and adrenergic stimuli. In patients with hypercholesterolemia, atherosclerotic plaque, diabetes, and smoking, vasodilatation may not occur, and in some instances, the vessel may actually undergo constriction. Vasoconstriction is controlled by the endothelium.[1, 2, 5, 8]

Coronary atherosclerosis is the most commonly encountered cause of CAD. As low-density lipoprotein (LDL) enters the endothelial cell wall, it is taken up by macrophages to form foam cells. Rupture of these foam cells, along with debris from cellular death, forms the atheromatous lesion. Abrupt changes, such as fissure, disruption, or thrombus formation, increase the size of the lesion or completely obstruct the vessel. Blood flow through a vessel with a fixed stenosis is usually adequate until a 70–90% cross-sectional area of the lumen is affected. Once this degree of blockage is exceeded, distal flow may drop precipitously during exercise or at rest. Impaired vasodilatation or paroxysmal vasoconstriction may occur at the site of the lesion but is not always limited to the site of the stenosis. Angina, which results from the blockage, is said to be stable as long as the plaque remains stable and causes only mild to moderate obstruction. The most common cause of unstable angina is a nonocclusive thrombus on a fissured or eroded plaque. Disruption of the plaque releases aggregating platelets that, in turn, contribute to further thrombus formation.

Pediatric Issues

Preparticipation electrocardiograms are not recommended as part of the routine physical examination of asymptomatic children and adolescents. CAD is extremely rare in this population. Even those at risk for CAD do not have symptom onset until adulthood. Adopted children and children with a family history of familial dyslipidemias should be screened for these conditions.[9] For a child with signs and symptoms similar to angina in the adult, arteriovenous malformations, shunts, and steals, which manifest at age 6 months, on average, should be considered.[3]

Obstetric Issues

The premenopausal age group is usually protected from coronary disease by the presence of hormones; however, family histories of dyslipidemais should be obtained. Pregnant women are more susceptible to spontaneous intimal dissection, which manifests as acute myocardial infarction, during or after delivery. The dissection is not associated with CAD.

Geriatric Issues

Incidence of CAD increases with advancing age. Often, multiple factors are involved in the accumulation of plaques and development of coronary disease. Risk factors should continue to be addressed regardless of the patient's age.

Epidemiology

CAD remains the leading cause of death in men and women, affecting 58.8 million Americans, resulting in approximately 600,000 coronary bypass graft surgeries annually. An estimated 900,000 Americans suffer from myocardial infarction, with one-fourth of all cases terminating in a fatality. The cost of health care related to myocardial infarction approaches $147 billion annually in the United States.[6, 10]

Major determining risk factors for CAD include hypercholesterolemia, diabetes mellitus, age, gender, hypertension, smoking, and dietary factors. Other factors include socioeconomic status, obesity, physical inactivity, and regional differences (incidence is higher in the southeastern U.S. than elsewhere in the nation).

Treatment Options

The primary goal in treatment of CAD is to ameliorate symptoms and improve quality and length of life. Medical treatment includes control of hypercholesterolemia, hypertension, and diabetes, cessation of smoking, and improvement in diet and exercise. Myocardial reperfusion with thrombolytic therapy is effective for acute occlusion due to thrombus formation. Reperfusion must be given within the first 6–12 h of obstruction and is associated with hemorrhagic risks. Catheter-based intervention, such as percutaneous transluminal coronary angioplasty (PTCA) with stenting, has several advantages over thrombolytic therapy in the treatment of acute occlusion. It provides reperfusion without the risk of hemorrhage, exhibits higher patency rates, and results in more complete opening of the culprit lesion.[8, 11]

Coronary artery bypass grafting (CABG) is a surgical intervention utilizing either an arterial (internal thoracic artery, radial artery, gastroepiploic artery, internal mammary artery) or venous (greater or lesser saphenous vein) conduit. The culprit lesion(s) are bypassed, allowing unobstructed blood flow distal to the lesion. Proximal anastomoses on the ascending aorta allow blood to flow unobstructed through to the distal anastomosis. CABG is preferable in cases of left main coronary artery disease, left main equivalent disease (proximal left anterior descending artery and circumflex artery), multiple diffuse lesions, or significantly impaired left ventricular dysfunction defined as an ejection fraction of less than 40%.[12, 13]

Diabetic patients may also benefit more from CABG, owing to the diffuse nature of their disease and the propensity of patients with diabetes to have smaller blood vessels.

Antianginal therapy, including beta adrenergic blockade, nitrates, and angiotensin-converting enzyme inhibitors, has also been shown to reduce CAD-related mortality and incidence of myocardial infarction. Advances in CABG procedures, including minimally invasive techniques, beating heart surgery, all-arterial revascularization, antegrade and retrograde cardioplegia, and heparin-bonded cardiopulmonary bypass pump circuitry, provide the surgeon with options for patients with end-stage disease that was not amenable to surgery as recently as 1990.

Patient Education

Primary prevention remains the cornerstone of therapy in all patients. Primary screening includes blood pressure measurements, avoidance of tobacco use, cholesterol testing, increased exercise, and healthy diet. See Chapter 7, Exercise, Chapter 13, Nutrition Education in the Clinical Setting, and Chapter 26, Substance Abuse.

Secondary prevention also includes primary prevention strategies as well as continued follow-up and compliance with treatment modalities. Follow-up and compliance are paramount in preventing progression of disease.

Enrollment in a cardiac rehabilitation program following myocardial infarction or surgical intervention may augment compliance. The goals of rehabilitation are to improve quality of life, reduce ischemic events, and reduce the incidence of subsequent cardiac sequelae, including myocardial infarction and life-threatening arrhythmias. Family members are also educated about cardiac risk factors. Exercise training should begin with structured physical conditioning, followed by an exercise test after 3 to 6 weeks, and then by gradually increasing exercise.

Prevention

Prevention of CAD is centered on avoiding or controlling hypertension, diabetes, and hypercholesterolemia, on avoiding smoking, and on exercise. Recent advances in medical treatment, including hydroxy-methylglutaryl coenzyme A (HMG-CoA) reductase inhibitors, anti-thrombin agents, and antiplatelet agents, play substantial roles in slowing the progression of CAD. Once the presence of CAD has been confirmed, primary prevention implementation may slow or reverse some forms of disease.

Screening Recommendations

Evidence is insufficient to recommend either for or against screening middle-aged and older individuals of either gender for asymptomatic CAD with an electrocardiogram (resting, ambulatory, or exercise). Screening asymptomatic high-risk individuals is indicated when the results will influence treatment decisions. Screening of asymptomatic individuals is recommended for certain populations that affect public safety (e.g., airline pilots and truck drivers). The method of screening is left to clinical decision.[6, 9]

C-reactive protein (high sensitive) is currently being researched as a predictor of myocardial infarction and may be recommended as a screening tool in the future. Certain medications have been shown to reduce C-reactive protein. Noninvasive testing, the use of high-speed electron beam computed tomography, has shown the ability to identify calcifications associated with atherosclerotic vessels and will be used more frequently as a routine screening tool in the future.

▬▬ PERIPHERAL VASCULAR DISEASE

Pathophysiology

The hallmark of clinically symptomatic peripheral vascular disease is atherosclerosis, characterized by extensive plaque in localized areas, including the carotid artery bifurcation and lower extremity arteries. Arterial bifurcations are common sites for plaque formation due to hemodynamic factors such as hypertension, changes in wall shear stress, low-flow velocity, and turbulence. Atherosclerosis may also occur at bifurcations as a result of increased contact time between atherogenic factors and inflammatory agents and the vessel wall. Common clinical scenarios include transient ischemic attacks, cerebral vascular accidents, claudication, rest pain, and gangrene.[14, 15]

Pediatric Issues

As with coronary disease, this disease is not seen in the pediatric population unless there exists a disorder of lipid metabolism. Adopted children and children at risk owing to family history of peripheral vascular disease should be screened.[3]

Obstetric Issues

The premenopausal age group is usually protected by the presence of estrogen. Family history of dyslipidemias should be obtained.

Geriatric Issues

Incidence increases with advancing age. Risk factors are the same as those for coronary disease.

Epidemiology

Clinical manifestations include intermittent claudication, rest pain, skin ulceration, gangrene, and impotence. Claudication is a clinical syndrome of pain and fatigue in large muscle groups of the leg exacerbated by exercise and relieved with rest. The natural history of claudication is generally progressive but with only a 5% risk of major amputation for gangrene within 5 years of diagnosis, according to the Framingham study. Rest pain indicates a more severe form of ischemia. Left untreated, 50% of patients with rest pain will require amputation for intractable pain or complications such as gangrene.[14, 15]

Cutaneous ulcers are common and may be the first sign of peripheral vascular disease. Ischemic arterial ulcers are found on the lower third of the leg and on the foot. Pain is severe, persistent, and increases at night. Venous ulcers are located around the ankle, particularly the bony prominences such as the medial and lateral malleoli. They tend to be less painful than arterial ulcers. Diabetic ulcers are usually located on the plantar or lateral surface of the foot. They may resemble arterial ulcers in appearance but are characteristically painless, a direct result of diabetic neuropathy.

Gangrene involves tissue death. "Dry" gangrene occurs as mummification of tissue, while "wet" gangrene indicates active infection with cellulitis.

Acute arterial occlusion, a surgical emergency, is caused by in situ thrombosis, emboli, vascular trauma, or thrombosis of an aneurysm. Patients typically present with acute onset of pallor, pain, paresthesias, pulselessness, and change in limb temperature (poikilothermia).

Differentiation between arterial and venous disease is essential, as outcomes vary significantly.

Treatment Options

Treatment begins with control of risk factors such as smoking, sedentary lifestyle, diabetes mellitus, hypertension, and hypercholesterolemia. Medical treatments including agents to dilate vessels and lower blood viscosity are often ineffective. Transluminal balloon angioplasty may be used in incidences of severe, focal stenosis of the iliac or proximal superficial femoral arteries. Results vary, depending on the site of dilation. A success rate of approximately 90% can be achieved in the iliac artery, with a 75% success rate in the superficial femoral artery. Surgical intervention is palliative but not curative.[16]

Endarterectomy is a standard treatment for severe, symptomatic carotid artery disease. Carotid artery plaques tend to be localized, whereas lower extremity disease is usually extensive without discrete margins.

Bypass procedures remain the standard of care for lower extremity occlusive disease. Inflow procedures (aortobifemoral bypass graft) are used for aorto-iliac obstruction. Prosthetic grafts yield a 90% patency rate 5 years after the surgery. Outflow procedures (femoral bypass) are used for superficial femoral and popliteal arterial obstruction. Conduit choices include the patient's own greater saphenous vein or a synthetic graft. A 70% patency rate can be expected at 5 years after the surgery with femoral-popliteal grafting, while femoral-tibial grafting has a lower patency rate, approximately 50%.

Gangrene requires amputation of the affected part and may be used in conjunction with any of the above procedures.

Patient Education

Peripheral vascular disease has a gradual onset and takes years to develop. It is imperative to stress the importance of caring for the skin, recognizing symptoms, and seeking early intervention if symptoms arise. The importance of controlling hypertension to reduce plaque accumulation, along with compliance with prescribed treatment modalities, cannot be overemphasized.

Prevention

Primary prevention includes avoiding smoking, controlling hypertension, screening for hypercholesterolemia, controlling diabetes mellitus, and exercising. However, prevention of peripheral vascular disease may not be entirely possible. Nevertheless, many steps may be taken to slow its progression. These include avoidance of risk factors and meticulous care of the legs and feet. HMG-CoA reductase inhibitors and anticoagulation are also beneficial.

Screening Recommendations

Screening is primarily aimed at identifying contributing factors. Screening for the presence of hypercholesterolemia is recommended for all men ages 35–65 and women ages 45–65. Early detection and control of hypertension and diabetes mellitus and participation in a less sedentary lifestyle are key in preventing or reducing the severity of peripheral vascular disease.[9]

Screening for peripheral vascular disease should be part of the total evaluation in patients at risk because of associated conditions.

■ BLEEDING DISORDERS

Pathophysiology

The normal hemostatic system is designed to stop leakage from a vessel only at the site of epithelial injury, without progression along the endothelial cell lining. Clots form only where and when needed, and the clot dissolves when normal epithelial cells are re-established. This system relies on vasoconstriction, platelet adhesion and aggregation, fibrin formation, vitamin K-dependent factors, the coagulation cascade, and fibrinolysis. Alterations in any of these processes may significantly affect the hemostatic system's ability to prevent either thrombosis (minor or major) or exsanguination. Thrombotic disorders include deep venous thrombosis, pulmonary artery embolism, and arterial embolism. Failure to form a clot produces bleeding disorders, including inherited and acquired hemorrhagic disorders.

Pediatric Issues

Acute idiopathic thrombocytic purpura (ITP) is the most common bleeding disorder, frequently occurring in children between ages 2 and 5, often following a viral infection. Thrombocytopenia is defined as a platelet count less than 150,000 per milliliter and should be investigated in any newborn with purpura.

Von Willebrand's disease is the most common inherited bleeding disorder (X-linked). Hemophilia A is a rare disorder of bleeding due to deficient or defective factor VIII. Factor IX deficiency, also known as hemophilia B or Christmas disease, is clinically indistinguishable from hemophilia A. It is important to elicit family history in children with bleeding disorders.

Sickle cell disease is an inherited disease that can cause acute thrombosis. Family history should be obtained for children (especially in those with Central African or Mediterranean ancestry) who experience acute thrombosis. Sickle cell disease affects one of every 400 African American infants. Eight percent of African Americans have sickle cell trait.

Deficiencies of protein C, protein S, and antithrombin III, which normally facilitate bleeding, will manifest in adolescence as venous thromboembolism. These hypercoagulable disorders are rare and of autosomal-dominant inheritance.[3]

Obstetric Issues

An increased risk of deep venous thrombosis and pulmonary embolus accompanies pregnancy or oral contraceptive use, in combination with smoking. Patients who smoke and are older than 35 years should not use oral contraceptives owing to the risk of deep venous thrombosis.

A history of bleeding disorders should be obtained from a patient before she becomes pregnant or as early in the pregnancy as possible.

Geriatric Issues

Many patients in this population are on warfarin for treatment of atrial fibrillation or following stroke. Falls and other trauma can cause serious complications owing to the hypocoagulable state. Careful monitoring of prothrombin time and international normalized ratio is important.

Epidemiology

Disorders of coagulation and bleeding are common. Hypercoagulability occurs when an underlying genetic predisposition is exacerbated by a specific stress, such as myocardial infarction, immobilization, direct injury, or pregnancy. Other causes of the hypercoagulable state include resistance to activated protein C, antithrombin III deficiency, protein C and protein S deficiencies, drugs (oral contraceptives), homocystinuria, and abnormalities in fibrinolysis.

Disorders of bleeding include thrombocytopenia (decreased platelet production, increased platelet removal, or platelet sequestration in the spleen) and platelet production defects (aplastic or hypoplastic anemia or drug toxicity, including heparin toxicity).

Acquired hemorrhagic disorders include vitamin K deficiency; drug induced disorders (caused by heparin or warfarin use, and can occur with any dose); dysproteinemias (myeloma, macroglobulinemia); and disseminated intravascular coagulation due to massive tissue damage, extensive alteration of vascular endothelium, shock, or impaired liver function. Hemorrhagic disorders may also occur in the context of circulation inhibitors and lupus.

Venous thrombosis affects 2.5 million people annually. Pulmonary embolism affects an estimated 700,000 patients annually, and 200,000 die as a result. The diagnosis is not made clinically in 40–60% of deaths. Pulmonary infarction occurs in 10% of patients with clinical evidence of pulmonary embolism. The incidence of the various bleeding disorders is unknown.

Treatment Options

Treatment is dependent on an accurate diagnosis of the disorder. Treatment for diseases of hypercoagulability includes heparin, warfarin, antiplatelet agents, or combinations of these drugs. Unfractionated heparin is inexpensive and may be given intravenously (bolus and infusion) or subcutaneously. It is easily titrated and does not cause paradoxical thrombosis because of unopposed depletion of protein C or protein S. Low molecular weight heparin has the advantage of improved bioavailability and prolonged half-life, reacts less with platelets (it has a decreased incidence of throbocytopenia compared with unfractionated heparin), and avoids costly monitoring. Warfarin, a vitamin K antagonist, is taken orally, is inexpensive, and must be closely monitored to prevent bleeding. Platelet inhibitors such as aspirin and ticlopidine exert their effects by making platelets "less sticky." For acute myocardial infarction or unstable angina, glycoprotein IIb/IIIa receptors may be employed.

Treatment of the hemorrhagic disorders is directed toward the cause. Elevated partial thromboplastin time from heparin may be reversed with protamine, and elevated prothrombin time/international normalized ratio from warfarin is reversed with vitamin K or fresh frozen plasma. Hemorrhagic disorders due to insufficient or inactive platelets are treated with platelet transfusion. Aprotinin is a useful adjunct during cardiopulmonary bypass to improve hemostasis. Specific factors are replaced in those individuals with hemophilia or von Willebrand's disease. Acquired hemorrhagic disorders, including dysproteinemias and disseminated intravascular coagulation, require rapid recognition and reversal.

Patient Education

Patient education can be an important deterrent for potential complications. The purpose of anticoagulation and its benefits, risks, and potential complications should be explained to the patient and applicable family members. Frequent follow-up is crucial to preventing bleeding disorders from excess anticoagulation or embolic events from insufficient anticoagulation.

Prevention

Prevention of bleeding disorders is achieved by avoiding iatrogenic excessive anticoagulation, careful monitoring of all therapies instituted, and discontinuing anticoagulation when possible. Patients with thrombocytopenia, platelet production defects, and acquired platelet function disorders, including von Willebrand's disease and the hemophilias, should be referred to a hematologist. Familial genetic counseling may be indicated for appropriate patients.

Identification of the genetic predisposition and avoidance of specific stressors, along with appropriate anticoagulation, can prevent untoward embolic events.

Screening Recommendations

Preoperative evaluation may include a screening prothrombin time and partial thromboplastin time to evaluate for occult bleeding disorders.

Family histories should include a history of bleeding disorders to identify patients at risk for a hypercoagulable state or for bleeding.

▬▬ CONGESTIVE HEART FAILURE

Pathophysiology

Congestive heart failure (CHF), in its simplest terms, is defined as the inability of the heart to circulate the quantity of blood required under the prevailing conditions of the body. CHF is better described as congestive heart insufficiency. Two basic pathophysiologic mechanisms can lead to CHF. The first is a reduction in systolic function leading to decreased forward flow because of reduced myocardial contractility. Causes of this type include decreased myocardial blood flow or ischemia, dilated idiopathic cardiomyopathy, myocarditis, or valvular insufficiency.

The second major type of CHF is diastolic heart failure, which occurs when the muscle within the right or left ventricle becomes extremely stiff and, during the relaxation period, is unable to expand properly. The relaxation period is the time within the cardiac cycle during which energy is required, and changes in diastolic function lead to significant pressure increases within the left ventricle and to inability of the ventricle to expand and increase its ejection of blood with each contraction. This impaired or inadequate ventricular filling is seen frequently in left ventricular hypertrophy, both secondary to hypertension and idiopathic varieties, as well as in infiltrative cardio-myopathies such as amyloidosis. Impaired filling can also be seen in acute myocardial ischemic situations.

Frequently, patients exhibit a combined pattern of both systolic and diastolic dysfunction, leading to their clinical syndrome of CHF. Two clinical variables are affected by systolic and diastolic function. The first variable is forward flow, where cardiac output can be reduced either by decreased systolic or by decreased diastolic function. This condition manifests with signs of low cardiac output, such as cool extremities and marked reduction in exercise capacity. The second variable is pressure within the ventricles, which can be increased either by diastolic dysfunction and impaired relaxation or by systolic dysfunction with increasing pressures. Increased pressure leads to backward failure with fluid retention and congestion in the lungs if the left ventricle is involved.

Pediatric Issues

Most CHF begins during the first year of life in children who develop the disorder. Causes include outflow obstruction, coarctation of the aorta, AV shunts, and acquired myocarditis.[3]

Obstetric Issues

Volume overload caused by pregnancy can cause CHF in a heart with underlying pathology. Peripartum cardiomyopathy is a potentially life-threatening problem.

Geriatric Issues

New onset of shortness of breath in an elderly smoker should not be dismissed as reactive airway disease. CHF is very common in this population.

Epidemiology

CHF affects 1–2% of Americans, and it consumes approximately 3% of the national health care budget. It is one of the most common reasons for hospital admission of Medicare patients. In addition to being a common and potentially costly illness, it is associated with a significant morbidity and mortality. Approximately half of all patients with chronic heart failure expire from sudden death. The annual mortality for patients in the New York Heart Association (NYHA) class I category is 5%. The rate increases to 10% in NYHA class II patients and to 20% in NYHA class III patients, and it significantly increases to 50% in NYHA class IV patients (Table 18–1).

Treatment Options

The principal goals in treatment for CHF are to reduce symptoms, reduce progression of left ventricular dysfunction, and prolong survival. Traditional treatment, with vasodilators and diuretics, is directed at relieving the symptoms of congestion. Drugs such as angiotensin-converting enzyme (ACE) inhibitors and ACE receptor blockers are used to slow or stop the progressive left ventricular dysfunction. Recently, beta blockers have been shown to improve the left ventricular function over time in patients with systolic dysfunction.

Progressive heart failure may require hospitalization for intravenous inotropes to offset hypotension induced by aggressive diuresis and afterload reduction. Patients with progressive heart failure are also at a significantly higher risk for ischemia and malignant tachyarrhythmias.

Table 18–1. New York Heart Association Functional Classification

Class	Description
I	Patients with cardiac disease but without resulting limitations of physical activity. Ordinary activity does not cause undue fatigue, palpitation, dyspnea, or anginal pain.
II	Patients with cardiac disease resulting in slight limitation of physical activity. They are comfortable at rest, and ordinary physical activity results in fatigue, palpitation, dyspnea, or anginal pain.
III	Patients with cardiac disease resulting in marked limitation of physical activity. They are comfortable at rest. Less than ordinary physical activity results in fatigue, palpitation, dyspnea, or anginal pain.
IV	Patients with cardiac disease resulting in inability to carry on any physical activity without discomfort. Symptoms of cardiac insufficiency or anginal syndrome may be present at rest. If activity is undertaken, discomfort is increased.

From Goldman L, Hashimoto B, Cook FF, Loscalzo A. Comprehensive reproducibility and validity of systems for assessing cardiovascular functional class. Advantages of a new specific activity scale. Circulation 1981;64:1227. Copyright American Heart Association, 1981. With permission.

As such, continuous telemetry monitoring is required, as is therapy (amiodarone, implantable defibrillator) to prevent sudden death.

Diastolic heart failure is best treated with volume control and ACE inhibitors to control hypertension and provide some (but not aggressive) degree of afterload reduction. It is also advantageous in this patient group to slow the heart rate to prolong diastolic filling and to maintain normal sinus rhythm, to benefit from atrial contribution (atrial "kick") to ventricular filling, which is especially needed in the presence of a stiff left ventricle.

For patients with end-stage heart failure on maximum inotropic support, an intra-aortic balloon pump or ventricular assist device may be required to rest the ventricle or as a bridge to cardiac transplantation.

Future treatments, including long-term implantable ventricular assist devices, recombinant gene therapy, and advances in cardiac transplantation, provide hope for patients with an otherwise poor prognosis.

Patient Education

Patient education should include counseling to discuss the cause or probable cause and symptoms of CHF. Instructions should also include the patient's potential for function and survival, life expectancy, self-monitoring, dietary recommendations, medications and their purposes, and recommendations for activity. Compliance cannot be overemphasized. Aggressive treatment of the underlying cause combined with lifelong treatment and compliance with prescribed medications is beneficial in all but the most refractory cases.

Prevention

Prevention of CHF is centered on identification and amelioration of underlying causes. Systemic treatment for hypertension and angina should be initiated. Ischemic heart disease and valvular or congenital lesions may need surgical intervention. Correction or control of underlying causes is crucial to reducing the risk of sudden death.

Screening Recommendations

Patients should be screened for factors that contribute to or cause CHF (see the sections on Coronary Artery Disease and Hypertension).

▬ HYPERTENSION

Pathophysiology

Hypertension is defined as a systolic blood pressure equal to or greater than 140 mmHg or a diastolic measurement equal to or greater than 90 mmHg. Hypertension results in increased pressure of the blood against the arterial wall. The heart has to work much harder to pump blood against a high-pressure gradient. The most common manifestation of hypertension is essential, or primary, hypertension, the cause of which is unknown. Essential hypertension may be seen with increased sympathetic activity due to epinephrine or norepinephrine spillover, increased sodium intake, decreased potassium and calcium intake, increased or inappropriate renin secretion, reduction in vasodilators, insulin resistance, obesity, or increased vascular growth factor activity. Other factors that are related to hypertension include genetics, water and sodium retention dependent upon renal function, and inherited cardiovascular risk factors including hypercholesterolemia. Causes of secondary hypertension include renal and endocrine disorders.

Pediatric Issues

Systolic hypertension in children is a greater problem than may be suspected. Blood pressure should be routinely obtained during office visits by pediatric patients. The upper limit of normal is 110 mmHg for children ages 6–10, and children aged 11–14 should have an average systolic blood pressure of 120–130 mmHg. For the patient older than 15 years of age, adult guidelines apply.[9]

Obstetric Issues

Hypertensive patients who become pregnant should review medications with their health care provider to assure there is no risk of teratogenic effects. Medications should be changed if necessary, but hypertension should always be treated. Blood pressure screening should be done at each visit.

Preeclampsia is acute hypertension that occurs after week 20 of pregnancy, accompanied by edema and proteinuria. Patients may be treated with medications, if necessary. Preeclampsia can also occur postpartum. Preeclampsia with seizures is called eclampsia and necessitates delivery of the fetus.

Geriatric Issues

Control of systolic hypertension in this age group is very important. Decreasing systolic pressure can prolong and improve quality of life (SHEP study).[9a] Single-drug therapy is frequently not sufficient to maintain control.

Epidemiology

Approximately 15–18% of Americans have hypertension, accounting for more than 50 million cases. Hypertension is one of the most common reasons for physician visits. The Framingham study showed a strong relation between blood pressure, heart attack, and stroke. As such, hypertension is a risk factor that affects the likelihood of developing these diseases, but it is not a cause of these diseases. Because prolonged hypertension ultimately results in vascular deterioration and is insidious in nature, it is necessary to treat it before symptoms or signs of damage are present.

Treatment Options

In western societies, blood pressure increases with age. While the ultimate goal of treatment is to prevent vascular complications, the immediate goal is to reduce blood pressure to provide both short- and long-term cardiovascular protection. The Veterans Administration Cooperative Study provided definitive evidence to show that early treatment reduces cardiovascular events.

Nonpharmacologic treatment includes weight loss, sodium restriction, potassium supplementation, exercise, smoking cessation, and reduction of excess alcohol intake. Control of other risk factors, including diabetes and hypercholesterolemia, is imperative.

Pharmacologic choices include diuretics, ACE inhibitors, calcium channel blockers, and centrally and peripherally acting antiadrenergic agents. Calcium channel blockers and diuretics are more effective in African American populations and in patients who have received blood volume expanders. Beta blockers and ACE inhibitors are more effective in Caucasians and in patients with vasoconstriction.

Patient Education

Hypertension is often called the silent killer. Patients must be counseled that lifetime treatment is required. While most patients do not have symptoms directly related to hypertension, it should be emphasized that treatment is directed to avoid future complications. Ultimate vascular complications, including coronary artery disease, carotid artery disease, aortic aneurysm and dissection, and peripheral arterial occlusive disease, can be controlled or prevented with consistent blood pressure control and lifestyle modifications. Compliance should be stressed and may be enhanced by a team approach using therapists to focus on the nature and consequences of the disease, lifestyle changes, and social support.

Prevention

Because hypertension is insidious and can exist for years without symptomatic evidence of vascular consequences, prevention may be very difficult. Careful attention must be paid to routine clinic visits to detect its presence, and early intervention with continued follow-up to ensure compliance is essential. Contributing factors such as diabetes and hyperlipidemia must also be controlled.

Screening Recommendations

Blood pressure measurements are recommended in all age groups using sphygmomanometry. The diagnosis of hypertension should not be made until more than one elevated reading is obtained on each of three separate visits over a period of one to several weeks.[9]

VALVULAR HEART DISEASE

Pathophysiology

Stenosis and insufficiency (regurgitation) are the two mechanisms responsible for the primary damage from valvular heart disease. They can occur together or independently in any of the cardiac valves.

Valvular stenosis is manifest as a reduction of the area of the valve's orifice in its opened position, and it results in a pressure overload state with accompanying changes to the chambers of the heart. Valvular stenosis may occur as a result of fusion of the valve commissures, as a congenital abnormality (including an abnormality in the number of valve leaflets), or as a result of a thickening of the leaflets to the extent that they cannot fully open. Each of these mechanisms constricts motion of the valve leaflets and restricts flow during emptying. Aortic stenosis (AS) is the most common valvular heart disease. An estimated 1% of the population is thought to have a congenitally bicuspid aortic valve. In the early stages, the patient is asymptomatic. As stenosis progresses, an increase in left ventricular pressure is required to empty the left ventricle in systole, resulting in a pressure gradient between the left ventricle and the aorta. To compensate, the left ventricle hypertrophies. As a result of left ventricular hypertrophy and an increased pressure gradient, left ventricular work is increased. Because this takes place, the quantity of blood ejected through the stenotic valve during systole is reduced. This can ultimately produce the classic symptoms of angina, syncope, and CHF, but the patient remains asymptomatic until the hemodynamic consequences are severe.

Mitral stenosis most commonly occurs as a consequence of rheumatic heart disease, producing both thickening of the valve leaflets and fusion of the commissures. Stenosis of the mitral valve obstructs flow and produces a pressure gradient between the left atrium and the left ventricle. This obstruction to flow decreases left ventricular filling and increases left atrial pressure. As a result, reduced cardiac output and pulmonary congestion combine to produce the classic symptoms of CHF without discernible left ventricular dysfunction. As pulmonary pressures increase, right ventricular output decreases, and right-side heart failure may follow.

Insufficiency, or regurgitation, connotes flow reversal through the valve while closed and results in a volume overload state and subsequent changes in the heart. The flow reversal is due to failure of the valve leaflets to close completely and seal. This failure may be a result of prolapse (movement of the leaflet beyond the valvular annulus), damage to a leaflet, or alteration in normal leaflet motion. Aortic insufficiency may result from pathology of the leaflet (vegetation) or damage to the aortic root (dilatation, dissection), which separates the leaflets. With progression of disease, left ventricular dilation occurs in response to volume overload. Each relaxation phase of the heart must receive more blood to compensate. As an increased blood volume is ejected from the enlarged left ventricle, the pulse pressure is increased, as with exercise. This increase is responsible for wide pulse pressure (the difference between systolic and diastolic blood pressure). Acute aortic insufficiency, most often a result of infective endocarditis or aortic dissection, is a medical emergency.

Mitral regurgitation may result from an alteration of the annulus, the leaflets, the chordae, or the papillary muscles (primary mitral regurgitation), or from left ventricular dilatation or other changes of left ventricular geometry (secondary mitral regurgitation). Regurgitation results in a volume overload in the left ventricle. Although the left ventricular ejection fraction remains elevated, a portion is ejected back into the left atrium. The left atrium enlarges to accommodate the added volume and pressure, with atrial fibrillation and increased pulmonary congestion as potential consequences. Mitral valve prolapse is a subset of mitral regurgitation, defined as having one or both leaflets prolapsing above the plane of the valvular annulus during systole. The clinical significance is related only to the degree of mitral valve leakage.

Pediatric Issues

Most congenital heart disease is due to septal defects.

Pulmonary valvular disease, causing right ventricular outflow obstruction, accounts for 10% of all congenital heart disease. Pulmonary valvular disease and distal pulmonary stenosis are frequently accompanied by septal defects.

Aortic stenosis accounts for approximately 5% of congenital heart disease. Distal aortic stenosis (e.g., coarctation of the aorta), accounts for 6% of congenital heart disease. Age of presentation with these disorders varies depending on the severity of the defect.

Mitral valve prolapse is rare in young pediatric patients but is estimated to range from 2% to 20% in young adolescents, especially in thin females. Mitral stenosis and tricuspid stenosis are very rare in this population.[3]

Children who are born without a right pulmonary artery or who have conditions such as atrioseptal defect, ventriculoseptal defect, or patent ductus arteriosis (left to right shunts) are at much greater risk for the development of high altitude pulmonary edema.[17]

Obstetric Issues

Patients with mechanical valves require treatment with warfarin, which is absolutely contraindicated in pregnancy owing to its teratogenic effect.

Geriatric Issues

Quality of life rather than age is the predominant consideration in deciding whether or not to perform valvular replacement surgery. Aortic stenosis is more prevalent in the elderly.

Epidemiology

Approximately 5 million Americans are thought to have some form of valvular heart disease. Only a small percentage have disease on the right side of the heart, leaving the greatest majority of disease to occur on the high-pressure left side of the heart. Aortic stenosis is the most common form of valvular heart disease. Symptoms may occur in patients as young as age 20 or 30 if the stenosis occurs in a bicuspid aortic valve, but usually they do not occur until after age 50. Mitral stenosis is much less common, with a 4:1 female to male ratio. The condition usually manifests in the fourth or fifth decade of life. Aortic insufficiency usually manifests later in life; however, acute aortic insufficiency may be seen in young patients with annuloaortic ectasia or Marfan's syndrome. Mitral regurgitation may be asymptomatic in young women, or it may develop as a result of a ruptured papillary muscle as a complication of acute myocardial infarction.

Treatment Options

Treatment of valvular heart disease is dictated by the severity of the symptoms and by the valve affected. Regardless of the valve involved, all patients should be treated prophylactically for endocarditis. The goal of surgical intervention in valvular heart disease is three-fold: to restore or replicate normal valvular function, to provide a long-term solution to the disorder, and to avoid chronic anticoagulation when feasible. Patients with symptomatic aortic valvular disease require valve replacement. Two major types of valves may be used. Mechanical valves can last many decades but require lifelong anticoagulation with warfarin. Tissue, bioprosthetic (stented or stentless) valves, and homografts do not require anticoagulation unless the patient is in atrial fibrillation but may deteriorate within the first decade after replacement. If aortic root dilatation exists, it must be addressed. In younger patients, the native pulmonic valve may be moved to the aortic valve position, with a homograft used to replace the native pulmonic valve (the Ross procedure). The choice of valve is based on considerations such as duration, need for anticoagulation, ease of placement, availability, infection risk, and noise of valve while functioning, after thorough review with the patient.

Repair rather than replacement is the preferred treatment for mitral valve disease, particularly mitral regurgitation. Repair entails reconstruction of the incompetent leaflet(s), restoration of the mitral annulus, reconstruction of the chordae, or any combination of the above. Repair of the aortic valve is usually not performed, as there has been little long-term success in doing so.

Advances in bioprosthetic valves, including the stentless valves, are showing promise, with increased duration.

Patient Education

Patient education centers on explanation of the pathophysiology of the specific disease. It is imperative that patients understand which symptoms to watch for and what these symptoms mean. Because aortic insufficiency and mitral regurgitation should be treated prior to the development of irreversible left ventricular dysfunction, patients must understand why they are referred for surgery when their symptoms are not limiting their activities. Education with regard to valvular repair versus replacement, and as to valve choices should also be carefully reviewed.

Prevention

Because valvular heart disease is a structural phenomenon, prevention is difficult at best. The only definitive treatment for symptomatic aortic stenosis, aortic insufficiency, mitral stenosis, and mitral regurgitation is surgery. Avoidance of rheumatic fever and endocarditis, while possible, is not possible in certain patient populations. All patients with known valvular heart disease should undergo endocarditis prophylaxis during any invasive procedure involving mucosal surfaces to reduce the risk of bacterial seeding of the diseased valve. Management of atrial fibrillation, if present, and prevention of volume overload may also be of benefit. While most valvular heart disease may be asymptomatic for prolonged periods, patients should be followed closely, as timing is critical to prevent irreversible changes. Transthoracic and transesophageal echocardiography remains the gold standard in assessing the severity and progression of disease.

Screening Recommendations

Heart auscultation for the presence of murmurs should be performed during all routine physical examinations.

▬ VARICOSITIES

Pathophysiology

Three anatomically distinct sets of veins exist in the lower extremity. The superficial system consists of the greater and lesser saphenous veins, which lie within the subcutaneous tissue. The deep venous system typically accompanies the named arteries. Communicating branches perforate the deep muscular fascia, linking the superficial and deep venous systems. Each of these systems possesses bicuspid valves that direct blood flow from the superficial to the deep venous systems. As such, approximately 90% of the venous return to the heart from the lower extremity occurs through the deep venous system. The most distinctive feature of the valves is their contribution to venous capacitance. In the foot, the hydrostatic pressure approaches 100 cm H_2O. This pressure is overcome by muscular contractions, which compress the deep veins, augmenting blood flow back to the heart. Intact valves prevent backflow and venous stasis.

Veins become varicose when they are dilated, elongated, and tortuous. Two mechanisms are responsible for these changes: venous valvular incompetence and weakened vascular walls. Valvular incompetence, the predominant finding, occurs in the main saphenous trunk or communicating vessels, producing higher venous pressures with localized dilatation. This, in turn, weakens the walls of the veins, producing further dilatation. Venous dilatation may also occur in the setting of normal pressures, and this condition appears to be an inherited trait. In these individuals, valves become incompetent as a result of wall dilatation.

Pediatric Issues

This condition does not occur in the pediatric population.

Obstetric Issues

Varicosities increase with pregnancy owing to increased weight bearing.

Geriatric Issues

Incidence increases in the geriatric population because of volume overload situations and incompetent valve systems caused by aging.

Epidemiology

Varicose veins occur in 10–20% of the population. They are most common in the lower extremities but may also manifest as hemorrhoids or esophageal varices, or as a varicocele. The incidence is higher in women and with prolonged standing and sitting, obesity, constrictive clothing, and following pregnancy.

Treatment Options

Treatment options are directed at reducing pain, preventing complications, and improving appearance. Common complications of lower extremity varicosities include small vessel rupture as well as superficial and deep venous thrombophlebitis. More serious complications include deep venous thrombosis and pulmonary embolism. Cosmetic concerns arise from the "bag of worms" appearance, as well as skin hyperpigmentation from build-up of hemosiderin in macrophages.

Nonsurgical treatment is also preventative. Options include walking, avoiding prolonged sitting and standing, leg elevation (ankle higher than the level of the heart), elastic stockings, or a combination of all of the preceding. Elastic stockings must be fitted properly. Stockings that extend to just below the knee are usually adequate, as thigh-high stockings tend to fall.

Surgical treatment is reserved for severe symptoms. Sclerotherapy may be used to obliterate the lumen of smaller vessels and is best suited for small, unsightly veins, dilated superficial veins, and perforating veins of the lower leg below the knee. Vein stripping may be used to augment any of the preceding methods of treatment, or it may be used in isolation for the treatment of very large varices, hemorrhage, ulceration (from venous stasis), and repeated attacks of superficial phlebitis. Vein stripping involves complete removal of the varicose veins with ligation of any incompetent branches. Success is directly dependent on the thoroughness of the procedure. A recurrence rate of approximately 10% is due to failure to ligate all branches of the greater saphenous vein proximally, as well as failure to ligate all incompetent perforators.

Patient Education

Patient education centers on a careful explanation of the pathophysiology of this disorder in terms that each patient can comprehend. Although symptoms can be troublesome, the condition is rarely life-threatening. Education about the condition should be augmented with an explanation of the mechanism of action of each treatment option. In addition, ongoing monitoring of compliance is imperative to reduce the severity of symptoms as well as to halt progression of this disorder.

Prevention

Primary prevention of varicose veins is difficult, if not impossible, in patients prone to develop them. Avoidance of prolonged sitting and standing, regular exercise including walking, and support stockings may reduce the severity and symptoms. Following surgical intervention, these guidelines should be continued.

Screening Recommendations

Evaluation for varicosities is recommended during physical examination.

REFERENCES

1. Braunwald E. Heart Disease: A Textbook of Cardiovascular Medicine, 5th ed. Philadelphia, WB Saunders, 1997.
2. Hurst JW. Hurst's The Heart, 9th ed. New York, McGraw-Hill, 1998.
3. Hay WW Jr, Groothuis JR, Hayward AR, Levin MJ. Current Pediatric Diagnosis and Treatment, 13th ed. Stamford, CT, Appleton & Lange, 1997.

4. Garr D, Tolentino A. Electrophysiology evaluation of elderly patients with sinus bradycardia. Ann Intern Med 1979;90:24–29.

5. Topol EJ. Textbook of Cardiovascular Medicine. Philadelphia, Lippincott, Williams & Wilkins, 1998.

6. Lonn EM, Yusuf S. Evidence based cardiology: Emerging approaches in preventing cardiovascular disease. BMJ 1999;318:1337–1341.

7. Conti CR. What is structural heart disease? Clin Cardiol 2000;23:397–398.

8. Goldman L, Braunwald E. Primary Cardiology. Philadelphia, WB Saunders, 1998.

9. Report of the U.S. Preventive Task Force. Guide to Clinical Preventive Services, 2nd ed. Baltimore, Williams & Wilkins, 1996.

9a. Kostis JB, Daws BR, Cutler J, et al. Prevention of heart failure by antihypertensive drug treatment in older persons with isolated systolic hypertension. SHEP Cooperative Research Group. JAMA 1997;278:212–216.

10. Heart and Stroke Facts, 1998, Statistical Supplement, Dallas, TX, American Heart Association.

11. A clinical trial comparing coronary angioplasty with tissue plasminogen activator for acute myocardial infarction. . . . (Gusto IIb) Angioplasty Substudy Investigators. N Engl J Med 1997;336:1621–1628.

12. Buxton B, Frazier OH, Westaby S. Ischemic Heart Disease: Surgical Management. St. Louis, Mosby, 1999.

13. Varnouskas E. 72 Year Follow-up of survival in randomized European coronary surgery study. N Engl J Med 1988;319:332–337.

14. Schwartz SI. Principles of Surgery, 7th ed. New York, McGraw-Hill, 1999.

15. Sabiston DC Jr, Lyerly HK. Textbook of Surgery: The Biological Basis of Modern Surgical Practice, 15th ed. Philadelphia, WB Saunders, 1997.

16. Rutherford RB. Atlas of Vascular Surgery: Basic Techniques and Exposures. Philadelphia, WB Saunders, 1993.

17. Hacker PH, Roach RC. High altitude medicine. In Auerbach PA (ed). Wilderness Medicine. St Louis, Mosby, forthcoming 2001.

CHAPTER 19

Bone and Joint Disorders

Gerónimo Lluberas, MD, FACP,
Annette Bairan, PhD, RN, CS, FNP,
and Betty R. Nally, RN, MN, CS, ANP

INTRODUCTION

Bone and joint disorders such as rheumatoid arthritis, osteoporosis, osteoarthritis, gout, and fibromyalgia are relatively common and can have a significant impact on a patient's quality of life. The traditional acute care model of medical care is of little help either to practitioners or to patients in dealing with these disorders. Often there are few or no predictors of response, the medications exert their effect slowly and sometimes inconsistently, and the underlying pathophysiologic abnormalities are poorly understood. Further, treatment of many of these diseases is often delayed. Traditional prevention concepts are of some but sometimes limited benefit. In this context, patient education takes on a new urgency, and the relationship between a practitioner and a patient assumes greater importance. (For additional resources, see the Resources Appendix at the end of this book.)

RHEUMATOID ARTHRITIS

Pathophysiology

The primary pathophysiologic abnormality in rheumatoid arthritis (RA) is the activation of cellular and humoral immunity against antigens in synovial tissue (the membrane lining the joints). This process has both systemic and local consequences. Constitutional symptoms of RA are very common, including malaise, weight loss, and anemia of chronic disease. Extra-articular manifestations are relatively uncommon but can be serious. These include rheumatoid lung disease, pulmonary nodules, osteoporosis (as a consequence both of steroid therapy and of the disease itself), pericarditis, vasculitis, episcleritis, pancreatic insufficiency, and scleromalacia perforans (a particularly virulent form of scleritis that can result in perforation of the globe of the eye). The presence of splenomegaly and neutropenia in the context of RA denotes a particular subset of the disease called Felty's syndrome, which is often associated with more myelosuppressive manifestations than other types of RA.

Direct articular consequences of RA range from minimal inflammation in a few joints to a severe, destructive arthritis resulting in polyarticular joint failure within months of the onset of the disease. Most commonly, patients develop a slowly progressive, advancing pattern of disease. Spontaneous remissions are uncommon but not rare.

The diagnosis of RA is clinical. Laboratory studies such as rheumatoid factor, antinuclear antibody (ANA), and erythrocyte sedimentation rate are of some help, but ultimately the diagnosis depends on whether the patient fulfills the clinical definition of the disease. To determine whether a patient meets the clinical definition, consult published diagnostic criteria for correctly classifying a patient as having RA.[1] An important component of diagnostic criteria, as well as of clinical common sense, is the requirement that the articular symptoms be apparent for more than 6 weeks. Although treatment of disease of shorter duration ought to be undertaken for control of symptoms, the diagnosis of RA is problematic in this context. Many viral and allergic illnesses manifest in a similar fashion but are most often self-limiting. It should also be noted that RA symptoms are most often symmetric, although they need not be of identical intensity. X-rays are helpful in assessing the progression of the disease but not as a diagnostic tool. By the time radiographic changes are apparent, joint damage is inevitable.

Typical laboratory findings include a positive rheumatoid factor and an elevated erythrocyte sedimentation rate (ESR). A positive ANA is also seen in a minority of patients and does not mean the presence of systemic lupus erythematosus.[2] Conversely, about 15% of patients with otherwise typical RA have a consistently negative rheumatoid factor.

Articular complications of RA include joint failure with the need for joint replacement, arthritis mutilans (a particularly destructive syndrome in which the small joints of the hands and feet are totally destroyed, rendering them useless), and tendon rupture. Atlantoaxial subluxation—erosion of the odontoid process with marked instability in the C1–C2 junction—is a particularly serious complication and, if not appropriately identified and managed, may result in transection of the spinal cord at this level and almost certain death.

Pediatric Issues

Treatment of otherwise typical RA in adolescents is similar to treatment of adults. Juvenile rheumatoid arthritis (JRA), however, is an entirely different proposition from adult RA and should be managed by clinicians experienced in that disease.

Obstetric Issues

Many of the drugs used in the treatment of RA are contraindicated in pregnancy, and some are overtly teratogenic. Contraception must be part of the management of women taking these medications. Corticosteroids at modest doses are the safest drugs to use during pregnancy. Fortunately, clinical experience suggests that RA becomes somewhat less virulent during pregnancy.

Geriatric Issues

Management is not significantly affected by age.

Epidemiology

RA is a serious, systemic autoimmune disease of unknown etiology. It affects women three times as often as men. It has been described in patients of all ages but is most common in women of childbearing age. The disease has been described all over the world and in most ethnic groups. A number of immunogenetic factors have been identified that may render certain populations somewhat more susceptible to the disease than others. In addition, concordance in identical twins is known to be much higher than in nonidentical siblings.[3] Current estimates suggest a prevalence of approximately 5 million cases in the United States.

Treatment Options

Isotonic exercise maintains mobility, range of motion, and muscle strength and is strongly recommended. Vigorous exercise, however, should be undertaken gradually and carefully, as a sudden increase in activity can result in a very serious recrudescence of articular symptoms. Aspirin is no longer recommended for the treatment of RA because of its toxicity. Nonsteroidal anti-inflammatory drugs (NSAIDs) are universally accepted as appropriate initial therapy to reduce swelling, inflammation, and pain. The availability of COX-2 inhibitors (NSAIDs with minimal gastric intolerance) represents a welcome advance in the therapy of RA.

The realization that the course of the disease can be altered before bone erosions develop has prompted a more aggressive treatment stance with disease-modifying antirheumatic drugs (DMARDs) earlier in the course. Medications such as hydroxycholoroquine (Plaquenil), auranofin (Ridaura), and sulfasalazine (Azulfidine) are now used in earlier cases. Methotrexate is presently the standard drug for aggressive therapy. Azathioprine (Imuran) and cyclosporine are used when patients are intolerant of or fail to respond to methotrexate. Occasionally gold injections are used, although they have fallen out of favor owing to toxicity. DMARDs, particularly methotrexate, azathioprine, and cyclosporine are fraught with serious metabolic side effects and require expert and frequent monitoring. The choice of DMARD is not easily described and depends on such factors as severity of disease, comorbidities, concomitant medications, and extra-articular manifestations. Combinations of DMARD are currently being studied. Pregnancy contraindicates most antirheumatic drugs.

New DMARDs such as leflunomide (Arava) and etanercept (Enbrel) promise efficacy comparable or superior to methotrexate with less toxicity, but the experience with these medications is much more limited than with methotrexate. Intra-articular, or at times systemic, corticosteroids are necessary. In cases of imminent joint failure, surgery may be indicated. The various modalities used in physical and occupational therapy may be helpful to overcome specific regional musculoskeletal complications of RA.

The use of minocycline for RA warrants discussion. Infectious etiologies for RA have been sought unsuccessfully for more than a generation. At various times antibiotics have been advocated for treatment of RA. Most recently, several studies have suggested a modest remittive effect of tetracycline.[4-6] However, the rates of improvement compared to placebo varied depending on the response criteria used.[7] It should be noted that the largest of these trials included just over 200 patients. At this time, minocycline must be considered a second-line drug whose efficacy has not been thoroughly studied. It certainly does not represent a substitute for other treatments previously suggested.

Prosorbacol (Prosorba), the recently approved treatment for severe RA, represents a novel approach. Prosorbacol is an apheresis column using a staphylococcal protein A adsorption column that binds circulating mediators of inflammation and thus halts the autoimmune attack. It is presently approved for patients who are refractory to other treatments and requires a setup similar to that of hemodialysis.[8]

Finally, treatment of patients with severe RA requires consultation and coordination with a rheumatologist in the same manner that an oncologist is involved in the treatment of cancer with chemotherapy.

Patient Education

Every effort should be made to educate the patient regarding the nature of RA and its complications. Very often, the choice of one or another medicine is made as a team decision between practitioner and patient. Instructions regarding the use of correct body mechanics and joint protection is paramount. In addition, it is imperative that realistic expectations be developed. A comprehensive treatment plan must consider the slow nature of the disease and the weeks to months that it may take for some of the treatments to exert their effects.

Prevention

No specific primary preventive measures have been demonstrated to avert the development of RA. Secondary preventive techniques consist of the treatments previously discussed to improve and maintain function and prevent complications.

Screening Recommendations

Appropriate diagnostic measures should be performed in patients with signs and symptoms suggestive of rheumatoid arthritis so that treatment can begin in the early stages of the disease process.

OSTEOPOROSIS

Pathophysiology

Bone regulation is a complex process. Bone structure is maintained by the equilibrium between bone deposition and bone resorption. Osteoblasts are the cells in bone tissue responsible for bone deposition, while osteoclasts are involved in bone resorption. These two functions are tightly regulated by a complex set of factors that include vitamin D, calcium, calcitonin, gonadal steroids, and parathyroid hormone. Disruption of this tight balance results in osteoporosis.

Certain factors have been clearly identified as increasing the risk of osteoporosis. These factors include early menopause (prior to age 45); postmenopausal status; Asian or Caucasian ethnicity; a thin, small frame; a family history of osteoporosis; and tobacco use.[9, 10]

Two distinct types of osteoporosis have been identified. Type I osteoporosis occurs as a result of hypogonadism in men or women.[11] Hypogonadism leads to accelerated osteoclastic activity and active bone resorption. Patients with Type I osteoporosis predominantly experience fractures in areas rich in trabecular bone (vertebrae and forearms). Type II osteoporosis is more often associated with the aging process and is the result of decreased osteoblastic activity and decreased bone formation. It is seen in the elderly and is associated with a predominant preference for cortical bone loss and a risk for fractures in long bones.[11] It is easy to understand why postmenopausal women experience both trabecular and cortical bone fractures, as they are subject both to the decreased osteoblastic activity of the elderly, and thus to decreased bone formation, and to the accelerated osteoclastic activity of hypogonadism, with accelerated bone loss.

A recently recognized and disturbing subset of osteoporosis is that seen in young, athletic women who become amenorrheic from vigorous exercise. The associated development of rapid osteoporosis results in unexpected fractures.[12] This condition has been termed the "female athlete triad" and consists of an eating disorder, amenorrhea, and osteoporosis. This syndrome is incompletely understood.

Secondary osteoporosis can be the result of administration[14] or endogenous production (Cushingism) of corticosteroids, poorly controlled diabetes mellitus, thyrotoxicosis,[15] chronic renal failure, hyperparathyroidism, or hyperprolactinism. Multiple myeloma, breast cancer, and other malignancies can result in relatively rapid secondary osteoporosis. All these entities have in common a tendency towards accelerated bone loss.

The diagnosis of osteoporosis requires a high index of suspicion. Prior to the first fracture, symptoms are absent. A history of previous fractures and reports of mid-back pain are characteristic but represent late findings. The presence of risk factors should be ascertained. The first indication of the presence of the disease may very well be loss of height. Kyphosis and scoliosis occur at a later stage. Ancillary studies seldom reveal anything useful in an otherwise healthy postmenopausal woman but should be performed if clinically appropriate. Silent thyrotoxicosis is an occasional coincidental finding. Demonstrating bone mineral loss in a bone mass assay is the accepted method of making the diagnosis of osteoporosis and is the best predictor for subsequent fractures.[9] Dual energy x-ray absorptiometry (DXA) is the best-studied and most reliable method of quantifying bone mass. It should be noted that bone loss is reliably seen on routine x-rays only at advanced stages of osteoporosis and should not be used to assess its presence. Without intervention the factors that lead to bone loss are likely to continue, and the likelihood of fractures can be accurately (statistically) predicted based on the bone mineral density value.

Pediatric Issues

Osteoporosis does not occur in children except in the context of a serious underlying illness. Its presence in otherwise healthy adolescents generally signals the female athletic triad previously discussed.

Obstetric Issues

In general, osteoporosis occurs in women well past their childbearing years. When it occurs in young women, it appears in the context of amenorrhea. As a result, pregnancy and osteoporosis rarely coexist.

Geriatric Issues

Management is not significantly affected by age.

Epidemiology

Osteoporosis is "a systemic skeletal disease characterized by low bone mass and micro-architectural deterioration of bone tissue, with consequent increase in bone fragility and susceptibility to fracture."[9] It affects 25 million people, 80% of whom are women. At age 50, a woman is estimated to have a 40% chance of an osteoporotic fracture during her remaining lifetime. Osteoporotic hip fractures in particular occur in excess of 250,000 yearly and carry approximately an excess 20% mortality within a year after the fracture itself. Close to half of the patients who experience a hip fracture never fully recover.[16] As a result, osteoporosis is an enormous and growing public health problem.

Treatment Options

A distinction must be made between treatment and prevention. The former represents the interventions necessary to prevent fractures in patients with established osteoporosis (who may or may not have already experienced osteoporotic fractures.) The latter is an attempt to minimize bone loss in a person who exhibits risk factors for the development of osteoporosis but whose bone density measurement is nowhere near the definition of the disease and who has not experienced fractures.

Treatment for osteoporotic hip and Colles' fractures requires expert orthopedic intervention. Vertebral compression fractures can often be managed with analgesics and local therapy. Although the presence of a fracture denotes relatively advanced disease, prevention of subsequent fractures is an achievable goal with appropriate treatment.[17]

Calcium and vitamin D supplementation is the foundation on which additional therapeutic interventions are based for both treatment and prevention. Presently, only calcitonin (Miacalcin)[18] and alendronate (Fosamax)[17, 19] are indicated for the treatment of osteoporosis. Alendronate is orally administered, and calcitonin is an intranasal preparation. Sodium fluoride has been studied for years, but remains experimental because of consistently disappointing results.

Patient Education

Among musculoskeletal illnesses, patient education offers one of the best opportunities to have an impact on the disease. Education must begin in childhood, with the importance of adequate calcium and vitamin D intake and an understanding of the importance of supplementation. Weight-bearing exercise (but not in excess) strengthens bone and retards bone loss. During adulthood, education stresses that osteoporosis is not an inevitable consequence of aging. It also underscores that removal of risk factors (e.g., tobacco use) considerably decreases the likelihood of osteoporosis. Other matters that must be addressed are the benefits of estrogen administration after menopause and awareness by the patient of other family members who have the disease. Injury prevention, ways of making an early diagnosis, and suggestive symptoms should be discussed. Once therapy is undertaken, instruction regarding appropriate administration of medications is essential to ensure maximum efficacy.

Prevention

Prevention of osteoporosis begins in childhood and continues through middle age.[20] It is accomplished by providing adequate dietary calcium intake, appropriate nutrition, and exercise. While this appears obvious, since 1950 there has been a major decline in the consumption of milk by children and adolescents and a corresponding increase in their consumption of carbonated beverages, which are devoid of calcium and vitamin D.

Delaying menopause by estrogen administration is of great benefit,[21, 22] as there is a major decrease in bone loss in the years immediately after loss of the menses. Patients who cannot or will not take estrogens but who are at risk for osteoporosis should be offered raloxifene (Evista), a selective estrogen receptor modulator (SERM).[23] This drug also adds some of the cardioprotective effect of estrogen without an increase in endometrial proliferation.[24] Low dose alendronate is also useful in the prevention of osteoporosis. Finally, some studies have suggested that calcitonin may also be helpful for prevention.[25]

Screening Recommendations

All women should receive primary preventive counseling regarding calcium and vitamin D intake, weight-bearing exercise, and smoking cessation to reduce fracture risk. Pre- and postmenopausal women should receive counseling regarding the risks versus benefits of hormone replacement therapy. There are no indications for or against routine screening with bone densitometry in asymptomatic, postmenopausal females.[26]

▬ OSTEOARTHRITIS

Pathophysiology

Osteoarthritis is the most common type of articular disease. Also known as degenerative arthritis, osteoarthritis involves a progressive degeneration of articular cartilage. As cartilage deteriorates, some inflammation occurs as a result of the cartilage shed into the synovial space. In an attempt to increase the loading surface area, bone remodeling produces osteophytes. Inflammation is mild and a result of the disease rather than the cause of the disease, as is the case in rheumatoid arthritis. Osteoarthritis is best thought of as substance fatigue of articular cartilage. Factors contributing to the development of osteoarthritis include family history, joint trauma, aging, obesity, and occupational overuse.

The diagnosis of osteoarthritis, like other musculoskeletal illnesses, is clinical. The characteristic joint pain is of long duration and of insidious onset. Stiffness lasting approximately 15 min in the morning or following prolonged immobility is a common finding. As the disease progresses, the patient may experience joint enlargement or deformity, decreased range of motion, and crepitus. Radicular pain may occur when spinal osteoarthritis (degenerative spondylosis) impinges on a nerve root. Joints most often affected include the distal interphalangeals, posterior interphalangeals, bases of thumbs, knees, hips, cervical spine, and lumbar spine.[27]

X-rays are not very useful during the early stages of the disease but will subsequently reveal narrowed joint space, osteophytes, subchondral bony sclerosis, and subchondral cyst formation. Laboratory testing is typically unrevealing. An elevated erythrocyte sedimentation rate and an anemia of chronic disease should not be considered the result of osteoarthritis, and other explanations should be sought.

Pediatric Issues

With the occasional exception following severe trauma, osteoarthritis does not occur in children.

Obstetric Issues

Osteoarthritis rarely occurs in young women, and when it does, the symptoms generally are manageable with acetaminophen.

Geriatric Issues

Management is not significantly affected by age.

Epidemiology

Approximately 44% of Americans over the age of 40 have osteoarthritis.[28] The Centers for Disease Control and Prevention estimate that it affects over 16 million Americans over age 60.[29] Osteoarthritis predominantly affects both men and woman over the age of 40 equally. It is the most common form of arthritis and the second most common cause of long-term disability in the United States.[30] The incidence of this disease varies among different populations.[28]

Treatment Options

Managing the pain associated with osteoarthritis should start with nonpharmacologic approaches such as exercise, joint protection, and ergonomic adjustments. Patients should be educated that the pain associated with osteoarthritis is reversible and not related to an irreversible loss of ability to function.

Treatment includes local therapy with heat, cold, moisture, or ultrasonography. Analgesics such as acetaminophen may control minor pain. NSAIDs may be necessary when there is inflammation in the affected joints. Capsaicin, an analgesic cream, may be useful in combination with these oral medications in reducing symptoms. Intra-articular corticosteroid injections are useful in treating pain unrelieved by analgesic or anti-inflammatory medications. More recent approaches include the use of intra-articular hyaluronate, particularly in the knees, to decrease the symptoms of advanced osteoarthritis. This regimen has been shown to be at least comparable to long-term NSAID administration.[31, 32] Physical therapy may be helpful for joint strengthening to improve performance of activities of daily living. Ultimately, arthroscopic debridement or arthroplasty of the joint may be necessary.

The use of nutraceuticals is an emerging area of interest. Several studies have shown the anti-inflammatory effect of the cartilage derivatives chondroitin and glucosamine. A recent study showed that there is considerable improvement in pain scores after as little as 8 weeks of treatment with glucosamine.[33] A comparison between diclofenac and chondroitin sulfate revealed a similar improvement in symptoms, but the improvement was longer lasting in the chondroitin group.[34] Debate exists over the mechanism of action of these substances, and clearly additional studies are required.[35] Nevertheless, diclofenac and chondroitin are inexpensive and available over the counter.[36]

Patient Education

As with other rheumatic illnesses, an understanding of the nature of osteoarthritis is invaluable. Encouraging weight loss in the overweight patient, decreasing weight-bearing by reducing strenuous activities such as stair climbing or jogging, and promoting non-weight–bearing activities (such as water aerobics and quadriceps strengthening exercises) can decrease the progression of the disease. Proper use of medications (over-the-counter, such as acetaminophen or ibuprofen, and prescription) is imperative in preventing potential adverse reactions related to these medications.

Prevention

Nothing has been shown to be helpful in the primary prevention of idiopathic osteoarthritis. Avoiding traumatic activities such as football, wearing protective gear, and ergonomic modification of the workplace can minimize the development of posttraumatic disease. Measures useful in minimizing the impact of osteoarthritis once it has developed include control of body weight, routine exercise, and joint preservation. Although there is no explicit scientific literature to support it, in view of the studies previously mentioned, it stands to reason that patients who are at high risk for the development or progression of osteoarthritis may benefit from the combination of chondroitin and glucosamine.

Screening Recommendations

A history of prior injuries, occupational details, and level of physical activity are useful in identifying patients at risk for the development of osteoarthritis. Interventions can be undertaken to prevent further injury resulting in the worsening of physical function.

GOUT

Pathophysiology

Gout is the result of gradual accumulation of uric acid in the body. Prior to the first attack, there is already a considerable uric acid load (hyperuricemia), which then precipitates in a joint as a result of minor trauma. Gout is an inflammatory reaction caused by monosodium urate crystal deposits in a peripheral joint. The most common joint affected is the great toe, although an attack may occur in any joint.

Gout can occur as a result of overproduction or, more commonly, under-excretion of uric acid. Diseases with high cell turnover such as malignancies, Paget's disease of bone,[37] hemolytic anemias, glycogen storage diseases, psoriasis, and sarcoidosis can produce secondary gout. Renal insufficiency can also produce gout by virtue of the kidneys' inability to excrete uric acid. Alcohol is a notorious precipitant of gouty attacks. Other factors related to the development of gout include obesity, starvation, lead intoxication, and ingestion of drugs such as salicylates (including low dose) diuretics, pyrazinamide, ethambutol, and nicotinic acid.[38] The diagnosis of acute gout is clinical and is confirmed by the examination of synovial fluid under compensated polarized microscopy.[39] Synovial fluid examination need not be performed in the joint affected, as patients with gout often have crystals in asymptomatic knees.[40] Hyperuricemia alone is insufficient to make the diagnosis of gout. Because an acute monoarthritis may mimic a septic joint, and polyarticular gout may mimic rheumatoid arthritis, it is recommended that patients who carry the diagnosis of gout undergo an arthrocentesis and synovial fluid examination at least once to confirm the diagnosis.

Clinically, gout is described in stages: hyperuricemia without gout, acute intermittent gout, and chronic gout.[41] In over 50% of cases, the initial attack manifests in the first metatarsophalangeal (MTP) joint. Initial symptoms associated with gout include a sudden onset of warmth, marked soft-tissue swelling, and severe pain of the affected joint. Commonly, the joint is so tender that patients describe being unable to place a sheet over the joint. The initial attack usually occurs in the early morning or at night. Accompanying symptoms may include fever and chills. An elevated white blood cell count and erythrocyte sedimentation rate, and possibly hyperuricemia, may be expected during an acute attack. The presence of tophi indicates a massive uric acid load and signals the development of chronic gout.

Pediatric Issues

Except in the context of the Lesch-Nyhan syndrome, a rare and devastating genetic illness associated with mental retardation, gout is unknown in children.[42]

Obstetric Issues

Gout is uncommon in women and virtually unknown during the childbearing years.

Geriatric Issues

Management is not significantly affected by age.

Epidemiology

Gout is primarily a disease of adult men. In the U.S., gout has a self-reported prevalence of 13.6 per 1000 in men and 6.4 per 1000 in women.[43] The incidence increases with age. Certain populations, specifically Pacific Asians, have a higher incidence of gout and hyperuricemia.[44] Obesity also increases the risk of gout.

Treatment Options

Treatment of the acute attack is best achieved with NSAIDs. These both decrease pain and control inflammation. More severe attacks may be treated with corticosteroids or adrenocorticotropic hormone.[45] Colchicine is helpful for an acute attack but almost invariably produces diarrhea. Patients with recurrent acute gouty attacks require urate-lowering agents such as allopurinol or probenecid. Patients who already have tophi should not be given probenecid, however, as it increases the incidence of urate kidney stones. Untreated, chronic gout may become a destructive arthropathy as severe as rheumatoid arthritis. An acute attack is not the time to initiate uric acid-lowering therapy with allopurinol or probenecid. Several studies, as well as extensive clinical experience, have demonstrated that starting such treatment during an attack tends to worsen its severity and prolong its duration.[46]

Patient Education

Patient education has a major impact in the prevention of gout and its complications. It revolves around instructing the patient to avoid the precipitants mentioned in the following section on Prevention. An understanding of the length of treatment of chronic gout (which is often lifelong) is paramount. Resting the affected joint during the acute phase will aid in pain and inflammation reduction.

Prevention

Gouty attacks and chronic gout can be prevented. Preventive measures involve restricting intake of purine-rich foods such as organ meats, shellfish, and nuts. Alcohol consumption should be eliminated. Weight reduction and limiting the use of thiazide diuretics are also helpful. Salicylates should be avoided.

Screening Recommendations

Appropriate diagnostic studies should be instituted in symptomatic patients to confirm the presence of gout or a disorder that mimics a gouty attack.

FIBROMYALGIA

Pathophysiology

The etiology of fibromyalgia remains unknown, and its pathophysiology is poorly understood. Theories abound and are a source of heated debate. These theories fall into two major categories: neurochemical and behavioral. Evidence for a neurochemical mechanism includes the demonstration of decreased serotonin levels in patients with fibromyalgia[47] and abnormalities in other neurochemicals, including substance P, nerve growth factor, and dynorphin A.[48] Abnormalities in central pain pathways further support a neurochemical mechanism.[49] Proponents of the behavioral set of theories, however, point out that the incidence of generalized pain in the general population is high,[50] but that only a small fraction of these people ever decide to seek medical care. Several studies have shown that the differences between the "nonpatients" and those who seek medical care lie not in the severity of their pain but in the presence of previous physical or sexual abuse,[51] psychiatric illnesses,[52] or even the perception of physical or emotional trauma.[53] Finally, the American College of Rheumatology's (ACR) criteria for fibromyalgia and the accompanying recognition of the disease have virtually silenced those who proposed that fibromyalgia is not a legitimate clinical entity. While the argument has virtually disappeared from the literature, however, it is far from being eradicated in clinical practice.

Fibromyalgia is more than muscle pain. Patients typically experience many associated somatic complaints. In addition to generalized muscle pain, symptoms of irritable bowel syndrome, insomnia and other sleep disturbances, depression, and anxiety may be present. Some patients resist the diagnosis of fibromyalgia, which leads to additional confusion and frustration in an already frustrated patient.[54, 55] The course of the disease is variable, ranging from full recovery to symptoms that become so ingrained that the patient becomes disabled.

Pediatric Issues

Fibromyalgia is almost nonexistent in children, but its incidence increases in late adolescence. The treatment of adolescents with fibromyalgia is the same as that of adults.

Obstetric Issues

Pregnancy appears to have neither a protective nor an aggravating effect in fibromyalgia. Because the treatment of this illness revolves around the control of constitutional symptoms, there is no indication to continue the medications throughout pregnancy. Conservative treatment and avoidance of medications is the best approach to treating a pregnant woman with fibromyalgia.

Geriatric Issues

Management is not significantly affected by age.

Epidemiology

Fibromyalgia is the most common cause of chronic generalized pain. The reported incidence of this condition depends on the definition used as well as the population examined. A survey in Wichita, Kansas,[55] reports an estimated prevalence of 3.4% in women and 0.5% in men when the 1990 ACR criteria for the classification of fibromyalgia are applied.[56] On the other hand, a similar survey in England[50] revealed a prevalence of chronic widespread pain of 11.2%, of which 80% formally fulfilled the ACR's criteria. The Wichita study also revealed that the prevalence increased with age.

Treatment Options

No one treatment strategy is consistently helpful in fibromyalgia. Accepted treatments include non-narcotic analgesics, NSAIDs, muscle relaxants, and antidepressants. These offer some relief from pain, muscle spasm, insomnia, and depression, but there is evidence that some of these therapies become ineffective after several months.[57] Opioids should be strictly avoided. Dietary manipulations, megadose vitamins, and herbal supplements are advocated by some patients with the support of alternative medicine practitioners, but these modalities are poorly supported by the per-reviewed scientific literature. Perhaps the value of these interventions is that they are patient-initiated and illustrate some coping tendencies.[58] Cognitive therapy and behavioral and educational interventions are helpful in minimizing the impact of the disease.[59]

Patient Education

Education is valuable in stressing to the patient the benign nature of the illness. Reassurance that the pain does not represent a life-threatening illness often goes a long way in alleviating anxiety and insomnia. Health care providers should attempt to identify coping strategies that tend to reduce distress experienced by patients with fibromyalgia, and then teach these patients how to use these strategies in the home and workplace. A skillful practitioner steers the patient toward discovering underlying psychosocial issues that contribute to the impact of the disease. Very often, the most powerful therapeutic instrument in the care of these patients is the practitioner-patient relationship.

Prevention

To date, there is no data to support the notion that any one intervention can result in prevention of fibromyalgia.

Screening Recommendations

Fibromyalgia should be a part of the differential diagnosis in patients with signs and symptoms suggestive of the disorder.

REFERENCES

1. Arnett FC, Edworthy SM, Bloch DA, et al. The American Rheumatism Association 1987 revised criteria for the classification of rheumatoid arthritis. Arthritis Rheum 1988;31:315–324.
2. Harris ED. Clinical features of rheumatoid arthritis. *In* Kelley WN, Harris ED, Ruddy S, et al. (eds), Textbook of Rheumatology, 5th ed. Philadelphia, WB Saunders, 1997, 898–932.
3. Winchester R. The molecular basis of susceptibility to rheumatoid arthritis. Adv Immunol 1994;56:389–466.
4. O'Dell JR, Paulsen G, Haire CE, et al. Treatment of early seropositive rheumatoid arthritis with minocycline: Four-year followup of a double-blind, placebo-controlled trial. Arthritis Rheum 1999;42:1691–1695.
5. O'Dell JR, Haire CE, Palmer W, et al. Treatment of early rheumatoid arthritis with minocycline or placebo: Results of a randomized, double-blind, placebo-controlled trial. Arthritis Rheum 1997;40:842–848.
6. Tilley BC, Alarcon GS, Heyse SP, et al. Minocycline in rheumatoid arthritis. A 48-week, double-blind, placebo controlled trial. MIRA Trial Group. Ann Intern Med 1995;122:81–89.
7. Pillemer SR, Fowler SE, Tilley BC, et al. Meaningful improvement criteria sets in a rheumatoid arthritis clinical trial, MIRA Trial Group. Minocycline in Rheumatoid Arthritis. Arthritis Rheum 1997;40:419–425.
8. Caldwell J, Gendreau RM, Furst D. Pilot study using a Staph protein A column Prosorba to treat refractory rheumatoid arthritis. J Rheumatol 1999;26:1657–1662.
9. Consensus Development Conference. Diagnosis, prophylaxis and treatment of osteoporosis. Am J Med 1993;94:646–650.

10. Cummings SR, Nevitt MC, Browser WS, et al. Risk factors for hip fractures in white women. N Engl J Med 1995;332:767–773.

11. Riggs BL, Melton LJ III. Evidence for two distinct syndromes of involutional osteoporosis. Am J Med 1983;75:899.

12. Cumming DC. Exercise-associated amenorrhea, low bone density, and estrogen replacement therapy. Arch Intern Med 1996;156:2193–2195.

13. West RV. The female athlete. The triad of disordered eating, amenorrhea and osteoporosis. Sports Med 1998;26:63–71.

14. Adachi JD, Benson WG, Hodsman AB. Corticosteroid-induced osteoporosis. Semin Arthritis Rheum 1993;22:375–384.

15. Mundy GR, Shapiro JL, Bendelin JG, et al. Direct stimulation of bone resorption by thyroid hormones. J Clin Invest 1976;58:529.

16. Fogelman I, Ryan P. Osteoporosis: A growing epidemic. Br J Clin Pract 1991;45:189–196.

17. Black DM, Cummings SR, Karpf DB, et al. Randomized trial of effect of alendronate on risk of fracture in women with existing vertebral fractures. Lancet 1996;348:1535–1541.

18. Overgaard K, Hansen MA, Jensen SB, Christiansen C. Effect of salcatonin given intranasally on bone mass and fracture rates in established osteoporosis. BMJ 1992;305:556–561.

19. Lieberman UA, Weiss SR, Broll J, et al. Effect of oral alendronate on bone mineral density and the incidence of fractures in postmenopausal osteoporosis. N Engl J Med 1995;333:1437–1443.

20. Kulak CA, Bilezikian JP. Osteoporosis: Preventive strategies. Int J Fertil Womens Med 1998;43:56–64.

21. Cauley JA, Seeley DG, Ensrud K, et al. Estrogen replacement therapy and fractures in older women. Ann Intern Med 1995;122:9–16.

22. Horsman A, Gallagher JC, Simpson M, et al. Prospective trial of oestrogen and calcium in postmenopausal women. BMJ 1977;2:789–792.

23. Ettinger B, Black DM, Milak BH, et al. Reduction of vertebral fracture risk in postmenopausal women with osteoporosis treated with raloxifene. JAMA 1999;282:637–645.

24. Delmas PD, Bjarnason NH, Mitlak BH, et al. Effects of raloxifene on bone mineral density, serum cholesterol concentrations, and uterine endometrium in postmenopausal women. N Engl J Med 1997;337:1641–1647.

25. Reginster JY, Deroisy R, Lecart MP, et al. A double-blind, placebo-controlled dose-finding trial of intermittent nasal salmon calcitonin for prevention of postmenopausal lumbar spine bone loss. Am J Med 1995;98:452–458.

26. Report of the U.S. Preventive Services Task Force. Guide to Clinical Preventive Services, 2nd ed. Baltimore, Williams & Wilkins, 1996.

27. Hochberg MC. Osteoarthritis: Clinical features and treatment. *In* Klippel JH, Primer on the Rheumatic Diseases, 11th ed. Atlanta GA, Arthritis Foundation, 1997, 218–222.

28. Peyron JG, Altman RD. The epidemiology of osteoarthritis. *In* Moskowitz RW, Howell DS, Goldberg VM, et al. (eds), Osteoarthritis: Diagnosis and Medical/Surgical Management, 2nd ed. Philadelphia, W.B. Saunders, 1992, 15–36.

29. Centers for Disease Control. Arthritis prevalence and activity limitations—United States, 1990. MMWR Morb Mortal Wkly Rep 1994;43:433.

30. Fife RS. Osteoarthritis: Epidemiology, pathology and pathogenesis. *In*

Klippel JH, Primer on the Rheumatic Diseases, 11th ed. Atlanta GA, Arthritis Foundation, 1997, 216–218.

31. Altman RD, Moskowitz R. Intraarticular sodium hyaluronate (Hyalgan) in the treatment of patients with osteoarthritis of the knee: A randomized clinical trial. Hyalgan Study Group. J Rheumatol 1998;25:2203–2212.

32. Adams ME, Atkinson MH, Lussier AJ, et al. The role of viscosupplementation with hylan G-F 20 (Synvisc) in the treatment of osteoarthritis of the knee: A Canadian multicenter trial comparing hylan G-F 20 alone, hylan G-F 20 with non-steroidal anti-inflammatory drugs (NSAIDs) and NSAIDs alone. Osteoarthritis Cartilage 1995;3:213–225.

33. Pujalte JM, Llavore EP, Ylescupidez FR. Double-blind clinical evaluation of oral glucosamine sulphate in the basic treatment of ostearthrosis. Curr Med Res Opin 1980;7:110–114.

34. Morreale P, Manopulo R, Galati M, et al. Comparison of the antiinflammatory efficacy of chondroitin sulfate and diclofenac sodium in patients with knee osteoarthritis. J Rheumatol 1996;23:1385–1391.

35. Deal CL, Moskowitz R. Nutriceuticals as therapeutic agents in osteoarthritis. Rheum Dis Clin North Am 1999;25:379–395.

36. Kelly GS. The role of glucosamine sulfate and chondroitin sulfates in the treatment of degenerative joint disease. Altern Med Rev 1998;3:27–39.

37. Lluberas-Acosta G, Hansell JR, Schumacher HR. Paget's disease of bone in patients with gout. Arch Intern Med 1986;146:2389.

38. Kelley WM, Wortmann RL: Gout and hyperuricemia. In Kelley WN, Harris ED, Ruddy S, Sledge CB (eds), Textbook of Rheumatology, 5th ed. Philadelphia, WB Saunders, 1997, 1313–1351.

39. Gatter RA. A Practical Handbook of Joint Fluid Analysis. Philadelphia, Lea & Febiger, 1984, 1–2.

40. Bomalaski JS, Lluberas G, Schumacher, HR. Monosodium urate crystals in the knee joints of patients with asymptomatic nontophaceous gout. Arthritis Rheum 1986;29:1480–1485.

41. Edwards NL. Gout: Clinical and laboratory features. In Klippel JH, Primer on the Rheumatic Diseases, 11th ed. Atlanta, GA. Arthritis Foundation, 1997, 234–239.

42. Seegmiller JE, Rosenbloom RM, Kelley WN. An enzyme defect associated with a sex-linked human neurological disorder and excessive purine synthesis. Science 1967;155:1682–1685.

43. Terkeltaub RA. Gout: Epidemiology, pathology, and pathogenesis. In Klippel JH, Primer on the Rheumatic Diseases, 11th ed. Atlanta, GA, Arthritis Foundation, 1997, 230–234.

44. Darmawan J, Valkenburg HA, Muirden KD, et al. The epidemiology of gout and hyperuricemia in a rural population in Java. J Rheumatol 1992;19:1595–1599.

45. Pratt PW and Ball GV: Gout: Treatment. In Klippel JH, Primer on the Rheumatic Diseases, 11th ed. Atlanta, GA, Arthritis Foundation, 1997, 240–243.

46. Popp JD, Edwards NL. New insights into gouty arthritis. Contemp Intern Med 1995;7:55–64.

47. Wolfe F, Ross K, Anderson J, et al. The prevalence and characteristics of fibromyalgia in the general population. Arthritis Rheum 1995;38:19–28.

48. Russell IJ. Advances in fibromyalgia: Possible role for central neurochemicals. Am J Med Sci 1998;315:377–384.

49. Bendtsen L, Norregaard J, Jensen R, et al. Evidence of qualitatively altered nociception in patients with fibromyalgia. Arthritis Rheum 1997;40:98–102.

50. Croft P, Rigby AS, Boswell R. The prevalence of chronic widespread pain in the general population. J Rheumatol 1993;20:710–713.

51. Alexander RW, Bradley LA, Alarcon GS, et al. Sexual and physical abuse in women with fibromyalgia: Association with outpatient health care utilization and pain medication usage. Arthritis Care Res 1998;11:102–115.

52. Aaron LA, Bradley LA, Alarcon GS, et al. Psychiatric diagnoses in patients with fibromyalgia are related to health care-seeking behavior rather than to illness. Arthritis Rheum 1996;39:436–445.

53. Aaron LA, Bradley LA, Alarcon GS, et al. Perceived physical and emotional trauma as precipitating events in fibromyalgia. Associations with health care seeking and disability status but not pain severity. Arthritis Rheum 1997;40:453–460.

54. Lluberas-Acosta G: Pseudolupus. South Med J 1989;82:1589.

55. Sigal LH: Pseudo-Lyme disease. Bull Rheum Dis 1995;44:1–3.

56. Wolfe F, Smythe HA, Yunus MB, et al. The American College of Rheumatology 1990 criteria for the classification of fibromyalgia. Report of the Multicenter Criteria Committee. Arthritis Rheum 1990;33:160–172.

57. Carrette S, Bell MJ, Reynolds WJ, et al. Comparison of amitriptyline cyclobenzaprine and placebo in the treatment of fibromyalgia: A randomized, double-blind clinical trial. Arthritis Rheum 1994;37:32–40.

58. Martin MY, Bradley LA, Alexander RW, et al. Coping strategies predict disability in patients with primary fibromyalgia. Pain 1996;68:45–53.

59. Nicassio PM, Radojevic V, Weisman MH, et al. A comparison of behavioral and educational interventions for fibromyalgia. J Rheumatol 1997;24:2000–2007.

CHAPTER 20

Gastrointestinal Disorders

Amy J. Cofer, PA-C, MMSc,
Alison Ann Lauber, MD,
Genie E. Dorman, RN, PhD, CS, FNP,
and Troy Spicer, RN, MS, CS, FNP

■ INTRODUCTION

Disorders of the gastrointestinal (GI) tract are among the most common conditions encountered by the primary care provider. Manifestations of GI disorders are quite variable and can involve any portion of the alimentary tract or abdominal organs. The GI tract extends from the mouth to the anus and is involved in the ingestion, propulsion, digestion, and absorption of nutrients, and in the elimination of waste. These processes occur in conjunction with the accessory organs, the liver, the gallbladder, and the pancreas.

From a primary preventive standpoint, a balanced diet containing adequate fiber and antioxidants, hepatitis vaccines, and the avoidance of high-risk behaviors compose the primary advice for preventing GI disorders.

Patient education can greatly assist patient self-care and reduce exposures to foodborne illnesses (see also Chapter 5, Environmental Health and Sanitation), thus reducing hospitalization for complications. Screening programs can facilitate early detection of malignancies and improve outcomes (see also Chapter 23, Neoplastic Conditions). Vaccination, prophylaxis, and special diets may help to modify symptom severity and reduce morbidity. This chapter primarily deals with disorders that are not malignant. However, it is important to understand that identification and treatment of benign disorders and/or lifestyle modifications may have an impact on the frequency of occurrence of neoplastic conditions. For additional resources, see the Resources Appendix at the end of this book.

■ GASTROESOPHAGEAL REFLUX DISEASE

Pathophysiology

The underlying pathophysiology of gastroesophageal reflux disease (GERD) is the hypofunctioning of the lower esophageal sphincter (LES) and/or persistent increases in intra-abdominal pressure.[1] The hypofunctioning LES allows acid to reflux into the esophagus, causing symptoms of heartburn, retrosternal pressure, nausea with or without vomiting, water brash, and sometimes bronchospasm. Reflux tends to worsen with intake of dietary fats, chocolate, peppermint, caffeine, alcohol, and tobacco, when lying flat on one's back, and with lying down within 1 h of eating.

Although the role of hiatal hernia in GERD is controversial, this condition has re-emerged as a possible contributing factor. Gastroparesis caused by disorders such as diabetes or viral infection may contribute to reflux of acid and food contents into the esophagus because of increased gastric pressure. Irritation of the esophageal tissues by gastric acid due to GERD leads to cellular changes in the esophageal mucosa (Barrett's esophagus) and thus to increased risk for esophageal cancer.

Pediatric Issues

Significant reflux occurs in 18% of all infants and is more common in those who are premature. Since 90% of these infants experience spontaneous resolution of the disorder by the ages of 12–18 months, management is aimed at reassuring parents, and at instructing them in correct postural and feeding techniques.[2]

Obstetric Issues

In pregnancy, chronic increased abdominal pressure is associated with the development or worsening of pre-existing GERD. The primary etiology for GERD in pregnancy is a decreased lower esophageal sphincter resting tone due to high levels of progesterone and estrogen. Treatment is focused on control of symptoms throughout the term of the pregnancy.

Geriatric Issues

Patients with long-standing disease may be at risk for Barrett's esophagitis, changes in the epithelium from squamous to columnar tissue that may lead to adenocarcinoma formation.

Epidemiology

Ten percent of adults experience daily symptoms of reflux, while 30% have symptoms at least once a month,[5] and 85% of all patients respond completely to nonsurgical interventions.

Treatment Options

The goals of treatment are to minimize long-term complications by decreasing gastroesophageal reflux, lessening its harmful effects, and promoting esophageal clearance. In mild cases, treatment includes

* Weight reduction
* Elevation of the head of the bed by 15 degrees
* Avoidance of lying down after meals
* Taking medications with sufficient amounts of water
* Dietary modifications that include eating smaller meals, limiting fat intake, and avoiding symptom-producing substances such as tobacco, alcohol, chocolate, peppermint, and coffee

In moderate cases, treatment includes reinforcement of the measures utilized in mild cases along with the addition of anti-acids after meals and at bedtime or H_2 blocker medications to reduce the amount of acid produced by the stomach. In more severe cases, the use of proton pump inhibitors, such as omeprazole (Prilosec), to block excess acid production, and prokinetic medications, such as metoclopramide (Reglan), may be considered. (Cisapride [Propulsid] was removed from the market in 2000.)

Drugs generally to be avoided include anticholinergics and calcium channel blockers; however, these may prove useful when LES spasm is a component of the overall problem.

Specialty referral for endoscopy and possible biopsy is elective with mild, recurrent GERD but is mandatory if abnormalities are demonstrated on upper GI series studies, if symptoms appear refractory to conservative management, or if there are complicating associated factors. Advanced cases refractory to the preceding treatments may require surgical intervention, including fundoplication or crural tightening.

Patient Education

Patients should be instructed in dietary modifications that include eating smaller meals, decreasing fat intake, and avoiding substances such as alcohol, chocolate, peppermint, coffee, and citrus fruits that produce symptoms. The patient should also be instructed to elevate the head of his or her bed 15 degrees (using 4- to 6-in firm blocks, not pillows or foam wedges), and to avoid the ingestion of food or fluids within 1 h before retiring. Weight reduction and smoking cessation plans should be included if applicable.

Prevention

Effective treatment of GERD diminishes the risk of complications such as bronchospasm, esophageal stricture, and Barrett's esophagus.

Many patients with asthma suffer from asymptomatic GERD that compromises their asthma control. Frequently an asthmatic patient's personal best peak air flow may be improved with effective GERD treatment.

Screening Recommendations

There are no primary preventive strategies other than treatment for mild disease. Severe and refractory forms of disease require endoscopy and biopsy to screen for complications such as Barrett's esophagus or strictures.

▰▰▰GASTRITIS AND PEPTIC ULCER DISEASE

Pathophysiology

Gastritis is defined as the inflammation of the gastric mucosa by excess acid, infection, or toxins (e.g., alcohol). Peptic ulcer disease (PUD) refers to ulceration of the stomach or duodenum. Both gastritis and PUD cause symptoms of epigastric pain, bleeding (often subclinical), and scarring that may lead to the obstruction of outflow. Episodes of gastric ulcer pain typically occur in clusters with symptom-free intervals. Pain is often relieved with antacids and precipitated by food, and it often radiates to the back. Duodenal ulcer pain may awaken a patient at night, is classically relieved by food, and resumes 2–3 h after ingestion of a meal.

Most peptic ulcers occur in the stomach or duodenum, with about 80% occurring in the duodenum. The precise mechanism for ulcer development is incompletely understood, but acid production, pepsin secretion, and decreased mucosal defense mechanisms play a role. Excess acid production tends to correlate more strongly with duodenal ulcer formation than with gastric ulcer formation.[1, 2]

Helicobacter pylori infection is associated with 95% of duodenal ulcers. The exact role of *H. pylori* in the pathogenesis of PUD is unknown, but it is believed that the organism causes the mucosa to be more susceptible to injury by acid and pepsin. Over two thirds of the world's population is infected with *H. pylori*, but most people do not exhibit symptoms.

H. pylori is a bacterial infection that has been associated with some ulcers, chronic gastritis, and iron deficiency anemia. It may be associated with an increased incidence of gastric malignancies. Although breath screening and serologic tests are available, treatment should be based on definitive biopsy cultures. Multiple drug regimens exist, and the health care provider's choice of treatment should be guided by cost, safety, patient compliance, and efficacy. Current recommendations may be found in the *Sanford Guide to Antimicrobial*

Therapy or at the Centers for Disease Control and Prevention web site, cdc.gov.

Nonsteroidal anti-inflammatory drugs (NSAIDs) also play a role in the development of gastritis and PUD through two mechanisms. First, NSAIDs are potent inhibitors of gastric mucosal prostaglandin synthesis, which normally protects the mucosa. Second, they cause direct erosion of the mucosa. However, the most common cause of upper GI bleeding due to NSAIDs is gastritis rather than PUD.

Other precipitants or risk factors of gastritis and PUD include

* Increased stress levels
* Tobacco use
* Excess alcohol and coffee intake
* Age over 50
* Heredity and type A blood

High stress levels cause an increase in acid production that increases the chance of ulcer formation. The number of cigarettes smoked correlates directly with the risk of gastric ulcer formation. Coffee stimulates acid production more than other beverages containing caffeine. Alcohol compromises the gastric mucosal barrier in addition to causing acid hypersecretion. Heredity may cause some individuals to have higher levels of food-stimulated gastrin release and pepsin secretion, and heredity certainly contributes to whether a person tends to internalize stress.

Duodenal ulceration does not correlate highly with carcinoma formation; however, *H. pylori* infection and gastric ulcers have been linked to the formation of gastric carcinoma.

Pediatric Issues

While GERD and functional bowel disease are much more common in the pediatric population, children may develop gastritis and ulcers. *H. pylori* infection may be diagnosed as part of a work-up for refractory iron deficiency anemia.

Obstetric Issues

GERD is the most common GI symptom in pregnancy after the nausea of morning sickness resolves. Acute gastritis and PUD are relatively rare but are treated in much the same manner as GERD, with antacids and H_2 blockers.

Geriatric Issues

Increased age is a risk factor for gastritis and PUD. The older individual is at increased risk for symptoms and GI bleeding due to gastritis and PUD because older patients are more likely to be on chronic treatment with NSAIDs for other conditions, and because natural tissue protective factors decrease with aging.

Epidemiology

PUD affects up to 10% of the United States population at some time during their lifetime. Male to female ratio in the past was 2:1; however, this gap is narrowing.[3] Peak prevalence of ulcer formation in men is between the ages of 45 and 64 years.

Treatment Options

Many ulcers heal within 4 weeks, especially with support of H_2 blocking medications and antacids. However, recurrences are common, and patients must be made aware of the potential for future symptoms. Regardless of the medications used for treatment, all patients with PUD should discontinue use of NSAIDs, eliminate tobacco and alcohol use, and develop coping strategies to reduce stress. NSAIDs, especially the newer cyclooxygenase (COX-2) inhibitors such as Celebrex and Vioxx, may be reintroduced after an ulcer heals if the benefits outweigh the risks.

No standard treatment regimen has been developed. Antacids are safe and may be used in frequent doses to neutralize acid. If symptoms are unrelieved, H_2 receptor blockers may be instituted to decrease 50–80% of acid formation. Proton pump inhibitors block 90% of acid production and should be reserved for refractory symptoms or disease owing to their relatively higher costs.

Sucralfate suspension is dosed frequently and binds to the gastric mucosa, forming a protective barrier and inhibiting pepsin activity. This medication is especially useful in the patient who continues to smoke, or in the patient in the intensive care unit (ICU) who will require a nasogastric (NG) tube. NG tubes break the natural esophagogastic barrier and thus increase the risk of aspiration. Sucralfate for ICU "stress ulcers" is superior to H_2 blockers in patients who require an NG tube, as this medication does not alter the gastric pH. Although neither medication affects the risk of aspiration, aspiration pneumonia is less likely when normal gastric pH is preserved.

Misoprostol helps to counteract the prostaglandin inhibition of NSAIDs and is usually given in conjunction when NSAIDs are absolutely necessary in high-risk patients. This medication unfortunately has been associated with GI intolerance and is expensive.

For *H. pylori*-induced disease, triple medication therapy is indicated (see the preceding discussion of pathophysiology).

Routine imaging or endoscopy is not necessary in all patients; however, endoscopy with biopsy is recommended for patients with refractory symptoms and/or recurrences, especially those over age 40. Symptoms of outlet obstruction or bleeding also require endoscopic investigation. Refractory cases should be evaluated to rule out Zollinger-Ellison syndrome, especially if there are multiple ulcerations.

Patients with an active GI bleed should be hospitalized for proper management. Surgical treatment may be necessary for recurrent bleeding, perforation, or outlet obstruction, or in the most medically refractory cases.

Patient Education

Patients should be counseled to eliminate tobacco and alcohol use, reduce stress, and avoid use of NSAIDs. Patients should be aware that recurrences are possible, and they should notify their physician for any persistent symptoms or evidence of GI bleeding. Although some patients may have problems complying with the multidrug therapy for the treatment of *H. pylori* infection, the risks associated with incomplete eradication of the bacteria must be communicated to them and the cost of the treatment course weighed against the patient's probable compliance problems.

Prevention

Lifestyle modifications such as eliminating tobacco and alcohol use, stress reduction, and the avoidance of NSAIDs may decrease the probability of developing gastritis or ulcer and certainly decreases the risk of recurrence. Treatment of *H. pylori* gastritis and instituting the preceding prevention measures will reduce the risk of complications such as development of subsequent ulcers, upper GI bleed, perforation, pancreatitis, and obstruction.

Screening Recommendations

There are no screening recommendations for gastritis or PUD. Screening all individuals within a community for the presence of *H. pylori* and providing subsequent treatment is not a realistic expectation owing to cost, compliance problems, and the probability of reinfection.

▬ GALLBLADDER DISEASE

Pathophysiology

The biliary tree consists of a duct system that drains bile and other liver byproducts from the liver into the small intestine. Gallstones can occur within the gallbladder itself or within the ducts leading to and from the gallbladder. The majority of gallstones in Americans are composed of cholesterol and bile salts.[1, 4]

Acute cholelithiasis symptoms occur when a gallstone becomes lodged in the duct system, preventing proper drainage. The ensuing pain is known as biliary colic, an acute onset, right upper quadrant, or epigastric pain that is stabbing in nature and radiates to the right or left scapula. Symptoms typically last 2–4 h and are associated with nausea and vomiting and dyspepsia. Fatty or spicy food intolerance may precipitate attacks of biliary colic. Untreated disease may lead to complications such as jaundice, cholangeitis, or pancreatitis in approximately 20% of patients.

Acute cholecystitis, inflammation from an infection of the gallbladder, causes classic biliary colic without dyspepsia. Patients often have an elevated white blood cell count and fever, and may have coexisting cholelithiasis and/or pancreatitis.

Pediatric Issues

Children with hemoglobinopathies (such as sickle cell disease or thalassemias) frequently develop gallbladder disease. Any infant who develops jaundice, has an increased level of hepatic enzymes, and has decreased stool production must be evaluated for improper ductal development (i.e., biliary atresia).

Obstetric Issues

Gallstones develop frequently in pregnancy but usually do not become symptomatic until after delivery. Pain and elevated transaminase levels during pregnancy must be distinguished from more critical conditions such as preeclampsia and acute fatty liver. Pregnancy is not a contraindication to acute surgical intervention.

♣

Geriatric Issues

The classic symptoms of postprandial colicky pain located in the right upper quadrant and radiating to the flanks and shoulders may be minimal or absent in the elderly, making diagnosis difficult. This population is more at risk for cholecystitis, especially in association with diabetes mellitus. Because gallstones may be occult or atypical in presentation, an abdominal sonogram should be considered as part of any evaluation of GI complaints, abdominal discomfort, abdominal mass, or sepsis of unknown etiology.

Epidemiology

Gallbladder disease affects over 20 million Americans each year, with over 475,000 cholecystectomies performed for surgical cure. An estimated 25% of all persons over 50 years of age will develop gallstones.[5]

Treatment Options

In most cases, symptoms of gallstones are mild or absent. Asymptomatic disease may be left untreated, since the majority of patients do not develop complications. Cholecystectomy is not indicated in individuals incidentally discovered to have stones.

Once an individual has symptomatic disease, recurrence of symptoms is common, and treatment should be tailored to the individual. Patients with recurrent attacks should be counseled to undergo elective surgical evaluation and cholecystectomy. Laparoscopic methods have decreased mortality and morbidity and have shortened recovery time, so that the benefits of this procedure far outweigh the risks in the average patient. Patients unwilling or too fragile to undergo surgery may elect lithotripsy or dissolution by cholesterol stone solubilizing agents such as Actigall (ursodiol) or Chenix (chenodiol).

Patients with acute cholecystitis require hospitalization for diagnosis, intravenous fluids, bowel rest, parenteral antibiotics, and surgical consultation. Pain control is essential. Opiates, such as morphine, should be avoided in favor of synthetic opiates, such as meperidine or fentanyl, as opiates can worsen or trigger spasm in the sphincter of Odi.

Patient Education

Women on oral contraceptives need to be aware of their increased risk of developing gallstones and should be taught the signs and symptoms of gallbladder disease. Weight reduction is helpful in decreasing the risk of developing disease. The importance of early surgical treatment in symptomatic disease should be emphasized.

Prevention

Risk factors associated with the development of gallstones include

* Use of oral contraceptives
* Female gender
* Obesity
* Multiparity

* Age greater than 40 years, especially patients with diabetes
* Native American ancestry
* Hemoglobinopathy

Gallstones are associated with acute and chronic cholecystitis, empyema of the gallbladder, cholangeitis with infection of the biliary tree, and pancreatitis. Treatment and prevention of gallstones can minimize long-term complications. While gallbladder cancer is more common in patients with long-term stones, it is such a rarity that prophylactic removal of the gallbladder in cases of asymptomatic disease is not recommended.

Screening Recommendations

There are no primary screening measures for gallbladder disease. A high index of suspicion should be maintained in patients with the risk factors previously described, so that atypical presentations are not overlooked.

■■■ PANCREATITIS

Pathophysiology

The pancreas is both an endocrine (insulin- and glucagon-producing) and exocrine (proteolytic enzyme-producing) gland. Approximately 90% of the pancreas must be damaged before the maldigestion of fat and protein is manifested. Acute pancreatic damage is the result of inflammation that causes the release of proteolytic enzymes that autodigest the gland. Pancreatic pseudocysts and abscesses due to infection are common sequelae of inflammation.[1, 3, 4]

Pancreatitis can be acute, relapsing, or chronic. Chronic pancreatitis follows a course of acute, recurrent attacks. Often, chronic disease is seen in alcoholic individuals and in patients with hemochromatosis. The manifestations of chronic pancreatitis are related to the degree of endocrine and exocrine insufficiency from pancreatic destruction. Patients may exhibit weight loss and steatorrhea from pancreatic insufficiency.

Pediatric Issues

Children with cystic fibrosis are at greater risk for developing pancreatitis. The etiology in children is unknown in 25% of cases. Infectious processes such as mumps, hemolytic uremic syndrome, Kawasaki disease, Coxsackie virus, *Mycoplasma,* viral hepatitis, influenza, and Reye's syndrome have been implicated. The use of valproic acid, acetaminophen, and sulfonamides is also associated with the development of pancreatitis.

Obstetric Issues

The incidence of pancreatitis in pregnancy is unknown but is thought to be less than in the population at large. However, mortality is higher with occurrences in pregnancy owing to delay in diagnosis and treatment. Preterm labor is more common in women with pancreatitis than in women without disease. Inpatient treatment is the same as for nonpregnant patients, with the exception that parenteral nutrition is considered sooner because caloric requirements are higher.

Geriatric Issues

Delay in diagnosis due to atypical or muted presentations in this population is a special problem. Almost all etiologies of pancreatitis increase with aging.[5]

Epidemiology

Five thousand new cases of acute pancreatitis occur in the U.S. every year, with a 10% mortality rate.

The incidence of chronic pancreatitis in the U.S. is largely unknown but is estimated at 8.2 new cases per 100,000 population each year, with a prevalence of 26.4 cases per 100,000.

Treatment Options

Approximately 50% of all acute pancreatitis cases are self-limited, and patients will recover with fluid replacement, bowel rest, and pain medication. Medications commonly used to decrease pancreatic stimulation include H_2 receptor antagonists, antacids, and anticholinergics. Sometimes prolonged bowel rest, requiring parenteral nutrition, is necessary to allow pancreatic recovery. Low-fat diets are generally advisable in the acute recovery phase despite the primary etiology. Any identifiable causes, including alcohol abuse, stones, hypertriglyceridemia, or hypercalcemia, should be identified and treated.

Patients with chronic disease may usually be managed with outpatient therapy.

Medication interventions depending on the degree of endocrine and exocrine deficiency include:

- Pancreatic enzyme replacement
- Insulin

* H$_2$ blockers or proton pump inhibitors
* Bicarbonate
* Tricyclic antidepressants for chronic pain management
* Cautious use of narcotics for exacerbations of pain

Severe pain, vomiting, and volume depletion may require hospitalization. Surgical procedures have been tried with limited success for patients with intractable pain associated with chronic disease.

Patient Education

The patient with pancreatitis must abstain from all alcohol and recreational drugs. Recurrences are uncommon if the precipitating cause is identified and treated. Patients should limit fat in the diet if they suffer from steatorrhea. A patient with chronic pancreatitis should be carefully instructed concerning the abuse-potential of any narcotic pain medications.

Prevention

Please see the preceding discussion of patient education.

Screening Recommendations

No screening is currently recommended.

APPENDICITIS

Pathophysiology

The appendix is located distal to the junction of the ascending colon and ileum. It is a cylindrical cavity that opens into the ascending colon and has no apparent function. Acute appendicitis is inflammation, and often obstruction, of the appendix cavity. In approximately two thirds of all acutely inflamed appendices, obstruction of the proximal lumen by fibrous bands, fecaliths, parasites, or lymphoid hyperplasia can be identified. In the remaining third, obstruction is not demonstrated.[4] Fecaliths and calculi are considered causative agents of obstruction, with fecaliths being five times more common.[4]

Appendicitis may become complicated by abscess formation, with distention of the lumen by pus. Although the timing is variable, gangrene and perforation generally occur within approximately 24 h of the beginning of the acute process.[1, 3, 4, 6]

The location of the appendix and the location of the inflammation and pain make the differential diagnosis of appendicitis challenging, especially in the female patient. Classic appendicitis is characterized by periumbilical pain that becomes localized to the right lower quadrant, usually within the first few hours of onset. Pain precedes other symptoms such as peritoneal irritation and spasm of the abdominal wall musculature, which produces involuntary guarding by the patient. Approximately 85% of patients experience associated emesis. Leukocytosis can support the diagnosis but is nonspecific; if the patient is immunocompromised, the white blood cell count may be normal or subnormal. Differentiation of appendicitis from a variety of common diseases affecting women can be challenging. These diseases include pelvic inflammatory disease, ruptured tubal pregnancy, twisted ovarian cyst, and endometriosis.

After perforation occurs, pain may transiently disappear, to be followed by more generalized pain, fever, and signs of sepsis.

Pediatric Issues

Appendicitis is often seen in children but is relatively less common before puberty. The risk of perforation may be greater because of more rapid culmination of disease and the younger child's difficulty in communicating history. Ultrasonographic studies frequently aid in the difficult diagnosis but are operator dependent. A relatively new imaging technique, computed tomography with rectal contrast (CTRC), used when the sonographic study is negative, can increase the accuracy of diagnosis to 94%.[7]

Obstetric Issues

Appendicitis is the most common nonobstetric surgical emergency during pregnancy, and prompt diagnosis and treatment are paramount to the safety of the mother and the fetus. Diagnostic delays can occur because of the displacement of the appendix from its usual location by the enlarging womb. Delays in surgery may result in perforation and generalized peritonitis owing to the omentum being less available to contain infection.[4] The differential diagnosis can include placental abruption, complications associated with preeclampsia, pyelonephritis, ovarian pathology, and acute cholecystitis.

Geriatric Issues

Presenting signs and symptoms may be atypical in this age group, making the diagnosis difficult. Appendicitis tends to fulminate more rapidly in the elderly, and prompt surgical intervention is necessary.

In adults, the CTRC scan is 98% accurate and should be considered when a diagnosis is unclear.[7]

Epidemiology

Peak incidence occurs between the late teens and early twenties. Men are more frequently affected than women at a ratio of 3:2. During the remainder of life, this condition affects the sexes equally.[1] An estimated 7% of the population in Western countries develops appendicitis some time during their life. Approximately 200,000 appendectomies are performed every year in the U.S.[4] Incidence is rare at the extremes of age; however, perforation is more common in infancy and in the elderly, resulting in a greater mortality in these age groups.[1]

Treatment Options

Accurate assessment and prompt referral to a surgeon are crucial for a favorable outcome. Serial abdominal examinations usually clarify diagnosis. If there is any suspicion of appendicitis, laxatives and enemas should be avoided until appendicitis is ruled out.

Antibiotics are avoided if appendicitis is suspected because antibiotics may mask early perforation.

Traditional open and laparoscopic surgical techniques are commonly employed in appendectomies.

Patient Education

Patients need to be told of incidental appendectomies performed during other abdominal surgeries and should ideally communicate this information to their primary care providers to lessen the chance of future diagnostic dilemmas. The patient with possible early appendicitis must clearly understand the importance of the surgical referral, as early intervention greatly lessens the probability of postoperative complications.

Prevention

There is no primary prevention, but prompt surgical care is essential to prevent the complications of perforation. Perforation in women of childbearing age may contribute to future infertility. Incidental appendectomies are commonly performed during other abdominal surgeries to prevent the risks of undiagnosed appendicitis.

Screening Recommendations

There are currently no screening recommendations for primary prevention of appendicitis. Secondary prevention is accomplished by incidental appendectomy during other abdominal procedures.

▄▄▄▄FUNCTIONAL BOWEL DISEASE

Pathophysiology

Functional bowel disease accounts for a great majority of general and specialty office visits for GI problems. The disease is defined as "a variable combination of chronic or recurrent GI symptoms not explained by structural or biochemical abnormalities."[2] Both irritable bowel syndrome and non-ulcer dyspepsia are included in the category of functional bowel disease. Irritable bowel syndrome is characterized by large bowel pain, difficult defecation, abdominal distention, and episodic constipation and/or diarrhea. Dyspepsia is characterized by bloating, nausea, and abdominal discomfort or pain. Both syndromes seem to be largely linked to emotional factors.[2, 4, 6]

No identifiable defects cause the symptoms of irritable bowel syndrome or non-ulcer dyspepsia. Rather, it is theorized that symptoms are caused by functional disturbances of motor activity or visceral sensation. Functional disturbance can be triggered by either emotional factors or luminal irritants. Patients with irritable bowel syndrome have an increase in non-propulsive bowel contractions compared with the general population. If the increased contractions occur in the small bowel, the patient exhibits symptoms of diarrhea. If contractions occur in the colon, the patient exhibits primarily symptoms of constipation. Patients with irritable bowel syndrome have lower thresholds for reflex motor activity when tested via balloon manometry, indicating a greater sensitivity to luminal irritation.

Stress levels have also been implicated in worsening or precipitating symptoms of irritable bowel. Lactose intolerance, food allergies, sorbitol ingestion, and bile acid malabsorption have also been theorized to play a role.

Non-ulcer dyspepsia is believed to result from dysfunctional GI motility, with many patients exhibiting delayed gastric emptying. *H. pylori* has been considered to play a role in the origin of non-ulcer dyspepsia, but evidence has not substantiated this claim. Patients with this sydrome do not have increased acid production when compared with the general population, but they seem to benefit from H_2 receptor blocking drugs. Emotional factors influence dyspepsia, but not as greatly as with irritable bowel syndrome.

Pediatric Issues

Management is not significantly affected by age.

Obstetric Issues

Management is not significantly affected.

Geriatric Issues

Management is not significantly affected by age.

Epidemiology

Approximately 50% of all GI motility and discomfort complaints are due to irritable bowel syndrome. It is estimated that 20% of all patients suffer from some aspect of this disease on a continuous or recurrent basis.[2] Non-ulcer dyspepsia is twice as common as peptic ulcer disease.

Treatment Options

Treatment of functional disorders necessitates a supportive provider-patient relationship. No single regimen is most effective; rather, treatment must be tailored to individual symptoms. Appropriate testing must be conducted to rule out diseases such as inflammatory bowel disease, PUD, *H. pylori* infection, infectious diarrhea, carcinoma, bowel obstruction, and diverticulosis.

Patients with irritable bowel syndrome may benefit from tricyclic antidepressants (if prone to diarrheal complaints), selective serotonin reuptake inhibitors (SSRIs), or anxiolytics. Dietary modifications to increase fluids and fiber to restore propulsion may be beneficial. It is helpful to eliminate irritating foods such as sorbitol, caffeine, alcohol, citrus fruits, and any foods that trigger symptoms. Patients with constipation often benefit from the use of prokinetics. Patients who primarily have diarrhea may benefit from the use of loperamide. Anticholinergic medications may help patients suffering from abdominal distention.

The pathophysiology of non-ulcer dyspepsia is poorly understood; therefore, treatment of this syndrome is often not successful. Patients are often tried on antacids, H_2 receptor blockers, or proton pump inhibitors, but any positive outcomes are generally attributed to the placebo effect. Short-term use of metoclopramide has been shown to provide relief by promoting gastric motility. Unfortunately, the drug is not very useful for long-term use.

Patient Education

Patients must be well supported owing to the frustration that accompanies chronic, recurring symptoms. Dietary modifications mentioned previously, antidepressant therapy, and counseling to reduce stress may be beneficial. Somatization is common among patients with functional bowel disorders. Patients should be told that their mortality rates are no different from those of the general population, and that functional disease does not predispose them to develop more serious diseases in the future.

Prevention

Please see the preceding discussion of patient education.

Screening Recommendations

There is no recommended screening for functional bowel disease. The provider is reminded that this disease is a diagnosis of exclusion and that it may be necessary to perform testing to rule out more serious disease processes.

■ HERNIA

Pathophysiology

In general, a hernia is defined as an abnormal protrusion of intra-abdominal tissue through an anatomical defect in the musculofascial layer. The size and rigidity of the anatomical defect determine the characteristics of the hernia. Congenital factors and/or increased intra-abdominal pressure may contribute to hernia formation. The most common types of hernias may be classified as inguinal, ventral, or femoral.

The anatomic defect in inguinal hernias involves the abnormal development of the structures of the inguinal canal. Femoral hernias pass beneath the inguinal canal and through the femoral ring. Ventral hernias may be epigastric, umbilical (through the umbilical ring), or incisional (through the scar of a previous incision). A reducible hernia is freely movable through the anatomic defect. An incarcerated hernia is not freely movable through the anatomic defect. A strangulated hernia is an incarcerated hernia with severely limited or absent blood supply owing to edema and ischemia.[3, 4]

Inguinal hernias may be indirect, in which the anatomical defect is congenital, or direct, in which the anatomical defect is acquired.

Pediatric Issues

Indirect inguinal hernias are more common in males and premature infants. In infants, the repair of an uncomplicated, reducible hernia is indicated as soon as is practical to prevent complications of strangulation, bowel obstruction and necrosis, and testicular infarction. Ideally the procedure should be managed electively by practitioners with experience in the surgery and anesthesiology of the infant.

Obstetric Issues

Incisional or ventral hernias may become increasingly uncomfortable during pregnancy. A pregnancy girdle or "belly bra" can provide substantial support and comfort for the pregnant patient with a ventral or an incisional hernia. However, should an acute incarceration occur, surgery should not be deferred.

Geriatric Issues

The elderly generally tolerate hernia repair well. The risk of surgical complications in mild, elective cases is less than the risk of strangulated hernia repair under emergency conditions.

Epidemiology

Approximately 700,000 inguinal hernias are surgically repaired each year. Indirect inguinal hernias account for approximately 50% of all hernias, and are 8–10 times more frequent in men than in women. Femoral hernias are 3–5 times more common in women than in men. However, inguinal hernias are twice as common in women than in femoral hernias. The incidence of direct inguinal hernia increases with advancing age.

The rate of a first-time recurrence of an inguinal hernia is 10%. The rate for subsequent recurrence is 35%.[3] The relative risk of incarceration and strangulation of groin hernias, from lowest to highest, is direct → indirect → femoral.

Treatment Options

In infants, all inguinal hernias require prompt referral for surgical intervention, even in the absence of complications. However, uncomplicated reducible inguinal hernias in adults may be conservatively managed. Patients may elect to undergo surgery for symptomatic improvement, or may manage symptoms with lifestyle modifications such as careful lifting and the use of a truss. If signs of incarceration develop, gentle reduction (taxis) may be attempted while referral is made for urgent surgical evaluation. If a hernia has become strangulated, emergency surgery is necessary. In patients with respiratory disease such as emphysema, smoking cessation is important because chronic cough may cause the development or worsening of a hernia. Respiratory diseases also increase risks at the time of surgery.

Patient Education

As part of general health, patients should be instructed as to proper lifting techniques. The presence of a hernia may preclude certain physical duties if found during a pre-employment or athletic physical examination. Patients should be advised as to the signs and symptoms of incarceration if surgical consultation is deferred.

Prevention

Proper lifting posture and stance along with abdominal supports for persons engaged in heavy lifting can reduce back strain; however, evidence is equivocal in terms of preventing acquired hernias.

Screening Recommendations

Well child checkups and directed health examinations for adults should include abdominal palpation and maneuvers to screen for hernias. Most pre-employment examinations require hernia evaluation.

▬ INFLAMMATORY BOWEL DISEASE

PSEUDOMEMBRANOUS COLITIS

Pseudomembranous colitis (PMC) is a form of inflammatory bowel disease associated with antibiotic use and superinfection with *Clostridium difficile*. The initial presentation of another form of inflammatory bowel disease could be clouded by the fact that 10% of the population is known to have *C. difficile* occurring normally in the intestines. Stool cultures for *C. difficile* toxin and sigmoidoscopy usually clarify the diagnosis. The mucosa becomes denuded and hemorrhagic. While certain antibiotics seem to have an increased association with this disorder, any antibiotic may be linked to it.[1, 2, 6, 8]

ULCERATIVE COLITIS AND CROHN'S DISEASE

Ulcerative colitis and Crohn's disease account for most incidences of chronic inflammatory bowel disease. Both diseases tend to follow chronic, unpredictable courses of exacerbations and remissions. Exact etiologies are unknown, and often the diseases are diagnoses of exclusion. Both are likely to have a psychological or emotional component, as there is a temporal relationship between flare-ups of disease and major psychological stresses. Familial and racial tendencies in disease formation suggest possible genetic causes. Symptoms of both diseases include diarrhea, bleeding, tenesmus (a constant feeling of the need to empty the bowels, associated with pain, cramping, and involuntary efforts at straining), and vague abdominal pain. In severe cases, anorexia, weight loss, and fever are common with an acute exacerbation.

Ulcerative colitis is an idiopathic, diffuse inflammatory condition of the colonic mucosa. The inflammation is continuous along the mucosa without skipped areas, causing a tubular appearance and loss of haustral markings. Highly affected areas include the rectum and the sigmoid and descending colon. Sigmoidoscopy often demonstrates a loss of the appearance of the submucosal vessels and a granular-appearing, friable mucosal surface. If the case is advanced, pseudopolyps and discrete ulcers may be seen along the tubular, inflamed area. Biopsies and mucus smears reveal the presence of leukocytes. The disease is believed to be of autoimmune origins (antibodies to intestinal epithelial antigens are detected in many patients).

Signs and symptoms outside the GI tract are often associated with ulcerative colitis. A monoarticular, migrating arthritis can be seen in up to 10% of patients. Also, uveitis, aphthous ulcers, skin lesions, and GI bleeding may be present, especially during flare-ups. The risk of colon cancer is increased with ulcerative colitis and is related to the severity and duration of the disease. The risk of developing cancer increases after being afflicted by the disease for 8 or more years.

Crohn's disease, or regional enteritis, is also a chronic condition marked by exacerbations and remissions. This disease may involve the entire GI tract from the mouth to the anus and is characterized by skip lesions of granular inflammation affecting the entire bowel wall (not just the mucosa). The areas most involved include the distal ileum and the ascending colon.

In approximately 20% of cases, arthritis, uveitis, erythema nodosum, ankylosing spondylitis, or aphthous ulcers may be associated with Crohn's disease. Long-standing disease may lead to formation of abscesses, fistulas, or strictures, but there seems to be no increased risk of developing colon cancer.

Pediatric Issues

Most inflammatory bowel disease does not manifest until the adolescent years. Children and adolescents with inflammatory bowel disease are usually short in stature owing to the use of corticosteroids for treatment of their disease and the malabsorption of nutrients by their diseased bowels. Ampicillin is the antibiotic most commonly associated with PMC in children.

Obstetric Issues

In the pregnant or nursing patient who experiences a flare-up of inflammatory bowel disease, steroids and sulfasalazine are considered safe. It is very important to remember that sulfasalazine significantly decreases the bioavailability of folic acid, so that when a potentially fertile or pregnant woman must take this drug, folic acid supplementation is necessary.[8] Women with ulcerative colitis may suffer an exacerbation within the first trimester of pregnancy, and their spontaneous abortion rates are higher compared with the general population. Generally there are few exacerbations during the second and third trimesters. There is no increase in fetal mortality or premature deliveries.[8] Young women should be counseled to delay childbearing until they have been in remission for at least 1 year.

Geriatric Issues

As a person with inflammatory bowel disease ages, the risk of complications such as cancer, perforations, obstructions, and fistulas increases. A high index of suspicion should be maintained for these conditions.

Epidemiology

Inflammatory bowel disease occurs more often in whites than in persons of color. Prevalence is highest in the Jewish population, with an incidence 3–6 times greater than among the non-Jewish population.[1] Both genders are affected equally. Ulcerative colitis typically manifests in the adolescent or young adult age group, while Crohn's disease tends to present with peak incidence between the second and third decades of life. A secondary peak of incidence occurs in persons 50–80 years of age.[5, 7]

Treatment Options

The primary goals of therapy are to control the inflammatory process, to replace nutritional losses, and to provide psychological support. Since these diseases follow a pattern of exacerbations and remissions, treatment is adjusted to active clinical manifestations.

In ulcerative colitis, sulfasalazine has been the traditional drug of choice for initial treatment and prevention of recurrence. This medication is generally well tolerated but may cause hemolytic side effects. Serious problems of bioavailability can occur when a health care provider attempts to use this medication along with digoxin. If the patient has a sulfa allergy, olsalazine may be used. Corticosteriods frequently may be necessary to interrupt an acute episode of inflammation. Immunosuppressives may be used in order to decrease the use of steroids. Opiates are useful in controlling diarrhea. Nutritional supplements, such as multivitamins, and high calorie-high protein diets to counter malabsorption are very important. Parenteral nutrition may be necessary during acute exacerbations and has helped many patients to avoid surgery.

Surgical intervention may be curative in some cases, but it may also be palliative. Surgery is often elected in cases of high-grade dysplasia and in cases unresponsive to other, more conservative treatments.

In Crohn's disease, a diet with sufficient protein and calories is essential to maintain nutrition. Reduction in fiber and fat is often beneficial. Vitamin supplements are useful, and in extreme cases, parenteral nutrition may be required. Sulfasalazine is sometimes used but is less effective in Crohn's disease, especially in patients with primarily small bowel disease. Corticosteroids are used in patients who have not responded to sulfasalazine and are very effective in patients with small bowel disease. Steroids are ineffective in preventing relapses. Metronidazole is effective for treating patients with colonic involvement and abscesses. Immunosuppressive drugs such as 6-mercaptopurine and azathioprine have been effective in maintaining remissions. Patients are usually treated for approximately 1 year. Thereafter, medication is stopped and the patient closely observed for recurrences.

Surgical intervention in Crohn's disease is never curative, as it may be in ulcerative colitis. Surgery is therefore limited to patients with intractable disease, perforations, or obstructions.

Pseudomembranous colitis usually responds to the withdrawal of offending antibiotics, supportive care, and/or treatment with oral vancomycin.

Patient Education

It is important to emphasize that most patients with inflammatory bowel disease lead normal lives without significant increase in mortality. The importance of adherence to a medication regimen should be stressed. Actions and side effects of medications, especially of corticosteroids, should be explained.

The role of emotional and psychological health in inflammatory bowel disease is important, as exacerbations tend to occur during times of stress. Strategies for enhancing coping skills are important. It is also important to recognize early symptoms of depression. Patients should increase intake of calories, protein, and vitamins, especially during symptomatic episodes. Patients should also be taught to recognize early symptoms of exacerbations and should seek medical help as soon as possible.

Prevention

Treatment is aimed at symptomatic relief and prevention of complications such as malnutrition, anemia, bowel resection, fistulas, perforation, obstruction, arthropathy, gallbladder disease, and peritonitis.

Barium enemas are often insensitive for inflammatory bowel disease; therefore, flexible sigmoidoscopy and colonoscopy are periodically necessary for monitoring disease. Any patient who experiences new-onset chronic diarrhea and/or rectal bleeding must have an endoscopy and a biopsy to establish or rule out the diagnosis of inflammatory bowel disease.

Screening Recommendations

Periodic screenings such as annual colonoscopy for early detection of cancer are recommended, especially in patients with long-standing ulcerative colitis. Active screening for complications of long-term use of corticosteriods, such as diabetes, hypertension, and osteoporosis, is recommended.

▬OTHER PERTINENT GASTROINTESTINAL DISORDERS

Owing to the extensive list of pathologies of the GI system, all conditions are not fully outlined. The following are a list of conditions of which the clinician should be aware to fully understand and provide effective patient education and preventive measures.

ESOPHAGEAL DISORDERS

Achalasia. This disorder is characterized by the reduced ability to move food down the esophagus and the inability of the lower esophageal sphincter to relax in response to swallowing. Etiologies can include nerve injury, parasitic infestations, and inheritance. Overall incidence is 2 out of 10,000 persons, but incidence increases with age.

Barrett's Esophagus. Irritation of the esophageal tissues by gastric acid due to GERD leads to cellular changes in the esophageal mucosa, presenting an increased risk for esophageal cancer.

Benign Stricture. This narrowing of the esophagus that causes swallowing problems occurs in 2 out of 1000 persons. Etiologies include GERD, ingestion of corrosives, viral or bacterial infections, treatment of esophageal varices, or the prolonged use of an NG tube.

Mallory-Weiss Tear. More properly described as a mucosal laceration at the cardioesophageal junction, this tearing, often accompanied by significant bleeding, is caused by forceful or prolonged vomiting or coughing. Predisposing factors include binge alcohol drinking, violent coughing episodes, or seizures. Incidence is 4 out of 100,000 persons.

Schatzki's Ring. This is a ring of tissue located at the junction of the stomach and the esophagus. While the most common etiology is a congenital defect, and the condition is most often diagnosed because of swallowing problems, some patients may develop this condition as a result of scarring from caustic material ingestions. Incidence is 4 out of 10,000 persons.

Varices. Esophageal varices develop owing to chronic liver disease or hepatobiliary obstruction and may be asymptomatic, rupture and bleed, or lead to swallowing problems (usually from scarring resulting from sclerosing treatments at the time of bleeding).

Web. Plummer-Vinson syndrome, or an esophageal web, is a disorder linked to long-term iron deficiency anemia. These "webs" may be easily broken and bleed, and can result in swallowing problems. Correction of the anemia results in resolution of the webs.

GASTRIC DISORDERS

Bezoar. Ingestion of hair, indigestible material such as plastic bags, or fuzzy materials can lead to the formation of a ball that collects in the stomach and fails to pass into the intestines. This condition is rare and is usually seen in mentally retarded or emotionally disturbed patients.[1, 2]

Gastroparesis. This condition is that of severely impaired emptying of the stomach unrelated to obstruction. Although definitive etiology is unknown, gastroparesis is usually associated with a diabetic autonomic neuropathy or surgical injury. Incidence is approximately 3 out of 1000 persons. Treatment usually is targeted at improving control of the underlying systemic condition and involves the use of prokinetic medications. Diabetic gastroparesis can be especially difficult to treat, as patients easily become resistant to promotility agents.

HEPATIC DISORDERS

Gilbert's Syndrome. This benign condition is a multifactorial inherited disorder in metabolization of bilirubin by the liver. It may manifest through jaundice, or it may be asymptomatic and identified only incidentally through laboratory work on the basis of chronic elevation of bilirubin. The condition affects approximately 2% of the general population. Jaundice may be precipitated by exertion, dehydration, stress, fasting, or infections.

Hemochromatosis. A condition caused by excess accumulation of iron within the liver, hemochromatosis causes liver enlargement, diabetes, skin pigment changes, heart disease, testicular atrophy, arthritis, and irreversible cirrhosis. Once cirrhosis has developed it is irreversible. Etiologies include a primary genetic defect or multiple transfusions leading to hemolytic diseases. Men are affected more often than women. The condition is usually detected between the fourth and the sixth decades of life. Rare cases in childhood have been described. Family history and alcoholism are established risk factors. Screening is best performed by the transferrin saturation blood test, and hemochromatosis may be suspected in the differential diagnosis of an elevated ferritin, a rapidly progressive degenerative joint disease, or congestive heart failure. Early treatment *before* liver damage occurs is associated with a normal life expectancy.

Hepatitis and Chronic Liver Disease. Many forms of infectious, inflammatory, and toxin-induced hepatitis lead to chronic liver disease and liver failure. The most significant of these include

* Hepatitis B
* Hepatitis C
* Autoimmune hepatitis
* Alcoholic hepatitis
* Drug-induced hepatitis

Primary prevention involves vaccination for hepatitis B, practicing safe sex, and avoidance of shared needles and blood product transfusions.

Especially important is the fact that an estimated 3 million Americans are infected with the hepatitis C virus, and most are unaware of the fact that they are infected. Hepatitis C may be present for 20–30 years before symptoms are first appreciated clinically, but liver damage occurs much earlier. There is no vaccine for prophylaxis of this viral hepatitis, so avoidance of any high-risk behaviors in which body fluids are exchanged is the only form of primary prevention. However, screening, diagnosis, avoidance of toxins (e.g., alcohol) and early treatment can significantly decrease the incidence of chronic liver disease, cirrhosis, and liver cancers (see also Chapter 21, Infectious Diseases).

Alpha-1 Antitrypsin Deficiency. This genetic defect results in a deficiency of a protein that exerts a protective effect on the liver and lung, resulting in an increased incidence of chronic liver disease, cirrhosis, and premature emphysema not associated with the more common causes.[1]

CONDITIONS AFFECTING THE COLON

Angiodysplasia. This condition of dilation and thinning or distortion of the arteriolar-venule connection within the tissue of the colon is associated with aging and vascular disease. Angiodysplasia is strongly associated with both symptomatic and occult GI bleeding. Seventy-five percent of such lesions are found in the right colon. Rebleeding is common, and surgical intervention may be indicated.[5]

Chronic Diarrhea and Malabsorption.[1–4] Most of the conditions in the following list are inherited forms of chronic diarrhea and malabsorption.

* Celiac sprue or gluten malabsorption
* Cow milk protein intolerance
* Cystic fibrosis
* Disaccharide malabsorption
* Lactose intolerance

Therapy is focused on avoidance of trigger foods and on using enzyme and/or food supplements to provide lost calories, vitamins, and minerals. Celiac sprue or gluten enteropathy is associated with an increased incidence of small-bowel lymphoma in patients who are chronically noncompliant with their dietary restrictions. Since forgoing all foods with even trace amounts of barley, rye, oats, and wheat is a formidable task, periodic screening with imaging (small-bowel follow-through) or endoscopy may be indicated.

Constipation and Fecal Impaction. Although many patients associate clock-like regularity as the only normal bowel elimination pattern, in fact, there is quite a wide variety of normal patterns. Some patients may have consistently firm stools but no difficulty with defecation, while others may have frequent, soft, large-quantity, infrequent stools. Constipation exists when the stool is harder and less frequent than the patient's norm and requires significant effort in elimination. Difficult passage of large-caliber stools may lead to problems with fissures, bleeding, and hemorrhoid formation. A new change in bowel habits is considered one of the seven danger signals of cancer. Therefore, along with treating the problem, the health care provider is obligated to investigate the etiology of new constipation and consider whether a cancer evaluation is warranted. Generally, constipation results from decreased fiber or water in the diet, inadequate exercise or immobility, medication effects, and/or behavioral/psychological problems. Some other etiologies include

* Congenital diseases, including meconium plug due to cystic fibrosis, Hirschsprung's disease, or meningomyelocele
* Cow milk ingestion
* Endocrine disorders
* Endometriosis and/or pelvic masses
* Functional ileus
* Neurologic diseases, including mental retardation, cerebral palsy, stroke, or paralysis
* Malignancies

Chronic constipation and/or abuse of laxatives create difficulties in management. Any fecal impaction should be removed before attempting to retrain a patient's bowel habits. Chronic constipation may lead to the accumulation of a large mass of stool within the rectum that becomes essentially impossible to pass. Loose stool may pass around this obstruction, potentially clouding the diagnosis. A combination of oil-retention enemas and manual disimpaction followed by a cleansing enema and/or a GoLYTELY preparation is usually effective. In more resistant cases a Gastrografin enema or surgery may be required.

Patients should be instructed in self-care for constipation. Dietary interventions should include increasing fiber and bulk in the diet by encouraging increased intake of fruits, vegetables, whole grains, bran, and/or fiber supplements. The intake of water should be a minimum of six to eight glasses per day; however, this may be increased as necessary (as in the case of an outdoor laborer), provided it is not contraindicated by cardiac or renal disease limitations. Ideally patients should not count soft drinks or caffeinated beverages in their daily total water consumption. For patients who express distaste for plain water, suggest unsweetened fruit juices or "flavored" water. Regular exercise is equally important to bowel regularity. Patients confined to bed or a wheelchair should be encouraged to change positions frequently and perform leg lifts and abdominal contraction exercises. A patient's medications should be reviewed to exclude constipating prescriptions if possible.[4] Stool softeners and bulking agents such as Metamucil or Citrucel can be added to the daily preventive routine. Suppositories, gentle laxatives (such as milk of magnesia), or enemas may be used during a bowel retraining program but should be avoided long-term if at all possible, as dependence occurs. Constipation due to primary and secondary effects of pregnancy and the constipating quality of iron supplements increases problems associated with hemorrhoids and fissures.

Diverticulosis and Diverticulitis. Diverticulae, or diverticulosis, simply describes the existence of small herniations of the mucosa through a defect in the muscularis layer of the colon. These miniature "pockets" develop in response to chronic constipation and are endemic in older Americans owing to the relatively lower fiber intake of Americans compared with the inhabitants of other developed countries.

Acute diverticulitis usually manifests with left, lower quadrant pain, fever, and leukocytosis ("left sided appendicitis"). A change in bowel habits may also be noted. Symptoms and signs may be muted in the older patient. Diagnosis is frequently made clinically, but contrast computed tomographic scans may be used to clarify diagnosis and/or rule out an associated abscess. Initial treatment requires antibiotic therapy and bowel rest with a clear liquid diet. A complete colonoscopy should be planned several weeks after symptom resolution to rule out additional factors, such as a constipation-associated malignancy. Recurrent or septic bouts may require parenteral antibiotics and nutrition. Surgery is usually restricted to refractory cases or cases of perforation with peritonitis or the formation of an abscess, fistulae, or strictures.[5] Diet recommendations include avoidance of small foodstuffs that are incompletely digested and may occlude the diverticula (e.g., peanuts or popcorn).

Ischemic Colitis.[1, 5, 7] Also known as acute interstitial ischemia, ischemic colitis is an inflammatory process caused by interference with circulation to the colon. It usually affects people over the age of 50 and those with a history of peripheral vascular disease. Other risk factors include oral contraceptive therapy and a previous history that includes aortic surgery, stroke, hypotensive shock, or abdominal radiation. Prompt diagnosis and surgery may be life-saving.

Bowel Obstruction. An intestinal obstruction, whether partial or complete, is a blockage that results in the inability of the intestinal contents to move through the bowel normally. Obstructions can be precipitated by a paralytic ileus (non-mechanical) or by mechanical cause.

Etiologies of paralytic ileus include

* Gastroenteritis
* Electrolyte disturbances
* Peritonitis
* Post abdominal surgery
* Abdominal circulation injuries
* Pneumonia
* Uremia
* Sepsis

Mechanical causes of bowel obstruction include

* Intussusception (the intestines telescopes on itself)

* Volvulus (the colon twists on itself)
* Adhesions
* Hernia
* Impacted stool or gallstones
* Tumor
* Granulomatous process
* Foreign bodies

Treatment for a paralytic ileus usually includes bowel rest and nasogastric decompression while the underlying cause is treated. Surgery is usually required to relieve mechanical obstructions.

Polyps. Intestinal polyps may be benign, cause bleeding, or progress to cancer. Polyps greater than 1 cm are associated with a greater risk of cancer. Regular monitoring colonoscopy and polyp removal are indicated in most instances. Occasionally prophylaxis with sulindac (Clinoril) or surgery may be indicated. Inherited conditions associated with polyps include

* Gardner syndrome
* Peutz-Jeghers syndrome
* Familial juvenile polyposis
* Familial adenomatous polyposis

Short Bowel Syndrome. This condition of malabsorption results from surgical removal or extensive disease of a large portion of the small intestine. Risk factors include inflammatory bowel disease and necrotizing enterocolitis (usually seen in premature or stressed infants).

Toxic Megacolon. This condition is a life-threatening complication of intestinal disease that is manifest by extensive damage to both the mucosa and the underlying cellular layers of the distal colon, resulting in tremendous dilation and systemic toxicity. Toxic megacolon is usually seen in association with inflammatory bowel disease, pseudomembranous colitis, dysentery, amebiasis, or congenital Hirschsprung's disease. Contributing factors may include hypokalemia, antidiarrheal treatments (opiates and anticholinergics), and laxatives. Mortality is very high, at 20–30%, and treatment is usually surgical.

ANORECTAL DISEASE

Hemorrhoids. Hemorrhoids are dilated or varicose veins in the anorectal area. They arise from increased venous pressure secondary to straining for bowel movements, arteriovenous fistulas, or loss of fibrous rectal and sphincter support. Constipation, hypertension, pregnancy, and diets low in fiber and/or high in fat tend to foster hemorrhoid formation. Hemorrhoids occurring above the dentate line are called internal, while those below are external. Hemorrhoids may also prolapse.[1–3]

Hemorrhoids may be treated with local anesthetics, cold packs, warm sitz baths, and stool softeners. Helpful medications include topical corticosteroid suppositories and over-the-counter preparations of benzocaine or pramoxine, and Preparation H. Long-term dietary modifications, to increase fluids and fiber intake, and regular exercise are helpful in preventing recurrence. Prolapsed, thrombosed, or actively bleeding hemorrhoids not responsive to the preceding therapies deserve surgical consultation. Options include

* Acute incision and drainage of thrombosed hemorrhoids
* Rubber band ligation
* Injection of sclerosing agents (rarely used today owing to scarring of the anal canal)
* Hemorrhoidectomy (last resort for refractory disease)

Fistula-in-Ano. A communication between the perianal skin and the anal canal, fistula-in-ano usually forms as a result of a previous abscess but may also be caused by other conditions, such as proctitis or cancer. There may be a single opening or multiple openings with granulation tissue and serous drainage.

Proctitis. Proctitis is an inflammatory disease of the rectum that may result from trauma, autoimmune (inflammatory bowel) disease, and both nonsexually- and sexually-transmitted infections. Sexually-transmitted infections that can cause proctitis include chlamydia, gonorrhea, herpes, lymphogranuloma venereum, and amebiasis. Engaging in anal intercourse and ano-oral sex increases the frequency of these forms of proctitis.[8]

Proctitis can also be caused by trauma from radiotherapy or by autoinoculation (scratching the rectal area with hands contaminated with nasal or oral secretions) from infections, including group A beta-hemolytic streptococcus. Streptococcal proctitis is usually a disease of children in conjunction with a strep throat when they autoinoculate themselves.

Anal Fissure. Most fissures can be treated with lubricants, stool softeners, sitz baths, and topical analgesics. If healing does not occur after several weeks, surgical consultation is advised. Abscesses require surgical drainage under anesthesia and antibiotic therapy. Fistulas must be surgically corrected.

PEDIATRIC CONDITIONS

Although it is beyond the scope of this chapter to deal with the specifics of neonatal GI problems such as imperforate anus, gastroschisis, necrotizing enterocolitis, duodenal atresia, and esophageal atresia, some common pediatric conditions should be briefly mentioned.[5–7]

Colic. Occurring in one fifth of all infants, colic usually begins at 3 weeks of age, peaks by 6 weeks and declines by 3 months of age. It is manifested by inconsolable crying (for hours), gaseous distention of the stomach, and drawing of the legs up to the stomach, accompanied by distressing facial contortions. Caring for an infant with colic can be very frustrating and exhausting to the parent or caregiver and can lead to shaking the child in desperation. There is no evidence to support the use of such medications as simethicone and dicyclomine. Burping followed by rocking or vibrating movements can be very calming to the baby. Activities providing vibrating movements include

* Riding in an automobile
* Placing the child, appropriately strapped into an infant carrier *and* under supervision, on the floor next to an electric vacuum cleaner with its power switch set to "on"
* Placing the child, again in an infant carrier and properly supervised, on top of an automatic washing machine or clothes dryer while the appliance is in use

If the mother is breast-feeding, she should omit cruciferous vegetables and/or chocolate from her diet. The bottle-fed infant may benefit from a change to a soy or a hydrolyzed milk protein formula. Treatment of GERD may also reduce symptoms.

Newborn Jaundice. Generally newborn jaundice is a physiologic condition due to immaturity of liver function combined with the destruction of red blood cells. This jaundice usually appears between days 2 and 5 of life and resolves by 2 weeks of age. Prematurity and sepsis may worsen the physiologic process. Hydration and ultraviolet light are the only treatments required. Nonphysiologic, prolonged, or pathologic jaundice requires an extensive workup focused on congenital infection, metabolic disorders, and hemolytic disorders.

Encopresis. Encopresis should be diagnosed only in children over the age of 4 years. Encopresis is the voluntary or involuntary soiling of clothing by stool. The most common form results from chronic constipation and fecal impaction that may have begun as early as infancy. A rarer form seems to be related to emotional conflict. Whatever the etiology, the child will suffer from shame and low self-esteem and may try to hide the evidence of the condition. Incidence is probably close to 1%, and males may be more commonly affected. Treatment involves removal of impaction, treatment of constipation, and bowel retraining.[7] Constipation and encopresis can lead to problems with anal fissures.[8]

Rectal Prolapse. The abnormal protrusion of the rectal mucosa down to or through the anus, rectal prolapse usually occurs before the age of 6 and may be associated with other conditions such as parasitic infestations, cystic fibrosis, or constipation, or with chronic malabsorptive disorders such as celiac sprue.

Failure to Thrive

Failure to thrive is a general term used to describe a child who is failing to maintain growth above the third to fifth percentile. A thorough history and physical examination focusing on feedings, diet, caregiver interactions, signs of neglect and/or abuse, and chronic illness is a necessary first step in the evaluation.

REFERENCES

1. Fauci AS, Braunwald E, Isselbacher KJ, et al. (eds). Harrison's Principles of Internal Medicine, 14th ed. New York, McGraw-Hill, 1998, vol. 2, pp 1633–1645, 1658–1660.
2. Goroll AH, May LA, Mulley AG Jr. Primary Care Medicine, Office Evaluation and Management of the Adult Patient, 3rd ed. Philadelphia, J.B. Lippincott, 1995.
3. Way LW (ed). Current Surgical Diagnosis and Treatment, 10th ed. Stamford, CT, Appleton & Lange, 1994, pp 712–724.
4. Noble J, Greene HL, Levinson W, et al. (eds). Textbook of Primary Care Medicine, 2nd ed. St. Louis, Mosby, 1996, pp 676–682.
5. Abrams WB, Beers MH, Berkow R (eds). The Merck Manual of Geriatrics, 2nd ed. Merck & Co., 1995, pp 660–668, 761–765.
6. Uphold CR, Graham MV. Clinical Guidelines in Family Practice, 3rd ed. Barmarrae Books, 1998, pp 533–535, 567–571.
7. www.adam.com
8. www.cdc.gov

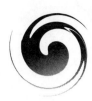

CHAPTER 21

Infectious Disease

Donna Gamero, PA-C,
Alison Ann Lauber, MD,
and Sharne Hampton, MD

INTRODUCTION

The advent of the 21st century triggers reflection on remarkable historical events, from catastrophic failures to marvelous accomplishments in the arena of infectious disease medicine and research. Deaths from infectious diseases have declined dramatically in the United States since the beginning of the 20th century (Fig. 21–1).[1] However, the last 100 years have witnessed two of the most devastating pandemics in recent human history: the 1918 influenza pandemic that caused 20 million deaths in less than 1 year and the current HIV pandemic which has, thus far, led to approximately 14 million deaths worldwide.[1]

In addition to the continued presence of such large-scale manifestations of infectious diseases, new pathogens continue to surface yearly (Table 21–1).[2] Infectious diseases in 1999 had a higher global mortality than all other causes combined.[1] Factors such as antibiotic overuse, the ability of a majority of microorganisms to evolve and experience adaptive mutations rapidly in response to their environment, and the globalization of human interactions play a role in the boundless nature of infectious diseases.

The pathophysiology and etiology of infectious diseases affect the human host structure from the cellular level to the organ and organ-system level, with all tissues potential targets of microbial pathogens. The normal, healthy patient is physiologically colonized with a myriad of beneficial microbial flora, such as bacteria and fungi, that play a role in protecting the host from infection. These include resident flora (microbes that colonize the body consistently and can re-establish themselves if disturbed) and transient flora (microbes that colonize the host for brief periods of time but are not permanently established). Infection occurs when normal body defense mechanisms (skin, mucous membranes, inflammatory mechanisms [i.e., macrophages and neutrophils] and specific immune reactions [i.e., antibodies]) are weakened, destroyed, or infiltrated by pathogenic microbial flora, leading to a cascade of events in which an infectious disease process can become initiated. Infection can also be established when the balance between beneficial microorganisms (resident or transient flora) and pathogenic microorganisms is disturbed. If the host is immunocompromised, the normal barriers to infection are no longer as effective, and the host is more susceptible to infections as well as an increased

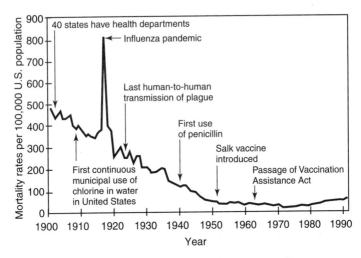

Figure 21–1. Crude death rate for infectious diseases—United States, 1900–1996. (From Achievements in public health, 1900–1999: Control of infectious diseases. MMWR Morb Mortal Wkly Rep 1999;48:621–629, adapted from Armstrong GL, Conn LA, Pinner RW. Trends in infectious disease mortality in the United States during the 20th century. JAMA 1999;281:61–66, with permission.)

risk of any infectious illness being of a more systemic and severe nature.

If the barrier defense systems of the host are breached, inflammatory cytokines mediate the inflammatory, nonspecific, acute-phase response by the body. The specific immune reaction next occurs as a late-phase response by way of antibody release. Invading organisms result in infection by a variety of factors. They are:

* Resistance to antibiotics
* Microbial resistance
* Release of toxins
* Virulence factors

As soon as the infection is initiated, the general symptoms experienced by the patient can include fever, chills, anorexia, fatigue, and/or myalgias. Leukocytosis, often with an accompanying increase in neutrophils and bands (immature neutrophils), thrombocytopenia, and anemia can be associated laboratory findings. Signs and symptoms can also be on a localized level, manifested by complaints of pain, localized edema, erythema and increased warmth, regional lymphadenopathy, and even lymphangitis (e.g., cellulitis).

Table 21–1. Examples of Newly Recognized Pathogens, 1970–2000

Microbe	Year Discovered	Disease
Bacteria		
Campylobacter jejuni	1977	Diarrheal illnesses
Escherichia coli 0157:H7	1982	Diarrheal illness; hemolytic uremic syndrome
Parasites		
Cryptosporidium	1976	Acute and chronic diarrheal illnesses
Cyclospora cayetanensis	1986	Diarrheal illness
Enterocytozoon bieneusi	1985	Diarrheal illness
Viruses		
HIV	1983	Acquired immunodeficiency syndrome
Hepatitis C	1989	Parenterally transmitted hepatitis
Hepatitis E	1988	Enterically transmitted hepatitis
Human herpesvirus-6	1988	Roseola subitum
Human herpesvirus-8	1995	Herpesvirus-like DNA sequence in AIDS-associated Kaposi's sarcoma

Adapted from Cohen M, Levy SB, Mead P. Infectious diseases: Still Emerging in 1998. Patient Care 1998;32(13):32–59.

Bacteria, fungi, parasitic agents, and viruses are the standard classifications used to categorize microscopic pathogens; however, there are also lesser known novel microorganisms, such as prions (proteinaceous infectious agents believed to cause a number of contagious neurodegenerative diseases) that can also cause a variety of diseases.

The Institute of Medicine defines emerging infections as "new, re-emerging or drug-resistant infections whose incidence in humans has increased within the past two decades or whose incidence threatens to increase in the near future."[3, 4] Furthermore, "The strides made in disease prevention, diagnosis, and treatment with modern technology and pharmaceuticals have lulled us into dangerous complacency. The public health problem of emerging infectious diseases is, unfortunately, flourishing."[3] Reasons for this trend encompass several, diverse factors[5]:

* Antibiotic resistance
* Changes in health care
* Changes in human behavior
* Changes in land use
* Evolution of existing pathogens

* Rapid propagation of infection through international travel and commerce

Refer also to Box 21–1 for further illustration of these factors.[7] Health care practitioners, particularly those involved in primary care and family practice, are often the first to recognize a potential infectious disease problem within a community. The ability to remain vigilant for possible infectious outbreaks and conveyance of the information in an expeditious manner to existing public health organizations can prove pivotal in infection control. Strategies recommended by the federal government are being implemented on both the federal and local levels to aid in controlling the emergence of new infectious diseases as well as in prevention and control of existing diseases.[5] Public health strategies for controlling infectious disease include:

* Application of research that incorporates laboratory and clinical science with epidemiology
* Improvement in detection and surveillance of emerging infections
* Prompt communication and execution of preventive health strategies
* Strengthening of local, state, and federal public health infrastructure

Immunizations

The effective use of vaccinations is imperative for optimal health. The goal of immunizations is to provide an effective public health instrument that allows for "safe, cost effective, and efficient means of preventing illness, death, and disability from infectious disease."[6] (See Chapter 11 Immunizations.)

Box 21-1–MAJOR FACTORS CONTRIBUTING TO THE EMERGENCE OF INFECTIOUS DISEASES

* Human demographics and behavior
* Technology and industry
* Economic development and land use
* International travel and commerce
* Microbial adaptation and change
* Breakdown of public health measures

From Institute of Medicine Report, Emerging Infections: Microbial Threats to Health in the United States. Public Health Image Library, 1997.

Blood Transfusions

The universal screening of all donated blood and blood products in the U.S., and the reliability of donor sources has dramatically decreased the incidence of infectious diseases transmitted via transfusions. The risk of HIV transmission is now 1/493,000; hepatitis B virus (HBV) and hepatitis C virus (HCV) transmission risks are 1/63,000 and 1/103,000, respectively.[7, 8]

Antibiotic Resistance

The resistance of microorganisms to antibiotics affects not only the treatment of bacterial infections, but antiviral and antifungal infections as well. The impact of bacterial resistance to drugs cannot be understated. The dreaded development of vancomycin-resistant enterococcal infections and resistance to other broad-spectrum antibiotics only serve to emphasize the potential hazards. Approximately 50 million of the 150 million antibiotic prescriptions dispensed in America (one in three) are unnecessary.[2] This statistic illustrates problems of antibiotic overuse and misuse. In these days of managed health care, and tightening of financial constraints on health care providers in conjunction with increasing demands on productivity, the antimicrobial options available may be limited and time pressures to expedite patient visits are building. Prescribing an antibiotic for an upper respiratory infection or bronchitis, especially if it is likely of viral etiology, can shorten the patient visit. Patient demands and insufficient time to explain why antibiotics are not warranted lead to the expeditious writing of unnecessary antibiotic prescriptions. However, the judicious use of antibiotics must be paramount in the management arsenal of infectious disease. Patients should be more aware of this problem through the news media; placing information and pamphlets on antibiotic resistance in patient waiting rooms can assist greatly in increasing their education and awareness.

If antibiotics are indicated, the focus of therapy must be on targeted antimicrobial management. Empirical therapy should be continued only until a causative agent can be identified; once a specific organism is identified, the medication can be switched to a more narrow-spectrum antibiotic.

ACQUIRED IMMUNODEFICIENCY SYNDROME

Pathophysiology

The human immunodeficiency virus (HIV) is the retrovirus responsible for the most infamous pandemic in the world today. This infection was initially and formally recognized in the U.S. in the June 1981 issue of *MMWR Morbidity and Mortality Weekly Report*[9] after four patients with *Pneumocystis carinii* pneumonia (PCP) were noted to have a strikingly diminished number of CD4 cells, a subset of T-lymphocytes.

Evidence now points to the fact that patients with primary HIV infection may be the force behind the continued spread of AIDS because the disease is spread before the person knows of the diagnosis and does not engage in universal safe sex practices.[10]

On exposure to HIV-contaminated blood or body fluids, if an adequate viral load is acquired by an individual, the retrovirus is incorporated into the recipient's cellular DNA. This occurs after the virus is transformed from the original RNA structure into "proviral" DNA copies via the reverse transcriptase enzyme. Once integrated into the host cell, DNA viral particles are replicated each time the host cell itself divides. The proviral DNA once transformed into HIV RNA then is converted into proteins that produce numerous reproductions of the virus ("virions"). The half-life of these virions in plasma is 6 h, allowing for rapid replication and dissemination of HIV throughout the host individual.[14] This primary infection results in establishment of long-lived reservoirs of replication-competent virus in resting memory CD4 T-lymphocytes (helper cells). The initial high-level viremia is associated with transient declines in the CD4 T-lymphocyte count and an increase in the CD8 T-lymphocyte count (cytotoxic/suppressor T-cells). The time between initial viral exposure and manifestation of symptoms of a primary infection is usually between 2 and 6 weeks following exposure. Studies indicate that the amount of HIV-specific CD4 T-lymphocytes produced during the primary infection ultimately orchestrates the patient's immune response to the virus (Figure 21–2).[10] The steady-state level of HIV RNA established in the blood during the first 6 to 12 months of infection is a direct indicator of disease progression.[10]

Pediatric Issues[11]

There are no set numerical criteria regarding CD4 counts in defining the presence of AIDS in children under 13 years of age. AIDS is classified by the CD4 T-lymphocyte count as relative to the patient's age (the normal T cell number is higher in infants than in older children and adults). The primary route of HIV transmission is via the perinatal route. HIV virus replicates faster in the immature, highly active, and rapidly developing immune system of children. It has also been noted that the immature neurologic system is uniquely vulnerable to HIV infection; therefore, careful monitoring for developmental delays is very important.

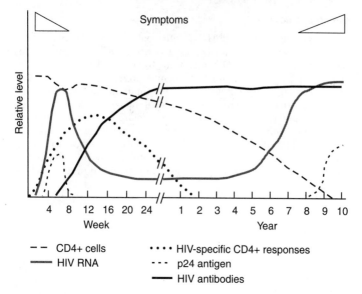

Figure 21–2. Virologic and immunologic patterns in primary HIV infection. HIV-specific CD4[+] responses persist in some patients in whom the disease is not progressing and in those who received treatment during primary HIV infection. (From Yu K, Daar ES. Primary HIV infection: Current trends in transmission, testing, and treatment. Postgrad Med 2000;107:119; adapted from Cordes RJ, Ryan ME. Pitfalls in HIV testing: Application and limitations of current tests. Postgrad Med 1995;98:178, with permission of McGraw-Hill, Inc.)

Obstetric Issues[11]

Becoming pregnant does not appear to affect the course of HIV-related disease. The risk of infection to a neonate born to an HIV-positive mother is estimated to be 13–39%. Zidovudine given during a pregnancy decreases the risk of transmission to the fetus by 68%. Protease inhibitors are still being evaluated for use during pregnancy. However, in many centers, if a patient is on this therapy at the time of conception, it is most likely continued. Elective cesarean-section has been shown to reduce the risk of vertical transmission independent of zidovudine use. Nevirapine as a single dose intrapartum and a single dose to the newborn has been shown to decrease vertical transmisson when antepartum prophylaxis had not been received. Breast-feeding should not be encouraged in the HIV-positive mother.

Geriatric Issues[12]

Greater than 10% of all HIV-positive patients are ≥50 years of age according to the Centers for Disease Control (CDC). There is a higher mortality in the older AIDS patient due to increased severity of illness at time of diagnosis, failure to recognize promptly the possibility of HIV infection, a greater likelihood of comorbid conditions, and the age-related decline of hepatic and renal function. There is an increased vulnerability to drug interactions and/or toxicities in the older population. With the increased use of protease inhibitors and their associated lipid disorders, the rising incidence of myocardial infarctions has begun to be apparent. Pravastatin (Pravachol) is the only "statin" drug that can currently be used in patients on protease inhibitors.

Epidemiology

Roughly 14 million people worldwide have expired from HIV-related infections.[1] As of the beginning of the year 2000, there were estimated to be about 40 million HIV-infected persons throughout the world.[9] Since the era of recognition of AIDS in the U.S., the impact of the HIV virus on a global scale has become progressively more apparent. In the U.S. the incidence has remained steady at 900,000 cases over the past few years while, conversely, many African countries now have a disease prevalence of 80% of the populace who are 20–49 years old. The U.S., over the past 5 years, has reported approximately 40,000 new cases annually. The mortality rate, as of 1998, is 21%. However, AIDS continues to have an increasing impact on women and minority groups.[9]

Treatment Options

The diagnosis of HIV infection is carried out by standardized antibody testing (ELISA with confirmation by Western blot). The p24 core antigen analysis has been the most common virologic load test used in the past. It is sensitive to the high levels of circulating virus generally present during a primary infection.[10] An even more sensitive molecular test that has come into routine use to assess the viral load in HIV-positive patients is the HIV RNA assay. In a patient with primary, symptomatic infection, the viral load generally exceeds 10^5 copies/mL.

Symptoms of primary HIV infection tend to be of a more nonspecific, influenza-like nature with fever, malaise, rash, arthralgias, and generalized lymphadenopathy that can last up to 2 weeks. Most frequently, the preliminary symptoms resolve, leaving the affected individual asymptomatic for a variable length of time. A person is considered to have AIDS if he or she is HIV-positive and has a CD4 count of < 200 cells/μL or has an opportunistic infection.[13]

The routine evaluation of the HIV-positive patient also includes a complete history and physical examination in addition to baseline laboratory and diagnostic studies.[14] Baseline laboratory tests should include:

* CD4 and viral load studies
* Complete blood count (CBC) and glucose-6-phosphate dehydrogenase (G6PD)
* Complete metabolic profile; amylase and lipase and lipid panel
* Hepatitis ABC panel, cytomegalovirus (CMV) and *Toxoplasma* titers
* Rapid plasma reagin (RPR) test
* Purified protein derivative (PPD) and chest x-ray

As soon as a diagnosis is made, patients should receive:

* Pneumovax
* Tuberculosis boosters
* Measles, mumps, and rubella (MMR) vaccine, if appropriate

Live vaccines (such as oral polio and varicella) are contraindicated. If the patient is nonimmune to hepatitis A or B, a vaccination series for hepatitis A (HAV) and HBV should be started. If the patient is hepatitis C-positive, he or she should be evaluated for interferon therapy.

The full spectrum of the manifestations of AIDS is extensive and frequently seems daunting. Due to the very nature of their immunosuppressed state, patients are significantly susceptible to any opportunistic infection. Even the most mundane or innocuous of infections in the immunocompetent individual can become life-threatening illnesses in the compromised patient. The absolute scale of AIDS includes not only the signs and symptoms of the disease itself, but also the signs and symptoms of any one of a number of possible opportunistic infections (Table 21–2). As the patient's CD4 cell count drops, these opportunistic infections become an increasing problem and prophylaxis may be indicated (Table 21–3). There are currently 16 licensed antiretroviral medications in the U.S. approved for treating and managing HIV/AIDS infections (Table 21–4).[9, 14] These drugs are divided into three main categories:

* Nucleoside reverse transcriptase inhibitors (NRTIs)—the first drugs used in HIV treatment with significant associated toxicity
* Non-nucleoside reverse transcriptase inhibitors (NNRTIs)—lower toxicity and improved side effect profile but greater probability of rapid development of resistance
* Protease inhibitors—their use has led to an overall decline in HIV-related mortality, with the disadvantages of complicated dosing

Table 21–2. Frequent HIV-Related Problems

	Symptom	Manifestations
Skin	Bruising	Folliculitis
	Lesions	Herpes zoster
		Kaposi's sarcoma
		Psoriasis
		Xerosis
Eyes/ENT	Odynophagia	Cotton-wool spots (retina)
	Oral lesions	Gingivitis
	Visual changes	Hairy leukoplakia
		Retinitis
CNS	Headache	Dementia
	Mental status changes	Encephalitis
		Peripheral neuropathies
Respiratory	Cough	Abnormal lung sounds
	Dyspnea	Pneumonia
		Tuberculosis
GI	Abdominal pain	Candidal esophagitis
	Anorexia	Hepatitis
	Diarrhea	Hepatosplenomegaly
	Nausea/vomiting	Colitis/proctitis
Genitourinary	Discharge (vaginal/urethral)	Candidal vaginitis
	Genital lesions	Genital HPV
		Genital HSV
General	Fever	Lymphadenopathy
	Malaise	
	Myalgia	
	Night sweats	
	Weakness	
	Weight loss	

CNS, central nervous system; ENT, ears, nose, and throat; HPV, human papillomavirus; HSV, herpes simplex virus.

schedules and long-term metabolic effects, especially lipid disorders and glucose intolerance

The rationale for treating HIV early in the primary infection is to prevent early disease and promote clearance of the HIV-infected CD4 cells. The presence of oral thrush, weight loss, or opportunistic disorders is an indication for instituting antiretroviral treatment at once. Conversely, drug management is instituted in asymptomatic HIV-positive patients when the CD4 count is below 500/μL and/or the HIV RNA viral load is greater than 10^4 copies/μL. The goal is to suppress plasma HIV RNA to imperceptible levels.[10, 14] Drug therapy in almost every case involves concomitant administration of a minimum of three to four medications (Table 21–5).[13–15] The overall choices in AIDS therapy are expanding rapidly; however, the cost

Table 21–3. Indications for Prophylaxis from Opportunistic Pathogens

CD4 Count	PCP	MAC	Toxo	Consider°
>600	+ History only	+ History only		
5–600	+ History only	+ History only		
2–500	+ History only	+ History only		
<200	Yes	+ History only	Yes	
<75–100	Yes	Yes	Yes	
<50	Yes	Yes	Yes	Yes

PCP: TMP-SMX, 1 double-strength tablet (TMP 160 mg/SMX 800 mg) 3×/week; dapsone 100 mg q.d., or pentamidine 300 mg nebulized each month are the most common regimens used; multiple alternatives exist.

MAC: Clarithromycin, 500 mg b.i.d.; azithromycin 1.2 g/week, or 500 mg 3×/week; or rifabutin 300 mg q.d.

Toxo: TMP-SMX, 1 double-strength tablet q.d. or dapsone 50 mg and pyrimethamine 50 mg/week.

°Consider *Candida albicans, Cryptosporidium,* or cytomegalovirus prophylaxis. PCP, *Pneumocystis carinii* pneumonia; MAC, *Mycobacterium avium* complex; Toxo, toxoplasmosis; TMP-SMX, trimethoprim-sulfamethoxazole.

associated with these drugs is significant. The actual drug costs, interactions, side effects, laboratory monitoring, and risk of resistance are all factors that must be taken into consideration. Additionally, the attention and time needed to manage these patients most effectively requires an appropriate level of expertise and experience.[16]

The highly active antiretroviral therapy (HAART) treatment concept is becoming the standard of care in the U.S. with many HIV specialists. This treatment concept involves use of the drugs listed previously, and has led to an overall decrease in mortality, with reduced drug resistance. It has been noted in a multicenter cohort study that CD4 cell counts decreased less rapidly and the time interval to the development of AIDS and death was lengthened among patients treated aggressively with antiretroviral therapy.[16] The downside to this therapy is a complicated drug schedule (with a greater probability of poor patient compliance and therefore of drug resistance), overall high cost of the drugs and laboratory monitoring, plus troublesome acute and/or long-term complications (pancreatitis, severe hyperlipidemias, insulin resistance, and marked body fat redistribution).[14, 17]

Patient Education

HIV is transmitted from person to person via blood and body fluid contact either parenterally or through disruptions in the skin or mucous membranes (inflamed or traumatized mucous membranes being the most vulnerable). The virus is found in blood products, breast

Table 21–4. Approved Medications for HIV Treatment

Medication	Typical Dosage	Adverse Effects
Non-nucleoside Reverse Transcriptase Inhibitors		
Delavirdine mesylate (Rescriptor)	400 mg p.o. t.i.d.	Rash
Efavirenz (Sustiva)	600 mg p.o. q.h.s.	Altered mental status
Nevirapine (Viramune)	200 mg p.o. b.i.d.	Rash
Nucleoside Reverse Transcriptase Inhibitors		
Abacavir sulfate (Ziagen) [ABD]	300 mg p.o. b.i.d.	Rash, fever
Didanosine (Videx) [ddI]	400 mg p.o. q.h.s.	GI upset, pancreatitis, neuropathy
Lamivudine (Epivir) [3TC]	150 mg p.o. b.i.d.	Rare
Stavudine (Zerit) [d4T]	40 mg p.o. b.i.d.	Neuropathy, mitochondrial abnormalities
Zalcitabine (Hivid) [ddC]	0.75 mg p.o. t.i.d.	Neuropathy
Zidovudine (Retrovir) [AZT]	300 mg p.o. b.i.d.	Anemia
Protease Inhibitors		
Amprenavir (Agenerase)	1200 mg p.o. b.i.d.	Nausea
Indinavir sulfate (Crixivan)	800 mg p.o. q8h	Nephrolithiasis
Nelfinavir mesylate (Viracept)	1250 mg p.o. b.i.d.	Diarrhea
Ritonavir (Norvir)	600 mg p.o. b.i.d.	GI upset, paresthesias
Saquinavir (Fortovase)	1200 mg p.o. q8h	Nausea

Adapted from Wolfe PR. Practical approaches to HIV therapy: Recommendations for the year 2000. Postgrad Med 2000;107(4), Table 1, p 132. With permission of McGraw-Hill, Inc.

milk, seminal and vaginal fluids, wound exudates, and saliva. Those who engage in unprotected sex, especially anal-receptive intercourse, those who are intravenous drug abusers, and/or others who engage in high-risk sexual behaviors (multiple partners or sex with IV drug abusers) are at highest risk. The rates of HIV transmission through needlestick injuries or from receiving blood transfusions or blood products have decreased noticeably. AIDS has evolved into a chronic medical condition that requires life-long management and therapy. Health care practitioners are now seeing AIDS patients who are surviving their disease long enough to experience non-HIV age-related diseases (e.g., atherosclerotic cardiovascular diseases, diabetes mellitus). All HIV-infected patients need primary care as well as specialized care. They experience the routine medical problems that non-HIV infected persons do, sometimes at earlier ages or with more severe presentations at diagnosis. Therefore, in addition to HIV-related patient education, these patients also require routine, standard preventive health care.[16] For this reason, the following modifications to

Table 21–5. Recommendations for Combination Treatment of HIV
Use at least 3 agents. Select one of the following:
Didanosine + lamivudine
Didanosine + stavudine
Didanosine + zidovudine
Lamivudine + stavudine
Lamivudine + zidovudine
AND add one of the following:
Efavirenz
Indinavir sulfate
Nelfinavir mesylate
Nevirapine

common preventive recommendations are suggested for the HIV-positive patient:

* Pap smear every 6 months; minor abnormalities should be evaluated more aggressively
* Annual ophthalmologic evaluations (retinal examinations every 6 months if CD4 count is <100)
* Annual RPR and *Toxoplasma* antibody titers
* Tuberculosis test every 6–12 months
* Annual chest x-ray
* Annual influenza vaccine
* Pneumovax booster every 5 years

Newly diagnosed HIV-infected individuals require counseling about decreasing risk factors and risk to their sexual contacts, managing and minimizing the effects of comorbidities, and the natural history and symptoms of the disease and opportunistic pathogens. The importance of educating these patients on their medication regimens and the significance of adhering to the drug schedule as closely as possible cannot be overstated. Recent studies have indicated that despite the success of current drug therapies, if drug therapy is discontinued, even in an asymptomatic patient who had attained an undetectable viral load, the disease will almost likely recur.[13] Due to the complexity of AIDS and HIV-related illnesses, it has been recommended by several physician groups that a specialty and board certification be developed for HIV disease management.[16]

Education of at-risk groups should continue, as recent studies have shown a small but significant increase in the number of AIDS cases in younger gay populations due to lack of safe sex practices.[9] Those who engage in high-risk sexual activities (adolescent sexual activity, multiple partners, anal-receptive intercourse, and failure to use barrier protection during any sexual activities) particularly require intensive education. Decreasing IV drug use or at least limiting the use of contaminated needles by improved access to sterile disposable syringes and sharps boxes also has been shown to decrease risks of contracting HIV. AIDS cases in developing countries are most frequently found in the heterosexual population. Although in the U.S. AIDS is more frequently detected in the homosexual and IV drug user populations, the heterosexual population rates of exposure are increasing as well.[9]

Prevention

The standard use of universal precautions in medical settings, the development of "operator-protective" and disposable medical equipment, and the usually small viral loads that are encountered via a needlestick injury have lessened the likelihood of disease transmission.

Continuing public health efforts in the U.S. to curb the proliferation of HIV include

* Counseling and testing of at-risk individuals
* Use of needle-exchange programs
* Improving the knowledge base among the general public about high-risk behaviors to avoid
* Early diagnosis

Vaccine development continues to be a major focus of AIDS-related research. Thus far progress has been disappointing, with continued difficulty in identifying a quantifiable indicator for immunity against transmission of the virus, and because the virus easily develops mutations and resistance. Also there has been a lack of practical animal models on which vaccines can be tested.[18] One study currently in progress hopes to demonstrate that the efficacy of existing genetic vaccinations can be enhanced through a variety of intracellular targeting and delivery mechanisms.[18] According to the National Institute of Allergy and Infectious Disease, there are at least eight ongoing, active studies targeting the development of an adequate and safe HIV vaccine.[18] Until that occurs, education and prevention by means of public health efforts and the primary health care provider are the most effective HIV prophylaxis available.

Screening Recommendations

Persons at risk for HIV/AIDS should be counseled and tested to obtain an early diagnosis and provide early treatment.

The mandatory screening of all donated blood has vastly reduced the chance of exposure to HIV-infected plasma and blood products.

ENCEPHALITIS

Pathophysiology

Encephalitis is an acute inflammatory process that is predominantly of viral etiology. This inflammation of the brain tissue results from direct invasion of the tissue by a virus or is due to an inflammatory reaction triggered by hypersensitivity to a virus or a foreign protein. Encephalitis is frequently accompanied by meningeal involvement. The most frequent viral etiologic agents include the arboviruses (RNA viruses that are spread mainly by mosquitoes and ticks), enteroviruses, and herpes simplex viruses (HSV-1 and HSV-2). Poliovirus is one of the more commonly recognized forms of epidemic encephalitis that crippled thousands in the U.S. through the 1960s. Recently, there has been an increasing prevalence of mosquito-borne encephalitic illnesses such as the St. Louis, eastern and western equine, and California serotypes. These arboviruses may account for up to 50% of all encephalitis cases in any given epidemic year.[19] Rabies, caused by a neurotropic virus, is a nearly always fatal type of encephalitis that is transmitted via the bite of an infected wild animal, especially bats. There are well over 100 viral agents that can cause encephalitis as well as other nonviral etiologies (Table 21–6).

Bacterial and other infectious agents can cause encephalitis; however, these microbes more commonly manifest as meningitis. Encephalitis as a direct result of HIV infection should always be differentiated from opportunistic infections that can stem from the depressed immune state of the HIV-infected patient.[20] Postinfectious encephalomyelitis can occur as serious sequelae of a nonspecific respiratory or

Table 21–6. Common Causes of Encephalitis		
Viral Infectious Causes	**Nonviral Infectious Causes**	**Noninfectious Causes**
Adenoviruses	*Borrelia burgdorferi*	CNS bleed
Arboviruses	*Brucella* spp.	Collagen vascular disease
Colorado tick fever	*Listeria monocytogenes*	Drug toxicity
Cytomegalovirus	*Mycobacterium tuberculosis*	Exposure to toxins
Enteroviruses	*Mycoplasma pneumoniae*	Inborn errors of metabolism
Epstein-Barr virus	*Rickettsia rickettsii*	Malignancies
HIV	*Treponema pallidum*	
HSV-1 and HSV-2	Various fungal species	
Human herpes virus-6	Various protozoal species	
Influenza		
Measles		
Mumps		
Rabies		
Rubella		
Varicella		

gastrointestinal illness. Acute cerebellar ataxia resulting from a postin-fectious encephalomyelitis due to a varicella infection is a relatively rare but dreaded complication.[19]

When encephalitis is the result of a direct viral infection of the brain tissue, the neural cells are infected, with subsequent surrounding gray matter inflammation and damage. Cerebral edema is often present; abundant petechial hemorrhages can be found scattered throughout the brain tissue and, occasionally, within the spinal cord. Direct viral invasion of the brain is likely to result in necrosis of the neurons. In postinfectious encephalomyelitis, conversely, the primary pathophysiologic process is perivascular demyelination.

Pediatric Issues[19]

Acute encephalitis is more common in infants.

HSV-2 encephalitis occurs predominantly in neonates; infants who survive the initial insult often go on to have permanent neurologic sequelae.

Very young children have a higher risk of morbidity and mortality due to encephalitis.

Presenting symptoms in infants and very young children are usually more nonspecific, such as lethargy and irritability, poor feeding, or anorexia.

Obstetric Issues

Treatment of the pregnant patient does not differ significantly, other than involving an obstetrician in the management of the patient.

Geriatric Issues[19]

The elderly have a higher risk of morbidity and mortality secondary to encephalitis.

Epidemiology

In the U.S., the occurrence of encephalitis is approximately 1/200,000 individuals annually.[19]

Treatment Options

Signs and symptoms of encephalitis are often preceded by a nonspecific prodrome. Headache, fever, malaise, nausea and vomiting, mental status and/or personality changes, neck pain, and photophobia are signs and symptoms associated with encephalitis. The development of seizures or focal neurologic symptoms is common. Diagnostic workup should consist primarily of an examination of the cerebrospinal fluid (CSF), in the absence of evidence of a space-occupying mass seen on neurologic imaging, or increased intracranial pressure. CSF analysis should consist of routine laboratory studies (i.e., glucose and protein, cell count and differential, Gram's, india ink and acid-fast bacillus (AFB) stains, veneral disease screenings, and opening pressures), appropriate cultures, and a variety of other antigens or special tests that are available to aid in the detection of certain viruses. Bacterial and viral cultures of blood, nasopharynx, rectum, and urine are also recommended. Routine comprehensive chemistry panels, CBC, HIV testing, and toxicology screening should also be included in the workup as indicated.

Imaging studies are also useful diagnostic examinations in the evaluation of encephalitis. Both CT and MRI are used, although MRI is the more sensitive and probably more valuable of the two. EEGs can also provide additional information, particularly in those with HSV encephalitis. Biopsy, while rarely indicated, is the gold standard for diagnosis.[19]

Empirical treatment of encephalitis should initially consist of antibiotics (recommended drugs usually include third-generation cephalosporins and/or vancomycin until a bacterial cause can be ruled out). Initial management using intravenous acyclovir has also been suggested.[21] In most cases, both therapies are often instituted until the etiology is determined. Supportive therapy is part of the management of the encephalitis patient. This includes placing the patient in a quiet, darkened room, and treating with analgesics and prophylactic antiseizure medications. Corticosteroid treatment has been advocated, although reports of its success have largely been anecdotal. Often, long-term rehabilitation is necessary after the initial illness is resolved.[19]

Patient Education

Patient education issues mainly focus on specific etiologies. For example, women with a known history of HSV genital infections must be carefully counseled to come in the labor unit at the first sign of labor or rupture of fluids. When active lesions are present, a prophylactic cesarean section reduces vertical transmission to the newborn. In patients who recover from encephalitis, long-term supportive care and rehabilitation is often required. The neurologic sequelae from these infections can include sensory and motor deficits, seizures, and permanent psychiatric and intellectual alterations. Many of these post-encephalitic complications can be of a more subtle nature. Audiometric and visual testing along with a complete neurodevelopmental evaluation should be instituted as part of the initial follow-up.

Prevention

The continuation of the successful rabies immunization program of domestic animals in the U.S. and the use of caution or avoidance on encountering wild animals makes rabies-related encephalitis a rare occurrence. Instituting the universal use of the varicella vaccine and continued universal administration of the MMR immunization also decrease significantly the incidence of these illnesses and the incidence of related encephalitis.[19]

Prevention of arboviruses is a focus of local government environmental and vector-control agencies, as the incidence of arboviral encephalitis has increased in some specific geographic areas.[19] Spraying of insecticides to deplete mosquito populations in areas where cases of mosquito-borne illnesses are reported has been one option. However, routine use of appropriate clothing and insect repellents in endemic areas should be encouraged.

Screening Recommendations

Identification of vectors carrying viruses with potential to cause encephalitis is the task of public health agencies.

▰▰▰ INFECTIVE ENDOCARDITIS

Pathophysiology

In 1646, the disease entity of "infective endocarditis" was first documented. Subsequently, in 1910, Dr. Emanuel Libman published a landmark article hypothesizing that the infective etiologies of endocarditis were more than just bacterial in nature—fungal and viral elements were causative agents as well.[22] Bacteria most commonly cause infective endocarditis, which is defined as an endocardial inflammation secondary to an infectious organism.

For endocarditis to develop, microbes must attach to an endocardial surface, survive, and be able to proliferate. This can occur if the subendothelial connective tissue is exposed secondary to endothelial damage within the endocardium. This most often occurs in the area of damaged or abnormal valves. Once the subendothelial connective layers are exposed, growth of a sterile platelet thrombus is promoted, leading to vegetation development, which serves as a nidus for bacterial growth. The sites in the heart most frequently affected are areas where blood flow strikes most forcefully as it circulates throughout the heart. Any transient bacteremia can lead to deposition of bacteria onto the nidi. Ultimately, the vegetative cluster is composed of alternating deposits of platelet-fibrin material and bacterial growth.

In most cases of non–intravenous drug use (IVDU)-related endocarditis, the left side of the heart is affected in 65% of patients with acute infection and in 85% of those with subacute infection.[22]

Gram-positive cocci are the most common cause of endocarditis; in native-valve (nonprosthetic valve) endocarditis, the most frequent bacteria are *Streptococcus viridans*. Other bacteria involved include Groups B, C, and G streptococci, and *Streptococcus pneumoniae*. *Staphylococcus aureus* occurs in approximately 20% of cases and enterococci in 5–10% of cases.[23] Gram-negative bacilli are infrequently implicated in endocarditis in native-valve, non-IVDU patients; they occur approximately in 5–10% of cases. Gram-negative bacilli are given the designation of HACEK organisms (*Haemophilus parainfluenzae, Haemophilus aphrophilus, Actinobacillus actinomycetemcomitans, Cardiobacterium hominis, Eikenella corrodens,* and *Kingella kingae*).[23] HACEK organisms should be considered if blood cultures are repeatedly negative for growth in a patient strongly suspected of having infective endocarditis.[23]

Intravenous drug abusers have a relatively different pathogenic profile; 50–73% of endocarditis secondary to IVDU involves highly virulent organisms, such as *S. aureus*. This group of patients also has a higher incidence of right-sided cardiac involvement, in contrast to non-IVDU patients. Patients who have undergone prosthetic valve placement also have a higher prevalence of *S. aureus* as the causative agent. In addition, there has been an increase in fungal-related endocarditis in prosthetic valve recipients; this has been attributed to the use of indwelling central lines and higher number of open-cardiac surgeries.[23]

Pediatric Issues

Infective endocarditis is primarily a disease of adults; however, there has been a gradual increase in pediatric cases due to the following:

* Improved survival in children with congenital heart disease
* Greater long-term use of central-line catheters
* Increased survival rates in children with immunodeficiencies
* Increase in IVDU

Obstetric Issues

Treatment of the pregnant patient does not differ significantly, other than involving an obstetrician in the management of the patient.

Antibiotic prophylaxis in those at risk for the development of bacterial endocarditis should still be used in the pregnant patient who is undergoing a genitourinary procedure that would put her at risk for bacteremia.

Geriatric Issues

More than half of all cases of infective endocarditis occur in persons >60 years of age.

The underlying cardiac lesions in the elderly are different from those in younger patients, with the higher incidence of atherosclerosis in the geriatric population postulated as a reason.

There is a higher prevalence of enterococcal infections, especially in older men, thought in part to be secondary to the increase in urinary tract infections seen in this patient group as well as the more frequent incidence of prostatic procedures.

Epidemiology

In the U.S., the patient groups who are most at risk of developing infective endocarditis include those with the following conditions: congenital cardiac lesions; history of rheumatic heart disease; presence of prosthetic cardiac valves (bioprosthetic or mechanical); history of intravenous drug use; predisposing valvular or cardiac abnormalities, including mitral valve prolapse; and most recently, history of appetite suppressant use (particularly fenfluramine and dexfenfluramine).[23] Even high-level close contact and exposure to certain animals and birds can predispose a person to developing infective endocarditis.[22] However, in 25–50% of patients, no predisposing factors are discovered.[23]

Treatment Options

The presenting signs and symptoms of acute infectious endocarditis can often be vague and nonspecific. Although the onset of symptoms in acute disease often occurs over a period of hours to a few days, the symptoms often mimic those of an influenza-like disorder: chills, fever, myalgias, arthalgias (which can even appear as acute-onset arthritis), headache, malaise, and fatigue. Signs to be evaluated on the physical examination are new-onset regurgitant murmurs and sinus tachycardia. The classic physical findings of Janeway's lesions (flat, nontender, irregular lesions found on the palms and soles), Osler's nodes (painful, erythematous nodules on the extremities), petechiae, splinter hemorrhages, and conjunctival and retinal hemorrhages are most commonly seen in the more chronic forms of infectious endocarditis.

In the subacute form of this disease, symptoms include even more vague complaints of weight loss, sleep disturbances, headache, malaise, anorexia, fatigue, dyspnea, and/or nonproductive cough. These symptoms can be intermittent and can last for months at a time. Physical examination findings can comprise any of the above-mentioned "classic findings" of endocarditis, but also include focal neurologic deficits, splenomegaly, new-onset murmur, sinus tachycardia, or evidence of congestive heart failure (CHF). These patients also have a greater risk of myocardial infarction, CHF, embolic events, and myocarditis. IVDU patients with endocarditis are at 300 times greater risk of sudden death than the general population.[22]

Blood cultures are positive for the causative bacteria in 95% of cases.[22] CBC and erythrocyte sedimentation rate (ESR) are useful and supportive, albeit nonspecific, laboratory tests that are also part of the workup. The diagnostic test of choice is still the echocardiograph; however, transesophageal echocardiography is found to be 86–100% sensitive in contrast to the more traditional transthoracic echocardiography, which has a sensitivity of 28–68%.[22] The Duke diagnostic criteria are used as the foundation of establishing the diagnosis of infective endocarditis (Table 21–7).[22, 24]

If infective endocarditis is suspected, it is necessary to begin empir-

Table 21–7. Diagnosis of Infective Endocarditis. Criteria Developed By Duke University	
Diagnosis	Can be made if one of the following is present: 2 major criteria 1 major and 3 minor criteria 5 minor criteria
Major criteria	2 blood cultures = for a microorganism commonly found as infectious cause of endocarditis Echocardiographic evidence of endocardial involvement Development of a new regurgitation-type murmur
Minor criteria	Presence of a predisposing condition Fever >100.4°F Embolic disease Presence of immunologic phenomena + Blood cultures, but major criteria not met + Echocardiographic findings, but major criteria not met

Adapted from Durack DT, Lukes AS, Bright DK. New criteria for diagnosis of infective endocarditis: Utilization of specific echocardiographic findings. Am J Med 1994;96:200–209, with permission from Excerpta Medica; Harris GD, Stemle J. Compiling the identifying features of bacterial endocarditis. Postgrad Med 2000;107(1):75–83, with permission of McGraw-Hill, Inc.

ical therapy promptly. The usual regimen consists of nafcillin or penicillin plus gentamicin while culture results are pending. Vancomycin is an alternative that is used, particularly if a resistant *S. aureus* infection is suspected.[22, 23] Once a specific causative organism is discovered, the antibiotic treatment can be more specifically targeted to that particular organism. Treatment is usually 4–6 weeks in duration. In those who are hemodynamically and clinically stable, are considered compliant, and have a good support system, consideration can be given to treatment on an outpatient basis; options include home IV therapy, once-daily ceftriaxone injections (if appropriate), or even oral ciprofloxacin (as applicable). Operative management is usually reserved for those who do not respond to medical treatment. Surgery is also considered in cases in which there is acute cardiac failure due to significant valvular regurgitation, or in cases of infected prosthetic valves, a fungal or gram-negative bacillus etiology, or in recurrent infection.[22, 23]

Patient Education

In patients with endocarditis infections, compliance with the medication regimen, close follow-up, and control of any preventable risk factors (such as IVDU), are the mainstays of patient education. These individuals also need to be made aware of their increased risk of contracting this illness if they have already had it or if they have moderate- to high-risk cardiac conditions. Meticulous detail to good oral hygiene on a daily basis is also essential. However, one of the most important concepts in prevention and patient education in infective endocarditis is antibiotic prophylaxis.[25] All patients must inform other health care practitioners and their dentists of the need for antibiotic prophylaxis if applicable.

Prevention

The American Heart Association (AHA) made their most recent recommendations for endocarditis prophylaxis in 1997. These guidelines are recommended for individuals who have a history of endocarditis, those who have what are considered to be "predisposing cardiac lesions," and those who have any type of prosthetic valve. The recommendations have been broadened to include mitral valve prolapse, particularly if associated with valvular regurgitation and/or thickened mitral valve leaflets. (Tables 21–8 and 21–9 detail the AHA 1997 guidelines for infective endocarditis prophylaxis).[26]

Table 21–8. Recommended Prophylaxis for Dental, Oral, Respiratory Tract, or Esophageal Procedures

Patient Status	Agent	Regimen*
Not allergic to penicillin and able to take oral medications	Amoxicillin	Adults: 2 g (peds: 50 mg/kg) p.o. 1 h before procedure
Unable to take oral medication	Ampicillin	Adults: 2 g (peds: 50 mg/kg) IM or IV within 30 min
Allergic to penicillin	Clindamycin or	Adults: 600 mg (peds: 20 mg/kg) p.o. 1 h before procedure
	Cephalexin or cefadroxil or	Adults: 2 g (peds: 50 mg/kg) p.o. 1 h before procedure
	Azithromycin or clarithromycin	Adults: 500 mg (peds: 15 mg/kg) p.o. 1 h before procedure
Allergic to penicillin and unable to take oral medication	Clindamycin or	Adults: 600 mg (peds: 20 mg/kg) IV within 30 min before procedure
	Cefazolin†	Adults: 1 g (peds: 25 mg/kg) IM or IV within 30 min before procedure

*Total pediatric dose should not exceed adult dose.
†Avoid using cephalosporins in persons with immediate-type hypersensitivity reaction to penicillin.
Adapted from Dajani AS, Taubert KA, Wilson W, et al. Prevention of bacterial endocarditis. Recommendations by the American Heart Association. JAMA 1997;277:1794–1801, and Prophylaxis guidelines for infective endocarditis. Consultant 2000;40:627–628.

Screening Recommendations

The clinician should remain vigilant to potential signs and symptoms in patients at high risk for infective endocarditis.

GASTROENTERITIS (FOODBORNE ILLNESSES)

Pathophysiology

Gastroenteritis as it relates to foodborne illnesses is the focus of this section. Food poisoning "denotes conditions that are limited to gastroenteritis (excluding enteric fevers or dysenteries) caused by bacterial multiplication or exposure to soluble bacterial exotoxins within the gastrointestinal (GI) system."[26a] Foodborne causes of gastroenteritis are numerous and broad in scope. In the U.S., the vast majority of infectious gastroenteritis cases are viral in origin; in nonindustrialized countries, up to 80% of these illnesses are due to bacterial infection.[27] In industrialized nations, most cases of nonviral infectious gastroenteric illnesses are acquired through travel to less developed countries.[28] Traveler's diarrhea is discussed in Chapter 15, Health Planning and Illness Prevention for International Travel.

Table 21–9. Recommended Prophylaxis for Genitourinary and Gastrointestinal* Procedures

Patient Status	Agent	Regimen°†
High risk	Ampicillin + gentamicin	Adults: Amp, 2 g IM or IV, + gent, 1.5 mg/kg (not to exceed 120 mg), within 30 min of starting procedure; 6 h later, give amp, 1 g IM or IV, or amoxicillin, 1 g p.o. Peds: Amp, 50 mg/kg IM or IV (not to exceed 2 g) + gent, 1.5 mg/kg, within 30 min of starting procedure; 6 h later, give amp, 25 mg/kg IM or IV, or amoxicillin, 2.5 mg/kg p.o.
High risk and allergic to ampicillin or amoxicillin	Vancomycin + gentamicin	Adults: Vanco, 1 g IV over 1–2 h, + gent, 1.5 mg/kg IM or IV (not to exceed 120 mg); complete injection/infusion within 30 min of starting procedure Peds: Vanco, 20 mg/kg IV over 1–2 h, + gent, 1.5 mg/kg IM or IV; complete injection/ infusion within 30 min of starting procedure
Moderate risk	Amoxicillin or ampicillin	Adults: Amox, 2 g p.o. 1 h before procedure, or amp, 2 g IM or IV within 30 min of starting procedure Peds: Amox, 50 mg/kg p.o. 1 h before procedure, or amp, 50 mg/kg IM or IV within 30 min of starting procedure
Moderate risk and allergic to ampicillin/amoxicillin	Vancomycin	Adults: Vanco, 1 g IV over 1–2 h; complete infusion within 30 min of starting procedure Peds: Vanco, 20 mg/kg IV over 1–2 h; complete infusion within 30 min of starting procedure

*Total pediatric dose should not exceed adult dose.
†A second dose of vancomycin or gentamicin is not recommended.
(Adapted from Dajani AS, Taubert KA, Wilson W, et al. Prevention of bacterial endocarditis. Recommendations by the American Heart Association. JAMA 1997;277:1794–1801, and Prophylaxis guidelines for infective endocarditis. Consultant 2000;40:627–628.)

Improved public sanitation and water systems in industrialized countries have dramatically decreased most outbreaks of dysentery-type illnesses, although there is a small but perceptible increase noted even in the U.S.[9, 27, 29] Many recent outbreaks have been due to traditional pathogens, but there are also new pathogens that are a source of increasing concern (calicivirus, *Cyclospora*, *Listeria monocytogenes*, *Campylobacter jejuni*, and *Escherichia coli* O157:H7).[29] The factors believed to be responsible for the increasing incidence of infectious gastroenteritis in the U.S. are[29]:

* Diet: overall change in eating habits
* Global food distribution: acquiring traveler's diarrhea may require only a trip to the local grocery store
* Expansion of commercial food services
* New methods of large-scale food production
* Increasing demand for fresh produce year-round
* Eating outside the home more often

Due to the changes in food consumption and distribution in this country, the potential for countrywide outbreak has become greater. Most foodborne diseases are transmitted via contaminated water supplies or food that is tainted through fecal contamination, improper hand washing by food handlers, or consumption of undercooked foods such as beef, pork, and poultry.[29]

When the GI tract becomes colonized with pathogenic organisms, a variety of changes is precipitated, leading to the development of symptoms, usually diarrhea. This is due to increases in intestinal fluid and electrolyte secretion, nonabsorption of intraintestinal elements, and altered intestinal motility.[28] These changes are caused by direct microbial invasion and subsequent colonization of the GI tract, or they can result from inflammation secondary to toxin production from pathogenic bacteria. Symptom onset from heat-stabile, toxin-forming bacteria such as *S. aureus* or *Bacillus cereus* is usually 1–6 h after exposure; symptom-onset from the heat-labile toxin produced by *Clostridium perfringens* is typically 8–16 h. In contrast, most bacterial or nonbacterial infections lead to symptoms that occur 16 h after initial contact.[27] Most of these gastroenteric illnesses resolve within 3–5 days; however, very young infants, malnourished or immunocompromised patients, and the elderly are at increased risk of a more severe, persistent disease course.[27]

E. coli O157:H7 has a 2–3 day incubation, and normally lasts no more than a week in uncomplicated cases. In any patient presenting with bloody diarrhea and the hemolytic-uremic syndrome (HUS), this serotype must be strongly suspected. This particular serotype is not the only producer of shiga toxin (toxins that are indistinguishable from the potent cytotoxin produced by *Shigella dysenteriae* type 1); other *E. coli* serotypes can cause similar symptomatology.[2]

Numerous other microbial etiologies must always be considered in working up a patient with acute-onset gastroenteritis. *Cyclospora* is a coccidian-like organism, which produces a prolonged course of watery diarrhea and is undetectable on routine ova and parasite (O&P) testing; its incubation period is routinely longer than a week.[29] The protozoal microorganisms *Entamoeba histolytica*, *Giardia lamblia*, and *Cryptosporidium parvum* must always be suspected in gastroenteritis that is unusually prolonged and is unresponsive to routine antibiotic therapy.[21] There are still other microorganisms involved that can survive conventional cooking methods; these include *L. monocytogenes*, *Vibrio vulnificus*, *Cryptosporidium cayetanensis*, the Norwalk virus, *Vibrio cholerae*, and *Yersinia enterocolitica*.[2]

Pediatric Issues [30, 31]

Rehydration. Dehydration is one of the greatest problems associated with gastroenteritis in children, particularly the very young; maintaining adequate hydration and correcting any dehydration is the most crucial treatment goal in children, and is often the only treatment necessary.

The American Academy of Pediatrics issued recommendations in 1985 regarding the appropriate hydration of children:

* Infants and young toddlers—rapid rehydration within the first 4–6 h with an oral glucose-electrolyte solution, followed by diluted milk or formula
* Older children—rapid rehydration with a similar type of rehydration solution, followed by institution of a BRAT-type diet (nonlactose, carbohydrate-rich foods such as bananas, rice, potatoes, etc.)

If severe vomiting and diarrhea persists or oral rehydration is unsuccessful, IV fluid therapy must be seriously considered; children should not go without adequate nutrition for more than 1–2 days.

Bacterial Infections. The peak incidence of shigellosis is within the first 4 years of life; children may present with severe dehydration and weight loss.

G. lamblia, which typically presents as acute, watery, persistent diarrhea, often has concomitant symptoms of recurrent abdominal pain, weight loss, and growth retardation. Asymptomatic "carriers" of *G. lamblia* are usually not treated with antibiotics.

Children are at greatest risk of developing a diarrheal illness within the first 2–3 months that they are in day care. Given the large number of children within a particular facility, the presence of diapered children, and the inherent poor hygiene and propensity of young toddlers to put items in their mouths, it is not surprising that diarrhea is such a prevalent problem in the day care setting. *G. lamblia* and *Shigella* infections are common etiologic agents that are found in outbreaks of diarrhea in day care facilities.[33]

Obstetric Issues

As is the case in treating gastroenteritis in pediatric patients, maintenance of hydration is a key component in treating pregnant patients with gastroenteritis.

If the pregnant patient requires antibiotics or other medications to treat infectious gastroenteritis, one must be cognizant of the safety profile of the drug in regard to fetal effects.

Geriatric Issues[27, 28]

The elderly are at increased risk of more severe, life-threatening courses of gastroenteritis, and are more prone to complications secondary to the illness.

If geriatric patients with gastroenteritis become hypovolemic, the resulting hemoconcentration puts those patients at greater risk of experiencing a stroke or other major ischemic event.

Epidemiology

Gastroenteritis is a particularly devastating and common problem in many less developed countries. Three million children alone die of gastroenteritis worldwide every year.[30]

Campylobacter fetus (also referred to as *C. jejuni*), currently exceeds *Salmonella* spp. as the most common foodborne pathogen in the U.S.[29]

E. coli O157:H7 is now the leading cause of diarrhea associated with HUS; 10,000–20,000 seek medical treatment for this disease in the U.S. annually. HUS develops in 3–7% of patients overall and 10% of children and the elderly who are infected with this particular type of *E. coli*.[2] *E. coli* O157:H7 was originally found in hamburger, but has since also been identified in lettuce, alfalfa sprouts, apple cider, and unpasteurized apple juice. *E. coli* O157:H7 must always be considered in the patient who presents with bloody diarrhea and/or HUS.

In *Salmonella enterica* serotype Typhimurium infections, the incidence of resistance has doubled over the last 15–20 years; this is suspected to be due to the routine antibiotic supplementation of animal feed. One of these Typhimurium subtypes is resistant to at least five antibiotics.[2] Shigellosis is also common in the U.S., and is most problematic if acquired in a day care setting or other crowded institutional settings, as only a very small amount of inoculum is necessary to infect a contact. Resistance is also becoming a problem with *Shigella* infections, especially if acquired in a crowded institutional setting (i.e., day care) or during international travel.[30]

Treatment Options

The general symptoms of infectious gastroenteritis include one or more of the following: diarrhea, nausea, emesis, abdominal pain and cramping, tenesmus, increased intestinal gas, and fever. A more dysentery-like presentation would consist of these symptoms in addition to very frequent, watery stools (most often containing blood and/or mucus), frank abdominal pain, and dehydration. Findings on physical examination may be few or include signs of dehydration, tachycardia, fever, and nonspecific abdominal abnormalities.

For any patient who is dehydrated (especially in children whose dehydration is ≥5%), measurement of serum electrolytes and blood urea nitrogen and creatinine should be considered.[30] Any patient with acute-onset diarrhea who appears toxic with high fever and blood or mucus in the stool should have the stool tested, at least for the presence of leukocytes, particularly in pediatric patients. If leukocytes are present, up to three fresh stool specimens should be cultured and tested for the presence of O&P and *Cryptosporidium* sp.[28, 30] *E. coli* O157:H7 can be readily identified using commercially available media, but is not routinely tested for unless specifically requested.[2] O&P testing should also be done in patients with diarrhea persisting for >2 weeks, or whose illness originated while traveling to less developed countries; this should also be done if the patient is from a day care setting or is immunocompromised.[28] Blood cultures should also be obtained in patients hospitalized with severe diarrhea associated with fever, especially if typhoid, nontyphoid *Salmonella, C. fetus,* or *Yersinia enterocolitica* is suspected; often the diagnosis in these cases can be made by blood culture alone.[28]

Other diagnostics that can be of use in certain situations[28]:

* Stool cultures
* *Clostridium difficile* toxin assay
* Viral examination
* Duodenal aspiration or carbon 14 D-xylose breath test
* Intestinal biopsy

Often, maintenance of adequate hydration is the only treatment needed. If antimicrobial therapy is warranted, the drugs used should be specifically targeted at the infectious microorganism involved.[27, 28] For mild to moderate traveler's diarrhea, judicious use of antimotility agents and maintaining adequate hydration is often the only treatment recommended; nevertheless, the use of antimotility agents should be approached with caution in infectious gastroenteritis. Bismuth subsalicylate can also be used in mild to moderate cases.[27, 28] Fluoroquinolones are used in more severe cases of traveler's diarrhea or if frank dysentery is present; the use of antimotility medications in dysentery is contraindicated.[27] Avoidance of antibiotics is often suggested in cases of *Salmonella infection*[2]; a fluoroquinolone or third-generation cephalosporin can be used in severe *Salmonella infection*. *Campylobacter* infections have been treated predominantly with fluoroquinolones, but resistance to this antibiotic class has developed rapidly; since 1997, fluoroquinolone resistance has been at 13%. Alternative drug treatments consist of macrolide antibiotics.[2, 28] With *Shigella* infections, antibiotic administration is not always necessary unless the patient has a severe case or is from a day care situation. Outbreaks of shigellosis are best managed by exceptionally strict hygiene measures.[2, 27, 28, 31]

Patient Education

Patients who become ill with infectious gastroenteritis must be educated about their illness as well as precautions they need to take to avoid spreading disease to others. Infected day care workers, in particular, should be kept from the workplace until their infection has resolved.

Prevention

With certain types of infectious gastroenteritis, the illness must be reported to the state public health department. Often the patient cannot return to the work setting until certain criteria as established by the public health department are met (such as three consecutive cultures negative for growth in shigellosis). The same criteria may be true for children who attend day care facilities.[31]

Future options in treating and preventing infectious gastroenteritis involve the use of nonabsorbable antimicrobials such as furazolidone, aztreonam, or rifaximin. In addition, the use of "biotherapeutic" agents made up of microorganisms that stem the growth of pathogens is being investigated, although the research results have so far shown only variable success with this type of treatment. Another alternative is using oral vaccines. Many are already in use, such as typhoid, cholera, and enterotoxigenic *E. coli*.[27]

The establishment and maintenance of high-quality public water and sewage treatment systems are pivotal in decreasing and controlling the incidence of infectious gastroenteritis. The appropriate processing, handling, and packaging of food is also critical in avoiding transmission of foodborne pathogens.[2, 27, 29] Outbreaks can be prevented (or at least decreased) by testing food for the presence of pathogens; there are in place extensive testing procedures on the state and national level involving identification of pathogens on foodstuffs by way of molecular subtyping. One method currently under investigation is a pulsed-field gel electrophoresis subtyping system, which is being coordinated by the CDC. The use of ionizing radiation has already been demonstrated to substantially lower the incidence of foodborne disease, particularly when used in processing red meats and poultry. The World Health Organization, the American Medical Association, and many other medical and public health groups have endorsed this method of food processing. Consumer fears have been the main hindrance in instituting ionizing radiation as a standard food treatment process.[29]

Screening Recommendation

It is important to obtain a history of potential sources of infection from a patient presenting with infectious gastroenteritis. It is also imperative to determine the prior or future potential for infecting others (e.g., day care workers).

HEPATITIS

Pathophysiology

There are five specific viral etiologies of liver disease, namely hepatitis A, B, C, D and E (HAV, HBV, HCV, HDV, and HEV, respectively); these encompass five different viral families. Each of these viruses is composed of RNA except for HBV, which is a DNA-containing virus that initially requires RNA transcription. Parenteral conduction is the mode of transmission for HBV, HCV, and HDV; HAV and HEV are spread via the fecal-oral route. In the U.S., 48% of viral hepatitis cases are attributable to HAV, 34% to HBV (including HDV infections), 15% to HCV, and the remainder are due to HEV.[32] Risk factors for acquiring a viral hepatic illness include:

* History of blood transfusion or organ/tissue transplant
* Intravenous drug use
* Employment in a patient-care setting or clinical laboratory
* Exposure to a sexual partner or close household contact with hepatitis
* Multiple sex partners

HAV is usually associated with epidemics and as sporadic cases; common sources of occurrence are contaminated water supplies or food. It is transmitted person to person via the fecal-oral route, although there have been some rare cases of parenteral transmission.[32] Due to recent outbreaks in the U.S., immunization against HAV may become standard, particularly for those employed in the food industry. Hepatitis B, once the bane of the blood transfusion sector of medical care in the U.S., now is most frequently contracted via heterosexual contact. Approximately 1–2% of those with acute HBV go on to develop chronic hepatitis infection (in immunocompromised individuals, the rate is higher).

HCV is the most common blood-borne, chronic infectious disease in the U.S. HCV is parenterally transmitted. HCV is an important contributing factor to developing primary hepatocellular carcinoma, and is the leading cause of patients needing liver transplantation in this country.[33, 34]

HDV is an entity that acts as a "virus satellite" to HBV. It is also parenterally spread, and is found only in the setting of HBV. HDV is usually acquired either as a primary coinfection with HBV or as a superinfection in a patient with pre-existing chronic HBV.

HEV is a waterborne virus spread through the fecal-oral route. It is most commonly found in underdeveloped countries, particularly after flooding.

Viral hepatitis causes hepatic inflammation and necrosis. The exact mechanism of the liver damage is unknown, as the specific viral agents themselves do not directly damage hepatic cells. The incubation period and duration of viral shedding or viremia vary among the different viral families (Table 21–10). The typical course of viral hepatitis also differs for each of these families. Chronic hepatitis is defined by the presence of persistently elevated alanine aminotransferase (ALT) for ≥ 6 months. HAV is characterized by an estimated 2-week period of clinical illness paralleled by a rise in ALT; there is a low mortality rate for HAV, and there is no chronic carrier or disease.

HBV has a much different clinical and immunologic profile.[8] Acute HBV infection generates three different antigen-antibody systems: (1) viral surface coating antigen (HBsAg) and antibody to HBsAg (anti-HBs); (2) viral core antigen (not detectable in the serum; only detectable in infected hepatic cells) and its antibody (anti-HBc); (3) e antigen — a soluble protein derived from the viral core (HBeAg) and antibody to HBeAg (anti-HBe). The presence or absence of any of these markers can help establish the stage and degree of HBV infection. The risk of a chronic carrier or disease state is much greater with HBV infections. Recent studies have demonstrated that the

Table 21–10. Incubation Period and Duration of Viral Shedding

Virus	Incubation Period*	Period of Viral Shedding or Viremia
HAV	4 weeks	4 weeks (fecal shedding) [? Period of transient viremia]
HBV	10 weeks	Several weeks to years (viremia)
HCV	5 weeks	Weeks to years (viremia)
HDV	10 weeks	Transient or chronic (viremia)
HEV	6 weeks	Several weeks (fecal shedding) [? Period of transient viremia]

*Average length of time.

immune system eliminates most HBV without resorting to large-scale destruction of infected liver cells.[35]

HCV disease is noted for its chronic state and significant morbidity. The hepatitis C viruses belong to at least six different genotypes.[33] Antibody to HCV can be detected 2–4 months after exposure, and the HCV RNA levels are detectable usually within 1–2 weeks after viral contact.[8] ALT elevation corresponds with symptomatology, but there is a subset of patients with detectable serum HCV RNA who maintain normal ALT levels.[33, 34] Progress to chronic disease is often gradual, and can occasionally take up to 20 years.

HDV only occurs in the setting of HBV illness (see above). HEV is a virus related to the caliciviruses (a virus associated with epidemic viral gastroenteritis and certain forms of hepatitis); it is rare in the U.S. and is waterborne.[36]

Pediatric Issues[31, 32, 37]

Day care settings are associated with a somewhat higher risk of HAV infection.

Hepatitis B immunization is now a routine part of the primary immunization series; neonates born to hepatitis B-positive mothers need passive immunization at birth, followed by the full immunization course, as there is a significant risk of maternal-fetal transmission during the perinatal period.

Many pediatric cases of HCV are asymptomatic, despite development of chronic hepatitis.

Obstetric Issues[33, 36, 38]

Viral hepatitis is the most common cause of jaundice in pregnancy; the course of the disease is unaltered unless the obstetric patient contracts HEV, in which the fatality rate is very high at 10–20%.[35]

In HBV the risk of vertical transmission from mother to fetus is directly proportional to the maternal HBV DNA level.

In HCV the vertical transmission rate is much more variable than in HBV; there is no treatment or prophylaxis available to prevent transmission.

Interferon should not be administered to a pregnant patient with HCV owing to possible adverse fetal effects; ribavirin use is contraindicated because of its teratogenic and embryocidal potential (Category X).

Geriatric Issues

No specific considerations are noted in this patient population, although immunizations for HBV and HAV are recommended in high-risk individuals as for any patient age group.

Epidemiology

The hepatitis viruses account globally for 95% of acute viral hepatitis cases and 80% of chronic hepatitis.[22] IVDU is the single most frequent risk factor for parenterally acquired viral hepatitis in the U.S. There has been anecdotal evidence of intranasal cocaine use being implicated in types of hepatitis traditionally associated with parenterally acquired hepatitis, specifically HCV.[7, 31–34] It is estimated that up to 80% of those who inject illicit drugs will be HCV-positive within 12 months of their first injection. Eighty-five percent of patients with acute HCV develop persistent infection, and 70% develop chronic hepatitis. The annual rate of HCV has decreased from 230,000 in the mid-1980s to 36,000 by 1996.[32]

Industrialized countries have experienced an overall decrease in HAV incidence.

Chronic HBV is found in about one million Americans. Of this group, 25% go on to develop cirrhosis and 5% develop liver cancer.[32]

HEV is rare in the U.S. but 1–5% of healthy blood donors test positive for anti-HEV; preliminary studies implicate pigs and wild rats as possible vectors.

HDV occurs only in the setting of HBV.

Treatment Options

A significant percentage of viral hepatitis cases remain asymptomatic, despite detectable viral loads and development of antibody titers in the serum. In symptomatic disease, the presentation usually consists of a prodromal phase and a later phase. The prodrome consists of nonspecific, viral-type complaints (malaise, fatigue, headache, myalgias, arthralgias, anorexia, fever, upper respiratory symptoms, cough) plus symptoms of nausea and vomiting, alterations in taste or olfaction, or photophobia. Symptoms that occur later in the disease course include jaundice, abdominal pain, and complaints of dark-colored urine and/or clay-colored stools; complaints that are more unusual are rash, pruritus, or arthritis. Jaundice, splenomegaly, hepatomegaly, spider angiomas, nonspecific viral exanthems, and/or cervical adenopathy are signs that can be detected on the physical examination in an individual with viral hepatitis.

In addition to the presence of viral markers and antibody levels (although, for each viral family, the stage at which the specific antigen indicators and antibody titers are diagnostic differs significantly), the serum transaminases may be strikingly elevated. ALT and aspartate aminotransferase (AST) in particular can be indicative of the degree of disease activity. The remainder of liver enzymes experience varying levels of elevation, although they can also remain within normal parameters. Evaluation of the CBC may demonstrate a fairly typical viral pattern, with normal to decreased leukocytes, anemia, and thrombocytopenia. In any patient in whom viral hepatitis is suspected, or who has unexplained hepatic enzyme elevations (specifically ALT/AST), a viral hepatitis panel is indicated. A liver biopsy is the standard for ascertaining the degree of hepatic involvement, and ruling out other etiologies; it should always be undertaken if antiviral treatment is being considered.[34]

For a vast majority of patients with viral hepatitis, conservative, supportive measures are the only treatment necessary. Maintaining adequate hydration and nutrition, with diet and activity as tolerated, is essential. Serum transaminases should be monitored during the acute phase to ensure that fulminant hepatitis, though rare, is detected as early as possible. Specific antiviral treatment is considered in patients who go on to develop chronic viral hepatitis; this can be the result of HBV, HCV, or HDV infections.

In HBV, treatment is recommended if a chronic disease state is established. The standard of care, which was interferon-alfa alone, has recently been changed to include lamivudine (a synthetic nucleoside analog with activity against HIV) for up to 12 months. The use of lamivudine for periods longer than 12 months is presently being investigated. In patients with concomitant HDV infection, treatment with interferon is difficult, poorly tolerated, and relatively ineffective.[32, 40]

Interferon (recombinant alfa-2a, recombinant alfa-2b, and synthetic interferon) and ribavirin (an antiviral used to treat respiratory syncytial virus) are now the standard of care for HCV. Treatment is recommended for those with chronic HCV infection who are at greatest risk of progression to cirrhosis. Those for whom treatment is not advised are patients with persistently normal ALT, advanced cirrhosis, alcohol use or IVDU, major depression, cytopenias, hyperthyroidism, renal transplant, autoimmune disease, or pregnant patients. Ongoing research is focusing on using antifibrotics, such as interleukin-10, and use of suppressive therapy in those who have developed cirrhosis.[32–34]

Patient Education

Much of patient education in individuals with viral hepatitis is aimed at preventing further spread of the disease. In patients with HAV and HEV, strict hygiene concerning hand washing, not sharing their dishware and toothbrushes with others, and strictly avoiding food preparation are all recommendations that need to be made to these patients. If the patient is in the food industry, he or she must stay out of the workplace until antigen levels drop, ALT returns to normal, and a chronic disease (and carrier) state has been ruled out. HAV is a reportable disease, and all contacts must be notified. Passive immunization should be given to all contacts.[7, 32] There is no prophylaxis for HEV.[30, 36]

Patients with parenterally transmitted viral hepatitis should be advised not to donate blood or be organ donors (especially chronic disease carriers); they also must use barrier protection with all sexual activity. All patients with viral hepatitis need to be educated as to their disease process and prognosis, advised to avoid hepatotoxic medications, strictly avoid alcohol-containing products, and not, under any circumstances, use illicit drugs, particularly if injectable. If they are under antiviral treatment for chronic HBV, HCV, or HDV, close monitoring is necessary of their treatment progress with education as to the medications they are taking, side effects to watch for, and, in women of childbearing age, avoidance of pregnancy. Contraception should be used while on antiviral therapy, particularly with ribavirin; in fact, male patients on ribavirin are often advised to use condoms.[31–34, 37, 39]

Prevention

Effective sanitation and maintenance of safe water supplies are key in preventing the spread of viral hepatic diseases transmitted via the fecal-oral route. HAV still continues to sporadically occur in epidemics in the U.S., most likely due to changes in eating habits in which a significant percentage of Americans now eat outside the home. Recent well-publicized outbreaks have led some local and state governments to require active hepatitis A immunization in all food-industry workers, and in some areas, in day care personnel as well.[20, 31, 32]

The institution of the hepatitis B vaccine as part of the primary immunization panel for children in the U.S. will continue to decrease the incidence of HBV, particularly as a sexually transmitted disease. It has been recommended that all children who were born before the institution of hepatitis B vaccination as a primary childhood vaccination component should receive full hepatitis B prophylaxis. All health care workers, close contacts of HBV-infected persons, and those who potentially may be exposed to HBV should also be vaccinated.[7, 31, 32, 37]

There is no prophylaxis or prevention of HCV except in regard to avoidance of any circumstances in which potential exposure to hepatitis C virus may occur.[32–34]

Primary prevention includes

* Screening and testing of blood, plasma, organ, tissue, and semen donors
* Inactivation of potential viruses in plasma-derived products
* Risk reduction and counseling, especially risks associated with illicit drug use and unsafe sexual activity
* Implementation of infection control practices:
  * Vaccine development
  * Standard barrier precautions and engineering controls to prevent blood exposure

- Protocols and follow-up protocols for needlestick injuries and other hazardous exposures

Secondary prevention includes

* Counseling and testing of those at risk of acquiring HCV
* Screening of appropriate patient groups:
  - History of IVDU
  - History of receiving clotting factor products prior to 1987
  - History of long-term hemodialysis
  - Persistently elevated aminotransferase levels
  - Transplant recipients (transplant performed prior to 1992)
  - History of needlestick injury or known exposure to hepatitis C in health care workers
  - Children born to hepatitis C-positive mothers

Because there are no pre- or postexposure prophylaxis protocols available for HCV, the costs of interventions are still far less than the cost of treating the disease. Interferon treatment alone is expensive, organ transplantation even more so.[32, 34, 39] The National Institutes of Health has established a network of hepatitis C research centers with the ultimate goal of preventing and effectively curing this infection.[6a]

Screening Recommendations

The routine screening of all donated blood, tissue, and organs prevents HBV contagion. Counseling should be done on high-risk patients (see primary and secondary prevention).

▬▬ MENINGITIS

Pathophysiology

Meningitis is characterized by inflammation of the meningeal membranes associated with pleocytosis. The overall profile of community-acquired bacterial meningitis has changed since the institution of the *Haemophilus influenzae* type b conjugate as a routine part of childhood immunizations. As recently as 1986, the most common pathogen involved in bacterial, community-acquired meningeal infections was *H. influenzae*. By the end of the following decade, its incidence had decreased by over 6000%. The mortality rate associated with *H. influenzae* is 3–6%.[6a, 41]

The organisms now most commonly associated with community-acquired meningitis are *Streptococcus pneumoniae* and *Neisseria meningitidis*. Mortality rates for *S. pneumoniae* continue to remain elevated, despite advances in medical care and appropriate antibiotic therapies; this is highest in patients <6 months of age. The mortality and morbidity rates are both estimated to be up to 40%.[41, 42] *N. meningitidis* occurs primarily in infants; almost one half of cases are in patients <2 years of age. The mortality rate peaks at 15% in very young children, with an overall fatality in all patient age groups of 5–10%. *N. meningitidis* is more prevalent over the past few years, with outbreaks occurring more frequently, particularly those associated with the C serogroup.[5, 41]

Staphylococcus aureus and gram-negative bacilli are the most common etiologic organisms in cases of postoperative meningitis or CSF shunt placement; gram-negative organisms are also more likely to cause meningitis in neonates, the elderly, and immunosuppressed persons. *Listeria monocytogenes* causes disease in newborns, the elderly, and in the immunocompromised as well. Aseptic meningitis is a febrile meningeal inflammation characterized by CSF mononuclear pleocytosis, normal glucose, mild elevations in protein, and an absence of bacteria on examination and culture; it is typically viral in etiology, and is on the average less severe than bacterial meningeal infections in immunocompetent patients.[7, 41, 42] Cryptococcal meningitis, a fungal infection caused by *Cryptococcus neoformans*, deserves particular mention, as it is the most frequent lethal fungal infection found in individuals with AIDS. In AIDS patients who survive the acute fungal infection, life-long antifungal prophylaxis is necessary.[43]

S. pneumoniae and *N. meningitidis* possess outer polysaccharide capsules that promote the virulence of the bacterial organisms by preventing phagocytosis of the bacteria and activation of the complement pathway. Meningitis is established once the general virulent bacterial properties overwhelm the host defense mechanisms that normally maintain a sterile environment within the subarachnoid space of the central nervous system (CNS). The bacteria gain entry typically via colonization of the nasopharyngeal areas. Once colonization is established, local tissue invasion occurs, and the bacteria can gain access to the vascular system. The bacteria multiply and circulate through the blood, eventually accessing the subarachnoid space by crossing the blood-brain barrier. The overall inflammatory response and colonization within the subarachnoid space can lead to an alteration of CSF dynamics and cerebral perfusion. These mechanisms, as well as other changes that occur in the subarachnoid and CNS environment, can lead to potentially lethal or permanent neurological sequelae.[7, 41]

Pediatric Issues[5, 41, 42, 44]

The profile of organisms responsible for meningitis is somewhat dissimilar in infants and the very young as compared to older children and adults. Group B streptococcal infections are virtually exclusive to neonates, and occur secondary to vertical transmission; almost half of *N. meningitidis* infections occurs in the very young; and *Listeria* and gram-negative infections also pose a threat to this age group.

The typical signs and symptoms of meningitis are often lacking in the very young. They may have more nonspecific symptoms such as lethargy, irritability, vomiting, and poor feeding. The classic findings of nuchal rigidity or bulging fontanels are observed in less than 50% of affected infants.

The use of dexamethasone immediately before or concurrently with the initial antibiotic dose is only recommended in young children with meningitis who have not been immunized against *H. influenzae* in order to avoid the development of auditory loss or other neurologic sequelae. However, the general concept of corticosteroid treatment remains controversial.

Obstetric Issues

Treatment of the pregnant patient does not differ significantly, other than involving an obstetrician in the management of the patient.

Geriatric Issues[41, 42, 45]

Listeria and gram-negative organisms are more common etiologic agents of meningitis in this age group. Aseptic meningitis is less common in the elderly. Typical signs and symptoms are less prevalent in the aged; signs more likely manifest as confusion and obtundation.

The mortality secondary to meningitis in the elderly can range as high as 75% due to a higher incidence of debilitation, comorbid conditions, delay in diagnosis, and greater likelihood of more virulent organisms.

Epidemiology

In the U.S., community-acquired meningitis occurs in an estimated 2.5–3.5 individuals per 100,000.[41]

Treatment Options

Adults and older children with meningitis often present with complaints of fever, headache, and altered mental status. Signs include nuchal rigidity and change in level of consciousness; Brudzinski's and Kernig's signs are present in 50–60% of affected patients.[41] Seizures and focal neurologic signs are less common on the initial presentation, but can be found later as evidence of progressive disease or permanent sequelae. If meningitis advances unchecked, signs of increased intra-cranial pressure may appear (elevated blood pressure, bradycardia, or coma). Patients with *N. meningitidis* infection and accompanying meningococcemia may have a diffuse rash that is either petechial or purpuric in appearance.

Short-term consequences of meningitis range from subdural effusions and cerebral herniation to cranial nerve palsies. The long-term effects may be significant; patients may be left with seizure disorders, hydrocephalus, learning problems, or focal neurologic abnormalities. The most common permanent sequela is sensorineural hearing loss (found in approximately 10% of postmeningitis patients).[7, 41] CBC often demonstrates a significant leukocyte elevation with a left shift in bacterial meningitis in immunocompetent individuals. The gold standard for diagnosing meningitis is performing a lumbar puncture to evaluate the CSF. CSF is tested for opening pressures, white blood cell count (WBC), glucose levels, CSF–serum glucose ratio, protein level, and presence of antigens to *S. pneumoniae*, *N. meningitidis*, *H. influenzae*, and Group B streptococci (be aware that the absence of detectable antigen does not rule out bacterial meningitis). CSF should also be cultured and Gram-stained. The use of CT or MRI should be reserved for those patients who present with papilledema, focal neurologic findings, or new-onset seizures.

Empirical antibiotic management should be started as soon as bacterial meningitis is suspected. In adults and older children, this usually consists of a broad-spectrum cephalosporin such as ceftriaxone or cefotaxime with the addition of vancomycin if there is a high probability of penicillin resistance; rifampin may also be included in the empirical regimen. (There have been warnings against the use of rifampin in the acute treatment of meningitis due to fears of the development of organisms resistant to rifampin). Ampicillin may also be used in patients <3 months of age, in the elderly, or the immuno-compromised. If the patient is allergic to penicillin, the management should include chloramphenicol, vancomycin, and rifampin. Once the culture results are available, those results should guide the choice of specific antibiotic medications.[41, 42] The issue of corticosteroid treatment remains divisive. Theoretically, corticosteroids can inhibit the provocative host response evoked by rapid bacterial lysis in the CSF secondary to antibiotic effects; however, this has not been a consistent result. Therefore, indications for corticosteroid use are only for pediatric patients in whom *H. influenzae* is strongly suspected; in addition, to be most effective, corticosteroids are ideally given before the first antibiotic dose.[41, 42]

Patient Education

AIDS patients need educating on their risk of meningitis (in addition to their risk of acquiring *any* opportunistic infection).

Prevention

For bacterial meningitis contacts, the disease type that requires chemical prophylaxis is that associated with *N. meningitidis* infections; rifampin is still the drug of choice for close contacts of patients with meningococcal disease and in asymptomatic carriers of *N. meningitidis*. Alternatives to rifampin are ciprofloxacin and ceftriaxone.[41]

The advent of routine *H. influenzae* vaccinations has played a major role in the marked decrease of *H. influenzae* meningeal disease. The pneumococcal vaccine advised for all people >65 years of age as well as asplenic patients has proved to have some effectiveness in preventing streptococcal meningitis. The quadrivalent meningococcal polysaccharide vaccine is currently recommended, and is close to 85% effective.[5]

Screening Recommendations

Any HIV-positive patient who presents with fever, headache, and/ or focal neurologic signs needs immediate evaluation for meningitis, particularly testing for serum cryptococcal antigens.[43]

▬▬ INFECTIOUS MONONUCLEOSIS

Pathophysiology

The presence of abnormally elevated levels of mononuclear leukocytes in the blood is the fundamental characterization of mononucleosis. The infectious form of mononucleosis primarily involves the Epstein-Barr virus (EBV) as its etiologic agent, and is commonly known as "infectious mono."

EBV is a herpes-type virus that primarily involves B-lymphocytes and nasopharyngeal cells. In most EBV infections, the disease is asymptomatic. In adolescents or adults, EBV infections are usually subclinical or are manifested as infectious mono. Infectious mononucleosis is mainly spread by contact with saliva, and is characterized by fever, sore throat, lymphadenopathy and splenomegaly, as well as a leukopenia that becomes a lymphocytosis by the end of the second week of illness. Transmission occurs most often via oropharyngeal contact with an infected asymptomatic person; it can also be transmitted occasionally by contact with EBV-positive blood. In only about 5% of those infected with infectious mononucleosis is there known contact with an infected individual. Clinical hepatitis with jaundice is present in 5–10% of patients in association with EBV infections; rarely, hepatic granulomas can develop, although this is usually an incidental finding.[1, 8]

Another viral agent associated with mononucleosis is cytomegalovirus (CMV). Its main impact is on women who contract CMV while pregnant due to the risk of possible effects on the fetus (see Obstetric Issues later). Mononucleosis secondary to CMV infection is not as common and is less likely to be detected than EBV-related mononucleosis due to the innocuous, often asymptomatic nature of its disease course. When clinical symptoms are evident, they are often associated with hepatitis.[7, 8] Both EBV and CMV infections can occasionally lead to significant morbidity and, even more rarely, mortality (Table 21–11).[7, 8, 45] This can occur in immunocompromised patients.

On introduction to and initial replication of EBV in the nasopharyngeal cells, the virus then infects B-lymphocytes, which are induced to secrete immunoglobulins. These lymphocytes, termed "atypical lymphocytes," are large, abnormally shaped lymphocytes that resemble monocytes. Collections of these atypical lymphocytes can be found primarily in the lymph system (lymph nodes and spleen), but can also accumulate in other areas (brain, meninges, and heart). Heterophilic antibodies develop within the first 4 weeks after symptom onset. These are a diverse group of antibodies that aid in the detection of acute EBV infections; they are demonstrable via a sheep cell agglutination antibody test. The incubation period of infectious mono is 30–50 days.

CMV-mediated mononucleosis is characterized by a mono-like illness in some ways similar to EBV except the pharyngeal and respiratory symptoms are not present, and heterophilic antibodies are absent. CMV can also occur as a post-transfusion phenomenon.[7, 8]

Pediatric Issues[7, 8, 46]

Congenital CMV occurs in approximately 0.5–1.5% of babies born to mothers infected with CMV during the pregnancy; congenital CMV causes defects of variable severity, spontaneous abortion, or stillbirth. Ten percent of essentially asymptomatic neonates with CMV eventu-

Table 21–11. Mononucleosis Complications

Virus	Complication or Associated Condition
Epstein-Barr virus	African Burkitt's lymphoma
	Specific types of B-cell neoplasms in immunocompromised patients
	Nasopharyngeal carcinoma
Cytomegalovirus (CMV)	Congenital CMV effects, spontaneous abortion, or stillbirths in pregnant women with CMV
	Esophagitis, proctitis, colitis, pneumonia, retinitis, or central nervous system involvement in immunocompromised patients

ally display evidence of sensorineural hearing loss, chorioretinitis, or mild neurologic or dental defects.

Some premature infants and neonates can develop a secondary immunodeficiency syndrome similar to infectious mono resulting from a variety of viral agents.

Heterophilic antibodies are detectable in <50% of patients with infectious mono who are <5 years of age.

Obstetric Issues[7, 8, 46]

Pregnant women who develop CMV infection most often are asymptomatic or have a mild mono-like illness; the hazard lies in the possibility of fetal development of congenital CMV disease (see Pediatric Issues earlier).

Geriatric Issues

No specific considerations are warranted in geriatric patients, other than to avoid the development of dehydration due to the risks of hemoconcentration in the elderly (i.e., stroke, embolic events).

Epidemiology

Approximately 50% of children have had their first EBV-type infection by the age of 5.[44] Infectious mononucleosis primarily occurs in individuals aged 10–35 years of age. Ninety to ninety-five percent of infected patients have subclinical evidence of hepatitis.

Treatment Options

Pharyngitis, diffuse lymphadenopathy, fatigue, and fever associated with atypical lymphocytosis are hallmarks of infectious mono. Fatigue is a predominant feature during the first 2–3 weeks of the illness. Fever, which can attain a maximum temperature of 40.5°C (105°F), usually peaks in the afternoon or early evening. In the "typhoidal" form of infectious mono, where fatigue and fever predominate, onset and resolution of the illness may be much slower.[7] Other complaints associated with the infection can include a nonspecific rash, urticaria, malaise, or symptoms consistent with aseptic meningitis or viral hepatitis. Depression can also be found in patients with acute EBV infection.[7]

A maculopapular rash or urticarial lesions may be evident on examination, as well as exudative tonsillitis with hyperemic, edematous tonsils and micropetechiae of the soft palate. Occasionally there will be periorbital edema. Findings of mild meningeal irritation can also be evident. Splenomegaly is found in approximately 50% of cases; the spleen tip usually extends no further than just inferior to the left costal margin. Splenic rupture as a consequence of infectious mono is rare, although it can occur in the setting of fulminant EBV infections in which splenic enlargement is rapid; it can also occur if splenomegaly is present and the patient sustains relatively mild trauma to the area of the spleen. Findings of hepatomegaly and hepatic tenderness are also common in infectious mono; many patients present with jaundice and clinical findings consistent with acute hepatitis. In a patient who presents with acute jaundice, the presence of diffuse lymphadenopathy, sore throat, and marked atypical lymphocytosis argues for the probable etiology of hepatitis secondary to infectious mono.

The presence of atypical lymphocytosis, positive heterophilic antibody titers, and elevation of hepatic enzymes are characteristic laboratory findings. The WBC count may be normal or depressed; thrombocytopenia is also a frequent discovery. Occasionally, severe pancytopenia can transpire. The monospot test is a heterophilic agglutination test typically used to diagnose infectious mono secondary to EBV. It may be a week or more for the monospot test to become positive in an acute infection. In older children and adults, ≥90% have positive heterophilic titers in primary EBV-mediated infectious mono disease. This test is positive in ≤50% of younger children with the disease.[7, 8, 44]

The course of infectious mononucleosis is usually self-limited; treatment is primarily supportive care and symptom alleviation by the use of analgesics, fluid support, and rest as needed. Disease duration varies, with the acute phase lasting usually no more than 2 weeks. Patients can usually resume usual activities as tolerated once the acute phase is resolved, but full resolution of the fatigue may take several more weeks. In a small minority of cases (1–2%), fatigue can last for months. Death occurs in <1% of cases, generally due to complications of primary EBV infection (e.g., encephalitis, splenic rupture, airway obstruction).[7, 8]

Patient Education

Due to the very real, though relatively uncommon, risk of splenic rupture associated with infectious mono, all patients diagnosed with this infection are advised against participating in contact sports or lifting heavy objects for up to 2 months after initial disease presentation, even if splenomegaly is not clinically apparent. Patients should be advised to rest during the acute phase of the disease, but are encouraged to resume normal activities as tolerated after the fever, pharyngitis, and severe malaise subside.

Prevention

Patients who are immunocompromised, particularly those with AIDS, transplant recipients, or those on chemotherapy, are particularly vulnerable to significant morbidity secondary to CMV infections (see Table 21–11). Health care practitioners must be alert to the possibility of CMV infections in their immunosuppressed patients.[7, 8]

Screening Recommendations

There are no specific primary screening recommendations for infectious mononucleosis.

SEXUALLY TRANSMITTED DISEASES

Pathophysiology

The overall incidence of sexually transmitted disease (STD) has steadily declined within the U.S. over the past few decades; however, the increasing effortlessness of global travel may affect this general downward trend, particularly for HIV-related disease. HIV infection is closely associated with the persistent presence of STDs.[47, 48] The profile of STD has changed over the last 40 years as well—for example, syphilis was a significant sexually communicable disease threat in the early part of the 20th century, whereas chlamydia is now the most common STD in this country.[48]

According to a recent report from the Institute of Medicine, women are more often the "victims of the hidden epidemic" of STDs; this is probably due to the fact that STDs are more easily transmitted from men to women, and women tend to have more severe complications from their STDs than similarly infected men.[48, 49] The reasons for this continuing epidemic are not only the globalization of travel and the presence of HIV, but also the lack of cohesive, nationwide public health measures, the relative variability in existing systems, and the inconsistent management of STDs.[48, 49] The ability to effectively deal with the risk factors is also difficult, because of the variety of many risk factors for acquiring STDs.

Chlamydia. *Chlamydia trachomatis* is an obligate, nonmotile, intracellular parasite; there are 15 chlamydia serotypes. Certain serotypes are more pathogenic for causing pelvic inflammatory disease, specifically types D through K.[48]

Genital Herpes. There are two main strains, HSV-1 and HSV-2. HSV-2 causes most cases of genital herpes, although HSV-1 is also capable of causing genital infection. HSV is a double-stranded virus that first targets epithelial cells, and is then transported via neural tissue to the sensory ganglia where it establishes a permanent, latent presence. Local or systemic stimuli can trigger reactivation; however, it has been shown in a recent review that stress does not seem to elicit reactivation.[48] Transmission occurs from contact with the viral lesions, although it has been clearly demonstrated that viral shedding can occur during asymptomatic periods in an infected patient. Most HSV infections are acquired via sexual contact. Individuals who are HSV-2 antibody positive often give no history of ever having genital herpes.[50]

Gonorrhea. *Neisseria gonorrhoeae* is a gram-negative diplococci that is the causative agent of gonorrhea (GC), which is usually spread sexually, but can also be vertically transmitted. This bacterium infects columnar and cuboidal cells, penetrating the epithelium within 24–48 h of initial contact. The neutrophilic response leads to the purulent discharge that is a common symptom of GC. The locality of the infection is usually the cervix, but can also be in the urethra or rectum.

Human Papillomavirus (HPV). There are more than 80 HPV types: HPV-6 and HPV-11 are implicated in 95% of genital warts, and at least five types have oncogenic potential.[51] After contact with viral lesions or particles, through microtrauma during sexual activity, the virus enters the epithelium via microscopic abrasions. Although unprotected sexual activity is the main route of transmission, studies have demonstrated HPV fomites on underwear and medical instruments. Other unsafe factors are multiple partners and the initial sexual encounter at an early age.[51] External genital warts have been found to contain a large viral particle load.[51] Most HPV infections are controlled by the immune system, and never manifest as cervical dysplasia or genital warts. The perilous impact of HPV is its role in the development of cervical cancer, which is the second most common cause of cancer deaths in women worldwide.[51]

Pelvic Inflammatory Disease (PID). Although chlamydia and gonorrhea are the most common causes of PID, it often has a polymicrobial etiology.[48, 52] Lower reproductive tract infections have a greater chance of ascending the genital tract if the woman is < 20 years of age, has had previous PID, uses vaginal douches, or has a history of bacterial vaginosis (BV). If there is a delay in the treatment of PID, it can lead to increased risk of infertility, ectopic pregnancy, chronic pelvic pain and abscess, and abdominal surgery.

Table 21–12. HPV Clinical Manifestations

Form	Manifestation
Clinical	Visible warts in genital area
Subclinical	Warts visible only on cervical cytology
Latent	Normal skin appearance

Syphilis. The spirochete organism, *Treponema pallidum*, is transmitted by sexual contact and also by vertical transmission.

Miscellaneous. Chancroids are caused by the gram-negative bacillus, *Haemophilus ducreyi*. This lesion often coexists with other genital lesions. BV is now managed not only as a nonspecific vaginitis, but also as an STD. It is found to be a potential cause of PID; the CDC now includes BV in its 1998 guidelines for treatment of sexually transmitted diseases.[47, 53] The new CDC guidelines also include hepatitis A in its recommendations; in 1995, the highest rate of HAV transmission was in close household and sexual contacts of patients with HAV. Thirty to sixty percent of the new cases of HBV each year are sexually transmitted.[52] Nongonococcal urethritis (NGU) occurs in both sexes; the most common etiologic agents include *C. trachomatis* (approximately 50% of cases),[7] *Ureaplasma urealyticum*, *Trichomonas vaginalis* and, most recently recognized as an etiologic agent, *Mycoplasma genitalium*.[47, 58] Trichomoniasis, a protozoal infection, affects both men and women.[47]

Pediatric Issues[47]

There is a high risk of STD infections in teens (Box 21–2).

One in four teens will develop an STD before graduation from high school. Forty to sixty percent of teens are sexually active by the ninth grade.

Genital Herpes. Infection in the neonatal period, while uncommon, can result in death or severe neurodevelopmental disabilities. If disseminated infection occurs, the mortality rate is approximately 60%, even with antiviral treatment.[50]

Box 21-2–RISK FACTORS FOR TEENAGERS

Early age of sexual debut
Lack of condom use
Multiple sex partners
Prior STD
History of STD in partner
Sex with a partner 3 yr or more older

Other Risk-taking Behavior
Tobacco use
Alcohol use
Illicit drug use
Dropping out of school
Pregnancy

STD, sexually transmitted disease

Gonorrhea. In systemic disease in children weighing more than 45 kg, ceftriaxone q.d. for 10–14 days is recommended.[52]

Syphilis. Infants born to seroreactive mothers should not be treated unless there is evidence of congenital syphilis by laboratory or physical examination findings in the neonate, or if the mother was untreated during pregnancy or had advanced disease. If the diagnosis of congenital syphilis is made, the treatment of choice is aqueous penicillin.[52]

Obstetric Issues

Chlamydia.[48, 52, 54] Azithromycin, erythromycin, or amoxicillin are acceptable treatments for infected pregnant patients.

Infants born to women with chlamydia should be monitored closely for symptoms, but do not need to be treated empirically.

Genital Herpes. Any woman with HSV who becomes pregnant needs to notify her health care practitioner immediately.

Pregnant women with HSV have a miscarriage rate three times that of uninfected women.[47]

In pregnant women with recently acquired infection, about 80% have at least one recurrence during the pregnancy.[50]

Acyclovir use is recommended only during pregnancy if infection is severe.[48]

Overall risk of vertical transmission in women with any history of HSV infection is 1/2000–4000 births, regardless of lesion presence or absence.[48]

Cesarean section is recommended for all women with evidence of active disease.[48, 50]

Not all neonates born to women with HSV need empirical treatment with acyclovir.[50]

HPV.[51, 52] Genital warts tend to grow more quickly during pregnancy and the lesions are more resistant to treatment. Recommended treatment is trichloroacetic acid, bichloroacetic acid, or cryotherapy. The safety of imiquimod and podofilox during pregnancy is not established. Cesarean section is advised if there are extensive lesions because of the difficulty of suturing the perineum through the lesions. There is also a slight risk to the infant of developing laryngeal papillomata, a life-threatening form of neonatal HPV.

Syphilis.[52, 53] Routine screening should be done in all pregnant patients during their initial prenatal visit. Serology and sexual history should be repeated in high-risk patients at 28 weeks and just prior to delivery. Penicillin is the only approved drug for the treatment of syphilis during pregnancy. There is a definite risk of vertical transmission. Early symptoms include stillbirth, prematurity, anemia, or thrombocytopenia; deafness, mental retardation, seizures, or deformities are late findings.

Geriatric Issues

Screening for syphilis should be done in all older patients with new-onset dementia.[53]

Epidemiology

It is estimated that in the U.S. there are 12 million new STD cases each year.[48]

Chlamydia. *C. trachomatis* is the most commonly reported STD in the U.S.; there are currently four million new cases each year. A majority of women with this STD (70–90%) are asymptomatic, and may carry the infection for years. The highest predominance is found in urban women under 20 years of age.[47, 48] Other risks include age between 15 and 21, being unmarried, and having a new sexual partner or multiple sexual partners.[47, 48]

Genital Herpes. One third of the world's population is infected by the herpes simplex viruses[48]; 45 million people in the U.S. alone are infected.[50] The total, lifetime number of sexual partners, age <30, African American race, female sex, low socioeconomic status, and positive HIV status are all risk factors for the acquisition of genital HSV.

Gonorrhea. The rates of GC have consistently declined over the past two decades. GC is most frequently in females between the ages of 15 and 19; as is the case for some of the other STDs, the danger of contracting gonorrhea also lies in being an adolescent or young adult, or being African American.[47]

HPV. With one million new cases each year, HPV is now the most common viral STD.[47, 51, 52] The highest rate is found in the 18–28-year-old age group.[51] Cofactors in allowing HPV to achieve pathogenic expression are oral contraceptive use, poor nutrition, immunodeficiency, pregnancy, and smoking.

PID. Ten percent of women develop this upper reproductive tract infection during their reproductive years.

Syphilis. Syphilis rates have steadily decreased in this country to the point at which the CDC is planning a campaign of eradication of this once dreaded disease.[47] From 1990–1997, the incidence of syphilis fell 84% to an unprecedented low of 3.2 cases/100,000.[53] Similar to the other STDs, the risks for acquiring syphilis include minority or lower socioeconomic status, and illicit drug use.

Treatment Options

General. Any patient presenting with an STD should be strongly advised to be tested for HIV in addition to consideration of testing for the presence of other STDs. A significant percentage of patients presenting with an STD have at least one coexisting STD.[47, 48, 51, 53]

Chlamydia. Most women with this infection are asymptomatic, whereas men tend to display more symptomatology. The most common complaint is a mucopurulent discharge. Complications of untreated disease include PID, reactive arthritis, and perihepatitis (Fitz-Hugh–Curtis syndrome).[48] The gold standard for diagnosis is the cell culture (wooden swabs cannot be used for obtaining the specimen). Direct fluorescent antibody testing and ELISA are used for screening, but have lower sensitivities. The use of the DNA probe allows for nucleic acid identification; the ligase chain reaction (LCR) and polymerase chain reaction (PCR) tests use DNA or RNA amplification, which allows for almost 100% sensitivity and specificity of these tests.[48]

Thus far, there have been no reports of antimicrobial resistance in this infection.[47, 48] Doxycycline is the drug of choice for treatment of isolated chlamydia; azithromycin is also an acceptable alternative.[52, 54] Follow-up testing is only needed in high-risk or pregnant patients, or if the symptoms do not resolve after treatment.[48]

Genital Herpes. HSV has an incubation period of several days after initial contact, followed by a prodrome of local pruritus, burning, or erythema. The classic lesions are very painful, and can materialize on the cervix, vaginal introitus, or anywhere on the perineum. The primary presentation is almost always the most severe. Systemic complaints of fever, headache, myalgias, or abdominal pain can be present. Occasionally, there can be severe inguinal adenopathy, signs of meningeal irritation, neurologic abnormalities, hepatitis, or pneumonia.[50] Men are more apt to complain of symptoms and have more obvious lesions.

Diagnosis by clinical appearance is usually the only evaluation necessary. Laboratory verification should be used only for lesions in a patient without a history of HSV or with a suspected first-time recurrence of HSV.[48] Antigen detection and Tzanck's test are traditional methods used for diagnosing HSV, although they have lower sensitivities. The gold standard and diagnostic test of choice is viral isolation by tissue culture.[48, 50] PCR is also now available, and, although expensive, is most useful for the diagnosis of HSV CNS infections, and can also detect active viral shedding.[50]

The updated guidelines include the use of famciclovir and valacyclovir in addition to acyclovir for management of HSV. Treatment is most effective if begun within the first 24 h of symptom onset. If patients demonstrate six or more outbreaks per year, then suppressive or episodic therapy is indicated. Episodic treatment consists of starting medication immediately on symptom onset, and continues until the outbreak has resolved. Suppressive therapy is more often preferred; it requires that the patient take medication every day, even during asymptomatic periods; it has been shown to reduce the incidence of outbreaks by 75% and reduces asymptomatic viral shedding.[48, 50]

Gonorrhea. GC has a variable incubation period. If symptoms are present, the female patient may experience vaginal discharge, dysuria without urgency or frequency, and/or vaginal bleeding. Males are more apt to have symptoms with complaints of urethritis, dysuria, and penile discharge. Other manifestations can be symptoms and signs of ocular infection (usually through autoinoculation), perihepatitis, or systemic infection with associated arthralgias, asymmetrical polyarthritis, and dermatitis. Pharyngeal GC is frequently a possibility, although it is often asymptomatic.

Despite the fact that cell culture is the gold standard for diagnosing GC, the presence of gram-positive diplococci with polymorphonuclear leukocytes on a Grams stain of endocervical or other appropriate specimen is less costly and highly specific; also, results are available within minutes. DNA probes and LCR assays are other more recently developed tests currently in use.

The first-line treatment of ceftriaxone (250 mg IM one time) followed by 10–14 days of oral doxycycline (to cover the probability of concomitant chlamydia) is still the standard of care. Other treatment options include cefixime, ciprofloxin, ofloxacin, azithromycin, and doxycycline.[47, 52]

Fluoroquinolones can be used both IV and orally; however, this group of antibiotics should be used judiciously due to fear of resistance. Resistance to this drug group seems to develop rapidly, although there is still only an approximate resistance of 0.5% in the U.S.; in other countries, the resistance rate is much higher.

According to the CDC, tests of cure are not necessary for uncomplicated GC; usually, if infection is detected after treatment completion with the patient having improved, it is considered reinfection.

HPV. There are three different clinical presentations of HPV (Table 21–12); most HPV infections present in the latent form. If warts are evident, they are usually painless. However, a small percentage of warts are pruritic or tender, and patients may complain of discharge or postcoital bleeding. HPV lesions can be further classified in four descriptive groups (Table 12–13). Flat condylomata are visible only after acetic acid (3–5%) solution is applied to the epithelial surface.[51]

Table 21–13. Classification of HPV Lesions

Genital Wart Groups	Description
Condylomata acuminata	Usually in moist areas; "cauliflower" lesions
Keratotic warts	Usually on dry surfaces; appearance similar to common skin warts
Smooth, papular warts	Usually on dry surfaces
Flat condylomata	Subclinical lesions

The diagnosis of HPV, similar to HSV diagnosis, is most often achieved by clinical observation of visible lesions; if there is a strong suspicion of possible HPV and no lesions are visible, it is routine to apply acetic acid solution to likely areas in conjunction with colposcopy in order to visualize the flat condylmatous warts. Cytology is usually not necessary to make the diagnosis, but it can be used in combination with colposcopy if needed. Latent infections can be identified only by detection of HPV DNA by use of PCR. No data from the CDC support the use of viral subtyping in the routine diagnosis and management of HPV.[51] Biopsy of any lesions is indicated if there is a suspicion of malignancy, the lesions progress in spite of treatment or rapidly recur after treatment, or if the lesions are pigmented or >1 cm in diameter.[51]

The main goal in managing HPV is to treat the symptomatic noncervical lesions and prevent further transmission of the disease. Therapy does not change the natural disease course, decrease the risk of cervical cancer, or decrease contagion.[51, 52] No treatment can eradicate this virus. There are many therapy options. The recommended treatments consist primarily of podofilox 0.5% gel or solution, or imiquimod 5% cream. Intralesional injection of interferon is an effective option, but is not advised due to the high incidence of adverse effects associated with this treatment.[51, 52]

PID. In addition to the signs and symptoms associated with a lower reproductive tract infection, PID is often accompanied by systemic complaints of fever, nausea and vomiting, dyspareunia, and abdominal pain (mild to severe). In advanced disease, peritoneal signs may also be evident. The diagnosis is often made based on the clinical findings of mucopurulent cervical or vaginal discharge, cervical motion tenderness, and toxic systemic signs. Attempts to identify the specific etiologic agent should be made via culture, DNA probe, LCR, or PCR in order to specifically target the causative organisms. ESR, WBC count, and C-reactive protein are elevated. Ultrasound or exploratory laparoscopy can also demonstrate findings consistent with PID.

A majority of patients can be treated on an outpatient basis as long as they are available for follow-up care within 72 h and do not have any indications for hospital admission. Empirical therapy is advised until a specifc etiology can be diagnosed, if possible. Outpatient regimens include (most also add chlamydia coverage) ceftriaxone; ofloxacin plus metronidazole; or cefoxitin (one dose) plus probenecid (one dose) given concurrently[47, 52]

The treatment of inpatient PID is beyond the scope of this book, but indications for consideration of inpatient treatment include[47]:

* Inability to exclude a surgical emergency
* Failure to respond to oral therapy
* Existence of severe illness (nausea and vomiting, high fever)
* Immunodeficiency

* Pregnancy
* Presence of tubo-ovarian abscess
* Inability to follow or tolerate outpatient regimen

Syphilis. Syphilis has often been labled the "Great Pretender" due to its wide range of symptoms and signs. However, there is a certain pattern to its disease progression and the accompanying presentations (Table 21–14).[53] Primary infection usually becomes evident about 3 weeks after contact with the spirochete; one or more of the characteristic chancre lesions may appear at the site of inoculation. This stage usually resolves within 3–6 weeks. If left untreated, the secondary stage can then present within the next 2 weeks to 2 months after the primary infection. Systemic involvement can present at the secondary stage or at a more advanced phase of the disease. In 8–40% of untreated patients, tertiary syphilis develops, usually presenting as neurosyphilis.[51] As in many of the other STDs, men are more likely to have obvious signs of infection than women.

Screening for syphilis is carried out by one of the nontreponemal antibody tests (VDRL or RPR); however, these tests do not become positive until several weeks after the initial infection. These tests are useful for general screening and are practical in monitoring the treatment response. Specific treponemal tests are the microhemagglutination assay for the spirochete (MHA-TP) and the fluorescent treponemal antibody absorption (FTA-ABS); both of these can be positive early in the infection. If an RPR or VDRL test is positive, then

Table 21–14. Disease Progression of Syphilis

Stage	Signs and Symptoms of Syphilis
1st degree	Painless ulcer at inoculation site
	Regional adenopathy
2nd degree	Mucous membrane lesions
	Prodromal symptoms: malaise, fever, pharyngitis, headache, arthralgia/myalgias, lymphadenopathy
	Rash (particularly on palms and soles)
	Iritis with uveitis
	Meningitis with cranial nerve palsies
Latent	Asymptomatic
	+ Serology tests
3rd degree	Gummatous syphilis
	Cardiovascular syphilis
Neurosyphilis	Asymptomatic
	Tabes dorsalis (locomotor ataxia)
	General paresis
	Dementia
	Pupillary and deep tendon reflex abnormalities
	Tremors, seizures

confirmation must be obtained by ordering an FTA-ABS, as the screening tests can have false-positives. Because there are no effective means of culturing *T. pallidum*, visualization of the organism by use of darkfield microscopy can be used for genital lesions. If neurosyphilis is a possibility, examination of the CSF is necessary.

If syphilis is treated in the primary, secondary, or early latent stage, the risk of progression to tertiary syphilis is <10%.[53] After completion of treatment, serologic titers should be done at 6 and 12 months. If there is not an adequate decline in the titers or symptoms recur, then further treatment is indicated. In addition, treatment is considered as having failed if the follow-up titers are higher than the pretreatment titers.[53]

Miscellaneous. BV often reveals itself with a "fishy-odor" vaginal discharge. The presence of clue cells on the wet mount helps establish the diagnosis.

Chancroid presents as a single, painful lesion in the genital area with accompanying tender, regional lymphadenopathy; the diagnosis is usually made on the basis of the clinical findings. Nonspecific complaints of discharge and dysuria accompany the syndrome of NGU; testing for the specific etiologic organisms may help aid in the diagnosis, although often no specific organism can be identified. Uncomplicated infections are treated with oral administration of either azithromycin, ofloxacin, tetracycline, or doxycycline. Azithromycin has been added as a recommended antibiotic for the treatment of NGU.[52]

If trichomoniasis is present, it is often asymptomatic, even in men. The symptoms, if present, are often nonspecific. Demonstrating the presence of the motile, flagellated protozoan on microscopic urinalysis or wet preparation establishes the diagnosis.

Patient Education

Few individuals in this country recognize the numerous risks associated with reckless sexual behavior.[47] "Prevention of STDs must overall focus on changing the sexual behaviors of patients at risk."[47, 52] The main risk factor for acquiring any STD is having more than one sexual partner.[47]

Chlamydia. Prompt treatment of chlamydia infection decreases the risk of developing PID and infertility.[48] The CDC advises screening all sexually active adolescents during their routine gynecologic examinations every 6 months. Screening for chlamydia should be carried out in those who are 20–24 years of age and have a new sex partner, or in those individuals who do not use barrier contraception.[48, 54] When a patient is diagnosed with chlamydia, all partners who have had sexual contact with that patient within the past 60 days need to be tested and treated.[48]

Genital Herpes. Treatment of the infected individual does not decrease the risk of transmission to sexual contacts.[48] Prevention of HSV is the only current option. Infected individuals must limit their number of sexual partners; they must also be explicitly advised not to engage in sexual activity when lesions or symptoms are present. Instruction on the natural history of their disease and the fact that they can have asymptomatic viral shedding and can transmit this virus to the fetus if the woman becomes pregnant needs to be fully discussed. Condom use should be strongly recommended; however, the patient must be cautioned that condoms are only partially effective. Research regarding HSV disease is focusing on the development of vaccines, in particular on the development of a vaccine based on mucosal immunity.[48]

Gonorrhea. All sexually active female adolescents should be screened twice a year. Men have less likelihood of being asymptomatic, so the same recommendation does not apply. Patients with GC need to refer all sexual contacts they have had within the previous 60 days for evaluation and treatment. Infected patients should also abstain from sexual activity until treatment is complete and symptoms have resolved. The use of condoms is effective in preventing the transmission of GC; even the use of a diaphragm with spermicide can reduce the risk of GC, although not as completely as a condom.

HPV. Clinicians must educate HPV-infected patients on their risk factors, the prevention, and signs and symptoms of HPV. They also need to be instructed in genitalia self-examination in order to detect recurrences in a timely manner. Teach patients that having a healthy immune system (by following a proper diet, discontinuing any tobacco use, getting regular exercise, and decreasing stress levels) can decrease their chances of developing cervical cancer. Women should be instructed to get annual gynecologic examinations. Condom use is encouraged, although patients must be clearly advised that condom use does not offer full protection. Vaccines are being investigated to control HPV; the only real progress made thus far is on the development of subunit vaccines that are based on noninfectious HPV-like particles; these types of vaccines are promising candidates in the prevention of oncogenic HPV infections.[49]

Syphilis. Individuals who have had sexual contact within 90 days with those diagnosed with syphilis need to be informed and treated.[53] Patients need to be educated about their disease, the risks of noncompliance with treatment, and their need to modify any known risk factors. They should also be advised that their screening test, the FTA-ABS, will remain positive throughout their life, although a recent Canadian study demonstrated negative results in patients who were at least 3 years post-treatment.[53] The possibility of tertiary syphilis with signs, symptoms, and disability should be discussed with patients to assist with treatment compliance.

Prevention

Avoidance of STDs involves educating all patients at risk for STD, locating all patients who are unlikely to seek treatment, and providing effective diagnosis and treatment of those with STDs. In addition, there has to be tools in place for evaluating, treating, and counseling the sexual partners of those with STDs. Another means is providing immunizations for at-risk patients by available vaccines. One way to identify those at risk is to always include a thorough sexual history as part of any routine physical examination (Box 21–3).[47] Many health care practitioners do not question their patients regarding their sexual activity and many do not follow the consensus guidelines for the treatment of STDs. This is felt to lead to the inconsistencies across the country in the evaluation and management outcomes. In one study, 50% of primary care physicians were unsure of the CDC guidelines or simply did not follow the guidelines when treating PID in their patients.[48]

STD prevention must address a variety of critical issues in order to have a significant impact on the disease profile. Prevention should address patients' specific high-risk behaviors and include information about the actions patients can take to avoid acquiring or transmitting STDs. Dangerous behaviors are listed here:

* Multiple or casual sexual contacts
* New sex partner
* Sexual activity related to drug use
* Lower socioeconomic status
* Urban living

Box 21-3–QUESTIONS TO ASK DURING A SEXUAL HISTORY

Are you sexually active?

Do you have a monogamous relationship, or do you have multiple partners?

Are you involved with someone who has an STD or multiple sex partners?

Have you ever had an STD or PID?

Do you use barrier contraception during sex?

Are your sexual partners male, female, or both?

Do you participate in vaginal, oral, and/or anal sex?

Do you engage in "casual" sex?

Do you or your partner experience symptoms associated with intercourse or have existing symptoms, such as vaginal/penile discharge, lesions, etc.?

STD, sexually trasmitted disease; PID, pelvic inflammatory disease

If a patient is diagnosed with an STD, it is crucial in almost every case that notification of all contacts be achieved, either by the patient or by the local health department. In most cases, the option can first be offered to the patient to notify any contacts himself or herself, as it allows the patient some privacy and discretion in a matter that may have great psychosocial impact on the patient and any others. If this notification is not carried out in a timely manner by the patient, then the local health department must become involved. If the practitioner suspects that a patient is hiding critical information, the local health department can be contacted for assistance.[47]

Adolescents are also another high-risk group that poses special problems in managing the spread of STDs. In teens, a matter-of-fact discussion of the prevention, symptoms, and complications of STDs should be part of all routine well-child checkups. In addition, a sexual history should also be obtained from them in a nonconfrontational, straightforward manner. It is often preferable, if the teenager agrees, to ask the parent or guardian to go to the waiting room if he or she has been present in the examination room to allow the teenager to speak more freely. This type of situation also has to be handled with tact and common sense.

Screening Recommendations

Intensive screening of all links to a patient diagnosed with an STD is vital to STD prevention. There are "core transmitters"—persons with a history of repeated infections—who are believed to be responsible for the transmission of the preponderance of STDs in urban settings. Screening and prevention programs must be aimed at this group.

TUBERCULOSIS

Pathophysiology

TB is caused by *Mycobacterium tuberculosis*, an aerobic, nonmotile bacillus; *M. africanum* and *M. bovis* are two other *Mycobacterium* strains that also cause disease. The primary clinical manifestation of *M. tuberculosis* is a persistent, often recurring infection in the pulmonary system, although the bacterium can affect any organ or organ system in the body.

TB occurs when an individual inhales droplets infected with *M. tuberculosis*. These aerosolized, infected microscopic beads can stay suspended for several hours. It has been found that fomites play little if any role in the spread of this disease. When a person inhales these droplets, they are drawn into the pulmonary tree, and settle into the middle and lower sections of the lungs. If the bacteria are not eradicated by the host defense systems, then multiplication occurs, leading to lymphatic and hematogenous dissemination. Once the cell-mediated immune response develops, the infection usually becomes walled off in the lung. This primary phase is almost always asymptomatic. The infection most often remains in this state for months to years until reactivation occurs. If the infected individuals are immunocompromised, particularly secondary to AIDS, they may progress directly to symptomatic, primary pulmonary TB.

Pediatric Issues[7, 16, 44]

Symptoms of airway obstruction are common presenting complaints; this is due to the increased incidence of hilar adenopathy associated with TB in children. Exposure to an adult who is at high risk for TB is the most common risk factor for children. Symptoms usually develop within the first year after exposure, and then remain dormant until adolescence when reactivation most commonly occurs. If a child is diagnosed with active TB, hospitalization is initially recommended in most cases. When testing a child who has had possible exposure to TB or is in a high-risk group, the tuberculin skin test to use is the Mantoux; the tine test is an inadequate diagnostic tool in these children.

Isoniazid (INH) is a safe medication to use, as the risk of hepatitis in children secondary to this drug is much lower than in adults. Pyrazinamide can also be safely used due to the decreased incidence of resistance and the lower incidence of drug side effects in children (e.g., hyperuricemia).

Ethambutol should be used with caution in pediatric patients, and then only if an eye examination is carried out every 2 months due to the drug's side effects of optic neuritis and color blindness.

In children who present with life-threatening airway compression, acute pericardial effusion, massive pleural effusion, or miliary TB, corticosteroids may be used as part of the initial management.

Obstetric Issues[46]

The incidence of TB in pregnancy is very low. There have been <200 reported cases of congenital TB in the U.S.

Geriatric Issues

This patient group is at increased risk of active TB via reactivation of dormant infection. The disease presentation may be more subtle, and the possibility of TB may not initially be entertained, leading to a delay in diagnosis and treatment. Miliary and meningeal TB are more common in the elderly.[7] Patients in nursing homes are at risk of a TB outbreak if a fellow resident is infected with TB.

Epidemiology

On a worldwide basis, TB is the most common cause of death from infectious disease.[55] In the U.S., there were approximately 21,000 new cases reported in 1996.[7] Until the advent of the AIDS pandemic, TB rates in this country were on a steady decline; the presence of HIV has set in motion an increase in the incidence of TB as well as a rapidly growing threat of multidrug-resistant TB. The impact that HIV has on all facets of TB is profound. In an HIV-infected person who encounters *M. tuberculosis*, the rate of the development of clinical TB rises from a 5–10% probability in 1–2 years (as seen in an HIV-negative individual) to a 50% chance of developing clinical disease within the first 60 days of exposure.[7] The greater number of TB cases are seen in individuals from countries outside of the U.S who were exposed to disease before emigrating. In addition to HIV-positive patients, older people with disease reactivation compose a significant percentage of TB cases.

Currently, immigrants with the greatest likelihood of being TB-infected are from Mexico, the Philippines, and Vietnam.[116] Those infected with HIV, intravenous drug users, African-Americans, Hispanics, and/or those who live in urban areas are also at highest risk. These facets of TB disease in this country, along with the growing threat of drug-resistant TB, place an increasing burden on the health care system.

Treatment Options

Many patients with pulmonary disease are asymptomatic. The most common symptom is cough that may initially be nonproductive, but then gradually progresses to being productive of purulent sputum. The patient may complain of hemoptysis during advanced disease. There may be constitutional symptoms of weight loss, night sweats, fever, anorexia, and fatigue. The examination is often remarkable for only an ill-appearing patient and the lungs are clear to auscultation or may demonstrate rales. Adenopathy is another possible finding. The possibility of TB should always be considered when a patient presents with persistent fever, night sweats, and chronic cough, regardless of ethnicity or country of origin.

If a tuberculin skin test is performed, anyone who has been infected with the *M. tuberculosis* bacilli will demonstrate a positive reaction, unless the individual is anergic. The tuberculin skin test is performed by injecting purified protein derivative (PPD) solution intradermally—the Mantoux test (0.1 mL of intermediate-strength PPD). A positive skin test (≥10 mm of induration at the injection site) does not necessarily indicate the presence of active disease. Individuals who have received the bacille Calmette-Guérin (BCG) vaccine or have been treated in the past prophylactically or for active TB also have a positive skin test due to the presence of antibodies. If a patient has a positive tuberculin skin test, and has no history of treatment or ever receiving BCG, then a chest x-ray should be ordered, and subsequent management recommendations made.

In active pulmonary TB, the chest x-ray may show a pleural effusion, heterogeneous opacities (mainly in the apices and upper lung segments), and/or cavitary lesions; hilar or mediastinal adenopathy may be present. In miliary disease, there can be a diffuse, cavitary pattern seen on x-ray study. A sputum sample is collected for culture and an acid-fast bacillus (AFB) smear. If the patient is symptomatic and/or has an abnormal chest x-ray, but is unable to produce sputum, sputum induction should be carried out. At least three consecutive, first-morning specimens should be collected. If the suspicion for TB is high, but the sputum smears remain negative, bronchial washings can be obtained via bronchoscopy.

Other laboratory abnormalities include anemias, thrombocytosis, elevated gamma-globulin, hyponatremia, and abnormal liver enzymes.

Hospitalization should be considered in a very ill patient with pulmonary TB, in patients with disseminated disease, or if compliance with infectious disease precautions and/or treatment cannot be ensured. Consultation with a specialist and the local health department helps dictate the type of treatment regimen to use. The HIV status of the patient, the geographic locality in which the patient lives, the country from which the patient emigrated, and the presence of other comorbid diseases or high-risk behaviors affect the pattern of drug resistance, choice of treatment options, and patient compliance.

Patient Education

For the PPD-positive patient who is treated prophylactically, the indications for chemoprophylaxis and education on the medication regimen should be outlined. These patients need to be cautioned that any future PPDs will be positive, and advised not to have any done in the future; if screening is needed, a chest x-ray is appropriate.

The natural history of the disease, risk factors, review of the treatment options, and infection control issues should be reviewed for the patient diagnosed with TB. Information also is collected regarding the patient's contacts, socioeconomic status, social history (any illicit drug/alcohol use, sexual history), past medical history, and medications. Local public health sectors monitor the patient's progress and treatment regimen; in addition, they deal with any TB contacts.

Prevention

The issues most pivotal in preventing TB hinge on prevention of HIV spread, managing treatment of existing TB effectively in order to limit the development of drug resistance, and efficient screening programs, particularly in high-risk groups.

Referral to the local health department is necessary for anyone with a positive PPD (and no prior history of treatment, TB disease, or BCG vaccine) or anyone diagnosed with probable TB (a positive AFB smear is enough for referral).[16] The majority of city and county health departments have a designated specialist to whom referrals or consults are made. In many localities, public health authorities directly observe treatment to ensure compliance with the prescribed course of therapy. This arrangement has proved decidedly effective in restricting disease spread.[16] These departments also have the authority to detain those who are incapable of following a treatment plan or who refuse therapy, as long as this can be proved to the satisfaction of the courts.

The only available vaccine is the BCG, a vaccine containing live, attenuated *Mycobacterium bovis*; it is primarily used in developing countries that have a high prevalence of TB in young people. It is not used routinely in the U.S. except for certain specific indications. In this country, it is given only to children and newborns that have negative PPDs and are living in situations in which there is a high risk of TB exposure; these children also have to be HIV-negative and unlikely to be available to receive INH treatment or follow-up. BCG is also recommended for those who are at high risk of exposure to multidrug-resistant TB.[16]

Current research efforts are focusing on development of vaccines that are more effective, treatment options in multidrug-resistant TB, and the further study of "postprimary" TB. It has been proposed that a major cause of postprimary TB ("infection that occurs many years after a primary infection") is from exogenous reinfection, not reactivation of latent disease as has been commonly thought.[56]

Screening Recommendations

Screening by appropriate tuberculin skin tests is advised for the following groups[7, 17, 37]:

* Well-child checkup
  * Screening should be administered at 12-month checkups but is only indicated for children considered to be at risk; if results are negative but risk factors are unchanged, the test should be done annually.[57]
* General
  * HIV-infected individuals
  * Close contacts of those with known or suspected TB
  * Foreign-born individuals from countries with high TB frequency
  * Medically underserved low-income populations
  * Alcoholics and illicit drug users
  * Patients with chest x-ray abnormalities consistent with old healed TB
* Residents of long-term facilities
  * Correctional institutes, mental institutions, and other long-term care facilities
* Employees of
  * Any health care facility
  * Nursing home facilities and other long-term care facilities
  * Correctional institutions
* Patients with certain medical conditions
  * Chronic renal failure
  * Diabetes mellitus
  * Gastrectomy
  * Jejunoileal bypass
  * Leukemia or lymphoma
  * Malignancies
  * Prolonged high-dose corticosteroid therapy
  * Silicosis
  * Weight loss of $\geq 10\%$ below ideal body weight

REFERENCES

1. Achievements in public health, 1900–1999: Control of infectious diseases. MMWR Morb Mortal Wkly Rep 1999;48:621–629.
2. Cohen M, Levy SB, Mead P. Infectious diseases: Still emerging in 1998. Patient Care 1998;32–59.
3. Osterholm MT, Symposium Coordinator. Emerging infections: A three-article symposium. Postgrad Med 1999;106:86–89.
4. Lederberg J, Shope RE (eds). Emerging Infections: Microbial Threats to Health in the United States. Washington DC. National Academy Press, 1992.
5. Danila RN, Lexau C, Lynfield R, et al. Addressing emerging infections. Postgrad Med 1999;106:90–105.
6. Institute of Medicine Report. Emerging Infections: Microbial Threats to Health in the United States. Public Health Image Library, 1997. http://phil.cdc.gov/PHIL_Images/04021998/00007/2MG0006_lores.jpg.

6a. Testimony of Anthony S. Fauci, M.D., Director of NIAID before the U.S. Senate Labor and Human Resources Subcommittee on Public Health Safety. Global Health: The United States Response to Infectious Disease. March 3, 1998.

7. The Merck Medical Manual, 17th Ed. PDR Electronic Library. Ramsey, NJ, Medical Economics Co, 1999.

8. Tierney LM, McPhee SJ, Papadakis MA. Current Medical Diagnosis and Treatment. New York, Appleton & Lange, 1999.

9. Bowers DH. HIV: Past, present, and future. Postgrad Med 2000;107:109–113.

10. Yu K, Daar ES. Primary HIV infection. Postgrad Med 2000;107:114–122.

11. Church JA. HIV disease in children. Postgrad Med 2000;107:163–176.

12. Talarico LD. Uncharted territory: AIDS in the older patient. Patient Care 1998;32:84–96.

13. Starr C. The Latest Recommendations for Antiretroviral Therapy. Patient Care 1998;32:154–171.

14. Wolfe PR. Practical approaches to HIV therapy. Postgrad Med 2000;107:127–138.

15. Staszewski S, Morales-Ramirez J, Tashima KT, et al. Efavirenz plus zidovudine and lamivudine, efavirenz plus indinavir, and indinavir plus zidovudine and lamivudine in the treatment of HIV-1 infection in adults. N Engl J Med 1999;34:1865–1873.

16. D'Epiro NW. HIV disease, persistent fever, nonresolving pneumonia, tuberculosis. Patient Care 1999;33:28–50.

17. Cohan GR. HIV-associated metabolic and morphologic abnormality syndrome. Postgrad Med 2000;107:141–146.

18. Song R, Liu S, Huang J, et al. National Institute of Allergy and Infectious Disease. Effect of LAMP-Targeting and GM-CSF Microspheres on Cytolytic Response to HIV-1 Gag DNA Vaccine. http://www.niaid.nih.gov/aidsvaccine/meetings/formulation.htm. October 7, 1999.

19. Gutierrez KM, Prober CG. Encephalitis. Postgrad Med 1998;103:123–143.

20. Rachlis AR. Neurologic manifestations of HIV infection. Postgrad Med 1998:103:147–161.

21. Clinical Trials.gov: A Service of the National Institutes of Health. "A Study on the Use of Valacyclovir to Treat Herpes Simplex Encephalitis." http://clinicaltrials.gov/ct/gui/c/alr/ac...; 2000.

22. Harris GD, Steimle J. Compiling the identifying features of bacterial endocarditis. Postgrad Med 2000;107:75–83.

23. Giesel BE, Koenig CJ, Blake RL. Management of bacterial endocarditis. Am Fam Physician 2000;61:1725–1732.

24. Durack DT, Lukes AS, Bright DK. New criteria for diagnosis of infective endocarditis: Utilization of specific echocardiographic findings. Am J Med 1994;96:200–209.

25. Infective endocarditis: Keeping a killer at bay. A Q&A session with Donald Kaye, MD. Consultant 2000;40:622–626.

26. Prophylaxis Guidelines for Infective Endocarditis (Consultant Quick Take). Consultant 2000;40:627–628.

26a. Stedman's Medical Dictionary. PDR Electronic Library. Ramsey, NJ, Medical Economics Co., 1999, p. 17.

27. Juckett G. Prevention and treatment of traveler's diarrhea. Am Fam Physician 1999;60:119–124.

28. Sutjita M, Dupont HL. Acute infectious diarrhea in adults. Patient Care 1999;33:58–77.

29. Bender JB, Smith KS, Hedberg C, Osterholm MT. Food-borne disease in the 21st century. Postgrad Med 1999;106:109–119.

30. Eliason BC, Lewan RB. Gastroenteritis in children: Principles of diagnosis and treatment. Am Fam Physician 1998;58:1769–1776.

31. O'Connor DL. Common infections in child care. Patient Care 1998;32:60–84.

32. Bacon BR, Di Bisceglie AM. Liver Disease: Diagnosis and Management. New York, Churchill Livingstone, 2000.

33. Moyer LA, Mast EE, Alter MJ. Hepatitis C. Part I: Routine serologic testing and diagnosis. Am Fam Physician 1999;59:79–88.

34. D'Epiro NW. Hepatitis C: Containing an invisible epidemic. Patient Care 1998;32:96–111.

35. NIH News Release. Immune Response to Hepatitis B Spares Liver Cells. National Institutes of Health, April 29, 1999.

36. NIH News Release. Hepatitis E Virus Infection May Be Widespread in Rats. National Institutes of Health, August 19, 1999.

37. Hunt CM, Sharara AI. Liver disease in pregnancy. Am Fam Physician 1999;59:829–836.

38. Recommendations of the Advisory Committee for Elimination of Tuberculosis. Screening for tuberculosis and tuberculosis infection in high-risk populations. MMWR Morb Mortal Wkly Rep 1990;39(RR-8):1–7.

39. Rose VL. CDC issues new recommendations for the prevention and control of hepatitis C virus infection. Am Fam Physician 1999;59:1321–1323.

40. Clinical Trials.gov: A Service of the National Institutes of Health. Lamivudine for Chronic Hepatitis B. http://clinicaltrials.gov, 2000.

41. Phillips EJ, Simor AE. Bacterial meningitis in children and adults. Postgrad Med 1998;103:102–117.

42. Abramowicz M (ed). The choice of antibacterial drugs. Medical Letter 1999;41:95–104.

43. Uremovich GR. Cryptococcal meningitis. Physician Assistant 1999;23:36–43.

44. Hay WW, et al. (eds). Current Pediatric Diagnosis and Treatment. Norwalk, CT, Appleton & Lange, 1999.

45. The Merck Manual of Geriatrics, 2nd ed. PDR Electronic Library. Ramsey, NJ, Medical Economics Co, 1999.

46. Beckmann CR, Ling FW, Barzanski BM, et al. Obstetrics and Gynecology. Baltimore, MD, Williams & Wilkins, 1998.

47. Trotto NE. STDs: Are you up-to-date? Patient Care 1999;33:74–102.

48. Kirchner JT, Emmert DH. Sexually transmitted diseases in women. Postgrad Med 2000;107:55–65.

49. Institute of Medicine Committee on Prevention and Control of Sexually Transmitted Diseases. The Hidden Epidemic: Confronting Sexually Transmitted Diseases. Washington DC, National Academy Press, 1996.

50. Longenecker RL, Franson JK. Managing genital herpes infection in pregnancy. Family Practice Recertification 1999;21:61–76.

51. O'Neill-Morante M. Human papillomavirus: A review of manifestations, diagnosis, and treatment. Physician Assistant 2000;24(1):19–25.

52. Miller KE, Graves CG. Update on the prevention and treatment of sexually transmitted diseases. Am Fam Physician 2000;61:379–386.

53. Birnbaum NR, Goldschmidt RH, Buffett WO. Resolving the common clinical dilemmas of syphilis. Am Fam Physician 1999;59:2233–2240.
54. Centers for Disease Control and Prevention. 1998 Guidelines for treatment of sexually transmitted diseases. MMWR Morb Mortal Wkly Rep 1998;47(RR-1):1–111.
55. NIAID Spotlight on Infectious Diseases. NIAID workshop develops blueprint for TB vaccine development. NIAID Council News 1999;8
56. Van Rie A, Warren R, Richardson M, et al. Exogenous reinfection as a cause of recurrent tuberculosis after curative treatment. N Engl J Med 1999;341:1174–1179.
57. American Academy of Pediatrics Committee on Infectious Diseases. Update on tuberculosis skin testing in children. Pediatrics 1996;97:282.

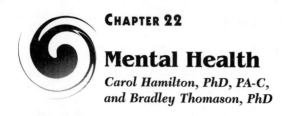

CHAPTER 22

Mental Health

*Carol Hamilton, PhD, PA-C,
and Bradley Thomason, PhD*

INTRODUCTION

Mental illness is one of the most prevalent and costly public health concerns in the United States, with associated behavioral or lifestyle factors that account for approximately 50% of premature death in the U.S. annually.[1] This statistic illustrates the enormous impact psychosocial and behavioral factors have on the health of the U.S. population. Given the high prevalence of both psychiatric illness and behavioral factors in chronic disease, it is paramount that non-psychiatric health care providers be educated in the assessment, diagnosis, and treatment of mental health issues that commonly appear in primary care settings.

Nearly one half of the population will experience some type of mental illness during their lifetime.[1, 2] As a group the most common mental health disorders are anxiety disorders (17%), followed by substance abuse (11%) and affective disorders (11%).[2]

The documented prevalence of mental health disorders in the U.S. represents a significant burden to society in terms of quality of life, lost productivity, and health care expenditures. Despite the ubiquity of mental illness, psychiatric disorders often are poorly understood and undertreated by non-psychiatric health care providers. Of those who experience a mental health disorder during their lifetime, less than 40% receive any type of treatment, as do less than 20% of those recently diagnosed with a mental health disorder.[2] Additional problems exist for those who do receive care. Societal stigma associated with mental illness remains high, resulting in shame and fear for these patients. Impaired emotions and cognitive processes may create difficulty in accessing and adhering to treatment. Moreover, third party reimbursements for mental health services are typically more restrictive than for standard medical services. These combined factors produce significant barriers to patients receiving optimal, or even adequate, health care for mental illness.

Major breakthroughs in recent years have afforded some positive changes in mental health care delivery. The development of the selective serotonin reuptake inhibitors (SSRIs) and other newer generation drug treatments has resulted in increased utilization of pharmacotherapies. The popularity of alternative therapies has offered additional treatment options. Psychotherapy remains a popular and empirically valid form of treatment. Recent legislation (e.g., the Patient's Bill of

Rights) being introduced at the state and federal level may improve mental health care delivery as well.

The majority of mental health care (pharmacologic and nonpharmacologic) is dispensed in primary care settings by non-psychiatric health care professionals.[3, 4] Approximately 24–50% of all primary care patients have a psychiatric illness.[3, 4] Twenty-five to seventy percent of all patient care visits are to address some psychosocial problem.[4, 5] Mood disorders, stress-related illnesses, psychosomatic problems, substance abuse, relationship and family dynamics, and obesity are among the most common psychological conditions treated in primary care.[3, 6]

Referral to a specialist in mental health care is medically indicated and appropriate if one or more of the following apply:

* Symptoms are severe (i.e., daily function is significantly impaired).
* The primary care clinician is not experienced in managing psychiatric illnesses.
* The toxicity of the indicated medication is significant (lithium, monoamine oxidase inhibitors [MAOIs], or anticonvulsants).
* The patient requests referral or consultation.

Perhaps the most compelling reasons to refer are to obtain a thorough diagnostic evaluation and to confirm the diagnosis. The patient will then be under the care of a team consisting of the mental health professional and the primary care provider, resulting in increased benefit to the patient. If the suspected diagnosis is not amenable to psychotherapy, referral for initial or periodic evaluation should be considered.

Patient education and effective communication skills generally increase the patient's acceptance of mental health treatment. It might be helpful to inform the patient that counseling is beneficial for a wide range of issues and concerns for a significant number of "regular" people who go to work and take care of their normal responsibilities every day. One effective patient education approach is to say that therapy does not "fix" people, but that it helps people develop tools to better deal with the stresses of life. Introducing the therapist and offering therapy in the same or in another geographically convenient facility may increase patients' access and adherence to treatment regimens because of decreased anxiety, increased comfort and familiarity, greater convenience, and decreased stigma.

When providing primary mental health care, basic treatment goals include:

* Ensure the safety of the patient and others.
* Carry out a complete diagnostic evaluation.
* Alleviate immediate symptoms.
* Address long-term well-being.

Hospitalization is indicated if the patient presents a risk to self or others. The risk may be active (suicidal or homicidal ideation) or passive (grossly impaired ability to secure food and shelter). The degree and imminence of risk are based on the patient's mental status, plan for inflicting harm, past medical history, and adequacy of family support. This judgment is often made in consultation with a mental health care professional. If immediate mental health consultation is not available and uncertainty regarding the imminence of risk remains, the provider should err on the side of caution and hospitalize the patient. The therapeutic relationship is best maintained if the patient agrees to hospital admission. Many patients with depression respond well to candid concern and voluntarily admit themselves. Patients with psychotic symptoms and grossly impaired judgment frequently lack insight into their condition and often refuse admission. If the patient refuses, most state laws provide a means by which certain health care providers can commit a patient. Familiarity with the laws and a standard plan for commitment procedures are necessary.

If a patient is hospitalized, it is financially and medically expedient to complete the diagnostic evaluation during the hospital stay. Patients with mental health disorders may have impaired capacity or motivation to follow up with outpatient appointments for diagnostic procedures. A thorough medical (including laboratory studies) and neurologic evaluation (which may include an electroencephalogram or a computed tomographic or magnetic resonance imaging scan of the brain) should be done as indicated.

Symptoms that are acutely distressing or disruptive of normal bodily functions can be alleviated with short-term pharmacotherapy. Medications can be prescribed to provide relief for sleep disturbances, agitation, fear, and acute emotional pain.

A combination of psychotherapy and pharmacotherapy has more long-term efficacy than either approach used alone to treat depression, anxiety, and most other mental health disorders. Many types of behavior therapy (e.g., relaxation training, breathing exercises, and systematic desensitization through in vivo exposure) have been shown to be effective in treating a variety of mental illnesses. Adding cognitive therapy (i.e., guiding the patient to change dysfunctional patterns of thinking) also improves treatment outcome.[2, 5, 7, 8] Electroconvulsive therapy (ECT) is used to treat refractory affective disorders. Phototherapy is a novel approach to treating depression with a seasonal component. Family counseling also can be done by the primary care provider, as family dynamics often contribute greatly to the onset or continuance of mental illness.

Primary care providers need to be well versed in dealing with psychosocial concerns and mental health disorders in the primary care milieu. Additionally, they should be aware of the demonstrated benefits of integrated primary care and mental health services, where behavioral scientists are situated in the same outpatient facility as primary care providers. This model, in which the primary care provider remains in charge of the patient's care and consults with the behavioral scientist, has been shown to result in improved outcomes and decreased health care costs.[9, 10] Having on-site psychiatric consultation allows primary care providers to improve their mental health interventions. Additionally, it aids in the management of patients with chronic psychosocial issues and high rates of utilization of medical services.

Most primary care providers develop a level of comfort in managing many psychiatric illnesses, such as mild to moderate mood disturbances and somatoform disorders. Providers may feel less at ease at treating more severe forms of mental illness. Psychosis, substance abuse, eating disorders, sexual dysfunction, and personality disorders may be identified first in a primary health care setting. It is beyond the scope of this book to outline conditions that require specialty intervention; however, the more common of these illnesses are outlined in Table 22–1.[9] (For additional resources, see the Resources Appendix at the end of this book.)

Table 22–1. Mental Illnesses Typically Requiring Specialty Care

Condition	Characterization
Schizophrenia	A disorder of thought marked by hallucinations, delusional beliefs, disorganized speech and behavior, and inappropriate affect. Subtypes: Paranoid, disorganized, catatonic, and undifferentiated
Substance abuse	Maladaptive pattern of drug use that results in negative consequences to physical, social, occupational, domestic, and legal well-being
Anorexia nervosa	Eating disorder in which the person fails to maintain normal body weight owing to body dysmorphism or fear of weight gain. Usually, the patient restricts and ritualizes the diet.
Bulimia nervosa	Eating disorder characterized by episodes of binge eating and compensatory purging behaviors (e.g., self-induced vomiting) to control weight. The patient feels a lack of control over the eating.
Sexual dysfunction	A disturbance in, or pain associated with the sexual response cycle. Subtypes: Hypoactive sexual desire disorder, sexual aversion disorder, female sexual arousal disorder, male erectile disorder, orgasmic disorder, premature ejaculation, dyspareunia, and vaginismus
Personality disorders	Patterns of experiences and behavior deviant from one's culture that cause impairment in cognition, affect, interpersonal functioning, and/or impulse control. The pattern pervades a broad range of interpersonal/social situations. Subtypes: Paranoid, schizoid, schizotypal, antisocial, borderline, histrionic, narcissistic, avoidant, dependent, obsessive-compulsive

■■■■MOOD DISORDERS

DEPRESSION

Pathophysiology

Depression typically has a consistent presentation with symptoms encompassing affect, biology, behavior, and cognition (Box 22–1). The

---

Box 22-1–THE A-B-CS OF DEPRESSION

Affective	**Cognitive**
Depressed mood	Guilt
Loneliness	Low self-esteem
Irritability	Attention, concentration, and
Anhedonia	memory problems
	Hopelessness
Biological	Helplessness
Sleep disturbance	Thoughts of suicide or death
Appetite/weight change	Indecisiveness
Decreased libido	
Fatigue	
Behavioral	
Social withdrawal	
Psychomotor retardation or	
agitation	
Suicide attempts	
Decreased activity level	

---

course of depression, however, is highly variable. Table 22–2 lists the different diagnostic subtypes of mood disorders (sometimes referred to as "affective disorders"). Mania is included as a disorder of (elevated) affect and is thought to be more endogenous or biological in origin than depression without mania. However, both biological and psychological theories have been offered to explain the origins of depression. The best supported theories are those that suggest an inherited potential combined with certain life events. Learned helplessness, lack of positive reinforcement, lack of self-control, and dysfunctional cognitions are among the chief principles underlying other empirically supported theories.[11]

Pediatric Issues

Depression is more common in children with a family history of chronic depression. Symptoms in children are essentially the same as in adults. Substance abuse and risk-taking behaviors are means by which the adolescent may deal with the depression. Suicidal and

Table 22–2. Common Mood Disorders

Mood Classification	Description
Major depressive episode	Mood symptoms occur nearly every day for at least 2 weeks and include a combination of: depressed mood, anhedonia, appetite or weight change, sleep disturbance, psychomotor agitation or retardation, fatigue, feelings of worthlessness or guilt, concentration problems or indecisiveness, thoughts of death or suicide
Manic episode	Abnormally elevated or irritable mood lasting at least a week (or until hospitalization). Symptoms include a combination of: inflated self-esteem/grandiosity; decreased need for sleep; pressured speech; racing thoughts; distractability; increased goal-directed acting or agitation; impulsive or risky behaviors (e.g., spending sprees, indiscreet sex)
Dysthymia	Chronic depressive disorder lasting at least 2 years with symptoms similar to a major depressive episode but milder in nature
Major depressive disorder	A major depressive episode manifesting once or recurrently
Bipolar disorder	A combination of manic and major depressive episodes
Cyclothymic disorder	A combination of hypomanic and low-level depressive symptoms

homicidal ideation must be taken seriously in youth, as suicide and homicide constitute two of the leading causes of death in people under 21 years of age. Whenever there is *any* concern that an adolescent may be a danger to her- or himself or to others, hospitalization is the standard of care.[12] When any childhood psychiatric disorder is suspected, the patient should be referred to a pediatric mental health specialist.

Obstetric Issues

Postpartum blues occurs in more than 50% of women after childbirth and is mild and self-limited. It consists of tearfulness, fatigue, anxiety, and irritability and lasts only a few days after childbirth.

Postpartum psychosis is a psychiatric emergency. It is characterized by depression, delusions, hallucinations, disturbed thought processes, agitation, florid psychotic symptoms, and ideation of harming the infant or the self. Up to 4% of patients commit infanticide, and 5% commit suicide. The mean onset of postpartum psychosis is between 2 and 3 weeks after delivery, and it rarely begins more than 8 weeks after childbirth. The disorder may be characterized by indifference to and reluctance to care for the baby, or by obsessive concern about the infant's health. The pathophysiology is incompletely understood, but the strongest data suggests that postpartum psychosis is an episode of a mood disorder. It is usually a bipolar disorder but can be a depressive disorder and may be hormonally mediated. The fact that two thirds of patients experience a second episode within 1 year supports its categorization as a mood disorder. Postpartum psychosis has a psychosocial basis as well, owing to its association with first births, stress, and marital discord. Certain medical conditions such as infection, eclampsia, hemorrhage, and drug intoxication are associated with increased risk of postpartum psychosis. However, stressors are known to precipitate expression of quiescent psychiatric disorders.

The incidence of postpartum psychosis is estimated to be between one and two per 1000 childbirths.[13] Between 50% and 60% of cases occur with first-born children, and 50% of cases occur in patients who have perinatal complications.[1]

Patients are treated with antidepressants and lithium, sometimes with an antipsychotic. None of these agents should be prescribed to the woman who is breastfeeding. Hospitalization with suicide precautions is warranted. Contact with the infant is usually beneficial but must be closely monitored. After the acute psychotic symptoms subside, psychotherapy addressing the areas of conflict should be undertaken. Usually, the conflict is related to the patient accepting and becoming comfortable with her mothering role. Family counseling directed at increasing support from the infant's father and other family members is also helpful. The chance of complete recovery from the acute episode is high. Early recognition of the disease and its potentially tragic outcomes will reduce the incidence of suicide and infanticide.

Patients may feel guilty about their "unnatural" emotional reactions to their infants and may need reassurance that they can be capable and loving parents. Patients should be educated concerning the symptoms of mood disorders so that they can recognize the return of the illness and seek treatment early. They should be informed that those who experience postpartum psychosis with a first birth have an increased risk of recurrence with future pregnancies.

Geriatric Issues

Depression can be misdiagnosed as dementia. *Generally*, if a patient complains of memory loss, then he or she is probably depressed and not demented. Depression can go unnoticed in the homebound geriatric patient. Poor health, chronic disease, and the loss of friends and family make the elderly prone to depression.

Recognition of depression by the primary care provider is imperative, as most geriatric suicide victims visited a primary care physician in the month prior to the suicide attempt. The highest rates of geriatric suicide are among white males over 85 years of age.[13]

Epidemiology

Depression is the most common psychiatric illness in the U.S. (equal in frequency to alcohol abuse). Lifetime prevalence of depression is estimated at 15–17%.[27] Clinical depression occurs twice as frequently in women and in over 40% of individuals with a chronic medical illness. When depression is untreated, approximately 15% of patients will commit suicide, and far more will make a suicide attempt.[8, 11]

Treatment Options

The primary treatment modalities for depressive illnesses are psychotherapy and pharmacotherapy. Studies have shown that a combination of these is more effective than either approach used alone. Electroconvulsive therapy (ECT) may be used to treat refractory affective disorders and may be particularly helpful in the elderly. Phototherapy is a safe and effective nonpharmacologic treatment modality for depression with a seasonal component.

Multiple psychotherapeutic approaches (e.g., psychodynamic, humanistic, gestalt) are used to treat depression. Cognitive-behavioral therapy (CBT) is perhaps the most empirically-based form of treatment. CBT utilizes a combination of behavioral and cognitive strategies that can easily be incorporated into primary care counseling. The goal of behavior therapy is to maximize behaviors that are positively reinforcing. Cognitive therapy attempts to change or restructure the patient's dysfunctional patterns of thinking. In addition to CBT, family counseling may be helpful because family dynamics often play a large role in the onset or continuance of depression.

Treatment with antidepressant medications significantly increases the chance of early recovery. The recently developed SSRIs are as effective as the older tricyclic, tetracyclic, or MAOI antidepressants and have substantially less toxicity and fewer side effects. Thus, SSRIs are the treatment of choice for depression and are frequently prescribed by primary care providers. Commonly prescribed SSRIs are fluoxetine (Prozac), paroxetine (Paxil), and sertraline (Zoloft). No one agent has been shown to be more effective than others; the fit between the side effect profile and the patient's symptoms should determine the selection. Any of the SSRIs may cause a variety of sexual dysfunctions in both men and women, most commonly delayed orgasm. Sexual dysfunction occurs in up to 30% of patients and is more likely to persist than other side effects. If sexual dysfunction is a problem for the patient, tricyclic antidepressants are a reasonable second choice. Nortriptyline (Pamelor), desipramine, and protriptyline (Vivactil) are among the better tolerated tricyclic drugs. Patients with high suicide risk generally should not be prescribed large quantities of tricyclics because of the potential for lethal overdose. In some cases, tricyclic or tetracyclic drugs (trazodone, alprazolam) may be useful but cause sedation. MAOIs are also helpful for some patients but are rarely used because their use entails dietary restrictions and the potential for dangerous drug interactions. Dosages of all antidepressants should begin at the low end of the spectrum and be slowly titrated upward.

Patient Education

Patients should be assured that having a mental illness is not a weakness or a lapse of moral character but a combination of genetic, biological, and psychosocial factors. Appropriate patient education regarding antidepressant medication is the key to acceptance and treatment success. The fact that both biological and psychological components of the illness benefit from antidepressant medication should be conveyed. Informing patients that antidepressants are not addictive improves adherence to treatment regimens. Couched in terms the patient can understand, an important message is that, while antidepressants cannot solve problems, they *can* alter neurochemistry and improve sleeping, memory, and concentration. Offering antidepressant therapy as a trial often makes the patient more comfortable. It should be explained that antidepressants typically take 3–4 weeks to exert optimal therapeutic benefits, and that antidepressants are not effective taken intermittently or as needed. Remind patients that most side effects of antidepressants are normally mild and transient. Finally, patients should understand that there are other effective treatments if the first-line medication is not effective.

Primary care providers should be candid in telling patients that the etiology of mental health disorders is not completely understood, but more is being learned all the time. Findings from medical research can be shared with patients (appropriate to their level of understanding), and they can be encouraged to learn more about depression on their own. (See the Resources Appendix at the end of this book.)

Prevention

The multifaceted causes of affective disorders, biological, genetic, and environmental, are not all amenable to primary prevention. The role of stress in the etiology of mental illness is supported by data showing that certain life events are predictive of major depressive episodes.[7] Given these predictors, the risk of mental illness may be reduced by helping people develop effective skills for coping with stress. Examples of programs aimed at increasing coping skills include parent education in child development and substance abuse education programs. Other programs, such as Outward Bound or Head Start, strengthen self-esteem and competency. Counseling around major stressful events, such as death and divorce, is also primary prevention. The primary care clinician is in an ideal position to practice anticipatory guidance for planned events as well as unexpected losses and traumatic events. Before a major stressful life event (marriage, birth of a child, remarriage), patients can receive counseling in the office or be referred for family counseling. Bibliotherapy (recommended reading that provides insight and self-management techniques) is a useful adjunct for affording insight and coping skills as well as patient education.

Regular exercise should be prescribed as a safe and effective means of alleviating stress and improving mood. Adequate sleep should be recommended. A nutritious diet and moderation in caffeine and sugar intake should be encouraged. Patients should be cautioned regarding the misuse of alcohol and mind-altering or sedative drugs (illicit or otherwise), as mood disorders have a high association with substance abuse.[7] Patients should be encouraged to build strong support systems and to talk about their feelings with their families and close friends. Studies have shown that single people who have pets are less likely to be depressed than others who live alone and do not have pets. If the patient's perceived stress is significant, specific stress reduction techniques should be encouraged or prescribed: meditation, yoga, visualization, and other relaxation techniques. Early referral for counseling to learn effective stress reduction techniques is recommended for patients with high levels of stress.

Treatment for diagnosed depression should not be delayed pending referral to a mental health professional. The rationale for immediate initiation of treatment by the primary provider is threefold:

1. Antidepressants take 3–4 weeks to reach therapeutic levels.
2. The patient may not follow through on the referral and thus will be untreated.
3. Receiving treatment may have the effect of creating some hope and preventing deterioration and even suicide (see Table 22–2).

Prevention of suicide begins with identifying patients at risk. Risk factors include

* A diagnosable mental health disorder
* Substance abuse
* Personal or family history of suicide attempt
* Adverse life events
* History of abuse (physical or sexual)

* Exposure to suicide of others
* Accessible firearms
* Incarceration

Attempts at suicide should be taken seriously. Underlying risk factors should be addressed and treated.[13]

Screening Recommendations

Current evidence does not justify screening asymptomatic patients for depression. A high index of suspicion should be maintained for adolescents, those with a past medical or family history of depression, and patients with chronic illnesses, recent loss, chronic pain, or multiple complaints. Referral or treatment is recommended for those with symptoms of depression. Alcohol and drug use should be ascertained. Queries regarding suicidal ideation are appropriate for those at risk. Those at risk should be referred or hospitalized.[14]

BIPOLAR DISORDER

Pathophysiology

Bipolar disorder (formerly referred to as manic-depression) is considered a biologically-based mood disorder in which there are episodes of both mania and depression (see Table 22–2). Manic episodes are typically more debilitating but are easily managed with medication. Psychotic symptoms may be present in either manic or severe depressive episodes and are usually congruent to the patient's mood (e.g., the person has a grandiose delusion during mania or demeaning auditory hallucinations during depression).[8]

Pediatric Issues

About 20% of patients will have onset of bipolar disorder before age 20. Substance abuse must be ruled out as a cause of mood swings. The manic episodes may lead to risk-taking behavior. These disorders are associated with a thirtyfold increase in successful suicide attempts.[12] When childhood bipolar disorder is suspected, the patient should be referred to a pediatric mental health specialist.

Obstetric Issues

Postpartum psychosis is an episode of mood disorder, usually a bipolar disorder. (See the discussion of Obstetric Issues in the preceding section on Depression.)

Geriatric Issues

Management is not significantly affected by age.

Epidemiology

The lifetime prevalence of bipolar disorder is 1%.[11] Although this is significantly lower than the prevalence of depression, the course of the disorder is less favorable, and the social and economic impact is substantial.

Treatment Options

Psychotherapy is of limited benefit in bipolar disorder. Family counseling to increase understanding and coping skills is helpful. For nearly all patients, pharmacologic management is necessary throughout their lifetime, although they may experience periods of remission when no medication is needed for normal function. Lithium has long been, and remains, the mainstay of treatment. Recent additions to the first-line agents used to treat bipolar disorder are two anticonvulsants, carbamazepine and valproate, that have been found to be as effective as lithium in treating the acute manic phase and appear to be preventive of both manic and depressive episodes. Additional drugs useful in controlling mania are clonazepam (Klonopin), lorazepam (Ativan), and haloperidol (Haldol). Antidepressants should be used with caution to treat depressive episodes because of the significant risk of precipitating a manic episode.

Patient Education

Patient education in bipolar disorder will address the same concerns surrounding the medications as with those for depression. Additionally, since many patients will have remissions and discontinue lithium use periodically, it is important to for patients to be able to recognize the return of signs and symptoms that require medication.

Prevention

There is no known way to prevent the occurrence of bipolar disorder. Since there is a more significant genetic component to bipolar disorder than to depression, patients should be given this information for family planning purposes. As with depression, the reduction of life stressors is almost certainly beneficial.

Screening Recommendations

See the recommendations in the preceding discussion of Depression.

ANXIETY DISORDERS

Pathophysiology

Both biological and psychological theories have been offered to explain the origins of the anxiety disorders. Anxiety has been observed in nearly every culture worldwide. However, the symptom expression often is culturally-dependent. Numerous theories have been offered to explain the origins of anxiety. Biological theories cite evidence for a genetic predisposition to clinical anxiety, as probands are four to seven times more likely to have a first degree relative with anxiety. Freud referred to anxiety as "neurosis," claiming neurosis was at the core of all human behavior, whether normal or pathological. Later researchers have provided support for behavioral theories (e.g., operant conditioning, classical conditioning, vicarious learning) to explain the development of anxiety.[8, 15]

The Diagnostic and Statistical Manual IV (DSM-IV)[8] defines over a dozen anxiety disorders, including phobias. In Table 22–3, characteristics of the more common anxiety disorders are outlined. Of note, panic disorder and agoraphobia are not considered diagnoses in and of themselves. They are combined to form three disorders, panic disorder with agoraphobia, panic disorder without agoraphobia, and (more infrequently) agoraphobia without a history of panic disorder.

Pediatric Issues

Anxiety disorders in children may manifest as school avoidance caused by separation anxiety, school phobia, or social fear. School-related problems are effectively treated by confronting the anxiety with the support of parents, teachers, and health care practitioners.

General childhood anxiety affects approximately 10% of children. It is characterized by developmental fears. Normal developmental fears include stranger anxiety (6–12 months), separation anxiety (18–36 months), and fear of the dark (3–6 years).[12] It is important to evaluate for issues in the home such as abuse, marital strife, or extreme emotion. The key is to not allow the anxiety to impair the child's life.[12]

Posttraumatic stress disorder (PTSD) is related to specific or ongoing traumatic events in the child's life. It is imperative to identify the traumatic event and to educate the caregiver and the child about the impact the event has on behavior. Strong support for the child is mandatory.[12]

Table 22-3. Common Anxiety Disorders

Anxiety Disorder	Essential Features	Common Associated Features	Typical Age of Onset	Lifetime Prevalence
Panic attack	Acute autonomic arousal that peaks quickly, accompanied by a sense of danger and/or fear of losing control; residual worry or concern about the episodes or significant behavioral changes secondary to the panic	Intermittent anxiety; demoralization; depression; comorbid anxiety disorders	Adolescence to mid-30s	1.5–3.5%
Agoraphobia	Fear and avoidance of places in which escape might be difficult	Typically occurs with panic disorder; anxiety manifests in environments outside the home, crowds, public transportation, bridges, elevators	Follows that of panic disorder	N/A
Specific phobia Subtypes: 1. Animal 2. Natural environment 3. Blood/injection/injury 4. Situational (e.g., travel)	Fear upon anticipation or exposure of a circumscribed stimulus (object or situation); avoidance of the stimulus	Anxiety expression may be a panic attack	1. Childhood 2. Childhood or early adulthood 3. Childhood 4. Childhood or early adulthood	10–11.3%

Disorder	Description	Features	Age of onset	Prevalence
Social phobia	Fear, anxious anticipation, and avoidance of performance situations	Can be general or specific (e.g., parties, public speaking); may take the form of panic; hypersensitive to evaluation, unassertive, poor social skills; low self-esteem; shy	Mid teens	3–13%
Obsessive-compulsive disorder	Persistent intrusive thoughts (obsessions) followed by a repetitive behavior or mental acts (compulsions) meant to neutralize the thought; the obsessions caused marked anxiety and/or are significantly time-consuming	Common themes include contamination/cleaning, ordering, checking, aggressive or sexual impulses; guilt and depression have a high comorbidity; hypochondriacal concern	Adolescence to early adulthood	2.5%
Post-traumatic stress disorder (PTSD)	Anxiety symptoms that follow exposure to an extremely traumatic event; symptoms take the form of re-experiencing the trauma; stimuli associated with the event are strongly avoided	Survivor guilt; dysregulation of affect; self-destructive behaviors; somatization; social isolation; personality change; dissociation	Any age	1–14%
Generalized anxiety disorder	Chronic uncontrolled worry about real-life stressors accompanied by persistent, low-level autonomic arousal	Somatization; other anxiety or mood disorders; substance abuse	Childhood to early adulthood	5%

When a childhood anxiety disorder is suspected, the patient should be referred to a pediatric mental health specialist.

Obstetric Issues

Anxiety regarding the unknown is common in pregnancy. Reassurance, education, and diagnostic testing may alleviate much of the normal anxiety. If the anxiety interferes with normal functioning, referral or treatment is necessary. Pharmacologic treatment should be evaluated for teratogenicity.

Geriatric Issues

Anxiety is more prevalent in the elderly because of fears associated with aging. These fears may include loss of independence, loss of income, and current or potential illness. Anxiety can manifest as panic or as withdrawal. A strong support network of family and friends helps reduce anxiety levels.

It is imperative to rule out a physical cause of the anxiety before administering sedatives. Hypoxia can cause significant anxiety, and sedation can prove fatal.

Epidemiology

As a group, anxiety disorders constitute the most prevalent group of psychiatric illnesses in the U.S., affecting an estimated 17% of the population *on any given day*,[2] in contrast to the prevalence of depression, which is slightly less on any given day but occurs in more people at some point in life. Anxiety disorders are diagnosed more frequently in women than in men. However, the gender ratio is comparable when the higher rates of substance abuse in men are considered (see the following section on Treatment Options).[8, 15]

Treatment Options

When treating anxiety disorders, it is imperative to rule out or treat underlying medical conditions that mimic anxiety symptoms (e.g., myocardial infarction, respiratory insufficiency). Treating substance abuse, if present, is important, as 25–50% of patients with alcohol abuse have an underlying anxiety disorder. After addressing possible organic causes of symptoms and substance abuse, a combination of pharmacotherapy and psychotherapy generally is recommended.

Psychotherapeutic approaches to treating anxiety are similar to those for depression, with CBT being the most empirically valid. Behavioral treatments for anxiety involve a combination of symptom management (e.g., progressive muscle relaxation, breathing exercises, guided imagery) and behavioral approach strategies to decrease avoidance of anxiety-producing stimuli. Specific CBT applications have been designed for each of the anxiety disorders (e.g., systematic desensitization for phobias, exposure with response prevention for obsessive-compulsive disorder, flooding for posttraumatic stress disorder). These treatments typically require referral to a behavioral therapist.

Pharmacotherapy is standard in the treatment of anxiety. In the acute management of panic attacks, benzodiazepines have the most rapid onset, often achieving relief within the first week. Alprazolam (Xanax) and lorazepam have been shown to be equally effective in treating panic disorder.[7] Because they impair cognitive function and carry significant risk of addiction and abuse (especially with long-term use), caution and the risk/benefit ratio need to be considered when prescribing benzodiazepines.

Benzodiazepines are typically effective in relieving the patient's acute symptoms while waiting for a long-term choice (e.g., SSRI, tricyclic antidepressant, or buspirone) to reach therapeutic levels. An SSRI is often the treatment of choice. After 4 weeks of SSRI therapy, the benzodiazepine can be tapered slowly over several weeks to prevent withdrawal symptoms. In addition to alprazolam, sertraline and paroxetine are FDA-approved for the treatment of panic disorder.[7] Other SSRIs are also useful in the long term, but the sedation commonly associated with paroxetine is useful in the immediate treatment of anxiety disorders. Other drugs less widely used than SSRIs for panic disorder are tricyclic and tetracyclic antidepressants and MAOI drugs. Although these may be effective, their side effect profiles and, in the case of MAOIs, dietary restrictions, limit their usefulness.

Patient Education

When diagnosing a patient with an anxiety disorder, providers need to maintain clarity about the meaning of the label "anxious." Lay definitions (e.g., eager, excited) differ from the clinical term *anxiety*. It is important that patients understand that their symptoms of anxiety, such as fast heart rate and shortness of breath, are accepted as credible and are real. It can be explained that the brain is sending a message to the body, and the body responds as though it is experiencing a life-threatening event. Providing patients with reading material that explains anxiety disorders can be a useful adjunct in education and treatment, increasing the patient's insight and providing him or her with tools for changing reactions to stimuli.

Prevention

In anxiety disorders there is much overlap between preventive measures and treatment, which usually includes therapeutic counseling and patient education. For example, the recommendation for patients to reduce stressors in their lives can be categorized as prevention, treatment, or patient education. Instruction in behavioral methods such as visualization and relaxation techniques can also fall under any of these categories. Making a formal written recommendation that the patient not work in a particularly stressful environment is both prevention (of poor outcomes) and treatment. General measures regarding stress reduction and augmentation of coping skills, as discussed with prevention of mood disorders, also apply to prevention of anxiety disorders.

Screening Recommendations

Mental health concerns should be part of a patient's general history in order to identify those with anxiety disorders.

SOMATOFORM DISORDERS

Patients often present with somatic symptoms of no known organic origin. The DSM-IV includes a classification scheme of circumscribed somatoform disorders.[8] These disorders usually present as medical syndromes but are primarily psychological in origin. Somatoform disorders differ from psychophysiologic disorders. Psychophysiologic disorders are medical conditions (e.g., asthma, rheumatoid disorders, chronic obstructive pulmonary disease) usually chronic in nature and highly susceptible to psychological influences such as stress, family dynamics, or mood changes.[10] The distinguishing features of the major somatoform disorders are as follows.[8]

SOMATIZATION DISORDER

Pathophysiology

Multiple somatic complaints that develop before the age of 30 and include a combination of pain complaints, gastrointestinal problems, sexual dysfunction, and/or neurologic symptoms.

CONVERSION DISORDER

Pathophysiology

Symptoms suggesting a neurologic problem associated with motor or sensory deficits. The dysfunction may mimic paralysis or seizures and is *not* intentionally produced.

PAIN DISORDER

Pathophysiology

The focus of the symptom presentation is pain. The pain may have an organic basis, but the severity of the complaint is incongruent with objective medical findings, and significant psychological factors are present.

HYPOCHONDRIASIS

Pathophysiology

A preoccupation or fear that one has a serious or terminal illness, despite medical reassurance. The patient often develops the concern by misinterpreting bodily functions or physical sensations.

BODY DYSMORPHIC DISORDER

Pathophysiology

Preoccupation with a defect in one's physical appearance. The defect is either imagined or exaggerated by the patient.

Pediatric Issues

Symptoms may occur in relation to family stressors and can mimic symptoms seen in other family members. Secondary gain (e.g., the child gaining attention or approval for imitating the parent's symptoms) is often present. Conversion symptoms seem to be associated with sexual abuse, so the child should be carefully evaluated for signs and symptoms of this form of abuse.[12] If the stressor is not identified or not understood, and if (nonorganic) symptoms do not resolve with reassurance, then referral is recommended.

Obstetric Issues

In adolescents who describe vague abdominal complaints, a pregnancy test is indicated because the patient may be in denial.[12] A serum human chorionic gonadotropin level test will accurately confirm or disprove a pregnancy.

Geriatric Issues

Organic disease is more prevalent in the elderly, sometimes with vague or nonspecific signs and symptoms. When the clinical findings do not match complaints, further probing may be necessary to elucidate potential nonorganic causes of the complaint.

Epidemiology

The epidemiology of somatoform disorders has not been clearly documented.

Treatment Options

Treatments for somatization disorder and hypochondriasis are similar and are most effectively achieved by ensuring continuity of care with one primary care provider. Visits should be scheduled on a regular basis (monthly is suggested), negating the tendency patients have to overutilize the health care system. Each new symptom should be attended to and a brief, directed physical examination performed. Further diagnostic studies should generally be avoided, as should prescription medications. The clinician's judgment determines the extent to which new complaints should be investigated and treated, as patients with somatoform disorders *can and do* develop organic disease.

Psychotherapy decreases the health care expenses of patients with somatoform disorder by 50%.[7] The indirect financial savings to society and the savings to clinicians of time and frustration are even greater. Antidepressants, particularly SSRIs, are useful in the management of pain disorder but should not be prescribed for somatization disorder or hypochondriasis without underlying mood or anxiety disorders. Referral to pain clinics or pain control programs can be useful for patients with pain disorders. These facilities offer a multidisciplinary approach to pain evaluation and treatment, utilizing cognitive, behavioral, and group therapies, as well as physical and occupational therapies. Psychotherapy is always indicated in conversion disorder, after thorough medical and neurologic evaluations have been completed.

Patient Education

Over time and repeated office visits, the primary care clinician should introduce the idea that psychological factors may be playing a part in the patient's symptoms, until the patient is willing to see a mental health clinician on a regular basis. Reassurance should be given that treatment will continue. In addition, the clinician should be clear that the patient is experiencing real symptoms and should validate the patient's symptoms. Suggesting by words or manner that the patient's symptoms are imaginary frequently worsens the symptoms.

Prevention

Primary prevention is aimed at reducing or identifying stress and family or social discord. The rationale for secondary gain can sometimes be identified with careful questioning. Conversion symptoms in children should be a warning sign for sexual abuse. Secondary preventive measures are aimed at getting the patient appropriate mental health treatment and are discussed under Treatment Options, above.

Screening Recommendations

Stress, coping skills, and family and social dynamics should be part of the history in any patient with symptoms that do not appear to have an organic basis.

ATTENTION DEFICIT HYPERACTIVITY DISORDER (ADHD)

Pathophysiology

Symptoms of attention deficit and/or hyperactivity disorder (ADHD) include developmentally inappropriate (decreased) attention and concentration abilities and increased levels of activity, distractibility, and impulsivity. ADHD is associated with significant difficulties in multiple settings (home, school, and social situations). It has long-term adverse effects on academic, vocational, social-emotional, and psychiatric outcomes. The pathophysiology of ADHD is incompletely understood, but there is evidence suggesting that genetics, neurochemical factors, and psychosocial factors play roles.[7, 17] The primary care provider should be aware that one type of ADHD (predominantly inattentive type) does not exhibit excessive motor activity. The diagnosis of ADHD should be made on the basis of thorough physical examination, mental status examination, and questionnaires completed by the child's parents and teacher. One commonly used instrument is Conners' teacher rating scale.[18]

Pediatric Issues

ADHD is a pediatric condition.

Obstetric Issues

Management is not significantly affected.

Geriatric Considerations

(Not applicable.)

Epidemiology

ADHD is the most commonly diagnosed pediatric behavioral disorder, affecting an estimated 3–5% of school-aged children.[8] Boys are between three and six times more likely to have ADHD than girls.[19, 20] It is estimated that 50% of those affected continue to manifest symptoms into adulthood.[21, 22]

Treatment Options

Pharmacotherapy with stimulants is the most common treatment for ADHD. Methylphenidate hydrochloride (Ritalin) seems to help 70–80% of children. Some physicians initiate therapy with a double-blind trial of methylphenidate hydrochloride alternating with placebo for a few weeks, during which the parents and teacher keep behavioral checklists. This method controls for parent and teacher expectations. Pemoline (Cylert) is beneficial in about 20% of patients who do not respond to methylphenidate hydrochloride. "Medication vacations" may be used during times when a child is not engaged in activities involving cognitive processes. Treatment is enhanced by the addition of behavioral management, including consistent rules and structure for the child. Using preplanned consequences and rewards rather than punishment is particularly effective.

Patient Education

In ADHD, patient education should be addressed to both the parents and the child. Parents and teachers should be counseled to depersonalize the child's behavioral difficulties. A warm and loving attitude should be maintained despite the fact that the child's behavior may be disruptive.

Prevention

There is no primary prevention for ADHD. Secondary prevention and control includes a structured home life, and adhering to a regular schedule of activities helps the family with an ADHD child. Providing the child with checklists and limiting instructions to one or two things at a time are also beneficial.

Screening Recommendations

It is crucial to differentiate ADHD from childhood anxiety disorder or depression. Both of these disorders may cause symptoms of restlessness, irritability, and difficulty concentrating. ADHD may also be confused with oppositional disorder and conduct disorder.

REFERENCES

1. U.S. Department of Health Education and Welfare. Healthy People: The Surgeon General's report on health promotion and disease prevention. DHEW (PHS) Publication No. 79-55071. Public Health Service. Washington, DC, U.S. Government Printing Office, 1979.
2. Kessler RC, McGonagle KA, Zhao S, et al. Lifetime and 12-month prevalence of DSM-III-R psychiatric disorders in the United States: Results from the National Comorbidity Survey. Arch Gen Psychiatry 1994;51:8–19.
3. Orleans CT, George LK, Houpt JL, et al. How primary care physicians treat psychiatric disorders: A national survey of family practitioners. Am J Psychiatry 1985;142:52–57.
4. Strosahl K. Mind and body primary mental health care: New model for integrated services. Behav Healthc Tomorrow 1996;5:93–96.
5. Farmer AE, Griffiths H. Labelling and illness in primary care: Comparing factors influencing general practitioners' and psychiatrists' decisions regarding patient referral to mental illness services. Psychol Med 1992;22:717–723.
6. McDaniel S, Campbell T, Sealsum D. Family-Oriented Primary Care. New York, Springer-Verlag, 1990, pp 248–262.
7. Goldman HH. Review of general psychiatry, 5th ed. New York, Lange/McGraw, 2000, p 280.
8. American Psychiatric Association. Diagnostic and Statistical Manual of

Mental Disorders Fourth Edition (DSM-IV). Washington, DC, American Psychiatric Association, 1994.

9. David AK, Johnson TA, Phillips DM, Scherger JE. Family Medicine Principles and Practice, 4th ed. New York, Springer-Verlag, 1993, p 1023.

10. Goldman LS, Weiss TN, Brody DS. Psychiatry for Primary Care Physicians. Chicago, American Medical Association, 1998, pp 19–71, 90, 120–133, 199–230, 257–259.

11. Klein DF, Wender PH. Understanding Depression: A Complete Guide to Its Diagnosis and Treatment. New York, Oxford Univesity Press, 1993, pp 87–102.

12. Hay WW Jr, Groothius JR, Hayward AR, Levin MJ. Current Pediatric Diagnosis and Treatment, 13th ed. Stamford, CT, Appleton & Lange, 1997, pp 127, 193.

13. National Institute of Mental Health. Suicide Facts, http://www.nimh.nih.gov/research/suifact.htm.

14. U.S. Preventive Services Task Force. Guide to Clinical Preventive Services, 2nd ed. Baltimore, Williams & Wilkins, 1996.

15. Barlow D. Anxiety and Its Disorders. The Nature and Treatment of Anxiety and Panic. New York, The Guilford Press, 1988, pp 219–234.

16. Fisher BC. Attention Deficit Disorder Misdiagnosis. New York, CRC Press, 1998, pp 121–126.

17. Searight HR, Nahlik MD, Campbell, DC. Attention-deficit/hyperactivity disorder: Assessment, diagnosis, and management. J Fam Pract 1995;40:270–279.

18. Conners CK. Conners' Rating Scales Manual. North Tonawanda, NY, Multi-health Systems, 1989.

19. Hales RE, Yudofsky SC, Talbott, JA. The American psychiatric press textbook of psychiatry, 3rd ed. Washington, DC, American Psychiatric Press, 1999, p 830.

20. Szatmari P, Offord DR, Boyle MH. Ontario Child Health Study: Prevalence of attention deficit disorder with hyperactivity. J Child Psychol Psychiatry 1989;30:219–230.

21. Leung AKC, Robson WLM, Fagan JE, Lim SHN. Attention-deficit hyperactivity disorder: Getting control of impulsive behavior. Postgrad Med 1994;95:153–160.

22. Weiss G, Hechman LT. Hyperactive Children Grown Up, 2nd ed. New York, The Guilford Press, 1993, p 22.

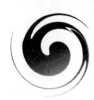

Chapter 23

Metabolic Conditions

Mary Byam-Smith, MS, PA-C,
Pamela L. Plotner, MD, Lee Lu, MD,
and Bich Nguyen, MD

■■■ INTRODUCTION

Metabolic conditions are broadly categorized as either congenital (due to an inherited enzyme abnormality) or acquired (due to disease or failure of a metabolically important organ). The scope of metabolic diseases that potentially affect the body is immense. However, prevention or early detection and treatment can result in decreased morbidity and/or mortality for several common disorders. These include dyslipidemias, diabetes mellitus, and disorders of thyroid, parathyroid, and adrenal hormones. (For additional resources see the Resources Appendix at the end of this book.)

Rather than being a clearly defined anatomic system, the endocrine system is composed of glands located throughout the body. The hypothalamic-pituitary axis forms a complex regulatory center that controls the function of each organ by a sensitive feedback system.[1]

THYROID

Synthesis and release of the thyroid hormones triiodothyronine (T_3) and thyroxine (T_4) are under the control of the anterior pituitary's thyroid-stimulating hormone (TSH). TSH is in turn regulated by hypothalamic thyrotropin-releasing hormone (TRH). This release of both TSH and TRH is regulated by negative feedback loops. Thyroglobulin, a glycoprotein formed within the follicular cells of the thyroid, combines with one or two iodine molecules to result in either of two discrete intermediate compounds. Coupling of these two intermediate compounds results in the formation of T_4 or T_3, depending on the number of iodine molecules added initially to the thyroglobulin molecule. T_4 may be converted to T_3 in the tissues outside the thyroid gland while predominantly bound to thyroxine-binding globulin (TBG) for transport to peripheral tissues. T_3 and T_4 affect carbohydrate, protein, and lipid metabolism and increase the body's oxygen consumption and heat production, which easily explains why patients are so frequently symptomatic, exhibiting changes of weight, energy-level, and temperature intolerance, at time of diagnosis.

PARATHYROID

The secretion of parathyroid hormone (PTH) is primarily regulated by blood concentration of ionized calcium. Increased concentrations of 1,25-dihydroxy-vitamin D and calcium inhibit PTH release. PTH acts to maintain normal serum calcium concentrations by inducing bone reabsorption and mobilizing calcium and phosphate, while also increasing vitamin D production within the kidney. Vitamin D increases gastrointestinal absorption of calcium, while PTH secretion increases renal tubular reabsorption of calcium and decreases the reabsorption of phosphate. Renal phosphate excretion allows the body to rid itself of excess phosphate (released from bone) that would otherwise further reduce calcium concentrations.

PANCREATIC ENDOCRINE

Three distinct hormones are produced in the pancreatic islets. Alpha cells produce glucagon, beta cells produce insulin, and delta cells produce somatostatin. Release of pancreatic hormones is regulated by chemical, hormonal, and neural controls. The blood glucose level is the major factor governing insulin release, with higher glucose levels triggering insulin release from the beta cells. Dropping blood glucose levels stimulate glucagon release. Parasympathetic stimulation initiates the discharge of acetylcholine and stimulates insulin release. Conversely, activation of the sympathetic nervous system releases epinephrine and norepinephrine, thereby inhibiting insulin release and stimulating glucagon release. Insulin facilitates the uptake and utilization of glucose by cells and prevents excessive breakdown of liver and muscle glycogen. It also favors lipid formation, inhibiting the catabolism and mobilization of stored fat, and protein synthesis. Glucagon decreases glucose oxidation and promotes increased blood glucose levels through stimulation of liver glycogen catabolism. It also stimulates carbohydrate formation in the liver from non-carbohydrate precursors and the catabolic lipid processes of the liver and adipose tissue. Somatostatin inhibits the release of both glucagon and insulin.

PLASMA LIPID METABOLISM

Triglycerides and cholesterol are transported within the plasma in the form of lipoproteins. There are four main lipoproteins, designated according to their density:
1. Chylomicrons
2. Very-low-density lipoproteins (VLDLs)
3. Low-density lipoproteins (LDLs)
4. High-density lipoproteins (HDLs)

Lipoprotein particles are composed of a central core of triglycerides and cholesteryl esters surrounded by a surface coat of phospholipids and apolipoproteins. Apolipoproteins are divided into five classes, A through E. Abnormal apolipoproteins are associated with defects of lipid metabolism.

Chylomicrons transport the converted dietary fat absorbed from the small intestine into the blood stream. The lipoprotein lipase (LPL) enzyme hydrolyzes the chylomicron's triglyceride into free fatty acids, which are then incorporated into adipocytes and muscle cells. Clearance of the remnant chylomicrons from the circulation occurs in the liver through the Apo-E receptor.

VLDL transports both triglycerides and cholesterol synthesized in the liver to the periphery. LPL hydrolyzes VLDL triglycerides to produce intermediate-density lipoproteins (IDLs). IDLs are then removed from the circulation by the ApoB-100 receptor within the liver or further metabolized into LDLs.

HDL, produced in both the liver and the intestine, takes up excess free cholesterol from peripheral tissues and transports it to the liver for disposal. This process, known as reverse cholesterol transport, is why HDLs are uniquely antiatherogenic.

ADRENAL

The adrenal cortex secretes three different types of hormones:
1. Glucocorticoids
2. Mineralocorticoids
3. Sex hormones

Release of glucocorticoids is controlled primarily by the pituitary's adrenocorticotropic hormone (ACTH). The secretion of ACTH is influenced by the release of hypothalamic corticotropin-releasing factor (CRF). Three factors appear to primarily regulate ACTH secretion:
1. High levels of circulating glucocorticoids suppress CRF and ACTH, while low levels stimulate their secretion.
2. A diurnal rhythm, with ACTH and cortisol levels peaking 3–5 h after sleep begins and declining throughout the day.
3. Stressful situations increase ACTH release and glucocorticoid secretion.

Glucocorticoid excess, triggered by physiologic stress or medications, causes shifts in

* Protein and carbohydrate metabolism
* Distribution of adipose tissue
* Electrolyte balance (indirectly due to osmotic shifts)
* Immune function
* Gastric secretion
* Erythropoiesis
* Brain function

Glucocorticoid excess also suppresses inflammatory processes.

The mineralocorticoid hormone of the adrenal cortex is aldosterone. Aldosterone excess stimulates proximal renal tubule reabsorption of sodium and triggers potassium and hydrogen ion excretion. Clinically these effects are

* Excess sodium water retention
* Expansion of intravascular volume
* Hypertension
* Hypernatremia and hypokalemia
* Metabolic alkalosis

While many sex hormone precursors are manufactured within the adrenal cortex, androgen excess is primarily associated with

* Cushing's syndrome
* Congenital adrenal hyperplasia
* Hyperplasia, with or without polycystic ovary syndrome
* Carcinoma

THYROID DISEASE

HYPERTHYROIDISM

Pathophysiology

Hyperthyroidism represents a condition in which an excessive amount of thyroid hormone (TH) is secreted by the thyroid gland. Diseases commonly causing hyperthyroidism include

* Graves' disease
* Toxic multinodular goiter
* Toxic adenoma
* Silent thyroiditis (lymphocytic and postpartum)
* Pituitary disorders with increased TSH secretion
* Excessive ingestion of thyroid hormone

Each disease has a specific pathophysiology. The most common cause of hyperthyroidism, Graves' disease, is thought to be a result of an autoimmune abnormality in which thyroid autoantibodies (or thyroid-stimulating immunoglobulins) stimulate the thyroid gland, directly increasing thyroid hormone production. Subacute thyroiditis, painful and self-limited, is due to the release of stored thyroid hormone from the inflamed gland. Silent thyroiditis is thought to be an autoimmune disorder with a self-limiting course similar to that seen with subacute thyroiditis.[1, 2] This disease causes symptoms in most of the bodily systems, especially cardiovascular, nervous, and gastrointestinal symptoms; as such, it has an important impact on health and behavior.

Pediatric Issues

Recommendations are unchanged in this population.

Obstetric Issues

Physiologic changes in pregnancy result in altered thyroid function testing. Changes of serum levels associated with estrogen-induced increases in thyroxine-binding globulin (TBG) include

1. Elevated total T_4
2. Elevated T_3
3. Decreased uptake of triiodothyronine (T_3RU).

Serum levels of T_3, free T_4, and TSH remain unchanged.

Hyperthyroidism occurs in 0.2% of all pregnancies, with more than 85% of these cases caused by Graves' disease. The remaining cases are associated with acute and subacute thyroiditis, chronic lymphocytic thyroiditis (Hashimoto's disease), toxic nodular goiter, and hydatidiform mole and choriocarcinoma. Treatment with propylthiouracil (PTU), an antithyroid medication, may result in neonatal hypothyroidism due to suppression of the fetal thyroid. Hyperthyroidism during pregnancy increases risks of adverse outcomes for both mother and child. While 90% of hyperthyroidism in fertile women is due to Graves' disease (which may improve due to immune system alterations in late pregnancy) many symptoms of uncontrolled disease may be overlooked or mistaken for normal physiologic changes of pregnancy. The primary maternal concern is uncontrolled disease or thyroid storm (usually provoked by stress), with an associated mortality rate as high as 25% even with excellent management. Fetal risks also include low birth weight, preterm labor, and stillbirth. Transient neonatal hyperthyroidism occurs in up to 10% of offspring of mothers with Graves' disease. Because the fetal thyroid concentrates iodine at a much higher rate in comparison to the mother's,[5] the use of radioactive iodine during pregnancy is contraindicated.

Geriatric Issues

Unrelated serious cardiac, pulmonary, or nervous system disorders often minimize or obscure the clinical presentations of hyperthyroidism (and hypothyroidism) in the elderly. The associated incidence of atrial fibrillation is eight times more frequent in the elderly hyperthyroid patient than in the young patient and therefore warrants TSH testing in any new-onset atrial fibrillation case. Achievement of a euthyroid state with antithyroid medications and propranolol prior to radioactive iodide ablation therapy minimizes the risk of thyroid storm.

Thyroidectomy rarely is required as a therapeutic intervention in the elderly.

Epidemiology

Thyroid disease, which affects approximately 10% of all Americans, is more common in women, the elderly, and persons with Down syndrome. The annual estimated incidence of hyperthyroidism in adults and adolescents is no more than 1:1000. Fatalities due to thyroid storm in hyperthyroidism are rare and usually associated with its impact on the central nervous system and the cardiovascular system. Hyperthyroidism during pregnancy increases the risk of adverse maternal and fetal outcomes. While overt disease is occasionally overlooked, the screening of asymptomatic individuals detects chemical hyperthyroidism in about 1%.

Treatment Options

Medical management with the thioamides, propylthiouracil or methimazole, commonly is the initial therapy. Radioactive iodine ablation of the overactive gland and surgery represent more definitive therapies. None of these therapies stops the production of autoimmune antibodies pathognomonic of Graves' disease. Systemic sympathetic symptoms (tachycardia, tremor, and heat intolerance) may respond to beta blockers pending normalization of thyroid hormone levels. Surgical thyroidectomy is an elective option when the patient's status is refractory to medical therapy or by patient preference (especially when conception is anticipated). Potential adverse side effects of long-term medical therapy include hepatitis and agranulocytosis. Iatrogenic hypothyroidism is a common complication of all forms of treatment, and its management will be discussed further (see the subsequent discussion of Treatment Options for hypothyroidism).[3]

Patient Education

An individual with hyperthyroidism should be counseled on the etiology of the disease and laboratory monitoring associated with disease control. Thorough explanation of treatment options is necessary. Specifically, patients using the antithyroid drugs PTU and methimazole should be aware of the potential leukopenia these drugs may induce and should agree to periodic blood monitoring. Patients need to recognize that pharmacologic treatment usually takes about 8 weeks to bring the symptoms under control but that they will likely need to continue taking the antithyroid medications for about 1 year. Patients with severe or prolonged symptoms requiring surgical removal or radioactive ablation of the thyroid gland need to understand that life-long thyroid hormone replacement is required. Patients with radio-active ablation must be able to reliably convey their treatment history to health care providers since it is not physically apparent, as is surgical removal.

Prevention

Although there is currently no way to prevent hyperthyroidism, this condition can be linked to preventable health consequences, including an accelerated rate of bone loss, cardiac muscle hypertrophy, and atrial fibrillation. Excessive thyroid hormone replacement, a common cause of subclinical hyperthyroidism, is easily prevented by the timely monitoring of hormone levels and adjustment of medication dosage.

Screening Recommendations

Although routine screening for thyroid disease is not recommended by most medical organizations including the U.S. Preventive Services Task Force working group, clinicians should remain alert for nonspecific or subtle symptoms of thyroid dysfunction. A low threshold for diagnostic evaluation of thyroid function, especially in high-risk individuals, will increase the clinical benefits of screening. The subgroups of individuals considered at high risk for developing thyroid disease include

* Patients with a history of other autoimmune diseases (e.g., diabetes mellitus or collagen vascular disorders)
* Individuals with a first-degree relative with thyroid disease
* Postpartum women
* Elderly patients
* Individuals with new-onset atrial fibrillation

The preferred test for screening is the measurement of TSH using a sensitive assay. Because fertile women are much more likely to have thyroid disease than significant lipid abnormalities, some authorities suggest that in this subgroup a TSH might be a useful screen. However, neither test is recommended by the U.S. Preventive Services Task Force for the general population before age 35.[3, 5, 6]

HYPOTHYROIDISM

Pathophysiology

Hypothyroidism, the most common thyroid dysfunction, is caused by a deficient secretion of TH by the thyroid gland. Primary causes include

* Abnormal hormone synthesis resulting from autoimmune thyroiditis, acute (bacterial infection of the thyroid gland) and subacute

(nonbacterial inflammation of the thyroid gland) thyroiditis, endemic iodine deficiency, or antithyroid drugs
* Congenital defects or loss of thyroid tissue after treatment for hyperthyroidism

The most common cause of hypothyroidism in the U.S. is chronic autoimmune thyroiditis (Hashimoto's thyroiditis). The destruction of thyroid tissue by circulating thyroid antibodies and infiltration of lymphocytes leads to a decreased production of TH. The response is an increased TSH secretion that leads to goiter. With the less common secondary hypothyroidism, causes include

* Insufficient thyroid gland stimulation, causing TSH deficiency from hypothyroidism of the pituitary or hypothalamus
* Resistance to TH in the periphery

Postpartum pituitary necrosis and pituitary tumors are the most common etiologies of secondary hypothyroidism, resulting in failure of the pituitary to produce adequate amounts of TSH.

Pediatric Issues

Congenital hypothyroidism is potentially associated with a number of causes, for example, endemic cretinism, agenesis or ectopic thyroid gland, genetic disorder of thyroid hormonogenesis, and hypopituitarism. Unidentified individuals who are not treated promptly suffer mental retardation and a variable degree of growth failure, deafness, and neurologic abnormalities in addition to the classic symptoms of hypothyroidism. Incidence is at least 1 out of 3600 births, occurring in females three times more often than in male offspring. Optimal screening tests include the determination of both T_4 and TSH levels. Treatment with oral levothyroxine at a dosage to produce a T_4 concentration within the upper half of the normal range is secondary prevention. Genetic counseling should be considered before subsequent pregnancies are planned.[3, 6]

Obstetric Issues

Undiagnosed hypothyroidism is rarely encountered in pregnancy, as it is associated with anovulation and infertility. Women already on replacement therapy when they conceive may safely continue their medication as long as it is monitored quarterly. Inadequate replacement has been associated with lower infant IQ.

Postpartum thyroiditis is a temporary form of (usually) painless subacute thyroiditis that occurs in 5–9% of postpartum women and usually is self-limited. The patient may transiently be hypo-, hyper-, or euthyroid. Prolonged postpartum depression should raise a high index of suspicion of hypothyroidism.[5]

Geriatric Issues

Subtle clinical manifestations of early hypothyroidism are often confused with the normal aging processes, thus explaining the recommendation for routine TSH screening annually in patients 60 years of age and older. Replacement TSH therapy is best approached with slowly titrated doses and careful monitoring of TSH. This is especially important in the geriatric patient with cardiovascular disease such as atherosclerosis or hypothyroid-induced cardiomyopathy, where excess replacement can precipitate a cardiovascular crisis. Starting doses of levothyroxine usually begin at 25 μg per day, adjusting doses every 4–6 weeks.[3]

Epidemiology

Overall annual incidence for hypothyroidism is estimated at 0.08–0.2%, with a higher incidence in elderly women. In fact, it is thought that subclinical hypothyroidism affects up to 20% of individuals over the age of 60. About 10% of adults have Hashimoto's thyroiditis, with a greater incidence in women than in men. Subclinical hypothyroidism is seen in 6–8% of adult women and 3% of adult men. Undetected subclinical hypothyroidism is suggested to have adverse effects on blood lipid profiles and on myocardial, gastrointestinal, and neuropsychiatric function.

Treatment Options

Medical management of hypothyroidism is tailored to the individual patient. Many health care providers will treat the goiter of chronic thyroiditis with levothyroxine, despite a normal TSH level. Treatment of clinical hypothyroidism is with daily oral levothyroxine. Controversy surrounds the treatment of subclinical hypothyroidism with levothyroxine. Most clinical endocrinologists, however, treat only the subclinical hypothyroid patient with high levels of thyroid autoantibodies. Although subacute thyroiditis is self-limiting, corticosteroid therapy is frequently used to decrease the associated pain in the thyroid gland and shorten the course.[3]

Patient Education

Patients must understand that when hypothyroidism is left untreated, it can lead to decreased concentration, depression, and even the loss of consciousness or coma. It is always important to review the laboratory results with patients so they will recognize the importance of these values in monitoring their treatment. Thyroid hormone replacement dosing depends on this monitoring. Health care providers must make patients aware of the potential for over-replacement and its attendant risks (bone and cardiovascular). This is especially true when the rare individual changes from a hypothyroid state to a non-suppressible euthyroid or hyperthyroid state. Since drug interactions also present a problem for maintaining therapeutic doses, patients should be warned about this possibility. Examples of drugs that interact with thyroid replacement medication include cholestyramine, ferrous sulfate, sucralfate, antacids containing aluminum hydroxide, and, to a lesser extent, dietary fiber. Patients should be advised to take thyroid replacement medications on an empty stomach 4–6 h prior to taking any of these medications.

Prevention

Most causes of hypothyroidism are not yet known to be preventable. One exception is the hypothyroidism induced by iodine deficiency. Iodine deficiency is rare in the U.S. owing to iodide fortification of table salt. Adverse health effects of hypothyroidism are easily reversed with oral replacement therapy.

Screening Recommendations

See the Screening Recommendations under the preceding discussion of Hyperthyroidism.

PARATHYROID DISEASE

HYPERPARATHYROIDISM

Pathophysiology

Causes of hyperparathyroidism are classified as either primary or secondary, and each has a somewhat different pathophysiologic mechanism. Primary hyperparathyroidism is a greater than normal level of PTH secreted by one or more of the parathyroid glands. Most cases of hyperparathyroidism are caused by solitary adenoma (80–85%), with the remainder caused by diffuse hyperplasia of all parathyroid glands. Parathyroid carcinoma is rarely the cause of hyperparathyroidism. Intrinsic PTH hypersecretion occurs when one of the normal negative feedback mechanisms, such as elevated serum levels of ionized calcium, fails to inhibit parathyroid secretion of PTH. Etiology of this is unclear. However, in studying a few familial clusters, evidence suggests that the disease is inherited as an autosomal dominant trait. Secondary hyperparathyroidism also results in excessive PTH but is secondary to a chronic disease state, such as chronic renal failure, that causes hypocalcemia. Hypocalcemia serves as a stimulus for increased PTH secretion and renal and gastrointestinal calcium absorption. Hypocalcemic individuals eventually become hyperparathyroid and develop hypercalcemia, a hallmark of hyperparathyroidism. Manifestations associated with the hypercalcemia of hyperparathyroidism can include pancreatitis; renal colic, nephrolithiasis, and nephrocalcinosis; peptic ulcer disease; bone disease; myalgia and muscle weakness; arthralgia and arthritis; hypertension; anorexia, nausea, and vomiting; constipation; polyuria and polydipsia; and neurologic and psychiatric problems, to name a few.[1, 4]

Pediatric Issues

Hyperparathyroidism is uncommon in pediatric patients; however, if it is diagnosed, multiple endocrine neoplasia (MEN) syndromes and hypothyroidism must be considered as important etiologies.

Obstetric Issues

Hyperparathyroidism is extremely rare in pregnancy. Occurrence during pregnancy results in significant perinatal morbidity and mortality risk for both mother and child. Parathyroid surgery is the treatment of choice.

Geriatric Issues

The frequency of elderly patients with primary hyperparathyroidism is increasing, with as much as 20% of patients with hyperparathyroidism being over age 60. This increase is due, in part, to routine measurement of serum calcium levels as part of chemical profiles. If an elderly patient exhibits hypercalcemia after starting a thiazide diuretic, this is a reflection of previously latent primary hyperparathyroidism. Mild, asymptomatic primary hyperparathyroidism is regarded as a factor that promotes bone demineralization, so it requires swift therapeutic intervention to decrease further bone density losses.[4]

Epidemiology

Routine use of biochemical screening has resulted in an overall increased incidence of primary hyperparathyroidism over the last 30 years, with approximately 100,000 new cases diagnosed each year in the U.S. Women are affected twice as often as men, and the incidence increases with age. Elderly women have an annual incidence of hyperparathyroidism of approximately 1 in 500. Asymptomatic hyperparathyroidism may have a benign course. The possibility, however, of progressive loss of bone mass and increased risk of fracture are the main concerns for an individual with undiagnosed hyperparathyroidism.

Treatment Options

The management approach to primary hyperparathyroidism depends on whether the patient is asymptomatic or symptomatic. Even with this designation, controversy surrounds the choice between medical observation and surgical intervention in the asymptomatic patient. Retrospective studies suggest significant long-term effects (bone loss, renal function, and hypertension) in untreated hyperparathyroidism. Criteria have been developed to delineate when surgical intervention is indicated in the asymptomatic patient with primary hyperparathyroidism. However, many clinicians believe that over 95% of patients are symptomatic even if symptoms are not overtly clear to the clinician. Parathyroidectomy is safe and effective with few complications, in curing more than 95% of patients.

Secondary hyperparathyroidism is treated medically by replacing the missing vitamin D metabolite(s). Intramuscular injection of ergocalciferol is used in cases of intestinal malabsorption. Oral calcium and phosphate supplementation as an adjunct to vitamin D metabolite therapy is essential for patients with symptomatic hypocalcemia and osteomalacia. Phosphate supplementation is added for only 4 to 6 weeks, whereas calcium and ergocalciferol are continued indefinitely. Adequate levels of phosphate binders and of dietary intake of calcium and vitamin D, in addition to supplements, are maintained through careful monitoring so as to prevent excessive levels of serum calcium and phosphate.[4]

Patient Education

See the Patient Education section under the succeeding discussion of hypoparathyroidism.

Prevention

Secondary prevention issues for hyperparathyroidism are directed primarily toward management of renal hyperparathyroidism. Preventive measures initiated in the early stage of renal insufficiency decrease the potential parathyroid hyperplasia that may require subtotal parathyroidectomy.

Screening Recommendations

Measurement of total serum concentration is a sensitive and cost-effective method for screening for primary hyperparathyroidism. Continued elevation of total serum concentration may necessitate ionized serum calcium determination in patients with decreased serum albumin. When hypercalcemia is confirmed, parathyroid hyperfunction can be established with immunoassays measuring the intact PTH molecule in serum.

HYPOPARATHYROIDISM

Pathophysiology

Most commonly, hypoparathyroidism is caused by damage to the parathyroid gland that results in abnormally low PTH levels. Hypocalcemia and hyperphosphatemia result when loss of PTH control of bone–calcium resorption occurs and impairs the regulation of calcium reabsorption from the renal tubules. Hypomagnesemia may also cause hypoparathyroidism by an unknown mechanism. However, once serum magnesium levels return to normal in a hypoparathyroid individual, PTH secretion stabilizes. Hypomagnesemia is often seen in chronic alcoholism, malnutrition, malabsorption, increased renal clearance of magnesium caused by use of aminoglycosides or certain chemotherapeutic agents, or prolonged magnesium-deficient parenteral nutritional therapy. Hypoparathyroidism is rarely seen as a familial disorder or associated with autoimmune failure of multiple endocrine glands.

Pediatric Issues

Sufficient PTH secretion is limited in normal infants; therefore, a relative deficiency of PTH can result in hypocalcemia in infants fed a high-phosphate formula such as cow's milk. Symptoms associated with pediatric hypocalcemia and hyperphosphatemia include tetany, convulsions, muscle cramps, laryngeal stridor, and paresthesias.

Infants with abnormal embryologic development of the third and fourth pharyngeal pouches (e.g., DiGeorge syndrome) often have PTH deficiency–induced hypocalcemia.[4]

Obstetric Issues

Hypoparathyroidism is rarely seen in the pregnant woman, and management remains unchanged.

Geriatric Issues

Recommendations are unchanged in this population.

Epidemiology

Hypoparathyroidism is most commonly caused by damage to the parathyroid glands during surgery. It occurs in approximately 1–3% of all individuals undergoing thyroid surgery, with the incidence increasing to 10% after repeated neck explorations.

Treatment Options

Acute management of hypoparathyroidism in patients with symptomatic hypocalcemia is accomplished with intravenous calcium gluconate immediately followed by additional dosing based on serum calcium measurements. If hypomagnesemia is present, it must be corrected to successfully treat the hypocalcemia. Long-term management requires calcium supplements and vitamin D or its active metabolites. Thiazide diuretics or chlorthalidone are used at times to increase phosphate excretion and decrease calcium excretion. The goal of treatment in either case is to achieve serum calcium levels between 8 and 9 mg/dL. Nephrolithiasis is a potential side effect of overzealous calcium replacement, and therefore serum and 24-h urinary calcium levels should be monitored every 3–6 months.[4]

Patient Education

Patient education in hyperparathyroidism and hypoparathyroidism is primarily focused on symptoms associated with the disorders so that a lower threshold for diagnosis is conferred on the clinician, especially in the case of hyperparathyroidism. It is important to review the common signs of hyperparathyroidism (weakness, muscle spasm, and cardiac irregularities) with the patient prior to surgery so that the patient can be motivated to return to the clinic if these symptoms occur subsequent to the surgery.

Prevention and Screening Recommendations

Currently there are no screening or prevention guidelines other than measurement of serum calcium and magnesium levels postsurgically as part of the postoperative management of thyroidectomy or parathyroidectomy.

DIABETES MELLITUS

DIABETES MELLITUS TYPE I

Pathophysiology

Diabetes mellitus Type I (DMI) is an autoimmune disease in which the body produces autoantibodies against the insulin-producing beta cells of the pancreas. Autoantibodies are produced in response to an unknown environmental trigger, such as a viral illness, imposed on a background of genetic susceptibility. The autoantibodies destroy the beta cells, resulting in a loss of insulin production. This process can take several years before the development of clinical symptoms, which appear only after a majority (more than 90%) of beta cells have been destroyed. The loss of insulin production results in excessive amounts of glucose circulating in the blood stream.

Excessive circulating glucose acts as an osmotic diuretic as the glucose load overwhelms the filtering capabilities of the kidneys. This leads to the symptoms of polyuria and subsequent polydipsia and the clinical sign of glycosuria. Without insulin, the body is unable to effectively use glucose and must begin to use fatty acids as an energy source, leading to increased ketone production and acidosis. The acidosis triggers deep, rapid breathing, known as Kussmaul's respiration, as the body attempts to correct the metabolic abnormality by ridding itself of excess carbon dioxide. This situation is known as diabetic ketoacidosis (DKA) and is fatal if left untreated. Prolonged exposure to hyperglycemia has long-term effects on the body, including retinopathy, nephropathy, and neuropathy. These effects are due to increased glycosylation and subsequent damage to the microvascular environment. Hemoglobin becomes glycosylated in the presence of glucose and is easily measured by blood sampling, thus making it a simple indicator of long-term glucose control.

One to two months after the acute onset of symptoms, a "honeymoon phase" occurs that is marked by a sudden decrease in exogenous insulin requirements. Over the next 2 to 24 months, a steady but gradual increase in the exogenous insulin requirement occurs as the remaining beta cells are destroyed. The term "dawn phenomenon" refers to morning hyperglycemia caused by an exaggeration of the natural rise in blood glucose in the early morning. The hyperglycemia is caused by growth hormones that are not sufficiently counter-regulated by the evening insulin dose. It is important to differentiate the dawn phenomenon from the Somogyi phenomenon, another cause of morning hyperglycemia, as the two are treated differently (see the subsequent Treatment Options section). The Somogyi phenomenon refers to rebound hyperglycemia due to early morning hypoglycemia induced by an excessive insulin dose the preceding evening. The body releases counter-regulatory hormones to correct the hypoglycemia, thus inducing the hyperglycemia.[1, 7]

Pediatric Issues

Poor glycemic control can delay puberty and slow linear growth. A poor psychosocial environment is associated with poor glycemic control. Parents need information on parenting a child with a chronic condition.

Most children are capable of taking partial self-care responsibilities, which will increase as they mature. This being said, as the child approaches adolescence, parents and the health care team should expect that previously attained goals may be lost, and that the teen may become noncompliant, prompting more frequent hospitalizations. Weight loss may indicate missed insulin doses and a distorted body image or a period of rapid growth. The teen's daily insulin requirements commonly increase because of increased growth hormone production. Dawn and Somogyi effects can become more pronounced and may be more difficult to regulate. Rapid weight gain may suggest the need to rule out the Somogyi phenomenon.

Obstetric Issues

Maternal complications are directly related to the duration and complications of DMI prior to pregnancy. About 15–25% of pregnant women with diabetes will have one or more of the following complications: progression of diabetic retinopathy, hypertension, frequent urinary tract infections, nephropathy, or polyhydramnios. Hypoglycemia is common during the first trimester, usually because of the effects of morning sickness. Hyperglycemia is common during the third trimester because of relative insulin resistance. The increased resistance causes insulin requirements to rise throughout the third trimester, which then precipitously drop after delivery. Often the dose required on the first postpartum day is only half of the term dose. Hypoglycemia and DKA significantly contribute to the twentyfold increase in maternal mortality among women with DMI.

Fetal complications are directly related to maternal glycemic control. Sustained hyperglycemia and DKA increase the risk of spontaneous abortion substantially. Hyperglycemia in early pregnancy contributes to a fourfold to tenfold increase in congenital malformations. Worsening nephropathy contributes to the increased risk of prematurity and intrauterine growth retardation.[5]

Geriatric Issues

Complications of DMI in the geriatric population are correlated to the duration of the disease. As one ages, the adrenergic response to hypoglycemia is blunted; thus, hypoglycemic events go unrecognized, leading to devastating results. Glycemic control becomes more difficult due to other confounding illnesses, making tight control an often unrealistic goal. Autonomic neuropathy leads to postural hypotension, neurogenic bladder, and erectile dysfunction.

Epidemiology

DMI accounts for only 10% of all cases of diabetes mellitus, but it represents up to 97% of pediatric cases (under 20 years of age). It is the most common metabolic disorder of childhood. It occurs in 1 in 500 people under the age of 20. Most people with DMI (up to 85%) have no other affected family members. First degree relatives, however, have an increased risk of developing DMI at approximately 1 in 20 (5%). DMI is 1.5 to 2 times more common in Caucasians, compared to the general population, especially those of Scandinavian descent. Up to 90% of people with DMI are positive for human leukocyte antigen (HLA) type DR3 or DR4. Annual incidence of DMI is 10 in 100,000 people under the age of 20. Although it can appear at any age, the peak incidence occurs at 12 years of age, with 80% of people with DMI developing the disease before 30 years of age. Gender differences are negligible.

Treatment Options

Insulin replacement is currently the only pharmacologic treatment for patients with insulin-dependent diabetes. Traditional sulfonylurea hypoglycemic medicines generally have no role in this type of patient. Total insulin dose is generally estimated for adults at 1 unit/kg/day. However, dosing may range from 0.5 units/kg/day in a child under 5 years of age up to 1.5 units/kg/day in an adolescent. Increased dose requirements occur during times of stress, illness, rapid growth, and in response to the dawn phenomenon. Decreased dose requirements occur during the "honeymoon phase" and in response to the Somogyi effect, improved dietary intake, and athletic conditioning. The benefits of exercise and adherence to the American Diabetes Association

(ADA) diet recommendations are found in Chapter 7, Exercise, and Chapter 13, Nutrition Education in the Clinical Setting, respectively.

Insulin analogs are available in rapid- (Humalog), short- (Regular and Semi-Lente), intermediate- (NPH, Lente), and long-acting (Ultra-Lente) formulations. The usual dosing regimen is to take two thirds of the total daily dose in the morning and one third in the evening, commonly before supper or bedtime. The morning dose is composed of two-thirds intermediate-acting and one-third short-acting insulin. The evening dose may be divided into the same ratio as the morning dose or may be divided 50:50.

Glucagon (IM injection) is used for hypoglycemic emergencies when oral intake is not possible. An ampule should always be kept available for severe emergencies. While epinephrine also stimulates the release of glucose from the liver, glucagon is preferred because it does not have the sympathetic activity of epinephrine.[3, 7]

Patient Education

Patients and their families need intensive education about the cause, treatment, and prognosis of DMI. A diabetic health care team that includes a primary provider, a diabetic nurse-educator, a podiatrist, a nutritionist and a consulting endocrinologist usually provides the best, most comprehensive care. Educational interventions should not simply include information about the disease but should empower patients and their families to take control of their disease. All patients should have a written protocol for management of intercurrent illnesses. This enables the patient to manage most illnesses and exacerbations at home. The protocol, however, must contain information on times when physician intervention is mandatory.

All patients should wear a medical alert tag stating that they have DMI.

Prevention

Currently no standard preventive strategies or screening recommendations exist, although several studies are now under way. See also comments about secondary prevention under Diabetes Mellitus Type II.

Screening Recommendations

See the screening recommendations under Diabetes Mellitus Type II.

DIABETES MELLITUS TYPE II

Pathophysiology

In contrast to DMI, diabetes mellitus Type II (DMII) is characterized by a relative insulin resistance at the level of the cell. Obesity increases cellular resistance to insulin, while exercise and weight loss decrease cellular resistance. The beta cells are intact and functional in DMII. Insulin production increases to overcome this cellular resistance to insulin activity. The systemic effect of increased circulating insulin levels may lead to acanthosis nigricans, especially over the nape of the neck; however, the effect is not enough to control the levels of circulating glucose, which leads to hyperglycemia and glycosuria. As with DMI, this state leads to the clinical symptoms of polyuria and polydipsia, although the onset is not as abrupt. DKA is rare in DMII. In some patients, the beta cells finally die after many years of increased productivity, which leads to a secondary form of DMI.

Patients with DMII are likely to go unrecognized for a prolonged period, incurring microvascular damage much as those with DMI, but seemingly in a shorter period of time owing to the typical delay in diagnosis. Because of the sustained hyperglycemic state, recurrent infection may be the first clinical clue to the presence of DMII.[1]

Pediatric Issues

The majority of children with DMII are obese and have other health problems related to their obesity, such as acanthosis nigricans, hypertension, sleep apnea, elevated triglycerides, depression, and eating disorders. Early intervention and anticipatory guidance is crucial to change the dietary and exercise habits of these children and their parents. Parental involvement is mandatory for this behavior modification to be successful. Frequent social and emotional support may be needed, especially for those who are morbidly obese, live in poverty, or live in a family of obese persons. Showing the patient and parents concrete information, such as a growth chart, current weight, and predicted future weight, often gives the family the sense of urgency required for change.

Obstetric Issues

Most of the obstetric concerns discussed under diabetes mellitus Type I are valid, to a lesser extent, in the patient with DMII. Patients with diabetes controlled with diet alone generally do well but may require insulin as the pregnancy progresses. Patients taking oral medication should ideally be transferred to insulin therapy before conception or as soon as the pregnancy is confirmed. All pregnant patients with diabetes have similar problems (although variable by degree) with increased strain on their kidneys, circulatory system, and vision. Complications of pregnancy such as prematurity, postmaturity, and preeclampsia occur more frequently in the pregnant diabetic patient. Prolonged hyperglycemia, especially in late pregnancy, leads to an increased risk of fetal macrosomia and predisposes to complications of shoulder dystocia, traumatic birth injuries, respiratory distress syndrome, and an increased rate of still birth. Carefully preplanned pregnancies, closer surveillance visits, and fetal welfare monitoring (e.g., biophysical profile [BPP], non-stress test [NST], oxytocin challenge test [OCT]) on strict schedules are needed to achieve a successful outcome of the pregnancy.[5]

Geriatric Issues

Complications of DMII are similar to those of DMI. In addition, those with DMII are at greater risk of infection, especially fungal and bacterial skin infections. These infections require prompt antimicrobial therapy and control of concomitant hyperglycemia.

Epidemiology

DMII accounts for the majority of cases (90%) of diabetes mellitus. In the pediatric population, however, it only accounts for 2–3% of all cases. This situation appears to be changing dramatically because of the increasing trends of youthful obesity and society's sedentary lifestyle. Studies show that the risk of developing DMII doubles for every 20% increase in excess body weight.

The risk of first degree relatives developing DMII is currently reported to be 10–15%. This is probably a result of complex environmental, societal, and dietary influences that have led to increased obesity and decreased activity. Among such a high-risk group as the Pima Native Americans, a genetic tendency toward the "thrifty genotype" may explain their exceptionally high diabetes prevalence of up to 40%.

Treatment Options

Appropriate diet, exercise, and weight loss are the cornerstones of treatment (see Chapter 7, Exercise, and Chapter 13, Nutrition Education in the Clinical Setting). Many patients will also need adjunctive therapy with oral hypoglycemic agents, such as the sulfonylureas (e.g., glipizide and glyburide) or the newer agents, metformin and troglitazone. A few patients will also need intermittent insulin therapy to control excessive hyperglycemia.[3, 7]

Patient Education

Appropriate diet, exercise, and weight loss are the cornerstones of patient education (see Chapter 7, Exercise, and Chapter 13, Nutrition Education in the Clinical Setting).

Explanation of routine monitoring of disease control should include both fingerstick analysis of blood glucose and hemoglobin A1C. Appropriate foot care by the patient is essential to avoid peripheral complications of microvascular disease. Likewise, routine ophthalmologic examinations are essential. All patients should wear a medical alert tag stating they have DMII.

Prevention

Appropriate diet, weight loss, and exercise have become the cornerstones of prevention (see Chapter 7, Exercise, and Chapter 13, Nutrition Education in The Clinical Setting). Primary prevention of childhood obesity with the establishment of appropriate dietary and exercise habits is fundamental (see the preceding discussion of Pediatric Issues). Prevention of respiratory infections is facilitated by careful attention to immunizations, especially pneumococcal and influenza vaccines.

Screening Recommendations

Currently, there is insufficient evidence to recommend either for or against universal screening for diabetes. However, many authorities recommend screening high-risk populations, including the obese, older persons, pregnant women, and those with a strong family history of DMII or an ethnic predisposition. The ADA currently recommends screening every three years with a fasting plasma glucose (FPG) owing to convenience and cost. An FPG greater than 126 is an indication for retesting on a different day to confirm the diagnosis of diabetes. Screening for gestational diabetes (GDM) is commonly accepted as standard care, despite its lack of evidence-based support in general populations. However, most authorities agree that such screening is the standard of care in those at increased risk, such as pregnant women

* Greater than 25 years of age
* Who are obese (body mass index [BMI] greater than 27)
* Who have a personal past or family history of GDM
* Who have glycosuria

In pregnant women, a plasma glucose level of greater than 140 mg/dL 1 h after a 50-g oral glucose load indicates the need for a diagnostic 100-g oral glucose tolerance test (OGTT).[6]

HYPERLIPIDEMIA

Pathophysiology

Genetic or environmental conditions may alter lipoprotein metabolism. Potential sites for genetic alterations include abnormal enzyme function and apolipoprotein and receptor defects. Environmental factors such as obesity or alcohol use tend to increase the amount and inhibit the disposal of lipoproteins, resulting in hyperlipidemia. Hyperlipidemia is a result of either a primary genetic or a secondary cause. Diabetes, excess alcohol intake, hypothyroidism, nephrosis, liver disease, steroids, diuretics, and beta-blockers are all common secondary etiologies. Primary etiologies include

* Familial hypercholesterolemia, an inherited defect in the LDL receptor gene leading to decreased clearance of LDL
* Familial combined hyperlipidemia, an autosomal dominant condition in which family members are at risk of premature coronary heart disease (CHD), regardless of an increase in VLDL, LDL, or both
* Familial dysbetalipoproteinemia, a defect in the Apo-E lipoprotein found in chylomicron and VLDL remnants disrupting binding to the Apo-E hepatic receptor necessary for remnant clearance
* Familial mixed hypertriglyceridemia, an autosomal dominant defect in which chylomicrons and VLDL are overproduced[8, 9]

Pediatric Issues

Hyperlipidemia in childhood increases the likelihood of hyperlipidemia in adulthood. Opinions vary about treatment approach, but there is a consensus that children whose serum cholesterol or triglyceride levels are beyond the 95th percentile for their ages and genders should be treated. Universal cholesterol and lipid screening strategies for children do not exist. Identification of a child with a family history of cardiovascular disease with events occurring before age 50 or a family history of hyperlipidemia warrants serum lipid analysis at regular intervals for that child. Children whose biological parents or siblings are found to have familial, and presumably genetic, hyperlipidemia are at increased risk for atherosclerosis of the coronary arteries and myocardial infarction in childhood, and therefore more aggressive lipid screening strategies should be followed.

Obstetric Issues

Currently there are no recommendations for screening pregnant women, and limitation of dietary fat and cholesterol intake during pregnancy and childhood may, in fact, be deleterious.

Geriatric Issues

Cholesterol levels are not reliable predictors of risk for symptomatic heart disease and generalized atherosclerosis after the age of 75. Also, in the elderly a very low cholesterol level (<120 mg/dL) may be predictive of significant morbidity and mortality. Therefore, decisions to treat or screen should be based on other risk factors, an individualized cost-benefit analysis, and the knowledge that evidence does not yet support routine interventions in these patients.

Epidemiology

There is a direct relationship between age and cholesterol level. The prevalence of serum cholesterol 240 mg/dL or higher increases from less than 9% for individuals under age 35 to almost 25% for men age 55 and nearly 40% for women over age 65. High-density lipoprotein-cholesterol (HDL-C) levels are low in approximately 14% of adults with desirable or borderline cholesterol levels. These levels increase approximately 18% in perimenopausal women along with decreased estrogen protection and increased weight. Studies have repeatedly shown a causal relationship between blood lipids and coronary atherosclerosis. Among persons with inherited lipid disorders, symptomatic heart disease and generalized atherosclerosis is seen at an earlier age than in those of the same age in the general population. This relationship seems less predictive in older women and is not consistent after the age of 75.[4]

Treatment Options

Clinical interventions for hyperlipidemia include both lifestyle modifications and pharmacologic therapies. Nonpharmacologic therapies include dietary modifications, weight loss targeting a body mass index of 27 or better, and increased physical activity. Dietary changes should be the initial intervention in all patients, and ideally a trial period of several months should ensue before drug therapy is considered. Graded modifications of diet are labeled as:

Step 1. (dietary fat <30% of total calories; <10% saturated fat and <300 mg/day cholesterol), or

Step 2. (dietary fat <30% of total calories; <7% saturated fat and <200 mg/day cholesterol)

Pharmacologic therapy should only be initiated when dietary and lifestyle changes have proved insufficient. Drug selection is based on lipoprotein analysis results (Table 23–1), cost, and the patient's acceptance.[3]

Patient Education

Pamphlets focused on a "Heart Healthy" diet or the Step 1 and Step 2 diets may be obtained from the American Heart Association. However, patient compliance will be substantially improved if adequate education is also provided as face-to-face contact time either in a class format or in individual counseling sessions provided by a trained educator or nutritionist.

Prevention

Reduction in cardiovascular morbidity and mortality by treating hypercholesterolemia aggressively, especially in individuals with known heart disease, is supported strongly by the literature. Multiple studies have shown regression of atherosclerotic lesions with aggressive lipid lowering. This regression is associated with significant declines in recurrent cardiac events.

Table 23–1. Drug Selection Based on Lipoprotein Analysis

Type of Intervention	Drug Classes Appropriate for Intervention
Lower LDL-C	Bile acid sequestrant resins (cholestyramine and colestipol)
	Nicotinic acid (niacin)
	HMG-CoA reductase inhibitors (lovastatin, pravastatin, simvastatin, fluvastatin, atorvastatin)
	Estrogen in postmenopausal women (conjugated estrogens, esterified estrogen)
Lower triglycerides	Nicotinic acid
	Fibric acid derivative (gemfibrozil and clofibrate)
	Selected HMG-CoA reductase inhibitors
Increase HDL	Nicotinic acid
	Estrogen

HMG-CoA: 3-hydroxy-3-methylglutaryl coenzyme A

Guidelines exist for both primary and secondary prevention of CHD based on the screening of total cholesterol and HDL-C levels. Regardless of results, providing education to the general population about ideal eating habits, physical activity, and additive risk factor reduction can be beneficial anytime that a serum cholesterol level is measured. When an initial cholesterol determination reveals any level above 200 mg/dL or an HDL-C <35 mg/dL, a complete lipoprotein analysis should be obtained following a fast of 9–12 h. When desirable levels of low-density lipoprotein-cholesterol (LDL-C) (<135 mg/dL) are noted, providing education and planning a repeat of total cholesterol and HDL-C measurements within 5 years is appropriate. If LDL-C is borderline high (130–159 mg/dL, confirmed by repeat determination) in an individual without risk factors, information on a Step 1 diet and increased physical activity should be provided. Re-evaluation of the individual's cholesterol status annually is advisable. In an individual with borderline or high LDL-C and two or more risk factors (men ≥45 years old, women ≥55 years old or premature menopause without estrogen replacement therapy, family history of CHD, current cigarette smoking, hypertension, low HDL [<35 mg/dL] or diabetes mellitus), the clinician should search for secondary causes and evaluate for a familial disorder. All individuals in this last category still need to initiate dietary treatment but will probably also require pharmacologic treatment. Initiation of drug therapy is essential when

* LDL-C > 190 mg/dL in an individual without CHD and with fewer than two risk factors, or
* LDL-C > 160 mg/dL without CHD, but with two or more risk factors, or
* LDL-C > 130 mg/dL with evidence of CHD

The goals of treating hyperlipidemia should be targeted toward achieving

* LDL-C < 160 mg/dL without CHD and fewer than two risk factors, or
* LDL-C < 130 mg/dL without CHD, but with two or more risk factors, or
* LDL-C < 100 mg/dL with evidence of CHD

Screening Recommendations

All men aged 35–65 and women aged 45–65 should have periodic screening for elevated blood cholesterol using specimens obtained in the fasting or non-fasting state. Individuals older than 65 years may benefit from cholesterol screening depending on other CHD risk factors (smoking, hypertension, diabetes). However, cholesterol levels are not reliable predictors of risk after age 75. In individuals who are at low risk, screening intervals of 5 years are reasonable. Decreased intervals are recommended for those individuals shown epidemiologically to have increasing cholesterol levels (e.g., middle-aged men, perimenopausal women, and individuals with weight gain). Selective screening in young adults with a history or physical examination suggesting a familial lipoprotein disorder or at least two other CHD risk factors is also advocated.[6]

ADRENAL DISORDERS

ADRENAL EXCESS (CUSHING'S SYNDROME)

Pathophysiology

The process is either ACTH-dependent or -independent. Causes of ACTH-dependent Cushing's syndrome include Cushing's disease (primary pituitary ACTH hypersecretion), secretion of ACTH from a nonpituitary source such as a lung cancer, and ectopic corticotropin-releasing hormone syndrome. Iatrogenic disease from the use of ACTH is rare. The ACTH-independent group of disorders involves primary adrenocortical masses (adenoma or carcinoma) and bilateral micronodular or macronodular adrenal hyperplasia. Exogenous administration of glucocorticoids, however, remains the most common cause.

Common physical findings in Cushing's syndrome are centripetal obesity with fat distribution mainly involving the face, neck, trunk, and abdomen; facial plethora; easy bruising; oily skin; acne; hirsutism; abdominal striae; and hyperpigmentation (only in ACTH hypersecretion). Other symptoms include glucose intolerance, proximal muscle weakness, impotence, amenorrhea, polyuria due to hypercalciuria and glycosuria, osteoporosis, and affective psychiatric disorders. However, cardiovascular complications such as hypertension and congestive heart failure account for the most frequent occurrences of mortality and morbidity.[1]

Pediatric Issues

Recommendations are unchanged in this population.

Obstetric Issues

Although Cushing's syndrome is exceedingly rare during pregnancy, it is associated with an increased risk of spontaneous abortion, preterm labor, and stillbirths. These patients require close fetal monitoring in addition to appropriate disease management.[5]

Geriatric Issues

Dose adjustments may need to be made as the patient ages; otherwise, recommendations remain unchanged.

Epidemiology

Incidence is probably underestimated due to unreported cases. Each year, about 10 million Americans require glucocorticoids. Incidence of ectopic ACTH syndrome is estimated at 600 per 1 million per year. The incidence of adrenal carcinoma is estimated by the National Cancer Institute to be two cases per 1 million population per year. For Cushing's disease, the incidence is 5 to 25 per 1 million population per year. Women are three to eight times more likely to have Cushing's disease, three times more likely to have adrenal tumors, and four to five times more likely to have Cushing's syndrome secondary to tumors when compared with male counterparts. Age of onset for ectopic ACTH syndrome is usually after age 50. Cushing's disease is usually diagnosed in women ages 25 to 45 years. Adrenal tumor occurrence is bimodal, with tumors occurring early in the first decade of life or later, in the fourth or fifth decades of life.

Treatment Options

The goal is to reduce the production of cortisol to normal. For pituitary adenoma, a trans-sphenoid microadenectomy is recommended. For other ACTH-secreting tumors, resection of the tumor is essential. In the case of exogenous glucocorticoids, tapering and subsequent discontinuation should be considered whenever possible. Medications may also be used in combination with surgical interventions. Mitotane, an adrenocorticolytic agent, can be used, but it is expensive and has many side effects, including nausea, vomiting, anorexia, rash, diarrhea, ataxia, gynecomastia, arthralgias, and leukopenia. Another class of medications are the adrenal enzyme inhibitors (aminoglutethimide, metyrapone, trilostane, etomidate, and ketoconazole). Mifepristone, an antiprogestational drug, competes with glucocorticoids at high doses and offers another pharmacologic option.[10]

Patient Education

Patients with Cushing's syndrome need education about the potential effects of excess cortisol, including impotence, transient infertility, menstrual irregularities, and hirsutism. Reassurance that treatment is available and that a majority of patients will respond within several months is essential. Cushing-induced obesity is more troublesome, developed over months to years and will likewise not resolve immediately even with treatment. Clinicians will need to educate patients about dietary modifications to assist in the treatment of their obesity. Education of patients with pituitary Cushing's disease must include the potentially poor prognosis associated with surgical resection alone. Routine follow-up appointments are necessary to decrease mortality and morbidity associated with the recurrence of pituitary tumors in over 30% of patients who undergo surgical therapy. Reviewing the clinical features of the most common diseases associated with Cushing's syndrome will provide the patient with insight into early detection of such diseases as frequent infections, hypertension, and diabetes.

Prevention

The only preventable cause of adrenal excess is the use of exogenous glucocorticoids. Corticosteroid alternatives are frequently available and should be considered whenever appropriate. Although the decision to use these drugs may involve a cost/benefit analysis, the medications should be used when appropriately indicated. If treatment with a glucocorticoid is necessary, then monitoring for glucose intolerance, hypertension, and osteoporosis should be taken into consideration. Supplementation with calcium and bisphosphonates should also be considered for osteoporosis prophylaxis.

Screening Recommendations

While there are no real indications for screening, if history or physical findings suggest Cushing's syndrome, a dexamethasone suppression test is the recommended first step.

ADRENAL INSUFFICIENCY (ADDISON'S DISEASE)

Pathophysiology

Adrenal insufficiency occurs when the adrenal gland is unable to secrete sufficient amounts of cortisol. This inability is caused by disorders of the adrenal glands themselves (primary adrenal insufficiency), or it occurs secondary to inadequate secretion of ACTH by the pituitary gland (secondary adrenal insufficiency). Addison's disease, a primary adrenal insufficiency, is caused by autoimmune destruction of the steroid-producing cells in the adrenal glands resulting in a cortisol deficiency and, occasionally, an associated aldosterone deficiency in the presence of elevated plasma ACTH. Symptoms of anorexia, weakness, nausea, vomiting, diarrhea, weight loss, and fatigue are often insidious and do not begin until at least 90% of the adrenal cortex has been destroyed. Other causes of adrenal cortex destruction include infections, hemorrhage, adrenalectomy, metastatic disease, congenital adrenal hyperplasia (CAH), and certain drugs (e.g., ketoconazole, phenytoin, and rifampin). Secondary adrenal insufficiency is traced to a lack of ACTH that subsequently causes a drop in cortisol production but not in aldosterone production. Causes include the abrupt cessation or interruption of glucocorticoid hormone therapy or the surgical removal of ACTH-producing tumors of the pituitary gland (Cushing's disease).

Pediatric Issues

Congenital adrenal hyperplasia (CAH) is a primary adrenocortical hypofunction caused by a deficiency in enzymes required for cortisol production. The most common enzyme defect is 21-hydroxylase deficiency, an autosomal-recessive disorder, resulting in increased serum concentration of 17-hydroxyprogesterone and salt wasting. This inborn error can be detected by neonatal screening by enzyme immunoassay or radioimmunoassay for measurement of 17-hydroxyprogesterone. Infants demonstrate severe hypotension, hyponatremia, and hyperkalemia, usually within 5–15 days of birth. These infants require aggressive fluid, electrolyte, glucocorticoid, and mineralocorticoid therapy for survival. Affected female infants, with or without clinically apparent salt loss, may exhibit varying degrees of ambiguous genitalia. Males who are not salt-losers often exhibit sexual precocity. Both conditions are caused by excess androgenic steroids. Clinical manifestation may be delayed into childhood in rare cases. Genetic counseling for the family and patient are necessary and advisable after the condition has been diagnosed.

Obstetric Issues

Addison's disease, like Cushing's syndrome, is exceedingly rare during pregnancy. Clinical manifestations of pregnancy, such as nausea, vomiting, fatigue, and weight loss, are common presenting symptoms for patients with undiagnosed Addison's disease. It is advisable, therefore, when a pregnant patient has persistent or worsening nausea and vomiting, with other symptoms of Addison's disease, to conduct further adrenal testing. Patients with adrenal insufficiency who experience nausea and vomiting early in pregnancy may need additional injections of glucocorticoid and mineralocorticoid to prevent adrenal crisis. During delivery, treatment is similar to that of patients needing surgery; gradual tapering of the dose to maintenance levels should not be achieved until about 10 days postpartum.[5]

Geriatric Issues

Recommendations remain unchanged in this population.

Epidemiology

Adrenal insufficiency is rare, affecting only about 1 in 100,000 people per year. Onset can occur at any age and affects men and women equally. Autoimmune-induced adrenal failure accounts for about 70–80% of all reported cases. Twenty percent of primary adrenal failure cases are caused by infections such as tuberculosis and histoplasmosis.

Treatment Options

Treatment of Addison's disease primarily is focused on substitution for the insufficiently produced adrenal hormones. Cortisol is replaced orally with hydrocortisone tablets or synthetic glucocorticoid in two divided daily doses. When aldosterone is deficient, it is replaced with an oral dose of the mineralocorticoid fludrocortisone acetate (Florinef) taken once daily. Adjustments to dosing are done on an individual basis. Patients requiring exogenous replacement of aldosterone are also encouraged to increase their salt intake. Acute adrenal crisis is treated with hydrocortisone sodium succinate (Solu-Cortef), 100 mg intravenously every 6 h for the first 24 h, along with full fluid and electrolyte resuscitation. Doses may be reduced by half each day as the patient improves. Oral doses can resume once the patient has recovered.[10]

Patient Education

Patients are well advised to display a medical alert tag and to be educated about emergency stress interventions, including knowledge of when to administer supplemental steroids and when to call their primary health care provider.

Prevention

There are no primary prevention strategies at this time. Secondary preventive measures include judicious use of corticosteroids in individuals with inflammatory diseases, and appropriate prevention, recognition, and treatment of infectious diseases such as tuberculosis, HIV, and histoplasmosis.

Screening Recommendations

There are no indications for screening.

REFERENCES

1. Wilson J, Foster D, Kronenberg H, Larsen PR. Williams Textbook of Endocrinology, 9th ed. Philadelphia, WB Saunders, 1998, pp 1–10, 517–664, 939–1060, 1172–1179.
2. Rudy DR, Tzagournis M. Endocrinology (Thyroid disorders). *In* Rakel RE (ed). Textbook of Family Practice, 5th ed. Philadelphia, WB Saunders, 1995, p 1103.
3. American Association of Clinical Endocrinologists: Evaluation and Treatment of Hyperthyroidism and Hypothyroidism. http://www.aace.com/clinguideindex.htm 1996; Medical Guidelines for the Management of Diabetes Mellitus. Endocrine Practice 2000;6:42–84; Medical Guidelines for Clinical Practice for Diagnosis and Treatment of Dyslipidemia and Prevention of Atherogenesis. Endocrine Practice 2000;6:162–214.
4. Mallette LE. Hyperparathyroidism and hypoparathyroidism. *In* Rakel RE (ed). Conn's Current Therapy, 50th ed. Philadelphia, WB Saunders, 1998, pp 624–631.
5. James DK, Steer PJ, Weiner CP, Gonik B. High Risk Pregnancy: Management Options. Philadelphia, WB Saunders, 1996.
6. U.S. Preventive Services Task Force, Guide to Clinical Preventive Services, 2nd ed. Washington, DC, U.S. Department of Health and Human Services, 1996, Chapters 2, 19, 20, 45.
7. American Diabetes Association. Clinical Practice Recommendations. Diabetes Care 2000;23(S1):20–23, 77–79.
8. Schoenfeld G. Inherited disorders of lipid transport. Endocrinol Metab Clin North Am 1990:19:229–257.
9. Grundy SM, Vega GL. Causes of high blood cholesterol. Circulation 1990;81:412–427.
10. Baker JT. Adrenal disorders. A primary care approach. Lippincott's Prim Care Prac 1997;1:527–536.

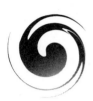

CHAPTER 24

Neoplastic Conditions

Kathryn Boyer, MS, PA-C,
and Emil J. Freireich, MD, DSc (Hon)

■ INTRODUCTION

Cancer is a group of diseases characterized by the uncontrolled development and proliferation of abnormal cells.[1] Cancer can occur anywhere in the body and often requires several injuries that result in genetic mutations that lead to uncontrolled cell growth. Current data indicate that changing lifestyles and modifying exposures can modify cancer risk.[2] A cell must undergo a series of changes before it realizes its potential for malignancy.

Cell reproduction and growth is normally an orderly and organized process regulated by several complicated feedback mechanisms. Rare errors are usually corrected and have no serious consequences. Sometimes an event or series of events goes uncorrected, leading to abnormalities in the cell's cycle of growth. Neoplastic conversion ultimately begins with an alteration in DNA, the genetic material necessary for all cell growth. If normal mechanisms do not repair this damage, a cancer may result.

Carcinogenesis is the process involving several progressive changes that transform a normal cell into a malignant cell.[1] Genes responsible for malignant transformation are divided into three groups:

* Oncogenes that, when activated, cause cancer
* Tumor suppressor genes that normally produce proteins preventing replication of tumor cells. When these genes are defective, tumor cells can reproduce uncontrollably, leading to cancer.
* Mismatch-repair genes that (to simplify) produce proteins that recognize and correct errors in replicating DNA

Activation of oncogenes and inactivation of tumor suppressor genes produce a series of genetic changes that lead to a malignant phenotype. A series of essential steps appear to be required for the malignant transformation of a cell, eventually resulting in a neoplastic tumor.

Carcinogenic agents implicated in malignant transformation include viruses, certain chemicals, electromagnetic radiation, asbestos, and hormonal factors. Cigarette smoking has been definitively implicated as a carcinogen, and, because many people who do not smoke develop cancer, other causes of malignancy must also exist.

Anecdotal evidence implicates a variety of factors in causing cancer. Based on this evidence, the mass media are quick to indict certain substances or behaviors as causing cancer. Because so many steps are involved in carcinogenesis, it is difficult to positively identify all cancer-causing agents and events.

Proving what prevents cancer is similarly difficult. Exercise and proper diet are felt to be preventive. Although both are necessary for optimal health, their role in the prevention of cancer is somewhat vague, so that while anecdotal evidence may suggest a preventive effect, definitive proof is elusive. The definition of exercise is broad, and it has not been proved to prevent cancer of any type (either primarily or secondarily). In fact, some factions of researchers theorize that exercise increases free radical formation and may thus contribute to the development of cancer.

Other cancers, such as Hodgkin's lymphoma, non-Hodgkin's lymphoma, and leukemia, do not lend themselves to preventive strategies and are not outlined in this chapter. Patient counseling is an important part of dealing with all forms of malignancy. Screening recommendations and leading cancer sites are listed later in this chapter, in Tables 24–3 and 24–4.

Often cancer results from activation of a dominant oncogene or deletion of a suppressor gene. Oncogenes can be activated by point mutations, chromosome translocations, or gene amplification. Removal of a suppressor gene can involve a small or a large deletion. Operationally, an agent can be considered carcinogenic when an alteration in the frequency or intensity of exposure to it is followed by a change in the frequency of occurrence of one or more types of cancer. The target for most carcinogens is, ultimately, the DNA. The steps of carcinogenesis include initiation, promotion, and progression (Fig. 24–1).

Initiation is the earliest stage of carcinogenesis and is the result of irreversible alterations to the genetic makeup of cells, usually induced by a specific agent or event. Initiation often may also include the transformation of a proto-oncogene into an oncogene and the inactivation of a tumor suppressor gene in a particular tissue. This process does not always result in cancer.

Promotion is the reversible propagation of the abnormality that has been created in the initiation step. Promotion increases the potential for malignancy and often includes exposure to cancer-causing agents (e.g., cigarette smoke or viral infection). It appears to be dependent on the dose and the duration of exposure of the cell to the exogenous agent. Promoters are essentially agents that cause clonal expansion of initiated cells.[2] The latency period, or the time between the exposure to a promoter and the development of a malignancy, seems to be critical but is extremely difficult to define.[1] Preventing exposure to promoters, or reducing the dose and duration of exposure, is likely to lower the probability of malignant expression of initiated cells.[1] Initiated cells respond differently to promoters than do normal cells.

Progression is the growth of the malignant clone cell, leading to

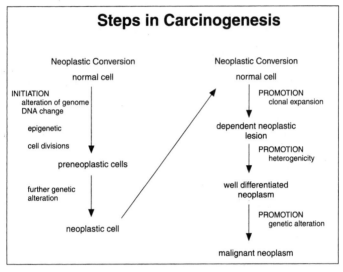

Figure 24–1. Most types of cancer stem from a complex sequence of steps, schematically outlined here. Naturally occurring chemicals related to lifestyle or carcinogens associated with occupational exposure must undergo metabolic activation (or, conversely, are detoxified biochemically). The resulting ultimate carcinogen, a reactive molecule (and also radiation or oncogenic viruses), interacts with cellular macromolecules and specifically with the heritable element, DNA. This altered DNA undergoes further changes during replication, leading to codon (oncogene) rearrangements and amplification. Also involved may be an effect on suppressor genes. This sequence of reactions is the result of "genotoxic" elements. Cells with such abnormal DNA must duplicate and develop, subject to the control of diverse factors at the level of the cell, organ, tissue, whole animal, or human being, and to external environmental elements. Factors bearing on growth promotion or inhibition may be involved. This sequence of reactions is the result of nongenotoxic, epigenetic events, which are highly dose dependent, with a threshold no-effect dose. (From Murphy GP, Lawrence W Jr., Lenhard RE Jr., American Cancer Society Textbook of Clinical Oncology, 2nd ed., 1995, p 19. Reprinted by the permission of the American Cancer Society, Inc.)

morbidity that is caused by local growth, systemic effects, and spread to distant organs.

Metastasis is the ability of malignant disease to spread from one organ or part of the body to another not directly connected to it. It most often occurs when malignant cells break away from the original or primary site and travel via blood or lymph to another site, most often the lymph nodes, the bones, the brain, the lungs, or the liver. Metastasis signifies advanced disease.

Although each cancer is unique, the etiology and basic mechanisms of alteration of DNA seem to be common for most if not all cancers. To determine the cause of cancer is a challenging task that minimally requires an accurate and thorough history and physical examination, extensive knowledge, and interpretation of current research data. As stated by Devita and colleagues, "Our current understanding of carcinogenesis and risk to human health comes from a variety of models and methods, including cell culture experiments, animal studies, and classic and molecular epidemiology. The goal is to elucidate etiologies, define cancer risks in individuals, and to identify cancer prevention methods."[2] (For additional resources, see the Resources Appendix at the end of this book.)

CAUSES OF CANCER

Viruses

Viruses are estimated to be involved in the development of approximately one seventh of all cancers. Eighty percent of virus-related cancers are sequelae of two viruses, hepatitis B and human papillomavirus (HPV). Oncogenic transformation requires DNA alterations in addition to infection with a virus in these cases.

Many human immunodeficient states result in a predisposition to malignancies of diverse cell lineages. Common neoplasms in HIV patients, usually those with end-stage HIV disease (or AIDS), are Kaposi's sarcoma, non-Hodgkin's lymphoma, and cervical and anorectal carcinomas.[2] Human T-cell lymphotrophic virus type I (HTLV-I) is thought to be involved in the genesis of leukemia.[2]

Hepatitis B virus (HBV) is a small DNA virus that can produce subclinical infection or acute hepatitis B in susceptible hosts.[2] Hepatocellular carcinoma (HCC), though rare in the United States, is a very common malignancy in Southeast Asia and sub-Saharan Africa, with approximately one million cases annually worldwide.[3] Distribution has been linked to chronic hepatitis B infection. Chronic hepatitis B infection is associated with a 100-fold increased risk of HCC. Other studies have shown a 250:1 relative risk for the development of HCC in asymptomatic hepatitis B surface antigen (HBsAg) carriers compared with noninfected controls.[3] Severe liver injury (cirrhosis or chronic active hepatitis) seems to be a necessary cofactor in the development of HCC.

Evidence linking cervical cancer to human papillomavirus (HPV) infection resulted from recognition that morphologic changes observed on Papanicolaou (Pap) smears interpreted as dysplasia were due to a papillomavirus infection.[2] However, infection with HPV is not alone sufficient to cause the development of cervical cancer (Table 24–1).

Table 24–1. Human Viruses with Oncogenic Potential or Properties

Virus	Human Tumor	Cofactor
Hepatitis B (HBV)	Hepatocellular carcinoma (HCC)	Aflatoxin, alcohol, smoking
Hepatitis C (HCV)	HCC	None known
Epstein-Barr virus (EBV)	Burkitt's lymphoma	Malaria
	Immunoblastic lymphoma	Immunodeficiency
	Hodgkin's disease	None known
Human papillomavirus–16, –18, –33, –39	Anogenital cancer	Smoking (?)

Adapted from DeVita VT Jr, Hellman S, Rosenberg SA, eds. Cancer Principles and Practice of Oncology, 5th ed. Philadelphia, Lippincott-Raven, 1997, pp 169, 175, with permission.

Chemicals

Observations of increased incidence of specific cancers in certain occupational groups led to the recognition of the chemical origin of some human malignancies. Chemical carcinogens are often organ specific, targeting epithelial cells and possibly causing genetic damage. Chemicals identified as human carcinogens have produced organ-specific tumors in laboratory animals.[2] Chemical carcinogens comprise several different classes with different mechanisms of action: DNA alteration or substitution, direct cytotoxicity, promotion, peroxisome proliferation, inhibition of cell death, and stimulation of proliferation.[4]

Asbestos

Asbestos includes a group of naturally occurring hydrated mineral silicates that form fibers when they crystallize.[2] The carcinogenicity of asbestos was first noticed in the 1950s, when an association of asbestos exposure with lung cancer and mesothelioma in asbestos miners was demonstrated. In the 1960s an association with lung cancer in shipyard workers, asbestos textile weavers, and pipe insulators was identified.[2] It appears that the latency period for the development of cancer from exposure to asbestos varies from 15 to 40 years after exposure and shortens as exposure levels increase. The latency period seems to lengthen for older workers.[2] It is postulated that radiation, cigarette smoking, and asbestos can act synergistically to increase cancer induction.

The mechanisms of asbestos carcinogenesis are not completely understood, but fibers accumulate in the perinuclear region of the cytoplasm of cells. The short fibers accumulate on the cell surface,

Table 24–2. Known or Suspected Chemical Carcinogens in Humans

Organ	Agents
Squamous cell cancer of oral cavity	Tobacco smoke, alcohol, nickel compounds
Squamous cell cancer of esophagus	Tobacco smoke, alcoholic beverages
Gastric adenocarcinoma	Smoked/salted/pickled foods
Colon adenocarcinoma	Heterocyclic amines, asbestos
Lung (all types)	Tobacco smoke, arsenic, asbestos, crystalline silica, beryllium, benzo(a)pyrene, coal tar, nickel compounds, soots, mustard gas
Pleural mesothelioma	Asbestos
Liver	Aflatoxin, vinyl chloride, tobacco smoke, alcohol
Renal cell carcinoma	Tobacco smoke
Bladder (transitional cell)	Tobacco smoke, benzidine, 4-aminobiphenyl, 2-naphthylamine
Prostate adenocarcinoma	Cadmium
Skin	Arsenic, benzo(a)pyrene, coal tar, mineral oils, soots
Bone marrow (leukemia)	Benzene, tobacco smoke, ethylene oxide, antineoplastic agents

Adapted from DeVita VT Jr, Hellman S, Rosenberg SA, eds. Cancer Principles and Practice of Oncology, 5th ed. Philadelphia, Lippincott-Raven, 1997, p 191, with permission.

the long ones in the nucleus of the cell. Animal studies suggest that asbestos fibers produce large, multilocus genetic deletions, leading to neoplastic transformation (Table 24–2).[2]

PHYSICAL FACTORS

Ionizing Radiation

A causal relationship was suspected between radiation exposure and skin cancer within 6 years of the discovery of x-rays.[2] Only a few years later, a similar relationship between radiation and leukemias was recognized. The important characteristic of ionizing radiation is the local release of large amounts of energy that causes breakage in biologically important chemical bonds. This breakage appears to be enough damage to eventually lead to malignancy. Radiotherapy substantially increases the risk of secondary malignancies, especially leukemias.[2] It has been proposed that radiation is effective at producing deletions and chromosome translocations, but is less effective at producing point mutations. Risk attributable solely to radiation treatment is difficult to assess because chemotherapy and radiotherapy are often given in combination to treat various malignancies.

All tissues appear to be at risk of developing a malignancy after exposure to radiation, but the susceptibility of different tissues varies widely. Radon is a naturally occurring radioactive gas that emanates from the soil and may accumulate in confined spaces, as in the basement of a house. Radon decays to short-lived radioactive progeny that ultimately aerosolize and, if inhaled, may become deposited in the tracheobronchial tree, increasing the risk of lung cancer.[2] Solar ultraviolet radiation is a potent DNA-damaging agent, and is thus a known inducer of non-melanoma skin cancers. Ultraviolet radiation probably also plays a promotional role in melanoma, possibly by altering the tumor suppressor gene p53. The use of cellular telephones has been proposed to contribute to an increased incidence of brain tumors; however, data to substantiate this assumption are sparse, and any conclusion as to causation is extremely premature.[3] Epidemiologic studies are currently ongoing worldwide.

Hormonal Factors

Hormonal factors appear to play a major role in the etiology of several human cancers. Some neoplasms are the consequence of excessive hormonal stimulation of the particular target organ. The best-understood hormone-related malignancy is endometrial cancer, which results from the cumulative exposure of the endometrium to unopposed estrogen.[4] Another risk factor for endometrial cancer is increased body weight, which is probably related to increased exposure of the endometrium to estrogens (obese postmenopausal women have increased plasma levels of estradiol, an estrogen).[2]

Ovarian cancer is another hormone-dependent malignancy whose epidemiology is also well-studied. The stimulus for ovarian cancer correlates with ovulation. It has been proposed that epithelial cells within the developing follicle are the cells of origin of ovarian cancer.[2] Therefore, any respite from ovulation would be protective against ovarian cancer. This seems to correlate with the fact that increased parity and combination oral contraceptive use seem to be protective against ovarian cancer.[2, 3]

Prostate cancer also appears to be hormone-dependent. Adenocarcinoma of the prostate can be induced in animals by increasing testosterone levels. The androgen is a requirement for tumor induction.[2]

Breast cancer is an additional well-studied hormone-dependent neoplasm. Estrogen (estradiol) is a primary stimulant for breast cell proliferation. The proliferation rate is probably further increased by the simultaneous presence of progesterone. The most consistently documented risk factors for breast cancer are early age of menarche, late age of menopause, late age of first pregnancy, and increased body weight.[1, 2] The increased risk appears to be shaped by effects of ovarian activity, with a major determinant of breast cancer being the cumulative number of ovulatory cycles during a woman's lifetime (Tables 24–3 and 24–4).

COUNSELING THE PATIENT

Certain cancers are amenable to therapy and are "curable." Other cancers, once discovered or after inadequate response to therapy, are terminal. Patients look to the health care provider to give them hope, guidance, and education. It is important to be honest about the prognosis while remembering that no one can predict the future. Sharing statistics with patients is one way to provide realism to the patient, reminding them that the statistics are nationwide historical

Table 24–3. The American Cancer Society Screening Recommendations for Early Detection of Cancer in Asymptomatic People

Location	Screening	Patient Age	Frequency	Patient Gender
Colorectum	Sigmoidoscopy,	50 and over	Every 3–5 years	Both
	Fecal occult blood test,	50 and over	Every year	Both
	Digital rectal examination (DRE)	40 and over	Every year	Both
Cervix	Papanicolaou (Pap) test	18 or sexually active	Every year	Female
	Pelvic examination	18–40	Every year	Female
		Over 40	Every 1–3 years	Female
Breast	Breast self-examination (BSE)	20 and over	Every month	Female
	Breast clinical examination	20–40	Every 3 years	Female
		Over 40	Every year	Female
		40–49	Every 1–2 years	Female
	Mammography	50 and over	Every year	Female
Prostate	Digital rectal examination (DRE)	50 and over	Every year	Male
Skin	Clinical cancer checkup	20 and over	Every 3 years	Both
		40 and over	Every year	Both

Adapted from Murphy GP, Lawrence W Jr, Lenhard RE Jr, eds. American Cancer Society Textbook of Clinical Oncology, 2nd ed., Atlanta, GA, American Cancer Society, Inc., 1995, pp 181–183.

Table 24–4. Number of Cancer Cases by Site, 2000 (Estimated Statistics)

Site	New Cases (Estimated) in 2000	Deaths (Estimated) in 2000
Lung and bronchus	164,100	156,900
Prostate	180,400	31,900
Breast	184,200	41,200
Colorectum	130,200	56,300
Bladder	53,200	12,200
Melanoma	47,700	7700
Oral cavity and pharynx	30,200	7800
Kidney	31,200	11,900
Leukemia	30,800	21,700
Pancreas	28,300	28,200
Ovary	23,100	14,000
Thyroid	18,400	1200
Esophagus	12,300	12,100
Liver	15,300	13,800
Stomach	21,500	13,000
Cervix	12,800	4600
Uterus and endometrium	36,100	6500
Childhood	12,400	2300
Non-Hodgkin's lymphoma	54,900	26,100
Hodgkin's disease	7400	1400
All Sites	1,220,200	552,200

Adapted from American Cancer Society: Cancer Facts and Figures 2000. Atlanta, GA, American Cancer Society, Inc.

data. The fact that cancer "cure" actually means 5-year disease-free survival should be explained. Patients who remain capable of understanding should be provided with the actual prognosis, if they desire, so that they can plan accordingly. This may mean that the patient will get his or her affairs in order, or take the vacation that he or she always dreamed of taking. There is often time to "say good-bye" to friends and relatives, in contrast to a rapid, traumatic death in which there may be unresolved family conflicts. An accurate prognosis also allows the patient to move beyond denial and attempt to enjoy what time remains.

Frequently, patients will spend their final months or years and significant resources attempting to find the cure for a terminal illness. Often, however, the only way a cure can ever be found is if patients and their health care providers participate in clinical trials, and if patients undergo therapy with investigational agents. The decision to participate in a trial is a personal one, as it deals with the time remaining in a person's life.

It is important to allow patients to speak freely about their religious faith, as faith is a significant issue for those facing a terminal illness.

Allowing the patient to discuss faith issues can help the health care provider to better understand human emotion and coping mechanisms associated with death and dying. Pastoral services should be involved if the patient desires.

Health care providers who share only the science with the terminal patient, or who are brutally honest, are, to a degree, shielding themselves from natural emotion. Objectivity should be maintained, but health care providers should remember that each patient is first and foremost an individual with a devastating disease. The provider should enlist the support of a hospice program for terminally ill patients. Hospice programs provide physical, psychological, social, and spiritual care to patients and their families. Referral to a hospice program should be viewed as an active, viable treatment modality rather than as abandoning the patient.[1]

Carcinogenesis is a multistep process involving both environmental and genetic factors that eventually can cause abnormal cell growth. Several viral, chemical, physical, and hormonal factors have been implicated in carcinogenesis, although other factors also play a role in the process. To identify environmental causes is difficult and takes several years. With the mapping of the human genome, genetic etiologies of carcinogenesis may soon be elucidated. Chemoprevention as a method of avoiding the development of cancer is gaining support at larger institutions, and studies investigating the potential of substances to prevent cancer are proliferating. Research continues and, when combined with the results of the human genome project and worldwide epidemiologic studies, may lead to the development of more cost-effective screening tests and more available prevention strategies. With ongoing collaborative efforts among basic scientists, researchers, clinicians, physicians, and epidemiologists, carcinogens will be identified and exposure to these agents prevented. Until all carcinogens are identified, we must increase preventive efforts, both primary and secondary, to decrease the individual's cancer risk and ultimately eliminate cancer.

BLADDER CANCER

Pathophysiology

Bladder cancer is the most common cancer of the urinary tract. Cigarette smoking seems to be responsible for the majority of cases. Chromosomal variations in patients with bladder cancer most commonly include abnormalities of chromosome 9 but also involve alterations of the p53 tumor suppressor gene on chromosome 17. Risk factors for bladder cancer include smoking, environmental chemical exposure (especially to aromatic amines), and abuse of phenacetin.[1] Smoking is associated with a sixfold increase in incidence of bladder cancer and is believed to contribute to approximately 50% of bladder cancers in men.[2] Aniline dyes used in the textile industry contribute to increased risk, although the latency period from exposure to tumor transformation is between 6 and 20 years in humans.[4]

Carcinogens and their metabolites are believed to be excreted in urine, where they act directly on the urothelial mucosal lining. Combustion gases have also been implicated in the development of bladder cancer.[2] The risks of consuming coffee and artificial sweeteners are controversial.

Pediatric Issues

Management is not significantly affected.

Obstetric Issues

Management is not significantly affected.

Geriatric Considerations

Peak incidence is in the seventh decade of life.[3]

Epidemiology

The American Cancer Society (ACS) estimates 53,200 new cases and 12,200 deaths from bladder cancer in the U.S. in 2000, with a male:female ratio of 2:1.5. Mortality rates have decreased significantly since 1970.[5]

Treatment Options

Treatment options are based on the extent of the disease. Surgical resection is curative to a point if local disease is present. Radiotherapy is seldom recommended. Intravessical chemotherapy or immunotherapy is indicated in patients with a high risk of recurrence. Systemic combination chemotherapy is another treatment option. A combined modality approach may be required depending on the stage of the cancer at diagnosis.

Patient Education

Smoking cessation or prevention should be strongly encouraged. Any hematuria with increased frequency of urination should be investigated immediately by a health care professional.

Prevention

Nothing can be done about occupational exposure to agents implicated in causing bladder cancer if the exposure has already occurred. Smoking cessation should be strongly encouraged. All patients who smoke should be referred to a smoking cessation clinic if one is available. Reduce exposure to known causative agents (aniline dye, combustion gases, phenacetin, cigarette smoke).

Screening Recommendations

Those at high risk and with symptoms should be screened on a regular basis with urine cytologies and possibly cystoscopies with biopsies.

▬ BREAST CANCER

Pathophysiology

Breast cancer is unique among tumor types in that it behaves differently in different patients, and it can have a relatively slow growth rate compared with other tumors. A tumor the size of 1 cm in diameter can be readily palpated, yet, conversely, a lesion may not be palpable.[2] Because of the relatively slow doubling time of some breast tumors, early detection is presumed to be beneficial and to lead to more effective treatment, which leads to an increased cure rate. A complete list of factors that have been shown to be associated with increased risk of developing breast cancer is immense.[2] Age is important, as risk increases with age. Familial aggregations are very common, but truly inherited breast cancers have been estimated to account for only 5–10% of the overall incidence rate.[4] Mutations of BRCA1, BRCA2, and p53 all carry a markedly increased risk of breast cancer.[2] (See Chapter 8, Clinical Genetics.)

Approximately 50% of affected women have no identifiable risk factors other than being a female and aging.[2] Breast cancer is clearly linked to hormones, as well as age of menarche, menopause, and first pregnancy. Most of these are nonmodifiable. Exogenous hormones (hormone replacement therapy and oral contraceptive use) have been extensively studied for links to breast cancer; however, the risk for each is not clearly established.[2]

Alcohol intake has been associated with an increased risk of breast cancer, as has smoking. Benign breast disease (such as fibrocystic disease) seems to carry a small increase in risk of cancer.[2] Exposure to ionizing radiation increases breast cancer risk, especially if the radiation has been secondary to nuclear explosions or medical procedures, with exposure early in life carrying the greatest risk.[2]

Pediatric Issues

This condition is not present in the pediatric population.

Obstetric Issues

Breast cancer may be diagnosed during pregnancy. If so, trials have shown that it can be safe to treat a patient for breast cancer during pregnancy, depending on the stage of the tumor and the stage of the pregnancy. Any pregnant patient diagnosed with breast cancer should be immediately referred to a specialty cancer institution prior to any treatment.

Geriatric Issues

No additional considerations have been identified, other than to screen for comorbid conditions that may contraindicate certain therapeutic options.

Epidemiology

Breast cancer is by far the most common cancer in American women, with an estimated 184,200 new cases and 41,200 deaths in 2000.[4] Less than 1% of breast cancer cases (1400) are diagnosed in men.

Treatment Options

Treatment is dependent on the stage of the cancer at diagnosis, the cell type, the location, and patient preference. Surgery is the mainstay of therapy. Radiotherapy is often used. Chemotherapy is being used frequently in hopes of preventing recurrence of disease. Hormonal therapy is also a common treatment modality and is being used as a preventive strategy in high-risk women or in those with significant risk of recurrence.

Patient Education

Breast self-examination should be taught to and performed by all women over the age of 20 on a monthly basis. Alcohol intake should be reduced or eliminated as a potential contributing factor. Smoking cessation is important as a possible contributing factor in breast (and other) cancers as well as for optimal health. Dietary fat intake should be decreased. Soy products contain some chemicals that are thought to have potential chemopreventive effects. Further investigation comparing the risks and benefits of plant estrogens with those of animal-derived estrogens is ongoing.

Prevention

The two most significant risk factors, gender and age, are nonmodifiable, so secondary prevention methods need to be addressed. Chemoprevention may be an important strategy in the future. Tamoxifen, a selective estrogen receptor modulator that blocks estrogen receptors in breast tissue, may be an important agent in breast cancer prevention. It has been shown to decrease risk in a primary prevention trial.[3] Trials with tamoxifen and raloxifene are continuing. Retinoids are also being studied and may show some promise in prevention. Dietary trials to determine the possible preventive role of a reduction of dietary fat to less that 20% of total daily caloric intake are also ongoing.[4]

Screening Recommendations

Early detection is important because of the slow-growing nature of most breast cancer tumor types. But to realize a survival benefit from treatment, breast cancer must be diagnosed prior to metastasis.

Breast self-examination is free and available to all women, and should be employed and incorporated into the lives of *all* women, regardless of age, diet, or presence of other risk factors. Any changes noted on breast self-examination should be brought to the attention of a health care provider for further evaluation.

Full screening recommendations, including mammography, are listed in Table 24–3.

CERVICAL CANCER

Pathophysiology

The exact mechanism of malignant transformation has not been identified, but risk factors include human papillomavirus (HPV) infection (especially with subtypes 16 or 18, herpes simplex virus subtype 2 [HSV-2] coinfection), genital warts, multiple sex partners, beginning sexual activity at an early age, and an immunocompromised state.[6] Other factors associated with increased risk include cigarette smoking, exposure to diethylstilbestrol (DES), and decreased intake of carotenoids, folate, and vitamins A, C, and E.[2] Cervical cancer is exceedingly rare in sexually inactive and nulliparous women.[4] Cervical cancer can be detected early by the Papanicolaou (Pap) smear, an inexpensive and effective screening technique. When detected early, cervical cancer can have a favorable prognosis.

Pediatric Issues

All sexually active women should have a Pap smear.

Obstetric Issues

Management is not significantly affected.

Geriatric Issues

An upper age limit for routine Pap testing should be individualized, as there is no sufficient evidence either to continue or to discontinue screening. Discontinuing routine testing after age 65 can be justified if the patient has had regular screening with normal results. Women who have had a hysterectomy in which the cervix was removed do not require further Pap testing unless the hysterectomy was performed because of cervical cancer.[7]

Epidemiology

Cervical cancer is the second most common malignancy among women worldwide, but it does not rank among the 10 most common cancers in women in the U.S.[1] The ACS estimates that in the U.S. there will be 12,800 new cases and 4600 deaths in 2000.[5] The largest reason for the disparity in worldwide incidence and incidence in the U.S. is the widespread use of the Pap smear for screening and early detection. Because of the use of the Pap smear for early detection, incidence rates in the U.S. have decreased steadily from 14.2/100,000 in 1973 to 7.4/100,000 in 1995.[5] Mortality rates have also declined.

Treatment Options

Treatment is dependent on the stage of the cancer at diagnosis; however, total hysterectomy with bilateral salpingo-oophorectomy with pelvic lymphadenectomy seems to be curative. Adjuvant radiotherapy is sometimes recommended, especially if the disease has spread or is more extensive. Chemotherapy is used if distant metastases are present.[1] Five-year disease-free survival is up to 70% for all stages, 91% for localized cervical cancers.[5]

Patient Education

The importance of the annual pelvic examination and Pap smear should be emphasized in any sexually active female, regardless of age. Reiterate the dangers of sexually transmitted diseases (STDs) and their long-term effects on reproductive organs. Some patients may need education on the causes of STDs and the availability and proper use of barrier methods of contraception. Stress the curability of cervical cancer if this malignancy is diagnosed at an early stage. Encourage young women to consider the consequences of having multiple sexual partners.

Prevention

Early detection can prevent most advanced-stage cervical cancer. Since smoking can contribute to carcinogenesis, smoking cessation should be strongly encouraged in all age groups. Prevention of STDs, especially HPV and HSV-2, by the use of barrier contraception, is extremely important. Delaying onset of sexual activity, practicing monogamous relations, and using condoms could dramatically reduce the rates of HPV infection, thus reducing HPV-related cervical cancer deaths. Reduction in the number of sexual partners to reduce HPV and other STD transmission should be stressed. A healthy diet with adequate intake of foods rich in vitamins A, C, and E, and folic acid may also contribute to prevention.

Screening Recommendations

Pap smear and pelvic examination should be performed annually in all sexually active women, beginning either at onset of sexual activity or at age 18, whichever comes first.[1] Any abnormalities should be closely followed and further investigated. Lesions should be diagnosed via colposcopy. Control of STDs is very important, as is early recognition of STDs and treatment of affected patients and all involved partners.

COLORECTAL CANCER

Pathophysiology

Because the colon and the rectum are anatomically contiguous, cancers of these organs are often classified together as colorectal cancers. Exact mechanisms of colorectal cancer development are not completely understood, but neoplastic transformation of colorectal cells seems to result from a complex interaction of dietary, environmental, and genetic events.

Diets low in fiber, fruits, and vegetables combined with intake of high-fat foods are thought to act synergistically to increase the risk of colorectal cancer.[2] Certain foods (fats) can promote abnormal cellular changes in the bowel mucosa. Fat slows the movement of food through the colon, leading to increased exposure of the bowel mucosa to carcinogenic substances. Tobacco use and a sedentary lifestyle are probable contributing factors.

Genetic predisposition for colorectal cancer is increased in those with polyposis syndromes (familial adenomatous polyposis [FAP], hereditary nonpolyposis colorectal cancer [HNPCC]), adenomatous polyps, or a family history of colorectal cancer.[2] Inflammatory bowel disease, especially ulcerative colitis, predisposes to colorectal cancer but is not in itself a cause.[4]

Pediatric Issues

Management is not significantly affected.

Obstetric Issues

Management is not significantly affected.

Geriatric Issues

Seventy-three percent of newly diagnosed colorectal cancers occur in patients over 65 years of age.[5] Incidence of colorectal cancer increases with age; however, outcomes are favorable when diagnosed and treated at an early stage. For this reason, screening is extremely important, especially in the older age groups.

Epidemiology

Cancer of the large intestine is the third most common cancer in the U.S. The ACS estimates 130,200 new cases and 56,300 deaths from colon cancer in 2000.[5]

Treatment Options

Surgery remains the primary therapy for all histologic types of colorectal cancer. Chemotherapy, either neoadjuvant or adjuvant, has been used in patients with metastatic or advanced disease; however, results have been less than optimal. The use of chemotherapy for metastatic disease has not yet been proved to offer a significant survival advantage.

Patient Education

Stress to patients that it is important to know their family medical history because some colorectal (and other) cancers are hereditary. It is also important to follow up with screening and immediately evaluate any abdominal pain or changes in bowel movements. Patients should be educated about the importance of early detection and the high curative potential if the malignancy is discovered at an early stage.

Prevention

Obesity has been associated with an increased risk of colorectal cancer in men.[5] A low-fat diet combined with a high-fiber diet rich in fruits and vegetables should help reduce the risk both of obesity and of colorectal cancer.

Chemoprevention aims to block the action of carcinogens on cells before cancer appears. Regular long-term use of aspirin (ASA) and other nonsteroidal anti-inflammatory drugs (NSAIDs) appears to decrease the incidence of colorectal cancer. Possibly these drugs inhibit colorectal carcinogenesis by reducing endogenous prostaglandin production. Controlled studies of the preventive effects of vitamins C and E, folic acid, and calcium have shown mixed results.[3] Hormone replacement therapy (estrogen) may decrease the risk of developing colorectal cancer in postmenopausal women.[5]

Screening Recommendations

Early detection of colorectal cancer is extremely important. Several methods for detection are available. The fecal occult blood test yields many false-positive and false-negative results; however, the test is very inexpensive, easy to use, and widely available, and the results are available almost immediately. Unfortunately, more than 50% of colorectal cancers go undetected because there is no bleeding at the time of testing.

Digital rectal examination is very simple to perform and can detect lesions up to 7 cm from the anal verge.[3] Sigmoidoscopy is relatively inexpensive and more comfortable for the patient since the development of flexible sigmoidoscopes. Fifty percent of neoplasms are within reach of the 60-cm flexible scope.

Colonoscopy has an extremely high sensitivity for tumor detection. However, the procedure is invasive and may be deferred by some otherwise asymptomatic people. Any suspicious polyps should be removed and sent for pathologic evaluation.

Recommendations for patients at low risk for colorectal cancer include digital rectal examination and fecal occult blood testing annually after the age of 40 and flexible sigmoidoscopy every 3–5 years after the age of 40.[3]

Recommendations for patients at high risk for colorectal cancer have shown no particular benefits, but annual fecal occult blood testing and colonoscopy every 5 years beginning at age 35–40 may be considered. Patients with HNPCC need even closer surveillance beginning at a younger age. These patients should consider enrolling in a clinical chemoprevention trial.

▰▰▰ ENDOMETRIAL CANCER

Pathophysiology

The exact cause of endometrial cancer is unknown, but certain oncogenes (HER-2/neu and c-myc) seem to play a role.[4] Estrogen stimulates cellular growth and glandular proliferation, which is cyclically balanced by the maturational effects of progesterone. Abnormal proliferation and neoplastic transformation of endometrium have been associated with chronic exposure to unopposed estrogenic stimulation.[2]

Risk factors for endometrial cancer include obesity, hypertension, diabetes, and nulliparity.[4] Other risk factors are irregular menses, chronic anovulation, unopposed exogenous estrogen therapy, pelvic irradiation, and late menopause.[4] Ingestion of a diet high in animal fat also may play a role.[4]

Pediatric Issues

Endometrial cancer does not appear in the pediatric population.

Obstetric Issues

Management is not significantly affected.

Geriatric Issues

Endometrial cancer is primarily a malignancy of postmenopausal women. Early diagnosis and treatment often lead to a favorable outcome, so screening and further surveillance must be continued in the geriatric population. Random endometrial biopsies in the elderly have been recommended by some for early detection; however, overall cost-effectiveness of this intervention has not been confirmed.

Epidemiology

Endometrial cancer has been extensively studied epidemiologically. It is the fourth most common cancer in women in the U.S., behind breast, lung, and colorectal cancer.[4] The median age at diagnosis is 60 years.[2] The ACS estimates that there will be 36,100 new cases and 6500 deaths in 2000, with incidence and mortality rates remaining constant since 1989.

Treatment Options

Surgery (total abdominal hysterectomy and bilateral salpingo-oophorectomy) is the treatment of choice for local disease. Adjuvant radiotherapy is sometimes incorporated into the treatment regimen. Some benefit has been seen with chemotherapeutic agents such as doxorubicin, paclitaxel, and cisplatin, but the addition of chemotherapy has not shown a significant survival advantage.[3] Hormone therapy with progestins has shown a good response if the primary tumor is progesterone receptor-positive.[3]

Patient Education

The benefits of a healthy diet and early treatment of hypertension and diabetes need to be stressed. The patient should be aware of family history of endometrial cancer. Patients with late onset of menopause need to be aware of their increased risk.

Prevention

Avoid, prevent, screen, and appropriately treat the associated conditions of hypertension, obesity, and diabetes. Avoid unopposed estrogen therapy in postmenopausal women.

Advocate a low-fat diet. Stress the importance of early detection through the use of regular Pap smears.

Screening Recommendations

Continue Pap smear screening even in postmenopausal patients.

■■■ESOPHAGEAL CANCER

Pathophysiology

Although uncommon in the U.S., esophageal cancer has the greatest variation in geographic distribution of any malignancy.[2] Risk factors appear to be alcohol ingestion and cigarette smoking. Sixty to eighty-six percent of esophageal adenocarcinomas may arise from Barrett's esophagitis; however, a variety of factors probably play a role in the etiology of esophageal cancer. Levels of nitrosamines and nitrosamine precursors (nitrates/nitrites) are high in food and water samples from areas of China with high incidences of esophageal cancer, and thus these substances are thought to contribute or to be causative of esophageal as well as gastric cancer.[4] Alcohol and tobacco are both also implicated in occurrence of esophageal cancer and may even act synergistically to produce a higher rate of cancer than each produces alone.[2]

Pediatric Issues

Esophageal cancer does not occur in the pediatric population.

Obstetric Issues

Management is not significantly affected.

Geriatric Issues

Management is not significantly affected.

Epidemiology

The ACS estimates 12,300 new cases and 12,100 deaths in the U.S. in 2000.[5]

Treatment Options

Treatment includes both surgery and radiotherapy. Supportive care is absolutely necessary. Chemotherapy is generally used palliatively but sometimes preoperatively or in combination with radiotherapy and surgery. Results remain dismal, with a suboptimal cure rate regardless of treatment modality.

Patient Education

The risks of smoking and alcohol abuse should be addressed with all patients. The fact that many cancers are already in the advanced stages at the time of diagnosis should forewarn the patient that behavior changes need to occur sooner rather than later.

Prevention

Patients should decrease intake of nitrosamines or only ingest with simultaneous vitamin C supplementation.[4] Reduction in alcohol intake and smoking cessation should be stressed in all age groups. Screening and appropriate treatment for Barrett's esophagitis are important in those with gastroesophageal reflux disease.

Screening Recommendations

A high index of suspicion should be maintained in at-risk patients. However, most esophageal cancers are advanced at the time of diagnosis.

GASTRIC CANCER

Pathophysiology

A genetic predisposition to gastric cancer may exist. For instance, Napoleon Bonaparte, his father, and his grandfather all died of gastric cancer.[2] Factors associated with increased risk are consumption of smoked and salted meat and fish, high nitrate consumption, drinking well water, smoking, and *Helicobacter pylori* infection. Gastritis is also considered a risk factor.[2] Consumption of raw vegetables, fruit, citrus fruit, and vitamins A and C, and a high-fiber diet are inversely related to increased risk of stomach cancer.[2]

Pediatric Issues

Gastric cancer does not occur in the pediatric population.

Obstetric Issues

Management is not significantly affected.

Geriatric Issues

Management is not significantly affected.

Epidemiology

In Chile and Costa Rica, gastric cancer is epidemic; Japan has the highest incidence in the world. The ACS has estimated 21,500 new cases of gastric cancer and 13,000 deaths will occur in the U.S. in 2000.[5] Mortality from gastric cancer in the U.S. has been decreasing for 50 years.[5]

Treatment Options

Surgery is the only potentially curative modality for local disease.[2] Some patients may be given postoperative chemotherapy. Adjuvant radiotherapy is also utilized. For advanced disease, palliation and supportive care are most important. Investigational treatments are being studied; however, no survival advantage has yet been shown.

Patient Education

Preventive measures listed in the next section should be followed. Patients with signs and symptoms of conditions such as gastroesophageal reflux disease should be treated appropriately.

Prevention

Decreased dietary intake of salted, cured, and smoked meats should be encouraged. A diet rich in vitamins A and C, fruits, and raw vegetables, and high in fiber should be advocated. Symptomatic patients should be screened for *H. pylori* infection and treated as appropriate. Smoking cessation should be encouraged for all age groups.

There appears to be a slightly increased incidence of gastric cancer in people with pernicious anemia; therefore, these patients should be followed closely.

Screening Recommendations

No effective screening methods exist for gastric cancer. A simple noninvasive test for *H. pylori* infection, the CLO-test, should be incorporated into patient examinations on a regular basis in primary care settings. If test results are positive, the patient should be treated with the most appropriate combination of bismuth or acid reducer and antibiotics for complete eradication of the bacteria.

▬ HEPATOCELLULAR CARCINOMA

Pathophysiology

One of the most common and most malignant tumors in the world's male population is hepatocellular cancer.[3] Hepatocellular cancer (HCC) essentially consists of three types, nodular, diffuse, and massive, and several histologic subtypes.[3] Risk factors include hepatitis B and C infection, alcohol-induced cirrhosis, aflatoxin exposure, ingestion of contaminated food, and use of anabolic steroids and immunosuppressive agents.[6] In the U.S., 60–80% of HCC patients have underlying cirrhosis associated either with hepatitis or with alcohol.[2]

Pediatric Issues

Hepatocellular cancer does not occur in the pediatric population.

Obstetrical Issues

Management is not significantly affected.

Geriatric Issues

Management is not significantly affected.

Epidemiology

In the U.S. in 2000, the ACS estimates 15,300 liver and intrahepatic bile duct cancers will be diagnosed, and 13,800 deaths from these malignancies will occur.[5] Only about a third of these are HCCs. HCC is relatively rare in the U.S.; however, it comprises almost 50% of all diagnosed tumors in the Far East and sub-Saharan Africa.[2]

Treatment Options

Eighty-five to ninety percent of HCC patients have disease so advanced at diagnosis that it is considered unresectable.[4] Surgery is the only form of treatment that offers potential for cure.[3] Several contraindications may exist that can preclude surgical resection. These include imminent clinical hepatic failure, ascites, renal insufficiency, hypoglycemia, elevated prothrombin time, and metastatic disease. Resection in the presence of cirrhosis often has increased morbidity. The noncirrhotic patient who has undergone surgery usually lives longer.[3] Liver transplantation is another option, especially for patients with cirrhosis.[6] Tumor recurrence is lower with transplant than with surgical treatment in all patients except for those with advanced-stage disease.[3] Radiation is often used for local disease. Arterial embolization is finding more favor as a form of treatment since the disease is often unresectable at diagnosis, or for patients who are not surgical candidates for other reasons, or if transplantation is not an option.

Chemotherapy is sometimes incorporated; however, no significant survival advantage has been demonstrated with current therapies, either single agent or in combination.[3]

Patient Education

Risks of anabolic steroids should be emphasized to teenagers (see the discussion of anabolic steroid use in Chapter 26, Substance Abuse). Significant hepatotoxicity can occur in the absence of symptoms.[9] Hepatitis infections should be treated as soon as possible when identified. Patients should be aware of the associated dismal prognosis of hepatocellular carcinoma.

Prevention

One method of prevention involves increasing immunizations for hepatitis B and reducing the incidence of cirrhosis. Preventing the ingestion of aflatoxins in Third World countries is difficult because of poor sanitation, lack of refrigeration, and other food storage problems. Alcohol consumption should be decreased overall to help reduce rates of cirrhosis.

Screening Recommendations

Alpha-fetoprotein (AFP) is produced by 85% of all HCCs. This test can be used as a screening tool. Hepatitis panels, liver function tests, and coagulation studies are often abnormal in HCC; however, they can often be abnormal for other, more common reasons, such as drug ingestion, alcoholism, malnutrition, and medical therapy. High-risk populations, defined as those who have chronic active hepatitis B, who are hepatitis B surface antigen (HBsAg) carriers, or who have cirrhosis should be screened with AFP every 4 months. This screening should ideally be combined with annual liver ultrasonography.[3] However, these screening recommendations are probably not cost-effective and are unavailable in Third World countries.

LUNG CANCER

Pathophysiology

There is no curative therapy for advanced lung cancer, which is the stage at which most lung cancers are diagnosed. This statement is essentially true for all histologic types of lung cancer (small cell, squamous cell, adenocarcinoma, and large cell). Tobacco smoke is the leading cause of lung cancer, but other factors that increase risk include exposure to asbestos, air pollution, benzene, radon, and radio-active dust.[2, 3] Occupational factors may be difficult to avoid; however, it is possible to avoid exposure to tobacco smoke.

Pediatric Issues

Lung cancer does not occur in the pediatric population.

Obstetric Issues

Management is not significantly affected.

Geriatric Issues

Advanced age and increased exposure to tobacco smoke increase the risk of lung cancer. Baseline cardiopulmonary performance status is an important factor in determining optimal management and treat-ment of a patient with lung cancer. Age alone may limit surgical resectability, possibly compromising treatment options in the geriatric population. Cardiovascular and pulmonary damage from long-term exposure to tobacco smoking also may limit treatment options, especially surgery.

Epidemiology

Lung cancer is the leading cause of cancer death in all adults in the U.S. In 2000, the ACS estimates 164,100 new lung cancer cases and 156,900 lung cancer related deaths will occur. Yet the cause of approximately 85% of lung cancer cases is well known—smoking tobacco.[1] Only about 10% of smokers develop lung cancer during their lifetime; however, other malignancies are also associated with tobacco smoking. The peak incidence of lung cancer diagnosis occurs between the ages of 50 and 75 years, with the mean age at diagnosis at 65 years.[1] Exposure to carcinogens may have occurred several years prior to diagnosis or onset of symptoms, as is usually the case with asbestos, owing to the long latency period. Cessation of tobacco use reduces the risk of cancer, and the longer a person is tobacco-free, the greater his or her risk reduction.

Treatment Options

Surgical resection, usually lobectomy, may be curative if the lung cancer is diagnosed at a very early stage. Only 25% of patients have disease limited enough at diagnosis to even consider complete surgical resection.[1] Often the cardiopulmonary status of long-term smokers prevents this modality of treatment, as the risks of surgery might possibly be greater than the benefit from the procedure.[1]

Radiotherapy must be aggressive and is often limited by toxicity to surrounding tissues. Chemotherapy is usually reserved for those with advanced disease, especially small cell lung cancer. Some new regimens are evolving, but results are still rather dismal. Combined modality regimens are currently the focus of research. Palliative and supportive care are very important in this group of patients, especially when widely metastatic disease is present, if disease progresses in spite of treatment, or if more chemotherapy would be too toxic to major organ systems.[1] At this point, risks of further conventional treatments may provide absolutely no benefit, and hospice care, investigational treatments, or comfort care measures should be considered.

Patient Education

The risks of tobacco smoking should be reinforced to all patients, especially adolescents. Smoking cessation clinics should be widely available. Occupational precautions should be strictly enforced, and employees should be educated on the risks of violating precautionary measures. (See the discussion of nicotine additiction in Chapter 26, Substance Abuse.)

Prevention

Smoking prevention/cessation and the reduction of exposure of everyone to tobacco smoke are the bases for improving outcome of lung cancer treatments. The primary goal is to prevent lung cancer. Occupational risks should be minimized for asbestos workers (and those who remove asbestos from buildings). Chemoprevention trials with retinoids and separately with beta carotene have apparently demonstrated no positive effect on the recurrence of lung cancers. However, studies are continuing, and other agents are currently being investigated.

Screening Recommendations

No cost-effective methods for lung cancer screening exist at the present time. The chest x-ray might possibly be used as a screening tool; however, considerable debate remains as to whether this is a cost-effective and sufficiently sensitive test to diagnose lung tumors at an earlier stage and thus further the goal of improving treatment outcomes. Screening with serial chest x-rays has proved to be costly and to have a low yield in early diagnosis.[1] The chest x-ray should be used to determine whether further workup is necessary. Any abnormality on the chest x-ray of a smoker should be closely followed and investigated expeditiously.

▄▄▄PANCREATIC CANCER

Pathophysiology

Smoking, high-fat diets, and eating meat appear to carry increased risk of pancreatic cancer. Incidence is twice as high in heavy smokers than in nonsmokers.[1] An inverse association has been found with consumption of a diet high in fiber, fruits, and vegetables.[4] Although several prospective studies have shown up to a fourfold increased risk in diabetic patients, no study has truly shown an association. There appears to be an increased risk in patients with chronic pancreatitis and cirrhosis. No definite etiology has been confirmed.

Pediatric Issues

Pancreatic cancer in the pediatric population is exceedingly rare and nonpreventable.

Obstetric Issues

Management is not significantly affected.

Geriatric Issues

Risk increases with increasing age.

Epidemiology

The ACS has estimated that 28,300 new cases of pancreatic cancer and 28,200 deaths will occur in the U.S. in 2000.[5] The rates in men have declined since 1980 and increased in women.

Treatment Options

Usual treatment is surgical resection (Whipple procedure or pancreatic duodenectomy) followed by chemotherapy (fluorouracil or gemcitabine) and radiotherapy. For unresectable tumors, combination chemo- and radiotherapy offers palliation from pain and may provide a survival advantage. Regardless of treatment, outcome is dismal.

Patient Education

The risks of smoking and alcohol abuse should be addressed with all patients. The fact that many cancers are already in the advanced stages at the time of diagnosis should forewarn the patient that behavior changes need to occur sooner rather than later.

Prevention

Smoking cessation should be encouraged in all age groups. A diet high in fiber, fruits, and vegetables might help; however, there are no proven preventive factors for pancreatic cancer.

Screening Recommendations

Currently there are no screening recommendations.

■ PROSTATE CANCER

Pathophysiology

The incidence of prostate cancer increases with age, especially with each decade of life after age 50. The cause is unknown, but environmental influences are important in prostate cancer. High-fat diets may increase androgen bioavailability, which may stimulate the prostate cancer.[1] Other risk factors are age, race, and family history of prostate cancer. All of these factors are nonmodifiable, so prevention efforts must focus on secondary means of prevention, screening, and early detection.

Age is the most important risk factor, with 70% of men over the age of 80 estimated to have some histologic evidence of prostate cancer.[2] Genetic predisposition has been proposed and may be responsible for 5–10% of all prostate cancers.[6] A Mendelian inheritance pattern has been postulated, with a higher risk if prostate cancer has been diagnosed in a first-degree relative.[1, 2]

Pediatric Issues

This disease does not occur in the pediatric population.

Obstetric Issues

(Not applicable.)

Geriatric Issues

More than 75% of all prostate cancers are diagnosed in men older than 65 years. It is very important to screen these men regularly and encourage them to see a urologist if they have any new or changing symptoms such as urinary frequency, retention, hesitancy, dysuria, or weak flow.

Epidemiology

The ACS estimates that 180,400 new cases and 31,900 deaths from prostate cancer will occur in 2000.[6] Median age at diagnosis is 66 years.[2] Mortality rates for prostate cancer have declined slightly since 1991.[5]

Treatment Options

Staging is very important; prostate cancer can be a slow-growing malignancy, so if the disease is confined to the organ, it may not have an impact on survival until 10–15 years after the original diagnosis (without treatment).[2]

What constitutes the best treatment method is a matter of controversy, and the patient's expected life span must be considered. Available options include observation, surgery, hormone therapy, radiotherapy, cryosurgery and chemotherapy.

Patient Education

It is important to educate the patient with regard to prostate-specific antigen (PSA). All elevated PSA levels do not indicate prostate cancer. Educate the patient and his family that he can live with prostate cancer. The prostate cancer may not affect his life span. Sexual function is a major concern of most men diagnosed with prostate cancer. Potency can be preserved, and most men over the age of 50 recover potency postoperatively. Advanced clinical stage is directly correlated with decreased potency.[4] Patients should be sent to a counselor or therapist specializing in sexual function related to prostate cancer diagnosis and treatments.

Prevention

The most important risk factors are nonmodifiable; therefore, early detection is important.

Screening Recommendations

Digital rectal examination (DRE) should be performed annually in all men over the age of 50.

Use of the PSA test is a complicated matter, as the PSA can be elevated by a number of conditions, including prostatitis, benign prostatic hypertrophy, and prostate massage. Men age 50 and older who have at least a 10-year life expectancy should have a DRE and PSA test annually.[5] Men at higher risk should consider annual testing at an earlier age.[5]

SKIN CANCER

Pathophysiology

The interaction between genetic and environmental factors is very important in the development of skin cancer. Skin cancers occur most frequently at low latitudes, in outdoor workers, on sun-exposed skin areas, and in light-skinned individuals with blond or red hair who tend to burn rather than tan.[1] Melanomas develop by malignant transformation of the melanocyte.[2] Non-melanoma skin cancers include squamous cell and basal cell carcinomas. Over 90% of squamous cell carcinomas of the skin in U.S. patients contain mutations to the p53 suppressor gene. Sunlight is directly implicated in the development of squamous cell carcinomas and melanoma.

Pediatric Issues

A long history of sun exposure puts anyone at an increased risk for a skin cancer. To prevent any and all skin cancers, children should avoid sunlight during the hours of 10 AM and 4 PM and wear sunscreen with at least a sun protection factor (SPF) of 15 during all outdoor exposure. Protective clothing should be considered beginning in infancy. The liberal use of sunscreen is always preferred to no sunscreen, but totally avoiding sun exposure is the best prevention.

Obstetric Issues

Management is not significantly affected.

Geriatric Issues

Older persons tend to have more sun-damaged skin and to have a higher rate of non-melanoma cancers than younger people. With the aging of the population, the incidence of skin cancers and melanoma will continue to increase. Sunscreen, protective clothing, and avoidance of sun exposure remain important prevention strategies in this (and all) age groups.

Epidemiology

More than 1.2 million new cases of non-melanoma skin cancer are estimated to be diagnosed in 2000.[5] The ACS estimates 47,700 new melanoma cases and 9200 deaths in 2000.[5] The incidence of skin cancer is increasing at a faster rate than that of any other cancer in the U.S.

Treatment Options

Over 90% of non-melanoma skin cancers are curable by local excision if diagnosed at an early stage. Several basic methods are used to treat non-melanoma skin cancers. Surgery is used successfully in 90% of all cases. Other treatments include radiation therapy, electrodesiccation, cryosurgery, laser therapy, and topical chemotherapy with fluorouracil (5-FU).

Melanoma treatment is more complicated. Local surgical excision is used for early-stage cancers; regional lymph node dissection is recommended for later-stage disease. Radiotherapy is effective primarily as palliative therapy (tumor shrinkage rather than eradication).[3] Chemotherapy results have been disappointing thus far in metastatic disease.

Immunotherapy results (alpha interferon and interleukin-2) are encouraging. Monoclonal antibody therapy, vaccines, and gene therapy are all currently being developed and hold some promise for this devastating neoplastic condition.

Patient Education

The proper use of sunscreen and the use of protective clothing are very important. People should be taught the dangers of sun exposure at an early age and also should be taught to avoid outdoor activities and sun exposure during the hours of most intensive sunshine (between 10 AM and 4 PM).[6] Self-examination should be taught at an early age and should be done at least annually, throughout each person's lifetime.

Prevention

The best prevention is to reduce and/or eliminate exposure to sunlight's ultraviolet radiation. All individuals should always use sunscreen and protective clothing when outdoors, especially at low latitudes. Immediate removal of any remotely suspicious lesion is imperative for diagnosis and treatment.

Screening Recommendations

A thorough skin examination by a dermatologist or other experienced health care professional is recommended, especially for fair-haired, light-skinned people who sunburn easily, every 3 years between the ages of 20 and 39 and annually for those over 40. Self-examination should be performed at least annually, observing for any changes in moles, freckles, or other skin lesions. Continued surveillance is imperative in the older population. It should be stressed that early removal of suspicious lesions can be curative, but ignoring the lesion can be extremely detrimental and may be fatal.

▬ TESTICULAR CANCER

Pathophysiology

The cause of testicular cancer is unknown. The condition usually presents with painless testicular swelling or severe testicular pain.[1]

Testicular cancer essentially consists of two types, nonseminomatous and seminomatous germ cell tumors. Seminoma is the most common subtype, representing 35–40% of testicular cancers. Embryonal carcinoma, yolk sac tumors, choriocarcinomas, and teratomas compose the remaining 60% of testicular cancers.[1] Testicular tumors do have serologic markers, but these are not used for routine screening. For seminomas, the level of the beta subunit of human chorionic gonadotropin (β-hCG) is increased, and with nonseminomatous tumors the level of alpha-fetoprotein (AFP) is elevated.[1]

Germ cell tumors are thought to arise from the precursors (totipotential germ cells) of spermatocytes. Abnormal embryologic development of the totipotential germ cells leads to germ cell carcinomas rather than spermatocyte formation.

Pediatric Issues

Cryptorchidism (undescended testis or testes) affects approximately 3% of term and 3% of preterm males. Within 2 months the testes descend in more than half of affected males. At 1 year of age about 80% of the testes have descended. If the testes do not descend after puberty, the incidence of testicular cancer increases.[7] Approximately 8.5% of men diagnosed with testicular cancer have a history of cryptorchidism.[1]

Some childhood seminomas, while rare, are hormone-producing (Leydig's cell, choriocarcinoma, dysgerminoma) and often manifest with sexual precocity. Teratomas of the testes may appear in childhood.[7]

Obstetric Issues

Certain genetic traits are associated with testicular cancer. These include Klinefelter syndrome, Down syndrome, true hermaphroditism, testicular feminization, Mullerian syndrome, and cutaneous ichthyosis.[1] Genetic counseling may be indicated for parents and affected individuals.

Geriatric Issues

Testicular cancer is a relatively rare condition overall (1% of cancers in men), with most cases being diagnosed in men between the ages of 20 and 34. It is exceedingly rare in the geriatric population.

Epidemiology

Testicular cancer is the most common cancer in young men between the ages of 20 and 34.[1] In this population, the incidence is 14/100,000, with an overall incidence of 6/100,000. Incidence among African American men is 0.7/100,000, for unknown reasons.[2] Disease-free 5-year survival ranges from 70% in patients with advanced disease to 92% in those who are diagnosed at an earlier stage.[8] Even patients with advanced disease at diagnosis can have a favorable prognosis with appropriate treatment.

Treatment Options

If a mass is identified via physical examination, testicular ultrasonography should be performed immediately and the patient immediately referred to a urologist. Tumor markers should be drawn to help confirm malignancy and to be used as baseline measurements. If the mass is consistent with testicular cancer, usually a radical inguinal orchiectomy is the surgery of choice, depending on the stage of the disease. Surgery via the scrotal route is contraindicated because of distinct lymphatic drainage of the scrotum and testes and the likelihood of lymphatic spread of tumor or local recurrence. In patients with early disease, retroperitoneal lymphadenectomy may be required if metastases are suspected or identified. Seminomas are radiosensitive, and adjunct radiotherapy may be applied to the areas of lymphatic drainage of the testes.[1]

Patients with intermediate or advanced disease are treated with surgical resection of the tumor and adjunct chemotherapy.

Patient Education

Patients with a history of cryptorchidism or atrophic testes are at increased risk of testicular cancer and should be instructed to perform self-examination and have professional screening. Patients who have a history of mumps orchitis, cancer in the contralateral testicle, inguinal hernia, or hydrocele should be apprised of their increased risk for testicular cancer.[8] The incidence of testicular cancer is also increased in men who have a first-degree relative with testicular cancer.[1]

Cancer survivors should be instructed to have regular follow-ups for serum marker evaluation, diagnostic studies, and physical examination to identify and treat any recurrent disease. Patients with a history of testicular cancer are at an increased risk of cancer in the contralateral testicle. Additionally, any cancer survivor who was initially treated with radiotherapy or chemotherapy is at a significantly increased risk of developing a secondary malignancy.

One very important fact to remember about testicular cancer is that 90% of malignant testicular masses are discovered by the patient himself. For this reason, education explaining the benefits of early detection should begin at adolescence and be positively reinforced throughout a man's lifetime.

Retroperitoneal lymphadenectomy may result in autonomic nerve dysfunction causing dry ejaculation.

Even patients with advanced disease can have a favorable prognosis. Patients should be educated to follow up as instructed for serologic marker evaluation, diagnostic studies, and physical examination to identify and treat recurrent disease. Two to five percent of men will develop cancer in the contralateral testicle during their lifetime, so regular examinations (self or professional) are necessary.

Prevention

Primary prevention includes orchiopexy prior to puberty in children with cryptorchidism. This is usually performed before the child reaches the age of 5 or 6 in an attempt to preserve fertility.[1] Once a tumor is found, aggressive treatment and follow-up are essential to prevent the secondary spread or worsening of disease.

Screening Recommendations

Any testicular mass is malignant until proved otherwise, and thus should be evaluated by a urologist immediately. Self-examination is easily performed and should be done monthly beginning at puberty. Any abnormalities or changes should be addressed by a health care professional without delay.

Any testicular abnormality should be screened for cancer, especially in young adult and adolescent males. The ACS recommends a cancer evaluation including testicular examination every 3 years in men over the age of 20 and an annual examination for those over the age of 40.

There is no evidence to recommend for or against routine screening in otherwise asymptomatic men.[9]

For additional resources, see the Resources Appendix at the end of this book.

REFERENCES

1. Boyer KL, Ford MB, Judkins AF, Levin B. Primary Care Oncology. Philadelphia, WB Saunders, 1999.
2. DeVita VT Jr, Hellman S, Rosenberg SA, eds. Cancer Principles and Practice of Oncology, 5th ed. Philadelphia, Lippincott-Raven, 1997.
3. Pazdur R, Coia LR, Hoskins WJ, Wagman LD, eds. Cancer Management: A Multidisciplinary Approach, Medical, Surgical, and Radiation Oncology. New York, PRR, 1999.
4. Murphy GP, Lawrence W Jr, Lenhard RE Jr, eds. American Cancer Society Textbook of Clinical Oncology, 2nd ed. Atlanta, GA, American Cancer Society, Inc., 1995.
5. American Cancer Society: Cancer Facts and Figures 2000. Atlanta, GA, American Cancer Society, Inc., 2000.
6. Beers MH, Berkow R, eds. The Merck Manual of Diagnosis and Treatment, 17th ed. White House Station, NJ, 1999.
7. Hay WW Jr, Groothius JR, Hayward AR, Levin MJ, eds. Current Pediatric Diagnosis and Treatment, 13th ed. Stamford, CT, Appleton & Lange, 1997.
8. Fuentes RJ, Rosenberg JM, eds. Athletic Drug Reference '99. Glaxo Wellcome, Inc., 1999.
9. Report of the U.S. Preventive Services Task Force. Guide to Clinical Preventive Services, 2nd ed. Baltimore, Williams & Wilkins, 1996.

RESOURCES

American Cancer Society
   Web site: www.cancer.org
   Telephone 1–800–ACS–2345

The University of Texas M. D. Anderson Cancer Center web site: www.mdanderson.org

The University of Texas M. D. Anderson Cancer Center Cancer Prevention clinic telephone number: 713–745–8040

CHAPTER 25

Neurologic Disease

Mark I. Harris, MD,
James B. Labus, BS, PA-C,
Heidi R. Meyer, MSN, C-FNP, CNRN,
and Amy J. Cofer, PA-C, MMSc

INTRODUCTION

The brain is the only entity in the universe that seeks to understand its own function. It is the brain rather than the heart that is the origin of emotion, personality, and behavior. Anatomy and neurochemistry may be tested by science, but the function of human emotion may never be known. Neurologic conditions are some of the most diverse disorders known. Neurologic disorders have an impact on essentially every other bodily system. These disorders influence endocrine (pituitary), musculoskeletal (e.g., radiculopathy, myelopathy, peripheral neuropathy), psychiatric (mood regulation and thought), cardiorespiratory, and gastrointestinal (autonomic nervous system) function.

The nerves of the central nervous system cannot be regenerated once destroyed, but the brain may be "retrained" to develop alternative nervous pathways that can allow for recovery of some function. Peripheral nerves have some ability to regenerate, albeit slowly (approximately 1 mm per month). Some neurologic conditions lend themselves somewhat to primary prevention with ischemic stroke being the most notable example. Other conditions are primarily degenerative (e.g., Parkinson's disease, multiple sclerosis), and require significant secondary preventive efforts to maintain or improve function and activities of daily living and prevent complications. Other conditions such as migraine can be prevented and/or aborted with medications and nonpharmacologic measures. Some conditions require additional education efforts aside from medical management to prevent injury (e.g., seizure causing motor vehicle accident). Due to the chronic nature of some disorders, patient education is paramount in helping the patient and family understand and accept the condition. The patient who is aware of the eventual changes can prepare both mentally and physically.

LOW BACK PAIN AND RADICULOPATHY

Pathophysiology

Low back pain (LBP) is a common malady affecting adults. Symptoms are usually transient, but occasionally the pain persists. In some cases, low back pain is accompanied by radiating lower extremity pain due to irritation or compression of the nerve root (radiculopathy). The pathogenesis of nonradicular back pain is poorly understood. Paraspinous muscles may be injured leading to facet joint strain. Disruption of the intervertebral disc may lead to pain due to irritation of the nerve fibers contained in the anulus fibrosus. Emotional factors can lead to vasoconstriction of the muscle vasculature, and pain may result after otherwise minor trauma. Subsequent muscle spasm can result in a cascade of muscle weakening of the involved muscles and reciprocal muscles. Compensation for the weakening results in restricted and painful spinal movement.[1]

The spine undergoes degenerative change that can be worsened by poor posture, incorrect body mechanics, inadequate physical fitness, and trauma. The degeneration (degenerative disc disease or osteophyte formation) can narrow the foramen through which the nerve root exits the spine.

Radicular pain is usually due to compression or irritation of a nerve root by a herniated disc or osteophyte as it exits the spinal canal via the foramen. The intervertebral disc is adjacent to the foramina and rupture of the disc can compress the nerve root. Disc herniations occur due to trauma, lifting, twisting, or other significant Valsalva maneuvers. Foraminal stenosis can cause direct compression or irritation of the nerve following trauma.

Nerve root compression can occur in the cervical, thoracic, and lumbar areas. Cervical root compression is frequently due to trauma or disc degeneration (most common in the C4–C5, C5–C6, and C6–C7 levels).

Thoracic root compression is uncommon due to the relatively rigid structure of the rib cage but can occur following trauma.

In the lumbar spine, the most common levels of nerve root compression are L4–L5, L5–S1, followed by L3–L4 due to the weight-bearing load that affects the lower lumbar spine.

Pediatric Issues

This condition is uncommon in children. Conservative treatment is the mainstay of therapy, and surgery is reserved for only severe cases with impending neurologic damage. Juvenile disc herniations are probably due to genetic factors.[2]

Obstetric Issues

Women frequently complain of low back pain and radicular symptoms in the later stages of pregnancy. This is due to the increased anterior and axial load on the lumbar spine. Symptoms frequently resolve after delivery. An exercise program should begin postpartum to prevent recurrent symptoms.

Geriatric Issues

There is an increased risk of herniated disc until the age of 45. After this age, radicular pain is more frequently due to spinal stenosis and osteophytic compression of the nerve root. Autopsy studies have revealed that almost 100% of people have disc ruptures by age 64 with a similar occurrence of osteophyte formation, facet joint osteoarthritis, and end-plate changes.[1, 3]

Epidemiology

Low back pain is the second most common reason for missed work. Forty to seventy percent of adults have a positive history of transient LBP with 14% reporting LBP of >2 weeks' duration. One percent of adults report a history of radicular symptoms.[2]

Treatment Options

Although the pain of radiculopathy can be excruciating, conservative treatment should be attempted in virtually all cases. The exception is with cauda equina syndrome or with cervical or thoracic spinal cord compromise (myelopathy).

Conservative therapy has traditionally consisted of bed rest, nonsteroidal anti-inflammatory drugs (NSAIDs), muscle relaxants, and/or analgesia. Bed rest may be less productive than sending the patient back to normal activities, provided the patient has a normal physical examination. Patients who are allowed limited or no bed rest return to work more quickly than those who are prescribed longer periods of bed rest.[4, 5] There have been some positive results with allowing the patient to continue with normal activities while avoiding aggravating factors such as bending, twisting, or lifting. Physical therapy is beneficial once the acute episode has resolved. The patient can improve paraspinous and abdominal strength and is taught appropriate lifting and back care techniques.

If radicular pain is present and the patient has failed initial conservative therapy, then epidural steroids may be considered to reduce nerve root inflammation. If the compression is minor or transient, then the pain may resolve and no additional treatment is required.

If significant compression by a herniated disc, fragment, or osteophyte is identified, and symptoms fail to resolve after conservative therapy, then surgical intervention may be required. Surgical techniques vary depending on the situation encountered. Removing the offending disc fragment or osteophyte may be all that is required. In some cases, when there is impaired mechanical function of the spine, fusion may be indicated.

A gradual return to normal activities is generally recommended. Ergonomic evaluation of the patient's job may be beneficial and changes are made to the extent possible.

Patient Education

Patients should be informed about the importance of attempting conservative therapy in the acute stage. Surgery, when indicated, is usually beneficial and safe. Patients frequently are informed by friends and coworkers only of back surgery "failures."

Lumbar degeneration is akin to developing gray hair and wrinkles. All individuals have some changes; it is the extent of change and impact on lifestyle that make a difference.

Patients frequently inquire about chiropractic care. This can be a viable conservative option provided there is communication between the chiropractic office and the medical office. Working as a team for the benefit of the patient is the best alternative.

Prevention

Risk factors for the development of low back pain include incorrect posture, poor body mechanics, reduction of soft tissue flexibility, poor physical fitness, and trauma.[1]

Sitting increases intradiscal pressures by more than 35% compared to standing. This may be due to posture with hips rotated forward and reduction in the lumbar spine lordosis. This pressure is reduced with the use of a back rest.[1]

The least amount of long-term degenerative changes are seen in patients who have maintained mixed activity of sitting, standing, and walking without heavy duties. Those individuals whose occupation requires heavy lifting experience the most degenerative change and increased risk of disc rupture.

Primary prevention consists of maintaining proper alignment and posture during lifting.

Formal back schools can teach an individual proper body mechanics and can customize the instruction to his or her specific job setting.

Screening Recommendations

Clinicians should make available to all patients information regarding proper back mechanics before an injury occurs. This is especially true of patients whose occupation requires frequent bending, twisting, or lifting.

DEMENTIA

Pathophysiology

Dementia may be defined as significant cognitive impairment that negatively impacts normal activities and function. The primary characteristic is a memory deficit combined with aphasia, agnosia, or disturbance of executive function.[6] Patients usually exhibit memory deficits and word finding difficulty early in the course of the disease. This is later followed by difficulty in organizing, sequencing, or planning more complex tasks; inappropriate judgment; and problems thinking in the abstract.

There are several etiologies of dementia, the most common of which is the Alzheimer's type. The diagnostic criteria for Alzheimer's dementia are listed in Box 25–1. Late in the disease, Alzheimer's patients display sundowning (increased confusion and agitation during the evening hours) and often have difficulty sleeping. Personality changes, irritability, agitation, psychotic symptoms, incontinence, gait dysfunction, and eventual progression to a bedridden state are part of the progressive symptoms. Average lifespan is 8–10 years after diagnosis.

Dementia is often noticed by a family member before the patient notices any deficit. Neuroimaging reveals either generalized or localized cerebral cortical atrophy and rules out structural pathology. Pathologic examination of Alzheimer's patients reveals neuronal loss, extracellular neuritic (senile) plaques, and intracellular neurofibrillary tangles. Pathologic diagnosis and clinical diagnosis concur 70–90% of the time.[6] The neuronal and resultant synapse loss is most pronounced in the hippocampus (memory) and adjacent structures.[7, 8] Cholinergic neurons are primarily affected.[8] The loss of functional synapse is directly correlated with disease severity.[7] Neuritic plaques and neurofibrillary tangles are widely distributed in the cerebral cortex.[6, 7] Neuritic plaques contain a core of amyloid, a protein fragment of amyloid precursor protein encoded by a gene on chromosome 21.[8] This is responsible for some cases of genetic Alzheimer's, but plaques can also be found in nondemented patients and most Alzheimer's is nonfamilial.[8] Therefore, neuropathologic criteria involve an adequate number of neuritic plaques within a patient of specific age range who has clinical features of dementia.[7] The amyloid protein can be measured in cerebrospinal fluid, although it should *not* be relied on for diagnosis. Neurofibrillary tangles are composed of helical filaments and can occur with other neurodegenerative processes as well as Alzheimer's.[7, 8]

Recently, the type 4 allele of apolipoprotein E (ApoE), a lipid transport protein on chromosome 19, has been identified as an independent risk factor for familial and sporadic Alzheimer's disease. A

---

*Box 25-1—*DIAGNOSTIC CRITERIA FOR DEMENTIA OF THE ALZHEIMER'S TYPE

The development of multiple cognitive deficits manifested by both memory impairment (impaired ability to learn new information or to recall previously learned information) and one (or more) of the following cognitive disturbances:
- Aphasia (language disturbance)
- Apraxia (impaired ability to carry out motor activities despite intact motor function)
- Agnosia (failure to recognize or identify objects despite intact sensory function)
- Disturbance in executive functioning (i.e., planning, organizing, sequencing, abstracting)

The cognitive deficits each cause significant impairment in social or occupational functioning and represent a significant decline from a previous level of functioning.

The course is characterized by a gradual onset and continuing cognitive decline.

The cognitive deficits are not due to any of the following:
- Other central nervous system conditions that cause progressive deficits in memory and cognition (e.g., cerebrovascular disease, Parkinson's disease, Huntington's disease, subdural hematoma, normal-pressure hydrocephalus, brain tumor)
- Systemic conditions that are known to cause dementia (e.g., hypothyroidism, vitamin B_{12} deficiency, niacin deficiency, hypercalcemia, neurosyphilis, HIV infection)
- Substance abuse–related conditions

The deficits do not occur exclusively during the course of delirium.

The disturbance is not better accounted for by another Axis I disorder (e.g., major depressive disorder, schizophrenia).

Reprinted with permission from the Diagnostic and Statistical Manual of Mental Disorders, Fourth Edition. Copyright 1994 American Psychiatric Association.

---

decreased age at onset has been associated with the ApoE allele.[6–9] Apolipoprotien E has been identified in neuritic plaques, amyloid, and neurofibrillary tangles, and it may promote amyloid filament formation.[7] Two copies of this allele have been found in cognitively normal individuals; therefore, the exact correlation is not yet understood. Testing for ApoE may be used to identify at-risk individuals, but should *not* be used for diagnosis or routine screening.[6, 9] In those with mild cognitive impairment, ApoE may be used to identify those at risk for progressing to Alzheimer's.[9] There is limited evidence that immunologic activation and free radical formation from metabolism may play a role in the degenerative process that leads to Alzheimer's.

Levels of acetylcholine, norepinephrine, serotonin, and other neurotransmitters are decreased in patients with Alzheimer's dementia. Reductions in acetylcholine and choline acetyltransferase are the most pronounced, and may justify treatment with cholinergic-enhancing drugs.[7]

Vascular dementia (multi-infarct dementia) occurs as the result of repeated ischemic insults on the brain. The decline in cognitive function is stepwise with each ischemic event. These events may be accompanied by focal neurologic deficits, positive history, and documented on cerebral imaging studies. Vascular and Alzheimer's dementia may coexist.

Approximately 20–60% of patients diagnosed with Parkinson's disease develop dementia.[6] Pathologically the dementia is due to either Lewy body inclusion or Alzheimer's changes.[7a] Lewy body disease has only recently been described and may account for a significant portion of dementia cases. Pathologically it is characterized by degeneration in the substantia nigra that leads to a reduction in dopamine production and symptoms of Parkinson's disease. There is also degeneration in the cortical regions of the brain causing symptoms similar to Alzheimer's disease. Surviving nerve cells contain abnormal structures called Lewy bodies, which are a pathologic hallmark. Shrinkage of the brain is particularly seen in the temporal lobe, parietal lobe, and the cingulate gyrus. Other behavioral changes include fluctuation in severity of the condition, and early development of visual hallucinations.[7b]

Other less common dementias include Pick's disease, Huntington's disease, and Cruetzfeldt-Jakob disease. Pick's disease primarily affects the frontal lobes and presents with personality, language, and social skill diminution early in its course. Huntington's disease is an autosomal dominant condition presenting with motor, behavioral, and cognitive symptoms. Cruetzfeldt-Jakob disease is due to slow virus infection and is rapidly progressive.

Pediatric Issues

Management is not significantly affected by age.

Obstetric Issues

Management is not significantly affected.

Geriatric Issues

Dementia is a disorder of the geriatric population.

Epidemiology

Dementia is an age-associated disease with a prevalence of approximately 3–11% at age 65. By age 85, 20–50% of individuals are affected.[6, 7, 9] Alzheimer's is responsible for 50–75% of dementias, and vascular dementia accounts for 5–20%.[8, 9]

There is a 12–17% average lifetime risk of developing Alzheimer's disease.[7]

From 21–72% of patients with dementia are not diagnosed, especially early in the course of the disease.[9]

The lifetime risk is 9% in patients with no family history and no ApoE 4 allele, increases to a 29% risk in patients with one ApoE 4 allele, and rises to 83% in patients with both alleles.[7]

Other Alzheimer's risk factors include advancing age, Down syndrome, and positive family history.[6, 7] Less definite and more controversial risk factors include head trauma, depression, personality disorder, and lower educational achievement.[9]

Treatment Options

The patient presenting with symptoms of dementia should be fully evaluated for reversible causes, as 10–20% of patients have a potentially treatable condition.[9] A comprehensive workup includes a full chemistry profile, complete blood count, VDRL, HIV testing, thyroid function tests, cerebral imaging (MRI), carotid vascular evaluation, vitamin B_{12} and folate, cerebrospinal fluid (CSF) analysis, and drug level/toxicology screen. Urine evaluation for heavy metals can be performed in select groups.[9] Psychiatric evaluation can identify underlying depression that is masked as dementia. Formal cognitive evaluation can be performed if the diagnosis is not clear. This is especially helpful in cases in which certain tasks and privileges must be withdrawn for reasons of safety (e.g., driving, career).[9]

Initial management is aimed at improving and maintaining function. Memory aids and labeling may be used if the patient is in familiar or supervised settings.

Pharmacologic treatment can be provided if the benefits outweigh the risks. Reductions in certain medications may improve mental status. There are no medications known to delay the eventual progression of dementia. Patients should wear a Medic alert bracelet. It should be mentioned that improvement in function or cognition actually means the absence of worsening. Untreated patients continue to worsen, while treated patients may maintain their baseline function with a small percentage exhibiting increased function.

Cholinesterase inhibitors include tacrine, donepezil, and rivastigmine. Useful in mild to moderate disease, they are felt to work by increasing the availability of intrasynaptic acetylcholine. Benefits are to improve or temporarily halt functional or cognitive decline.[6]

Vitamin E is thought to be beneficial due to its antioxidant properties. There appears to be no evidence of improvement with therapy, but functional decline may be postponed. Cognitive decline appears to be unaffected.[6]

Selegiline is a Parkinson's medication that affects catecholamine metabolism. Selegiline may delay poor outcome and improve cognition.[6]

Ergoloid mesylates may affect behavior in Alzheimer's, but has better evidence for efficacy on vascular dementias.[6]

NSAIDs, estrogen replacement therapy, melatonin, and ginko biloba may have some positive effect on dementia but require more definitive study. Chelating agents are quite toxic and are used for treatment of heavy metal exposure. Routine use is not recommended.[6]

Patient Education

Alzheimer's disease is a clinical diagnosis. It is only on postmortem examination that the definitive diagnosis can be made.

An important concern among patients and family members is the risk of developing Alzheimer's disease. Elderly patients who encounter memory problems or relatives of those affected by Alzheimer's may inquire as to the possibility of developing Alzheimer's.

Predicting those who will eventually develop the disorder is currently under study. The combination of a clinical dementia rating and functional questions shows promise in predicting eventual progression to Alzheimer's.[10]

Another classification has been developed termed "mild cognitive impairment." These patients do not meet the diagnostic criteria for Alzheimer's, but do exhibit memory deficits. These patients tend to progress to Alzheimer's at a greater rate than normal subjects, but do not have as rapid a functional decline as those with mild Alzheimer's.[11]

The importance of early identification is to begin pharmacologic treatment at an early stage and to define the boundaries between normal aging and pathologic decline in mental function.[10] The clinician should educate and assist with these discussions so the patient does not abandon hope. Patients and families can also plan for potential decline in function in a proactive fashion and discuss end-of-life issues with the affected family member.

The ApoE 4 allele is a risk factor, but the presence does not guarantee Alzheimer's progression and should not be used for diagnosis or screening.

Once the patient is diagnosed with dementia, the target of education becomes the family and/or caregivers. In the initial stages, a structured environment and routine are important with frequent checks by the family generally all that is necessary. As the disease progresses, full-time supervision is required. The family may be willing to supervise the patient or hire a full-time caregiver while the patient remains at home. If this is not a viable option, a skilled nursing facility (nursing home) may be the best option. The provider may assist the family with the choice of a facility and/or follow the patient in the facility. Referral to a caring medical director who is versed in geriatric care is an option for those practitioners who do not routinely visit nursing homes.

An important goal is to get the family to accept the inevitability of mental and physical decline. The patient should be kept comfortable with chronic and mild illnesses treated. Frequently, even more advanced medical care can be provided in the facility. Pharmacologic intervention may be required to control agitation and anxiety. However, as the patient may be unable to communicate effectively, medical conditions that cause agitation and anxiety (e.g., hypoxia) need to be ruled out.

Life-prolonging measures such as intubation, gastric tube, and full code status should be discussed with the family prior to the inevitable decline in status. In this way, the family can discuss among themselves a reasonable plan of care and choose one that all family members will support. Waiting until the patient is in cardiac or respiratory arrest will require a hasty and sometimes unreasonable request for care by the family. It should be brought to the family's attention that even treatment and cure of severe illness will not improve the patient's mental state and the best that can be accomplished is to return the patient to the premorbid state. Recent public education efforts have allowed patients to discuss end-of-life issues with their families before nursing home placement. This alleviates much of the dissonance within the family and makes the provider's job easier.

Prevention

There is no way to primarily prevent dementia. Neuroimaging in the appropriate-age population may demonstrate atrophy, but may not correlate with the severity of symptoms.

Secondary prevention involves maintaining safety for the patient and preventing injury. Items such as meal delivery versus cooking, assistance to administer medications, and removing the car and keys from the premises all prevent secondary injury. Finances should be managed by someone agreed to by the family. Medications may be required for agitation. Other medications should be routinely reviewed to assess for continued efficacy, necessity, and potential side effects.

Screening Recommendations

It is recommended that clinicians observe for signs of declining cognitive function in the elderly. Early recognition of mild cognitive impairment or dementia can allow for early intervention. Other conditions that may present with declining mental status should be investigated before a diagnosis of dementia is made. Cultural, language, and educational differences may artificially raise or lower mental status evaluation results.[12]

Amyloid protein that forms the core of neuritic plaques is secreted in varying amounts in demented and nondemented individuals, and may be measured in plasma or CSF; it should not be used as a screening tool. The ApoE 4 increases risk of progression to Alzheimer's but is not recommended as a screening tool.

MIGRAINE HEADACHES

Pathophysiology

Migraine is a distinct diagnostic headache type. Other common headache types include cluster, episodic tension type, and chronic tension type.

The diagnostic criteria for migraine headache according to the International Headache Society (IHS) are shown in Box 25–2.

Box 25-2–DIAGNOSTIC CRITERIA FOR MIGRAINE HEADACHE

Migraine Without Aura
A. At least five attacks fulfilling Criteria B through D
B. Headache lasting 4–72 hours
C. At least two of the following characteristics:
  1. Unilateral location
  2. Pulsating quality
  3. Moderate to severe intensity
  4. Aggravated by routine activities such as walking upstairs.
D. During the headache at least one of the following apply:
  1. Nausea or vomiting
  2. Photo/phonophobia
Migraine With Aura
A. At least two attacks fulfilling the following:
B. At least three of the following four characteristics:
  1. One or more fully reversible aura symptoms
  2. At least one aura symptom over more than 4 min or two or more symptoms occurring in succession
  3. No single aura symptom lasts more than 60 min
  4. Headache follows aura with a free interval of less than 60 min (headache may begin before or simultaneously with the aura)

From International Headache Society Classification, www.I-H-S.org, with permission.

For both migraine with aura and migraine without aura, the history, physical examination, and appropriate investigations must adequately exclude secondary disorders. If a secondary condition coexists, the migraine is considered primary only if the original migraine onset did not occur in close temporal relation with the other disorder.[7]

Most migraineurs have a positive family history of migraine. Clinically, the migraine can be divided into four phases: prodrome, aura, headache, and postdrome. The prodrome may occur several hours or days before the headache, and includes symptoms such as depression, irritability, euphoria, dysphasia, stiff neck, anorexia, diarrhea, or constipation. Approximately 60% of patients have a prodrome.

Aura consists of focal neurologic symptoms such as visual, auditory, olfactory, sensory, or motor phenomena. Visual aura is the most common aura. Auras may spread over the entire visual field and include flashing lights, shapes, or hemianopsia.

The headache itself is throbbing and usually unilateral. Pain is moderate to severe and is often accompanied by nausea and vomiting, photophobia, and phonophobia. Headache may last up to 3–4 days, but average length is 48 h.

During the postdrome phase, the patient experiences fatigue, irritability, problems concentrating, scalp tenderness, or depression.

There are many subtypes of migraines: migraine with aura, migraine without aura, basilar, hemiplegic, and ophthalmoplegic migraine. Basilar migraines are preceded by visual aura, then display features suggestive of vertebrobasilar ischemia such as vertigo, diplopia, paresthesia, syncope, and often a change in cognition. Hemiplegic migraines can be familial or sporadic, and are accompanied by hemiplegia which may last from 1 h to several days. Ophthalmoplegic migraines occur with third nerve palsy causing dilated pupil and unilateral eye pain. The attack may last for weeks. Hemiplegic and ophthalmoplegic migraines should be diagnosed only after neurologic pathology is ruled out.

The integrated hypothesis of the pathologic events that occur during migraine attacks include:

* Dilation of intra- and extracranial arteries (in migraine with or without aura) and cerebral blood flow alterations
* Neuropeptide release (calcitonin gene-related peptide (CGRP), neurokinin A, substance P) causing neurogenic inflammation, neuronal sensitivity, altered microvascular flow, and possibly meningeal inflammation
* Trigeminal nerve stimulated by neuronal and chemical activators (prostaglandins, serotonin and histamine)
* Serotonin (5-HT), a neurochemical pain modulator, is decreased

Several theories have been advanced regarding the pathogenesis of migraine. The oldest model is vascular, suggesting that the aura is due to intracerebral vasoconstriction and the headache is due to subsequent vasodilatation.

Another theory is that of neural origin. Reduced electrical activity in the brain causes the aura and neural-mediated vasodilatation is responsible for the headache.

A third theory is the trigeminovascular. Stimulation of the trigeminal nerve may cause a reverse conduction through the nerve, affecting cranial blood vessels. This triggers neurotransmitter release that causes neurogenic inflammation of the blood vessels leading to headache.

The most recent development and the theory that is receiving the emphasis in treatment is 5-hydroxytryptamine (5-HT) (serotonin). There are multiple 5-HT receptors with varying functions (5-HT 1D is implicated in the pathogenesis of migraine). In the vascular system, 5-HT can cause both vasoconstriction and vasodilatation. It also promotes platelet aggregation. The bodies of the major 5-HT neurons are found in the brain stem midline raphe nucleus. From here, pathways ascend to the basal ganglia, hypothalamus, limbic system, and cerebral cortex that affect mood, motor activity, hunger, thermoregulation, sleep, and endocrine control. Stimulation of the midline raphe nucleus can produce a 20% increase or decrease in cerebral blood flow. It is also involved in pain transmission, as neural pathways also project caudad to the pain gating system in the spinal cord.

Reserpine, a drug that decreases 5-HT, has been found to cause migraines in susceptible migraineurs. Tryptan drugs were developed to act as 5-HT agonists[13] and act as cranial vessel vasoconstrictors and inhibit proinflammatory neuropeptide release.

Rapid eye movement sleep affects serotonin release from the dorsal raphe nucleus and generally improves migraine pain.

Pediatric Issues

Approximately 4% of children[7] experience migraine, usually (85%) without aura. About 20% of adult migraineurs have a history of childhood migraine. Headaches are more frequently bilateral and associated with vomiting. Before puberty, male and female predominance is equal. Hemiplegic migraine typically begins in childhood and may end in adulthood. It may be preceded by head trauma. Hemiplegia may last for 1 h or less or days to weeks.[7] Basilar migraines should not be treated with tryptan drugs.

Obstetric Issues

Many migraineurs experience improvement in symptoms during pregnancy; however, a small percentage experience worsening, especially in the first trimester. Migraines seem to increase in frequency during the postpartum period. The risk of pregnancy complications are not increased, but treatment of migraine pain may be more difficult due to limitations in the use of some medications.[7] If migraines are infrequent, analgesic medication may be given. If the migraines are severe and/or frequent, prophylactic medication may be indicated. Table 25–1 lists pregnancy risk categories for migraine medications.

Geriatric Issues

In general, migraines tend to dissipate after age 50. In women, migraine tends to peak at age 40 and decrease as menopause approaches.[14] Disability (headaches requiring bed rest) decreases as age increases.[15]

New-onset headache in those greater than age 50 warrants interventional studies.[13]

Epidemiology

More than 10% of the general population experience a migraine within their lifetime. Migraines may occur at any age, but typically occur in the late teens or twenties. Approximately 18% of women and 6% of men are affected. Positive family history is common. Migraine

Table 25–1. Pregnancy Risk Categories* of Migraine Medications

Medication	Risk Category
Acetaminophen	B
Meperidine	B, D (third trimester)
Metoclopramide	B
NSAIDs	B†
Mefenamic acid	C
Triptans	C (pregnancy registry for sumatriptan is underway‡)
Barbiturates	C/D
Propranolol	C
Amitriptyline	D
Ergotamine	X

*Categories: A: safety established using human studies; B: presumed safety based on animal studies; C: uncertain safety; D: unsafe; X: highly unsafe.

†Avoid if possible because NSAID use could lead to premature closure of the ductus arteriosus.

‡Call the Sumatriptan Pregnancy Registry at (800) 722-9292, extension 39441, with questions concerning the use of sumatriptan during pregnancy.

NSAIDs, nonsteroidal anti-inflammatory drugs.

From Newman LC, Lay CL. Menstruation-Associated Migraine, Meniscus Educational Institute, www.meniscus.com. West Conshohocken, PA.

costs $13 billion per year in absenteeism and reduced work output and about $1 billion per year in direct medical costs.

Treatment Options

Appropriate treatment first depends on accurate diagnosis. Once a diagnosis is made, an accurate assessment of burden of suffering will guide treatment options (frequency, intensity, disability during headache).

Determine headache trigger factors (Table 25–2). These trigger factors may not be immediately apparent. A headache diary can be completed by the patient to accurately assess factors associated with the headache (i.e., occur during and around the headache) rather than attempting to recall events at a later date.

Treatment is abortive and prophylactic, nonpharmacologic and pharmacologic. Abortive therapy refers to treatment of an acute episode and is usually pharmacologic. Medications include acetaminophen, nonsteroidal anti-inflammatory drugs (NSAIDs), tryptan drugs (sumatriptan, zolmitriptan, naratriptan, rizatriptan), ergotamine, dihydroergotamine (DHE), and narcotics (not generally recommended). Basilar migraines should not be treated with tryptan drugs. It may be necessary to use adjunct therapy with antiemetics, neuroleptics, or corticosteroids if symptoms are severe. Nonpharmacologic treatment includes biofeedback (after training) or bed rest and sleep.

Prophylactic treatment is aimed at preventing the onset of migraine or reducing the frequency, duration, or intensity of repeated attacks. This is considered if a patient has two or more attacks per week, if attacks are debilitating or predictable (menstrual), or if headaches are associated with neurologic symptoms. Beta-blockers, calcium channel blockers, serotonin antagonists, antidepressants, anticonvulsants, and lithium are used for prophylactic treatment. Nonpharmacologic treatment includes avoidance of known trigger factors, biofeedback, and continued use of the headache diary (gives the patient a sense of empowerment). Hormone replacement therapy should be used cautiously, because these medications can exacerbate symptoms.

Patient Education

Patients do not need to suffer because they have "migraines." A headache does not have to be incapacitating to fulfill IHS criteria for migraine. Accurate diagnosis makes effective treatment possible. There have been significant advances in the understanding of migraine in the past several years and previous failure at treatment should not be an excuse for avoiding care.

Only one in 2000 migraineurs have a positive brain scan. Reassur-

Table 25–2. Selected Migraine Triggers

Environmental	Behavioral	Dietary	Physiologic	Pharmacologic
Odors or strong perfumes	Missed meals	Alcohol	Menstruation	Oral contraceptives
Changes in atmospheric pressure	Changes in sleep patterns	Tyramine*	Ovulation	Glyceryl trinitrate
Bright or flashing lights	Acute stress	Aspartame†	Ovarian cycle disorders	Theophylline
Acute stress		MSG‡		Reserpine
		Phenylethylamine§		Nifedipine
		Nitrates‖		Indomethacin
		Citrus		Cimetidine

*Present in aged cheese and fermented foods.
†Present in many diet soft drinks.
‡Present in flavor enhancers and some Chinese restaurant food.
§Present in chocolate.
‖Present in preserved meats, such as bacon, sausage, and bologna.
MSG, monosodium glutamate.
From Newman LC, Lay CL. Menstruation-Associated Migraine. Meniscus Educational Institute, www.meniscus.com, West Conshohocken, PA.

ance that the patient in all likelihood does not have a brain tumor (with a negative physical examination) may help alleviate symptoms.[13] Migraine is associated with depression, manic episodes, anxiety, panic disorder, epilepsy, stroke, mitral valve prolapse, and fibromyalgia.[7, 15] Depression is conversely associated with migraine.[7] Appropriate screening and treatment for concomitant conditions should be instituted.

It is important to instruct the patient to avoid narcotic analgesics for relief of the migraine headache to avoid a phenomenon called "rebound headache."

Prevention

There is essentially no primary prevention for migraine. Prophylactic (preventive) treatments can reduce the frequency and severity of headaches and may cause headaches to cease, but the disorder remains active. Secondary prevention is aimed at understanding events causing headache and treating attacks appropriately. Periodic re-evaluations are required to monitor response to treatment.

Screening Recommendations

Patients should have headache complaints classified according to the IHS criteria. Once the headache is appropriately classified, appropriate treatment measures can be prescribed.

MULTIPLE SCLEROSIS

Pathophysiology

Multiple sclerosis (MS) is one of the most common neurologic diseases affecting young adults. It is a demyelinating disease that is characterized by relapsing inflammatory exacerbations and chronic progressive deterioration.

The causes of MS are thought to be multiple. Potential causes include genetic factors coupled with viral exposure, environmental factors, and/or immune system events. The most probable scenario is that an individual has a genetic propensity to develop MS. When exposed to a viral or environmental trigger, an autoimmune process is initiated.

Twenty percent of MS patients have one or more affected relatives. There is a 26% incidence of concomitant disease for monozygotic twins and only 2.4% for dizygotic twins. MS has not been mapped to a specific gene locus and is likely polygenic.

MS is characterized by multifocal areas of demyelination due to an inflammatory, autoimmune process. The focal areas of chronic inflammation and demyelination are known as plaques. Plaques occur mostly in the white matter of the brain and spinal cord. Demyelination leads to decreased conduction velocity within the nervous system due to the loss of sufficient sodium channels. In most cases, plaques evolve over many years. Eventually, scar tissue called gliosis forms within the central nervous system (CNS), resulting in sclerosis and clinical deficit. There is some repair of the myelin with higher than normal sodium channels that allow for the resumption of conduction. In some cases the axon itself degenerates, leading to irretrievable loss of conduction.

Autoimmune disorders occur when cells become tolerant to antigenic cells. Myelin basic protein (MBP) in the CNS may be the primary autoimmune target. MBP-specific B- and T-cells have been found in cerebrospinal fluid, lending support to an autoimmune response. Although such findings exist in patients without MS, higher levels tend to correlate with presence of disease and the extent of injury.

There are many viruses known to cause demyelination in animals and humans. In humans, the JC papillomavirus, measles virus, and human T-cell lymphotropic virus type I have been suspected and studied. Serologic studies have been controversial and inconclusive for viral involvement. However, recent studies have found human herpesvirus-6 located in oligodendrocyte nuclei near plaques in MS patients. Human herpesvirus-6 is also found in normal individuals, but the virus exists in the oligodendrocyte cytoplasm. This finding may indicate persistent CNS viral infection as a trigger for disease.

Many soluble products of the immune response have been found to be toxic to myelin. Activated complement, tumor necrosis factor, reactive oxygen species, and arachidonic acid have been investigated as triggers in the development of MS.

The course of disease is extremely variable and survival may be only a few months from diagnosis, or >25 years after diagnosis. The condition may affect virtually any portion of the central nervous system, causing a wide variety of symptoms. Most commonly, the patient presents with sensory symptoms such as numbness, paresthesias, and/or dysesthesias (burning sensation). A common manifestation is Lhermitte's phenomenon, in which the patient experiences rapid tingling sensations shooting down the legs or arms with neck flexion. Also common is optic neuritis (30% risk of MS in patients with isolated optic neuritis), which is characterized by temporary blindness in one eye, lasting only a few days. Patients may also experience pain around the involved eye, blurred vision, decreased color vision, and visual field defects. Other presenting symptoms of MS include useless hand syndrome, poor balance, weakness of extremities, constipation, urinary frequency or urgency, alteration of vibratory or position sense in the extremities, spasticity, hyperreflexia, hemiparesis, or paraparesis. Often, these symptoms are worsened by exercise and increases in heat.

Patients with MS may experience cognitive decline, manifesting as memory loss, inattention, difficulty with complex reasoning and abstract concepts, and slow information processing. Depression and anxiety are more common in this population than in the age-matched general population. Fatigue is a persistent symptom, which may require decreases in activity and periods of rest. Sexual dysfunction is a common problem for both men and women affected with MS. Seizures can occur in up to 10% of patients.

MS can be classified into four major categories, depending on symptoms:

* Relapsing-remitting (RR) disease occurs in approximately 80–85% of patients. The patient may experience complete or incomplete symptomatic resolution after the episode. About 50% of RR patients enter into the next category.
* Secondary progressive MS involves a gradually advancing pattern of disability that may or may not include exacerbations.
* Primary progressive disease affects 10–15% of patients from disease onset. Symptoms are chronic and progressive and are not accompanied by exacerbations and remissions.
* Progressive relapsing MS is very rare and is characterized by progressive disease from the time of diagnosis.[16]

Pediatric Issues

MS rarely occurs in the pediatric population. Although subclinical disease may begin to develop at a young age (e.g., teenage years), symptoms rarely present until young adulthood.

Obstetric Issues

Pregnancy does not alter the risk of developing MS, but it does affect relapses and remissions. Relapse rates drop by approximately 30% in the second and third trimesters, but increase dramatically during the postpartum period. Studies have failed to demonstrate any long-term effect of pregnancy on the progression and disability of disease. It is very important for patients anticipating pregnancy to consult their health care provider before conception, as many medications used for control of MS may be toxic to the fetus.

Geriatric Issues

In the majority of cases, MS onset is before the geriatirc years. Maintenance of drug therapy is important for this population. Most geriatric patients with MS are dealing with progressive disease and disability. Often, spasticity and paresis limit activities of daily living, and permanent care may be necessary. It is important to thoroughly assess the patient's limitations and provide the necessary support for daily activities.

Epidemiology

MS affects 400,000 people in the U.S. alone, and millions worldwide. It affects women 1.5 times more frequently than men. Age of onset is usually between 20 and 40 years, with peak onset at 24 years. MS occurs most frequently in Caucasians, especially those of Northern European heritage. In other groups (e.g., Eskimos) the incidence is essentially zero.

Worldwide, MS occurs more frequently north of the 40th parallel, and in the U.S. it is more prevalent above the 37th parallel (Newport News, VA to Santa Cruz, CA).[17] The disease rarely occurs in those living in tropical climates near the equator. There is evidence that individuals who migrate from a high-risk area to a low-risk area before their midteen years carry the lower risk of their new residence. This supports the theory that an environmental exposure occurs within the first two decades of life which coupled with genetic predisposition may cause the development of MS. Data also reveal that there is a latent period of approximately 20 years between environmental exposure and clinical symptom development.

Treatment Options

There is no cure for MS, nor is there one specific treatment due to the wide range of symptoms. The goals of treatment are twofold: to prevent exacerbations, and to reduce the effect of relapses. Relapses are most commonly treated with IV methylprednisolone in 500 mg–1200 mg doses daily for a period of 3–5 days. Mild and moderate relapses are treated with oral prednisone. Long-term or chronic treatment with corticosteroids is controversial.

The goal of treatment is to prevent or prolong periods in-between relapses, and to delay progression of disease and disability. Immunosuppressant drugs such as cyclophosphamide, methotrexate, and azathioprine may be used if patients fail to respond to first-line treatments. Interferon-beta 1b and and beta 1a have shown a reduction in frequency of relapses and apparent stabilization of lesion volume on MRI. Disablity may be delayed with long-term treatment.[18] Glatiramer acetate (Copaxone) may also be used to decrease the frequency of relapses and number of exacerbations, decrease plaques (on MRI), and reduce disablility.

Because of the wide range of symptoms present in MS, many different drugs may be added to the treatment regimen. Spasticity is initially treated with a stretching program. This is followed with diazepam, baclofen, tizanidine, or dantrolene. Tremor may respond to clonazepam, isoniazid, or carbamazepine. Fatigue is difficult to treat, but amantadine, pemoline (Cylert), or methylphenidate (Ritalin) may be useful. Seizures are treated as in non-MS patients. Anticholinergics and self-catheterization may be useful in treating bladder disturbances. Depression is usually treated with tricyclics, and sometimes amitriptyline or dothiepin. Constipation is treated with stool softeners and bulk laxatives. If constipation is severe, osmotic agents and manual disimpaction may be necessary. Sexual dysfunction may be treated with vacuum devices, intracavernous injections of papaverine, prostaglandins, vaginal lubricants, or sildenafil (Viagra). Although pain is a rare symptom of MS, when present it is treated with carbamazepin tricyclics, or baclofen rather than chronic narcotics or other analgesics.

Some lifestyle choices are known to benefit MS patients. Exercise can maximize function by maintaining joint mobility, strength, and stamina. Patients should maintain a healthy diet, decrease smoking and excess alcohol intake, and prevent obesity. If disability is severe, physical and occupational therapy may help the patient regain some independence. Extreme cases may require surgical intervention.

Patient Education

MS patients tend to respond well to placebo suggesting that a positive attitude is very important, especially with MS. MS patients are also targets of charlatans. Due to the relapsing nature of the disease and response to placebo, therapies that are uncertain, expensive, and potentially dangerous may appear to show benefit. Conversely, clinical trials are necessary to determine future treatments, as the disease is not fully understood. The National Multiple Sclerosis Society is a good resource to research potentially beneficial versus bogus studies and therapies.

Trauma does not cause or exacerbate the symptoms of MS.[19]

MS is extremely variable in course and presentation, so each case and prognosis is individualized. In general, positive prognostic indicators include few attacks in the first years following diagnosis, long intervals between attacks, complete recovery following attacks, and pure sensory attacks. Poorer prognosis is associated with attacks that affect the cerebellum, and attacks with incomplete recovery.

Prevention

Since the actual cause of MS is unknown, it is impossible to prevent development of disease. However, it is important to prevent or delay relapses and progression of disease by maintaining a healthy lifestyle and proper drug treatment.

Screening Recommendations

Routine screening for MS is not recommended. MS is a clinical diagnosis that is supported by the finding of two or more separate plaques on MRI. CSF may demonstrate several nonspecific changes, including elevated protein levels and the more specific finding of oligoclonal bands by electrophoresis. The future may bring further understanding regarding mechanisms for developing disease that may lead to specific diagnostic testing or screening recommendations.

■■■ PARKINSON'S DISEASE

Pathophysiology

Parkinson's disease (PD) is a clinical diagnosis associated with multiple combinations of signs and symptoms. There is no specific clinical marker or radiologic finding to ensure the diagnosis.[20] The diagnosis requires a combination of bradykinesia, rigidity, resting tremor, and/or postural instability.[20, 21] There should be no identifiable cause and no evidence of other CNS disease.[20] Patients with Parkinson's *syndrome* may have an identifiable cause for their symptoms, such as neuroleptics, metoclopramide, or carbon monoxide. Other criteria for diagnosis include asymmetrical presentation and a positive response to levodopa.[20] However, the signs and symptoms are not necessarily distinct to PD, and early in the course of PD, all of the distinctive features have not developed.[21]

About 10% of patients with PD remain unrecognized by their physician,[22] and in early PD, the incorrect diagnosis is made in 24–35% of cases.[20] In patients who have been clinically diagnosed with PD, only 75% can be confirmed at autopsy.[21] Experience with PD aids in correct diagnosis. Even with experience, diagnosis should be amenable to change.[20] Frequency of symptoms are listed in Table 25–3.

Other features include festination, blink rate, micrographia, freezing while walking, blepharospasm, subtle speech abnormalities, autonomic dysfunction, and impotence.[21]

The origin of PD is unknown. Genetics are not a factor unless the disease occurs early in life (age <51 years).[22] Theoretically, PD is due to environmental toxins or factors, as there is increased risk with pesticide use, living in a rural area, drinking well water, herbicide exposure, and proximity of home to industrial plants and quarries. Certain environmental factors may cause a gene mutation. In certain

Table 25–3. Frequency of Symptoms

Symptom	Frequency
Tremor	79–90%
Rigidity	89–99%
Bradykinesia	77–98%
Postural instability	37%
Asymmetrical presentation	72–75%
Levodopa responsiveness	94–100%
Dementia	25–40%
Depression	5–40%
Psychotic features (nonmedication)	2–6%
Psychotic features (medication related)	20%

(rare) familial cases, the gene mutation is on the alpha-synuclein gene.[22]

Depigmentation and loss of neurons are found in the substantia nigra of patients with Parkinson's disease. Lewy bodies (eosinophilic inclusions) and pale bodies (neurofilament and vascular granules) are also found. The cells of the substantia nigra generally produce dopamine. As these cells degenerate, less dopaminergic activity is noted at the axonal projections in the striatum of the basal ganglia. It is estimated that between 60 and 85% of dopaminergic activity is lost by the onset of clinical symptoms.

Pediatric Issues

Parkinson's is a disease of adulthood, and symptoms in this population are generally attributed to another cause (e.g., medications, illicit drugs).

Obstetric Issues

Because the disease is generally a geriatric condition, obstetric concerns are few. However, it is possible for a woman of childbearing age to have Parkinson's. Women with PD should consult their physicians before becoming pregnant.

Geriatric Issues

Parkinson's is largely a disease of mid to late adulthood. Because the disease is progressive, patients should periodically be evaluated to determine interference with the normal activities of daily living.

Epidemiology

The prevalence of Parkinson's disease in the general population is approximately 1–2 per 1,000 people, with no gender preference. Actually, disease prevalence in persons aged >70 years is 1.5–2.5%.[22] Onset usually occurs after age 50.

Treatment Options

Treatment is centered on replacing deficient dopamine and alleviating symptoms. The most effective treatment of PD is levodopa, which is converted to dopamine by the dopa-decarboxylase enzyme. Carbidopa (an enzyme inhibitor) is often an adjunct to this therapy because it reduces side effects from dopamine in the periphery, allowing more levodopa to cross the blood-brain barrier. The levodopa-carbidopa combination medication is marketed as Sinemet.

After several years of treatment, patients may experience dyskinesias. Symptoms may occur immediately after taking the medication, but within 2 h symptoms improve. As the plasma levels decrease, patients again experience dyskinesia. This is alleviated by taking small doses of medications several times per day or taking a controlled-release formulation. Unfortunately, after treatment with levodopa for 2–5 years, the efficacy becomes limited. The wearing off may be in the form of the "on/off" or freezing phenomenon.

Other medications that have been used in treatment include monoamine oxidase inhibitors (deprenyl, selegiline), anticholinergics (trihexyphenidyl), and dopamine agonists (bromocriptine and pergolide). Anticholinergics may be useful in the early stages of disease but appear to have no long-term effect on disease. Bromocriptine and pergolide are drugs that stimulate dopamine receptors. They have long half-lives and help to smooth out motor fluctuations. Some advocate the use of these medications early in therapy, and others use them late in therapy to augment the effects of Sinemet.

Studies are underway to demonstrate the efficacy of new dopamine agonists such as pramipexole (Mirapex) and ropinirole (Requip) as first-line agents. The use of dopamine early in the disease process may provide better options later in the disease process. A new class of drugs, the catechol-O-methyltransferases (COMT), work by decreasing dopamine metabolism in the periphery, thereby increasing the bioavailability of dopamine. Selegiline may be used more in the future because of its potential neuroprotective role.

Surgical techniques may be necessary in some patients. Constructive surgery seeks to provide new cell sources for dopamine at the striatum through the implantation of mesencephalic fetal cells.[23] Destructive surgery seeks to ablate overactive pallidal or thalamic function to reduce motor dyskinesia. With all the new developments in the treatment of Parkinson's, survival is nearly equivalent to that of the age-matched populations.

Patient Education

Educate patients as to the natural history of PD so they may prepare for functional decline. After the patient falls and has an injury, it is too late to warn him or her of postural instability. Medication risks and side effects should also be discussed early so potential problems can be readily identified and prepared for.

Prevention

There is no current primary prevention. Until a definitive cause is found, there is no definite avoidance of environmental factors. Secondary prevention is aimed at reducing disability or injury. Patients with bradykinesia and tremor often have marked difficulty performing the activities of daily life (brushing teeth, feeding, bathing). Those with postural instability are more prone to falls. Evaluation and periodic follow-up with physical and occupational therapy is effective at maintaing quality of life.

Screening Recommendations

There are no routine screening recommendations, as this diagnosis is based on clinical symptoms and signs. Recognition of PD in the early stages may be difficult but may allow for earlier treatment. If the diagnosis is unclear, referral to a neurologist with substantial PD experience helps to optimize treatment for the patient.

STROKE (TRANSIENT ISCHEMIC ATTACK)

Pathophysiology

Stroke or "brain attack" is a complex pathologic process. Stroke occurs when there is an interruption of blood flow to the brain resulting in cellular death. Stroke may arise due to atherosclerosis with subsequent development of thrombus (50%) in the cerebral arteries. The blockage may also be due to an embolus (32%) from a cardiac or thrombotic source. Less commonly, stroke may be due to a hemorrhagic (17%) etiology.

The development of cerebrovascular and extracranial atherosclerosis that leads to acute stroke and subsequent cell damage is not completely understood. Atherosclerotic disease is a decades-long process that begins in childhood. The lumen of a blood vessel becomes narrowed by cellular and extracellular substances to the point of obstruction.[24] The progression to clinically significant lesions occurs with increased frequency in persons with risk factors. These modifiable risk factors include diabetes, hypercholesterolemia, hypertension, smoking, obesity, sedentary lifestyle, and heart disease.[25]

The main site for atherosclerotic disease is the inner lining of the wall of the blood vessel, the intima, which lies just below the endothelium. An accumulation of complex lipids, proteins, and carbohydrates as well as a proliferation of cells characterize atherosclerosis in the intimal layer of an artery. Smooth muscle also proliferates within the intima providing the bulk of the atherosclerotic lesion.[26] This lesion narrows the lumen of the artery causing either a temporary loss of blood flow to an area of the brain (transient ischemic attack [TIA]) or complete and permanent loss of blood flow to the brain (stroke).

Two major areas of injury include the core ischemic area and the surrounding ischemic penumbra. The penumbra contains viable cerebral tissue if blood supply is restored. The core ischemic area, once depleted of nutrients and oxygen, is no longer viable.

There are two different origins of embolus. An embolus can occur when a small clot breaks off a thrombus and travels through the blood stream until it lodges in and occludes a narrowed artery. This results in an ischemic infarct. More commonly, however, cerebral emboli originate from the heart. Atrial fibrillation is the most common cause of emboli, but any type of major functional or structural abnormality that allows for stasis of blood in the heart may cause emboli. Cardiogenic emboli lodge in the middle cerebral artery 80% of the time.[25]

Lacunar infarcts account for 20% of strokes. These are most commonly associated with hypertension and advanced age. Lacunar infarcts occur when there are occlusions of small deep penetrating arteries known as lenticulostriate arteries branching from the middle cerebral artery or penetrating branches of the circle of Willis, vertebral or basilar arteries.[27] Hemorrhagic stroke includes intracerebral hemorrhages and subarachnoid hemorrhages. Intracerebral hemorrhages most frequently occur secondary to hypertension. Aneurysms and arteriovenous malformations may be associated with intracerebral or subarachnoid hemorrhages. These types of strokes can cause necrosis of brain tissue due to the cytotoxins that are released when blood enters the brain tissue. Signs and symptoms of stroke include sudden weakness, paralysis, or numbness of the face, arm and/or leg, loss of speech or difficulty speaking and understanding speech, loss or dimness of vision, unexplained dizziness, unsteadiness and falls, severe headache, and loss of consciousness.

Pediatric Issues

Stroke is uncommon in the pediatric age group. The incidence is approximately 2.5/100,000. Children <2 years of age are affected more frequently than older children. Infants may present with seizures, coma, and hemiparesis. Etiology includes congenital heart disease, hematologic and clotting defects, genetic disorders, and unknown.

Obstetric Issues

Pregnancy can increase the risk of stroke 3–13 times. This is a relative increase, as overall, young women are at low risk for stroke. The incidence is about 8/100,000 women with 25% being fatal. Hemorrhagic strokes (subarachnoid and intracerebral), although uncommon, are the leading cause of maternal death in the U.S.

The risk of obstetrically related stroke is highest in the 6-week postpartum period. The overall risk of ischemic stroke is approximately 9 times higher and the risk of hemorrhagic stroke is >28 times higher for postpartum women than for nonobstetric women. The cause is unknown.

Geriatric Issues

Stroke is primarily a condition of the elderly.

Epidemiology

Stroke is the third leading cause of death and the leading cause of disability. More than 700,000 strokes occur yearly resulting in over 150,000 deaths.[28] Currently there are more than 3 million surviving stroke victims. Annual direct and indirect costs for health care expenditures and lost productivity have been estimated at $20–$40 billion.[29, 30]

Stroke is more prevalent in the elderly, male, African American population. In the southeastern states, stroke risk is approximately 1.4 times that of other regions.[31–33] Stroke risk doubles with every decade after age 55 years old. Men and African Americans increase their risk of stroke 1.3 and 2.0 times, respectively.

Hypertension, diabetes, heart disease, and current smoking are major risk factors for stroke in the young adult (Table 25–4).

Table 25–4. Increased Risk Factors for Stroke	
Diabetes	3 times
Previous TIA or stroke	10 times
Blood pressure consistently >140/90	6 times
Heart disease, atrial fibrillation, left ventricular hypertrophy	4–6 times
Carotid artery disease and peripheral vascular disease	3 times
Smoking	2 times
Male gender	1.3 times
African American	2 times
Hypercholesterolemia, excessive alcohol consumption, excessive weight, sedentary lifestyle (amount of increased risk unknown)	

Treatment Options

Acute stroke treatment can occur if the patient reaches the emergency room or other medical facility within 3 h of stroke symptom onset. After the patient is screened for possible hemorrhage with the use of CT of the brain and other screening tests, the patient may be a candidate for tissue plasminogen activator (TPA). TPA is a clot dissolving agent that can reverse the effects of a stroke by returning blood flow to the affected area. There is a 6% chance of bleeding if TPA is given within the 3-h window and increased greatly if given outside the 3-h window; therefore, the protocol should be strictly adhered to.

Unfortunately, <5% of patients with ischemic stroke present within the 3-h time period. These patients may wait days or weeks before seeking medical attention. In this case treatment focuses on preventing worsening symptoms and possibly reversing the damage. The use of heparin is controversial in acute stroke, unless there is a cardioembolic source (e.g., atrial fibrillation), as it may slightly increase the risk of intracerebral hemorrhage.

Patients should be evaluated for intracerebral or carotid stenosis with the use of carotid ultrasound and/or magnetic resonance angiogram of the brain. If symptomatic carotid stenosis is detected (>70%), carotid endarterectomy may be indicated. If a carotid endarterectomy is contraindicated for medical reasons or if intracerebral stenosis is detected, then medical management with antiplatelet medications or anticoagulants may be an alternative.

An echocardiogram should be performed to evaluate for thrombus. If further evaluation is needed, a transesophageal echocardiogram may be indicated. If the patient is found to have a cardioembolic source for the stroke, heparin is started and the patient is placed on warfarin (Coumadin) long-term therapy and the cardiac etiology is treated, if possible

If all tests are normal, a daily aspirin may be indicated. If the stroke occurred while on aspirin, another antiplatelet medication may be prescribed (e.g., ticlopidine, clopidogrel, and Aggrenox [aspirin and dipyridamole]). The patient may require a relatively elevated blood pressure, and intervention only counteracts the patient's hemostatic mechanisms. Patients may be allowed to autoregulate their blood pressure. If hypertension is treated, it should be done cautiously in the acute stroke phase. Reducing the blood pressure may cause cerebral damage due to hypoperfusion. Once the patient is stable, blood pressure should be maintained at <140/90 for the general population, and <135/85 for diabetics.

A fasting cholesterol and lipid profile should be obtained. If the total cholesterol is >200 μg/dL, then exercise and diet modification may be enough to lower cholesterol to within normal range. However, if after 3 months of lifestyle modifications, the total cholesterol is still >200 μg/dL, then medical management with cholesterol-lowering agents such as pravastatin or simvastatin are indicated.

Obesity must be identified and treated appropriately. Thirty percent above ideal body weight (IBW) places the patient at an increased risk of stroke. Diet and exercise must be discussed at every visit.

Smoking cessation should be discussed and encouraged at every visit. Offering bupropion hydrochloride (Zyban) or nicotine replacement may be of some benefit.

Patient Education

Educating patients on the pathophysiology of stroke and the signs and symptoms of stroke are just as important as educating them on reducing the risk of stroke. Patients must understand the importance of calling 911 at the first sign of a stroke symptom in order to obtain the best care. The incidence of stroke can be reduced, and public education is the answer.

Prevention

Emerging therapies are helping to reduce the morbidity and mortality of stroke. However, these advances need to be coupled with a greater emphasis on prevention. Stroke prevention strategies should be aimed at those who are at increased risk of stroke and modify those risks, if possible. Hypertension, cardiac disease, diabetes, hyperlipidemia, asymptomatic carotid stenosis, cigarette smoking, and alcohol abuse are all risk factors that may be modified to prevent stroke. Besides advancing age (>55 years), hypertension is the most powerful stroke risk factor. Thirty percent of Americans suffer from high blood pressure. Individuals with uncontrolled hypertension (BP > 140/90) are at seven times the risk of developing a stroke as those with normal blood pressure.[34] Antihypertensive treatment is highly effective in preventing stroke in all ages, genders, and races.

Various cardiac diseases have been shown to increase the risk of stroke. Atrial fibrillation is the most common and treatable cardiac cause. Atrial fibrillation incidence doubles with every decade after age 55. Fifty percent of all cardioembolic strokes are related to atrial fibrillation. Warfarin anticoagulation reduces the risk of stroke by 68% in a pooled analysis of atrial fibrillation trials. Left ventricular hypertrophy and myocardial damage are also prominent risk factors and need to be identified and treated appropriately.

Antiplatelet therapy has been shown to be a great benefit to prevent stroke. Antiplatelet medications include aspirin, ticlopidine, clopidogrel, dipyridamole, and sulfinpyrazone. Aspirin promotes protection against a second stroke in individuals who previously have had a stroke or TIA.[35] Clopidogrel has a relative risk reduction of 8% over aspirin for promoting protection against stroke in persons who have suffered stroke.[36] Ticlopidine has been shown to be more effective than aspirin alone in reducing stroke risk in persons who previously had a stroke or TIA, but it has increased side effects. Aspirin and dipyridamole combined have a relative risk reduction for stroke about 20% greater than aspirin.

Eighty percent of strokes are preventable. Learning what patients' risk factors are gives health care providers the ability to empower patients to make healthy choices. Teach patients what a stroke is, tell them repeatedly what the signs and symptoms of stroke are and to call 911 if they should experience symptoms. Explain the importance of taking their blood pressure medicine, aspirin, cholesterol-lowering medicine, and diabetic medicine daily. Allow them the chance to ask questions. Help them quit smoking. Get them involved in a new diet and exercise program.

Screening Recommendations

Risk factor screening is advised, as noted above.

References

1. Kirkaldy-Willis WH, Bernard TN. Managing Low Back Pain, 4th ed. Churchill Livingstone, 1999.
2. Wiesel SW, Weinstein SN, Herkowitz HN, et al. The Lumbar Spine, 2nd ed. Philadelphia, WB Saunders, 1996.
3. Videman T, Nurminen M, Troup JDG. Lumbar spinal pathology in cadaveric material in relation to history of back pain, occupation, and physical loading. Spine 1990;15:728–740.
4. Gilber JR, Taylor DW, Hildebrandt A. Clinical trial of common treatment for low back pain in family practice. BMJ 1985;291:791–794.

5. Deyo RA, Diehl AK, Rosenthal M. How many days of bedrest for acute low back pain? A randomized clinical trial. N Engl J Med 1986;315:1064–1070.

6. APA Online http://www.psych.org/clin_res/pg_dementia_2.html

7. Goetz CG, Pappert EJ. Textbook of Clinical Neurology. Philadelphia, WB Saunders, 1999.

7a. www.parkinson.org/pddement.htm

7b. www.ccc.nottingham.ac.uk/~mpzlowe/lewy/lewyhome.html

8. Adams RD, Victor M, Ropper AH. Principles of Neurology, 6th ed. New York, McGraw-Hill, 1997.

9. Mayo Clinic, Geriatric Medicine, Community Internal Medicine Division. http://www.mayo.edu/geriatric-rst/Dementia.1 ToC.html

10. Daly E, Zaitchik D, Copeland M, et al. Predicting conversion to Alzheimer disease using standardized clinical information. Arch Neurol 2000;57:675–680.

11. Peterson RC et al. Mild cognitive impairment, clinical characterization and outcome. Arch Neurol 1999; 56:303–308.

12. Guide to Clinical Preventive Services, 2nd ed. Report of the U.S. Preventive Services Task Force. Baltimore, Williams & Wilkins, 1996.

13. MacGregor A. Managing Migraine in Primary Care. Oxford, England, Blackwell Science, 1999.

14. Newman LC, Lay CL. Menstrual Associated Migraine. Continuing medical education activity sponsored by an unrestricted grant from Glaxo Wellcome. Meniscus Education Institute, West Conshohocken, PA, May 1999.

15. Hu XH, Markson LE, Lipton RE, et al. Burden of migraine in the United States: Disability and economic costs. Arch Intern Med 1999;159:813–818.

16. Anderson PB, Waubant E, Goodkin DE. Multiple sclerosis that is progressive from the time of onset: clinical characterization and progression of disability. Arch Neurol 1999;56:1138–1142.

17. National Multiple Sclerosis Society web site. Http://www.nmss.org/

18. Tselis AC, Lisak RP. MS therapeutic update. Arch Neurol 1999;56:277–280.

19. Hogencamp WE, Noseworthy JH. Demyelinating disorders of the central nervous system. In Goetz CG, Pappert EJ (eds). Textbook of Clinical Neurology. Philadelphia, WB Saunders, 1999, pp 971–983.

20. Jankovic J, Rajput AH, McDermott MP, Perl DP. The evolution of early Parkinson's disease. Arch Neurol 2000;57:369–372.

21. Gelb DJ, Oliver E, Gilman S. Diagnostic criteria for Parkinson's disease. Arch Neurol 1999;56:33–39.

22. Cummings JL. Understanding Parkinson's disease. JAMA 1999;281:376–378.

23. Hauser RA, Freeman TB, Snow BJ, et al. Long-term evaluation of bilateral fetal nigral transplantation in Parkinson's disease. Arch Neurol 1999; 56:179–187.

24. Breslow JL. Mouse models of atherosclerosis. Science 1996; 272:685–688.

25. Harrison's Principles of Internal Medicine, 14th ed. New York, McGraw-Hill, 1998.

26. Hajjar DP, Nicholson AC. Atherosclerosis. American Scientist 1995;83, No. 5.

27. The Stroke/Brain Attack Reporter's Handbook. Englewood, CO, National Stroke Association, 2000.

28. Sacco RL, Benjamin EJ, Broderick JP, et al. American Heart Association Prevention Conference IV. Prevention and rehabilitation of stroke: Risk factors. Stroke 1997;28:1507–1517.

29. Heart and Stroke facts: 1996 Statistical Supplement. Dallas, TX, American Heart Association, 1996.

30. 1995 Heart and Stroke Facts. Dallas, TX, American Heart Association, 1996.

31. Thom TJ. Stroke mortality trends: An international perspective. Ann Epidemiol 1993;3:509–518.

32. Lanska DJ. Geographic distribution of stroke mortality in the United States: 1939–1941 to 1979–1981. Neurology 1993;43:1839–1851.

33. Howard G, Evans GW, Pearce K, et al. Is the stroke belt disappearing? An analysis of racial, temporal, and age effects. Stroke 1995;26:1153–1158.

34. U.S. Public Health Service. Healthy People 2000: National Health Promotion and Disease Prevention Objectives. Publication (PHS) 91–50212. Washington, DC, U.S. Department of Health and Human Services, 1991.

35. Jonas S, Zeleniuch-Jacquotte A. The effect of antiplatelet agents on survival free of new stroke: A meta-analysis. Stroke Clin Updates 1998;7:1–4.

36. CAPRIE Steering Committee. A randomised, blinded trial of clopidogrel versus aspirin in patients at risk of ischaemic events (CAPRIE). Lancet 1996;348:1329–1339.

CHAPTER 26

Substance Abuse

Major William A. Mosier, EdD,
PA-C, USAFR,
and Joseph J. Altieri, MD

INTRODUCTION

When searching for an understanding of substance abuse disorders, one encounters a mountain of theoretical constructs derived from hypothetical ideas that have been tested on an overwhelming quantity of clinical data. Dopamine seems to intertwine with defense mechanisms like denial, serotonin reuptake seems to compete with symbiosis, and environmental factors like stress and divorce, on the surface, appear to be as influential in the development of substance abuse disorders as gamma-aminobutyric acid and the endorphins. Viewing substance abuse as an adaptive attempt to alleviate emotional suffering and repair self-regulatory deficiencies is a step toward understanding the psychology of addiction.[1, 2]

Much of what can be said about the pathophysiology of any addiction, with slight variations of mechanisms, can apply to all addictions, including alcohol, nicotine, caffeine, cocaine, benzodiazepines, prescription narcotics, or heroin.[3, 4] Substance abuse disorders are a syndrome with mixed biological, genetic, psychological, and social factors contributing to its origins. A family history of substance abuse remains the single greatest risk factor for developing a substance abuse disorder.[5, 6]

Changes in the expression of numerous genes occur with chronic drug exposure. Chronic ingestion of any substance of abuse produces a molecular rewiring of the brain.[7, 8] On a cellular level, dependency provokes a state of adaptation in which the presence of the substance of abuse is necessary for homeostasis. Withdrawal induces alteration of cell membranes, neurotransmitters, and receptor sites. Although these changes are the basis of withdrawal symptoms, there is also a significant psychological component to withdrawal. Environmental stimuli can trigger a withdrawal response. Persistent use of a substance of abuse has a direct effect on the neural substrates of motivation. This adaptive response results in sensitization, tolerance, and dependence.[9, 10] How the tissue changes are interpreted by the brain depends on the situation, expectations, and emotional state of the individual. The individual's reactions to the withdrawal experience produce feedback that either magnifies or reduces the withdrawal symptoms.[11, 12]

Chronic use of the abused substance produces persistent dysphoria, leading to craving and relapse even after prolonged abstinence. Addictive behavior is primarily the result of the activation of internal neuro-psycho-biological states striving for homeostasis.[13, 14]

A wide variety of psychological disorders are associated with substance abuse and/or substance dependence. Patients with a substance abuse disorder are more likely to have a comorbid mental condition. The highest rates of comorbidity are among patients with a bipolar disorder (40%) or an anxiety disorder (20%). Personality disorders are also commonly linked with substance abuse disorders. Individuals with a diagnosis of antisocial personality disorder have a 30-times greater risk of developing alcohol abuse and a 12-times greater risk of developing other substance abuse disorders than the general population. Substance abuse disorders often complicate the treatment of other mental health disorders owing to medication noncompliance. The successful treatment of substance abuse disorders is intimately tied to the successful treatment of any comorbid mental health conditions.[15, 16]

A Substance Abuse Screening Tool (SAST) (Table 26–1) has been modeled after the Epidemiology Catchment Area (ECA) Diagnostic

---

Table 26–1. The FIND Substance Abuse Screening Tool (SAST)

1. Referring to the list of substances identified below, have you ever used one of them more than six times in your life?
   * Amphetamines (e.g., speed)
   * Phenobarbital (e.g., quaaludes, Seconal)
   * Benzodiazepines (e.g., Librium, Valium)
   * Cocaine or crack
   * Marijuana
   * Opiates (e.g. codeine, Darvon, Demerol, heroin, morphine)
   * Hallucinogens (e.g., DMT, LSD, mescaline, PCP, peyote, psilocybin)

YES	NO
(1)	(0)

   If you answered NO to question number one, stop here. If you answered YES go on to the next question.

2. Have you ever found that you needed larger amounts, of any substance you identified above, in order to achieve the same effect that you were once able to get on a lower dose?

YES	NO
(1)	(0)

3. Have you ever experienced psychological effects from any substance that you identified above (e.g., feeling people are against you, a loss of pleasure of previously enjoyable activities)?

YES	NO
(1)	(0)

   A total score equal to 2 or 3 demonstrates a risk for substance abuse.

From The Florida Institute for Neurodevelopmental Disorders, 1997, with permission.

Interview Schedule. It can be used as a quick assessment tool easily completed by a patient prior to seeing a health care provider. If the SAST result is positive for substance abuse, the provider can utilize the tool to address the issues identified.

According to the *Diagnostic and Statistical Manual of Mental Disorders* (DSM-IV), the criteria for the diagnoses of substance abuse or substance dependence are the same for all substances of abuse (Boxes 26–1 and 26–2). If the behavioral criteria are met, an aggressive treatment intervention is indicated, even if the patient is in denial about his or her substance abuse.[17]

Seventy-five percent of all patients needing treatment for substance abuse go untreated. Brief intervention counseling can provide an effective first-line treatment. During brief interventions, it is most important to be direct—yet supportive.[20, 21]

Two misconceptions about when a patient is ready to accept treatment are common:

1. Substance abusers must "hit rock bottom" before they will accept help.
2. Individuals who are coerced into treatment are more likely to relapse than individuals who request help on their own. In fact, prompt intervention has the same efficacy as waiting for the individual to voluntarily undergo treatment or to be coerced by family, employers, or the court system.[22, 23]

Box 26-1–DSM-IV CRITERIA FOR SUBSTANCE ABUSE

A maladaptive pattern of use of a substance that has abuse potential leading to significant functional impairment in at least one of the following areas, occurring within a 12-month period.

1. Recurrent substance use resulting in nonfulfillment of important responsibilities (e.g., inadequate work performance or frequent absenteeism due to substance use, substance-use related school problems, neglect of children or household responsibilities).
2. Recurrent irresponsible use of a substance in situations that would be considered physically dangerous (e.g., operating a motor vehicle while under the influence of a substance).
3. Recurrent substance-use–related legal entanglements (e.g., arrest record for substance-use related violations, such as disorderly conduct or receiving a DUI).
4. Persistent substance abuse in spite of recurrent social problems caused by the effects of a substance (e.g., physical or verbal aggression exacerbated by the use of a substance).[18, 19]

Reprinted with permission from the Diagnostic and Statistical Manual of Mental Disorders, Fourth Edition. Copyright 1994 American Psychiatric Association.

Box 26-2–DSM-IV CRITERIA FOR SUBSTANCE DEPENDENCE

A maladaptive pattern of substance use leading to significant distress or functional impairment that is more profound than substance abuse. (This distress or impairment must be manifest by at least three of the following occurring together in the same 12-month period.)

1. Signs of tolerance
- A need for increased amounts of the substance to achieve a desired effect
- A significantly diminished desired effect with continued utilization of the same quantity of the substance, requiring larger amounts to recapture the desired effect
2. Signs of withdrawal
- Displaying at least two of the following characteristics of substance-use withdrawal syndrome (anxiety, sweating, pulse rate >100, insomnia, hand tremor, nausea or vomiting, psychomotor agitation, hallucinations, seizures)
- Substance is taken to relieve symptoms of withdrawal
3. Signs of abuse
- Substance is often taken in larger amounts or for a greater period than intended.
- Efforts to cut down or stop are unsuccessful.
- An inordinate amount of time is spent seeking the substance or in recovering from its effects.
- Substance use is disrupting to work, social, or recreational activities.
- Substance use continues, in spite of the realization that it is causing a health problem.[18, 19]

Reprinted with permission from the Diagnostic and Statistical Manual of Mental Disorders, Fourth Edition. Copyright 1994 American Psychiatric Association.

Brief interventions, for as short a time as a 10-min office visit, can be just as effective as intensive inpatient treatment. The essential elements of a successful treatment plan are long-term office follow-up, working with the patient and the family as a unit, and addressing comorbidities.[24, 25] The level of empathic communication demonstrated by the clinician is the one factor most directly related to a successful outcome. In fact, aggressive confrontation correlates with a less favorable outcome.[26, 27]

The elements of effective brief interventions are

1. Individualized and objective feedback regarding the patient's substance abuse habit

2. Emphasis on the patient accepting responsibility for deciding what to do about his or her continued substance abuse
3. Presenting clear recommendations for change
4. Providing the patient with specific intervention options for change from which the patient can choose
5. Helping the patient to develop specific goals for change
6. Emphasizing self-efficacy
7. Conducting interventions with an empathic style of communication
8. Encouraging the patient to enter a community-based program that reinforces the patient to remain clean and sober[28, 29]

Though substance abuse disorder tends to be chronic, manifesting with frequent relapses, it is highly treatable when managed correctly. There is no one best treatment. The key to effective intervention is to individualize the treatment for each patient.[30, 31]

Patient education related to substance abuse issues must be tailored to the specific needs of each patient. Self-help groups, such as Alcoholics Anonymous (AA) and Narcotics Anonymous (NA), can play a vital role in a patient's recovery from substance abuse and offer an infrastructure of continuous reinforcement for avoiding relapse.[32] For additional resources, see the Resources Appendix at the end of this book.

ALCOHOL ABUSE AND ALCOHOL DEPENDENCY

Pathophysiology

The oxidation of alcohol leads to many biochemical changes in the body. Chronic alcohol use impairs the ability of the liver and pancreas to adequately control the metabolism of carbohydrates. Alcohol can decrease cell sensitivity to insulin. This loss of insulin sensitivity can have a markedly adverse effect on glucose levels in the blood, posing a serious risk of diabetes. Abnormalities in carbohydrate regulation can also contribute to difficulty in maintaining a normal acid-base balance.[33] Alcohol-related disorders include cirrhosis, hepatitis, malnutrition, anemia, pancreatitis, gastrointestinal bleeding, cardiovascular disease, cardiomyopathy, and specific cancers.[34]

Persons with alcoholism may be genetically predisposed to produce larger than usual quantities of a morphine-like compound that is produced by the body in response to the ingestion of alcohol. Environmental factors may be the determiner of whether or not a biological tendency for alcohol dependency will manifest; however, heredity plays an extremely important role in the development of alcohol dependence.[35-37]

Pediatric Issues

Over 65% of young people in America have tried alcohol by the time they reach the eighth grade. Children of parents with alcoholism have four times the risk of developing alcoholism as children of parents who do not have alcoholism.[38]

Obstetric Issues

The mother who drinks alcohol during pregnancy risks fetal alcohol exposure that can lead to alcohol-related birth defects (ARBDs) or fetal alcohol syndrome (FAS), which causes physical or neurobehavioral anomalies.[39, 40]

Geriatric Issues

An estimated 10% of the elderly population in America abuse alcohol. The National Institute on Alcohol Abuse and Alcoholism recommends that in individuals under age 65, men should have no more than two drinks containing alcohol per day, and women should have no more than one drink per day. Over age 65, both men and women should avoid more than one drink of alcohol per day.[41–44]

Epidemiology

Alcohol is the most frequently abused drug in most countries. Excessive alcohol consumption is a cause of the type of reckless behavior that often leads to death. Blood tests for the presence of alcohol can be expected to be positive in approximately 50% of all deaths due to unnatural causes. Over 50% of all fatal automobile accidents involve drivers who were intoxicated at the time of the accident. Fifty percent of those who die from falls or in fires have been drinking alcohol. Suicide is 30 times more common among persons with alcoholism than in the general population. Alcohol-related disorders are present in as many as 30% of adult patients seen in primary care settings, a prevalence rate similar to chronic diseases such as diabetes and hypertension.[45, 46] Despite the magnitude of alcohol-related health problems, less than 20% of patients who meet the criteria are diagnosed with alcohol abuse, and the percentage who received the appropriate referral is even smaller. An estimated 18 million people with alcohol use problems in the United States need intervention, yet only one in four receives treatment.[47–49]

Men are three times more likely than women to develop alcoholism. Twenty percent of male patients and 10% of female patients in the average primary care practice will be at risk for medical, legal, or psychosocial problems related to alcohol abuse. Though it manifests more frequently in men, vulnerability to alcohol-related problems is probably equal in men and women.[50, 51]

Most ethnic groups demonstrate similar rates of alcoholism, with the exception of individuals of Asian extraction. A greater propensity for experiencing a discomforting flushing sensation from excess drinking of alcohol, caused by a presumed absence of adequate amounts of aldehyde dehydrogenase available in the liver, probably accounts for the markedly lower rate of alcoholism among Asians.[52–55a]

Fifty percent of Americans over the age of 18 admit to a family history of alcoholism among first or second degree relatives. One in four says that alcohol has been a major cause of trouble in his or her family. Susceptibility to alcoholism runs in families, whether the children of alcoholic parents are raised by the alcoholic family or not. Twin studies demonstrate that sons and daughters of alcoholic parents who are raised by non-alcoholic adoptive parents are predisposed to alcoholism even if they are raised in a happy, healthy, and stable adoptive setting. Individuals from broken homes are six times more likely to become alcoholic if one of their biological parents was alcoholic than if one of their adoptive parents is alcoholic. Twenty-five percent of sons of alcoholics become alcoholic, an incidence five times greater than in the general population. A family history of alcohol abuse in two or more relatives increases the risk of an individual manifesting alcohol dependency by a factor of three. The theory that a "dysfunctional" childhood is a predictor of future alcoholism has not been substantiated by research. Alcohol abuse appears to be independent of an individual's childhood environment. Family, twin, and adoption studies provide compelling evidence for the influence of genetic factors in the etiology of alcoholism. Although genetics do not explain the entire cause of alcoholism, there is no doubt that a predisposition for alcoholism is an inheritable trait in humans. For individuals who are genetically predisposed, vulnerability to alcoholism appears to be lifelong.[56–58a]

Treatment Options

Alcoholism is the most thoroughly studied substance-abuse disorder. Over 600 case studies or reports of clinical trials concerning the treatment of alcohol abuse and dependence have been published. Over 250 of these studies included control or comparison groups.[54–55a]

Once a patient is identified as being at risk for alcoholism, intervention can begin. Brief interventions are a good first step. To be successful, brief intervention strategies should include the following:

1. Combat patient resistance by maintaining focus on the relationship

Table 26–2. The FIND Alcohol Use Questionnaire (AUQ) (Circle the response that most closely applies to you.)

1. How often do you have a drink containing alcohol?

never	less than once a month	monthly	weekly	daily
(0)	(1)	(2)	(3)	(4)

   (If you circled the word <u>never</u> stop here—you are finished.)

2. On an occasion where you find yourself drinking alcohol, how many drinks will you typically have?

(1)	(2)	(3)	(4)	(5) or more

3. Have you ever awakened the morning after you have been drinking and not remembered part of the previous evening?

No	Yes
(0)	(1)

4. In the past 12 months, has anyone expressed concern about your use of alcohol?

No	Yes
(0)	(1)

5. In the past 12 months, have you gotten into trouble because of your use of alcohol?

No	Yes
(0)	(1)

6. In the past 12 months, have you driven a motor vehicle within one hour of drinking an alcoholic beverage?

No	Yes
(0)	(1)

7. Do you ever drink an alcoholic beverage on an empty stomach (without food)?

No	Yes
(0)	(1)

(Add up the numbers in parentheses ( ), reflecting the answer for each question. A score of 7 or more indicates an increased health risk from alcohol consumption.)

From The Florida Institute for Neurodevelopmental Disorders, 1997, with permission.

between the health complaint that originally brought the patient to the office and the patient's alcohol use, as revealed by the patient's responses on the Alcohol Use Questionnaire (AUQ) (Table 26–2). Avoid arguing. Remain tolerant of any denial or hostility. The more confrontational or directive the health care provider is, the more resistant the patient will be.

2. Be reassuring. Remind the patient that the problem has a genetic link (if the patient has a family history of alcoholism). Maintaining a supportive attitude will help a patient feel safe returning for follow-up visits, even after a relapse. If a relapse does occur, assure the patient that it will not disrupt the patient-provider relationship. Make honesty one of the ground rules for working together. The patient's desire to preserve the health care provider's trust can be

a motivating factor for the patient to return for follow-up even after a relapse. If a patient is not honest about reporting alcohol use, it is best to confront the patient and renegotiate the parameters of the relationship. A key element is to communicate unconditional positive regard for the patient.

3. Maintain the role of medical expert with knowledge to share about the potential negative health effects of the patient maintaining his or her current level of alcohol use. Share the data about what constitutes a heavy drinker. Most high-risk drinkers do not realize that their alcohol consumption is not "normal." Mention that the National Institute on Alcohol Abuse and Alcoholism (NIAAA) defines low-risk drinking as no more than two drinks a day for men and no more than one drink a day for women, with never more than four drinks per occasion.[1] Persuasive advice from the clinician is the cornerstone of effective brief interventions. The more the advice is integrated with health concerns, the greater is the chance of success with a brief intervention.

4. Help the patient to understanding that there are no safe levels of alcohol use for patients who meet the DSM-IV criteria for alcohol abuse or alcohol dependence, or for patients who are pregnant or are diagnosed with breast cancer or peptic ulcer disease. Total abstinence is the goal for these patients.

5. Be prepared for resistance and setbacks. There is no direct correlation between the severity of a patient's health risks from alcohol use and readiness to accept the importance of making a lifestyle change. It can be expected that most patients will initially express ambivalence or resistance.

6. When the patient indicates a readiness to attempt a lifestyle change, help the patient to establish realistic goals and strategies for reaching the goals. Patients will be more motivated to work toward goals that they themselves set, as opposed to following goals set for them by others. A written contract is often a helpful support tool, as is also a diary of daily alcohol consumption. Follow-up visits should be scheduled.[56–58a]

Alcohol consumption correlates directly with the number of brief intervention sessions. A brief intervention targeted on at-risk alcohol use is not the same as administering a single dose of medication to treat an infection. Repeated interventions may be needed in order to attain and maintain the patient's goal of sobriety. If the patient's alcohol abuse persists, brief interventions may serve as a springboard for convincing the patient of the need for more specialized treatment interventions.[56–58a]

When malnutrition is present, high doses of vitamins and minerals are not useful. However, when indicated, 50–100 mg per day of thiamine is adequate to prevent central nervous system damage from Wernicke's encephalopathy.[33] There is no convincing data supporting the use of benzodiazepines and hypnotics in alcohol rehabilitation.

Only about 5% of persons with alcoholism require intensive detoxification and withdrawal interventions utilizing medication.

The use of alpha-2 adrenergic receptor agonists, such as clonidine or guanabenz, and the use of beta blockers, such as propranolol or atenolol, are effective in suppressing symptoms of alcohol withdrawal. Clonidine at 0.2 mg t.i.d. is more effective than chlordiazepoxide (Librium) at 20 mg p.r.n. in lessening withdrawal symptoms, even in the first 24 h.[62]

Carbamazepine at 200 mg q.i.d. has also demonstrated superior efficacy to benzodiazepines for withdrawal symptoms and psychological distress. Carbamazepine is also useful for management because of its antikindling effects. The risk of thrombocytopenia is rare, and if it does occur, it will occur in the first 3 weeks of treatment. Stopping carbamazepine when a blood test demonstrates signs of thrombocytopenia will quickly reverse any hematologic side effects produced by the drug. There have been no documented cases of irreversible blood changes with this drug.[63]

Disulfiram, 250–500 mg, helps to increase abstinence and only rarely has been associated with serious side effects. Only about 25 cases of disulfiram-induced liver damage have been reported worldwide, compared to millions of doses prescribed without any adverse effects.[64]

Naltrexone, 50 mg daily, has demonstrated lower relapse rates in patients who receive concomitant cognitive behavioral therapy.[65, 66]

Delirium tremens (DTs) is an infrequent component of alcohol withdrawal syndrome. The DTs typically begin 2 to 3 days after drinking stops and subside within 1 to 5 days. When the DTs occur during withdrawal from alcohol, the clinician should watch for a concurrent medical condition such as hepatic decompensation, pneumonia, subdural hematoma, pancreatitis, or for bone fractures (due to dysequilibrium, and/or malnutrition secondary to alcohol use). The clinician should routinely screen patients undergoing alcohol withdrawal for signs listed in Box 26–3.

Box 26-3–SIGNS OF ALCOHOL WITHDRAWAL

- Agitation
- Anxiety
- Auditory disturbances
- Headache
- Nausea
- Disorientation
- Sweating
- Tactile disturbances
- Tremor
- Visual disturbances

If a patient is oriented and at least five of the other signs listed in Box 26–3 are absent, he or she can safely be managed without the need of specialized treatment.[67, 68]

Patient Education

The clinician can use brief interventions as "teaching moments" in which to address risk factors associated with the patient's alcohol consumption and to explore with the patient potential behavior change. Even a single 10-min patient education session about the risks of alcohol abuse can decrease alcohol consumption and its harmful consequences by as much as 50%. In fact, brief interventions that include offering patients self-help booklets have demonstrated the same efficacy, in terms of maintaining sobriety and avoiding relapse, as formal treatment programs.[69–71]

Prevention

The American Medical Association's guidelines for health care provider involvement in the prevention of alcohol-related disorders are as follows:

1. Recognize, as early as possible, through history taking and screening of patients, signs of alcohol abuse, medical complications from alcohol abuse, and dysfunction caused by alcohol abuse.
2. Match the patient's needs for ongoing assessment and treatment with the appropriate resources (e.g., abstinence support groups and/or more specialized treatment).
3. Assist patients to maintain sobriety and manage their withdrawal symptoms.
4. Provide patient education about the complications of alcohol abuse.
5. Assist the patient in formulating a plan for recovery and be available for nonjudgmental, ongoing support and medical management.
6. Involve the patient's significant others in interventions.
7. Ensure ongoing monitoring for the need for repeat referral, in case the patient relapses.[5, 72]

Acknowledging alcohol abuse and alcohol dependence as diseases rather than an indication of moral weakness legitimizes efforts to implement interventions.[73, 74]

Screening Recommendations

A useful tool for assessing a patient's use of alcohol is the Alcohol Use Questionnaire (AUQ). It can be given to patients for completion in the waiting room prior to seeing a health care provider[75] (see Table 26–2).

After completion of the AUQ a thorough medical, psychological, family, and social history should be taken. It is important to include questions about use of alcohol and other drugs by the patient's parents, grandparents, siblings, spouse or partner, children, and friends, as well as by the patient. It is also important to ask about a history of domestic violence, child abuse, treatment for alcohol abuse, driving under the influence (DUI), or other legal entanglements, and sexual history.[76, 77]

If the results of the AUQ indicate that the patient is at risk for alcohol abuse, consider obtaining a gamma-glutamyl-transferase (GGT) blood test to assess for liver disease. This test should not be used as a routine screening. Although GGT levels may be elevated in other conditions, such as hepatitis, pancreatic cancer, and diabetes, a rise in GGT levels has also been correlated with an increase in alcohol intake. Although GGT is an imperfect indicator of heavy alcohol use, it may be useful as a marker if the level is elevated.[78]

■■ NICOTINE ADDICTION

Pathophysiology

Addiction to nicotine involves the increased release of two central nervous system neurotransmitters: dopamine and norepinephrine. Nicotine ingestion stimulates an increased discharge of dopamine from the nucleus accumbens and of norepinephrine from the sympathetic ganglia. This discharge of dopamine and norepinephrine leads to a pleasurable response and reinforces the continuation of the behavior that produces the response.

The mechanism by which smoking causes cancer is the introduction of tars and other carcinogens into lung tissue. These foreign substances invade the lung tissue and precipitate a mutation within the DNA of lung cells. Some of these foreign substances confuse the body's immune system and deactivate the protein that normally recognizes and marks abnormal cells for destruction by the immune system.[64]

Pediatric Issues

Children exposed to cigarette smoke have a greater frequency of middle ear infections, lower respiratory tract infections, and asthma attacks than children not exposed to environmental tobacco smoke. One out of every five 17-year-olds attending high school in America smokes regularly.

Obstetric Issues

Two out of every three women who smoke cigarettes continue to smoke during pregnancy, either unaware of or in denial about the dangerous effect of cigarette smoke on the development of the fetal brain.

Geriatric Issues

Chronic obstructive pulmonary disease and emphysema can result from long-term cigarette use. In the diabetic patient, nicotine causes reduction of blood flow to the limbs. This contributes to death of tissue and eventual amputation if not corrected by abstinence from smoking. Individuals who stop smoking after age 70 will experience less wheezing, coughing, and sputum production and fewer respiratory infections than those who continue to smoke. Within 1 year after discontinuing smoking, the risk of myocardial infarction and coronary artery disease is cut in half. After 2 years of not smoking, the risk of having a cerebral vascular accident is significantly decreased. Compared to smokers who continue their habit, individuals who remain smoke free for 15 years can anticipate that they will eventually regain lung function similar to that of an individual who never smoked.[79]

Epidemiology

One out of every four Americans over the age of 18 smokes cigarettes daily. Cigarette smoking is responsible for one out of every five deaths in the U.S. In fact, smoking is the most modifiable cause of premature death in America. Close to half a million deaths annually are related to cigarette smoking.

Smoking accounts for approximately 150,000 cancer deaths each year. Annually an estimated 100,000 deaths from coronary artery disease and 20,000 deaths due to cerebrovascular disease result from cigarette smoking. Respiratory diseases such as chronic obstructive pulmonary disease and pneumonia account for over 80,000 deaths each year in America. Nonsmokers exposed to tobacco smoke have an increased risk of lung cancer; as many as 3000 deaths due to lung cancer per year may result from exposure of nonsmokers to "second-hand" cigarette smoke.[8]

Treatment Options

Nicotine chewing gum, patches, inhalers, and nasal spray have all demonstrated efficacy in helping patients to stop smoking. Proper instruction on the use of nicotine products is imperative in order for patients to use these products correctly. The use of bupropion (Wellbutrin or Zyban) has been found to be helpful to a significant number of patients. Evidence is ample that counseling and behavior modification combined with prescription nicotine products facilitates smoking cessation. Smoking cessation programs are more successful when the health care provider offers encouragement at each scheduled office visit.[80]

Patient Education

The value of encouraging smokers to stop should not be overlooked. Individuals who stop smoking by the age of 50 cut their risk of dying from a smoking-related cause in half. The cancers related to the use of tobacco, in order of frequency of occurrence, are lung, trachea, bronchus, larynx, pharynx, oral cavity, and esophagus.

Less frequently occurring cancers related to tobacco use include cancers of the pancreas, kidney, bladder, and cervix. Cigarette smoking promotes atherosclerosis and is a significant risk factor in myocardial infarction, coronary artery disease, and cerebrovascular and peripheral vascular disease. Research has demonstrated that counseling women on the dangers of smoking during pregnancy results in a significant decrease in smoking behavior during pregnancy. Providing patients with self-help materials, counseling them about the use of nicotine products to help break the vicious cycle of smoking, and encouraging them to select a "quit date" to stop smoking all tend to increase long-term abstinence.[13]

Helping all patients to avoid or discontinue tobacco use can best be facilitated by:

1. Using eye-to-eye contact while encouraging patients not to smoke
2. Providing verbal reinforcement about the dangers of using tobacco directly to the patient
3. Scheduling follow-up support visits to encourage continued abstinence
4. Posting signs in the office about the risks of tobacco use
5. Having self-help materials readily available in the office for patients to read and take home
6. Encouraging the use of medications to relieve withdrawal symptoms as an adjunct to counseling[4, 22]

Prevention

The clinician should take an active role in preventing health problems that stem from the use of tobacco products in both smoked and smokeless forms. Counseling children and adolescents to resist the social pressure to use tobacco produces should be considered a moral imperative.

Screening Recommendations

Clinicians often fail to discuss the problem of nicotine addiction with their patients. Even brief interventions (such as the technique described in the section on alcohol abuse) have been shown to be effective in helping patients to stop smoking. Use of tobacco products in both smoked and smokeless forms should be part of the routine history obtained from all patients.

ANABOLIC STEROID ABUSE

Pathophysiology

Anabolic steroids, synthetic forms of testosterone, promote the development of lean body mass by enhancing protein synthesis. When the body senses that it has too much of this hormone, it tends to shut down its own normal production of the substance. When this happens, serious health risks occur.[81]

Steroid use can result in many adverse effects such as elevated liver enzyme levels, angiosarcoma of the liver, hypertension and other cardiovascular diseases, trembling, severe acne, chronic halitosis, pedal edema, decreased testosterone production, decreased sperm count, decreased libido, impotence, increased low-density lipoprotein and decreased high-density lipoprotein levels, decreased glucose tolerance, rapid weight gain in the form of increased muscle mass, purple- or red-colored spots on the body, a jaundiced appearance, swelling of the lower extremities, an unexplained darkening of the skin, sudden onset of moodiness, or aggressive behavior.

Steroid use in men can result in enlargement of the prostate as well as in prostate cancer. Steroid use may cause accelerated male pattern baldness, testicular shrinkage, and gynecomastia.

The extended use of steroids can induce stroke and/or myocardial infarction. Since steroid use does not improve tendon strength, there is an increased risk of tendon rupture if muscles become too bulky for the tendons to support. In females, irreversible effects can include deepening of the voice, growth of facial hair, an increase in body hair to the chest, arms, and legs, thinning of scalp hair, irregular menstruation, breast shrinkage, and clitoral enlargement.[82]

The less obvious problems related to steroid abuse are psychological changes in personality caused by prolonged use. With initial use of steroids, the user experiences a euphoric sensation. However, with prolonged use there is an eventual lack of energy, mood swings, and increased irritability. These signs signal a withdrawal syndrome similar to that seen in other drugs of abuse. The use of androgenic anabolic steroids can impair judgment and lead to personality changes such as paranoia, to delusions of invincibility, and to suicidal ideation. The most pronounced sign of steroid abuse is displaying aggressive behavior that is often referred to as "roid rage." The most common psychiatric side effect of steroid use is major depression.[81]

Steroid use causes the body to retain salt and water. This water retention is what accounts for the "puffy" look that steroid users carry around the face, neck, and upper extremities. It is important to understand that steroid use does not enhance aerobic athletic performance or respiratory functioning, only anaerobic performance and the building of muscle strength. Although not everyone experiences life-threatening side effects from the use of steroids, these substances pose a very serious health risk to the average person.

Pediatric Issues

Approximately 7% of male high school students under the age of 18 use anabolic steroids either to enhance personal appearance or to improve athletic performance. Adolescent steroid users often use steroids in conjunction with other drugs of abuse. An irreversible effect of steroid use in young people is stunted growth because steroids promote premature closure of growth plates in bones.[81]

Obstetric Issues

Because of their masculinizing effects, steroids used during pregnancy may result in birth defects, especially in the unborn female.

Geriatric Issues

Management is not significantly affected by age.

Epidemiology

An estimated 300,000 people in America use steroids for nonmedical purposes. Though steroid abuse is much more prominent among males, a significant percentage of women athletes also abuse anabolic steroids. The injectable forms of steroids can carry an increased risk of contracting HIV/AIDS infection if the user shares needles with other users. Steroid abuse is most prevalent among adolescent and adult patients preoccupied with workouts and weightlifting. Since 1990 anabolic steroids have been a Schedule III controlled substance. The illegal possession and/or distribution of steroids is a criminal act.

Treatment Options

The primary treatment for steroid abuse is discontinuation followed by continued abstinence. Informing patients of the dangerous and potentially irreversible side effects may be all that is necessary to persuade patients to stop using steroids. It is important to inform males who abuse steroids that it may take as long as 3 years to reverse infertility problems resulting from use. Regular monitoring of hepatic function is vital in known users who refuse to discontinue use.

Patient Education

Scare tactics are not an efficient way to discourage steroid use. Education that includes discussion of the risk factors should be done in an objective and matter-of-fact manner. A key component is attending to the patient's underlying insecurity that has stimulated the obsession with steroid use. Most often the patient will have an as yet undiagnosed anxiety disorder, usually obsessive-compulsive disorder that is manifesting as a compulsion to use steroids. If brief office contact interventions are not successful, individuals who have been identified as steroid abusers should be referred for substance abuse counseling. The most successful approach is group counseling. The most effective group interventions include exercises where the participants actually practice drug-refusal role-playing. This is particularly important because the glamour of sports heroes who abuse steroids to gain fame and fortune can easily overshadow a patient's sense of commitment to discontinue use.[67, 81]

Prevention

When steroid use is discontinued, most of the increased muscle mass gained will disappear within 6 months because the intense workouts that usually accompany steroid use are usually not maintained. Because of this loss of muscle mass, relapsed steroid use is common. The best prevention of steroid abuse is to educate patients about the potential dangers of using steroids. The greatest effort should be made to dispel the myth that steroid use is harmless.[20, 81]

Screening Recommendations

Frequently, steroid use will be apparent in the young male athlete who has significant muscle bulk or in the female bodybuilder with a deep voice. Counseling these individuals can begin immediately. The counseling can commence as described in the preceding Patient Education discussion if there is an admission of steroid use. If there is no admission, a "generic" educational effort can be performed (e.g., tell the patient, "If you were to consider steroid use, the risks are. . . ."). Primary prevention can target groups of young athletes or coaches.

REFERENCES

1. National Institute on Alcohol Abuse and Alcoholism. The Physicians' Guide to Helping Patients With Alcohol Problems. NIH Pub.No. 95-3769. Rockville, MD, National Institute on Alcohol Abuse and Alcoholism, 1995.
2. Smith DE, Landry MJ. Psychoactive substance-related disorders: Drugs and alcohol. In Goldman H (ed), Review of General Psychiatry. Norwalk, CT, Appleton & Lange, 1992.
3. Friedman LS, Fleming NF, Roberts DH, Hyman SE. Source Book of Substance Abuse and Addiction. Baltimore, Williams & Wilkins, 1996, pp 109–137.
4. Institute for Health Policy, Brandeis University. Substance Abuse: The Nation's Number One Health Problem: Key Indicators for Policy. Princeton, NJ, The Robert Wood Johnson Foundation, 1993.
5. Dinwiddie SH. Genetic and family studies in psychiatric illness and alcohol and drug dependence. J Addict Dis 1993;12:17–28.
6. Institute of Medicine, Committee on the Future of Primary Care. Donaldson MS, Yordy KD, Lohr KN, Vanselow NA, eds. Primary Care: America's Health in a New Era. Washington, DC, Institute of Medicine, 1996.
7. Nestler EJ, Hope BT, Widnell KL. Drug addiction: A model for the molecular basis of neural plasticity. Neuron 1993;11:995–1006.
8. Karch SB. Drug Abuse Handbook. Boca Raton, FL, CRC Press, 1998, pp 307–538.
9. Widiger TA, Smith GT. Substance use disorder: Abuse, dependence and dyscontrol. Addiction 1994;89:267–282.
10. Grant BF, Harford TC, Dawson DA, et al. Prevalence of DSM-IV alcohol abuse and dependence: United States, 1992. Alcohol Res Health 1994;18:243–248.
11. McMicken DB. Alcohol withdrawal syndromes. Emerg Med Clin North Am. 1990;8:805–819.
12. Winger G, Hofmann FG, Woods JH. A Handbook on Drug and Alcohol Abuse (3rd ed). New York, Oxford University Press, 1992, pp 56–84.
13. Hyman SE. Molecular and cell biology of addiction. Curr Opin Neurol Neurosurg 1993;6:609–613.
14. Gardner EL. Brain reward mechanisms. In Lowinson JH, Ruiz P, Millman RB (eds), Substance Abuse: A Comprehensive Textbook. Baltimore, Williams & Wilkins, 1992, pp70–99.

15. Regier DA, Farmer ME, Rae DS, et al. Comorbidity of mental disorders with alcohol and other drug abuse. Results from the Epidemiologic Catchment Area (ECA) Study. JAMA 1990;264:2511–2518.

16. Anthenelli RM, Schuckit MA. Genetics. *In* Lowinson JH, Ruiz P, Millman RB (eds), Substance Abuse: A Comprehensive Textbook. Baltimore, Williams & Wilkins, 1992 pp 39–50.

17. Balfour WK. Psychotropic Drugs of Abuse. New York, Pergamon Press, 1990.

18. American Psychiatric Association. Diagnostic and Statistical Manual of Mental Disorders, Fourth Edition (DSM-IV). Washington, DC, American Psychiatric Association, 1994.

19. American Psychiatric Association. Diagnostic and Statistical Manual of Mental Disorders, Fourth Edition (Primary Care Version) Washington, DC, American Psychiatric Association, 1994.

20. Landry MJ. Overview of Addiction Treatment Effectiveness. Pub No.(SMA) 96-3081. Rockville, MD, Substance Abuse and Mental Health Services Administration, 1996.

21. Miller NS. Addiction Psychiatry: Current Diagnosis and Treatment. New York, Wiley-Liss, 1995, pp 71–80.

22. Sanchez-Craig M. Brief didactic treatment for alcohol and drug-related problems: An approach based on client choice. Br J Addict 1990;85:169–177.

23. Gerstein DR, Harwood HJ, eds. Institute of Medicine. Treating Drug Problems. Washington, DC, National Academy Press, 1990.

24. Center for Substance Abuse Treatment. Outpatient Treatment for Alcohol and Other Drug Abuse. Treatment Improvement Protocol Series, Number 8. DHHS Pub. No. (SMA) 94-2077. Washington, DC, U.S. Government Printing Office, 1994.

25. Gordis E, Archer LD, et al. Eighth Special Report to the U.S. Congress on Alcohol and Health. Bethesda, MD, National Institutes of Health, 1994.

26. Schuckit MA. Drug and Alcohol Abuse: A Clinical Guide to Diagnosis and Treatment, 4th ed. New York, Plenum, 1995, pp 55–117.

27. Fleming MF, Barry KI. Clinical overview of alcohol and drug disorders. *In* Fleming MF, Barry KI (eds), Addictive Disorders. Chicago, Mosby–Yearbook, 1992, pp 3–21.

28. Kahan M, Wilson L, Becker L. Effectiveness of physician-based interventions with problem drinkers: A review. CMAJ 1995;152:851–859.

29. Skinner HA. Alcohol/drug problems in primary care: Changing roles—changing practices. *In* Proceedings of the Secretarial Conference to Link Primary Care, HIV, Alcohol, and Drug Treatments. Washington, DC, February 26–28, 1992.

30. Sullivan E, Fleming M. A Guide to Substance Abuse Services for Primary Care Clinicians. U.S. Deptartment of Health and Human Services. Rockville, MD, DHHS Publication No. (SMA) 97-3139, 1997, p xvi.

31. Substance Abuse and Mental Health Services Administration. National Household Survey on Drug Abuse: Population Estimates, 1994. Washington, DC, U.S. Department of Health and Human Services, 1995.

32. Substance Abuse and Mental Health Services Administration. Percent of population with substance abuse, mental disorder, or both disorders in lifetime, age 15 to 54, 1991. *In* Rouse BA (ed), Substance Abuse and Mental Health Statistics Source Book, DHHS Pub. No. (SMA) 95-3064.

Rockville, MD, Substance Abuse and Mental Health Services Administration, 1995, p 37.

33. Lieber CS. Medical and Nutritional Complications of Alcoholism: Mechanisms and Management. New York, Plenum, 1992.

34. Helzer JE, Burnam A. Epidemiology of alcohol addiction: United States. *In* Miller NS (ed), Comprehensive Handbook of Drug and Alcohol Addiction. New York, Marcel Dekker, 1991.

35. McGue M. Genes, environment, and the etiology of alcoholism. *In* Zuchker R, Boyd G, Howard J. (eds), The Development of Alcohol Problems: Exploring the Biopsychosocial Matrix of Risk. NIAAA Research Monograph Series, Number 26. NIH Pub. No.94-3495. Rockville, MD, National Institute on Alcohol Abuse and Alcoholism, 1994, pp 1–40.

36. Aguirre JC, Del Arbol JL, Raya J, et al. Plasma beta-endorphin levels in chronic alcoholics. Alcohol 1990;7:410–441.

37. Cloninger CR. Alcoholism and alleles of the human D2 dopamine receptor locus. Arch Gen Psychiatry 1991;48:655–663.

38. Farrow JA, Schwart RH. Adolescent drug and alcohol usage: A comparison of urban and suburban pediatric practices. J Natl Med Assoc 1992;84:409–413.

39. Rouse BA, Carter JH, Rooriguez-Andrew S. Racial ethnicity and other sociocultural influences on alcohol treatment for women. *In* Galanter M (ed), Recent Developments. Vol 12, Alcohol and Women. New York, Plenum, 1995, pp 343–367.

40. Van Thiel DH, Galvao-Teles A, Monteiro E, et al. The phytoestrogens present in de-ethanolized bourbon are biologically active: A preliminary study in a post menopausal woman. Alcohol Clin Exp Res 1991;15:822–823.

41. American Medical Association. Alcoholism in the Elderly: Diagnosis, Treatment, Prevention. Guidelines for Primary Care Physicians. Chicago, American Medical Association, 1995.

42. Solomon K. Alcoholism and prescription drug abuse in the elderly: St. Louis grand rounds. J Am Geriatr Soc 1993;41:57–59.

43. Gupta KL. Alcoholism in the elderly. Postgrad Med 1993;93:203–206.

44. Gaziano JM, Buring JE, Breslow JL, et al. Moderate alcohol intake, increased levels of high-density lipoprotein and its subfractions, and decreased risk of myocardial infarction. N Engl J Med 1993;329:1829–1834.

45. Stinson FS, Dufour MC, Steffens RA, DeBakey SF. Alcohol-related mortality in the United States, 1979–1989. Alcohol Res Health 1993;17:251–260.

46. Van Gijn J, Stampfer MJ, Wolfe C, Algra A. The association between alcohol and stroke. *In* Werschuren PM (ed), Health Issues Related to Alcohol Consumption. Washington, DC, ILSI Press, 1993, pp 43–80.

47. Stoudemire A, Fogel B, eds. Alcohol and drug abuse in the medical setting. Psychiatric Care of the Medical Patient. New York, Oxford University Press, 1993, pp 139–153.

48. College of Family Physicians of Canada. Alcohol Risk Assessment and Intervention (ARAI): Resource Manual for Family Physicians. Ontario, Canada, The College of Family Physicians of Canada, 1994.

49. Blum K, Payne TE. Alcohol and the Addictive Brain. New York, Free Press, 1991.

50. Halvorson MR, Campbell JL, Sprague G, et al. Comparative evaluation

of the clinical utility of three markers of ethanol intake: The effect of gender. Alcohol Clin Exp Res. 1993;17:225–229.

51. Brown SA, Irwin M, Schuckit MA. Changes in anxiety among abstinent male alcoholics. J Stud Alcohol 1991;52:55–61.

52. Pichens RW, Svikis DS, McGue M, et al. Heterogeneity in the inheritance of alcoholism. Arch Gen Psychiatry 1991;48:19–28.

53. Gianoulakis C. Endogenous opioids and excessive alcohol consumption. J Psychiatry Neurosci 1993;18:148–156.

54. George SR, Roldan L, Lui Al, Naranjo CA. Endogenous opioids are involved in the genetically determined high preference of ethanol consumption. Alcohol Clin Exp Res 1991;15: 668–672.

54a. Galanter M, Kleber HD. The American Psychiatric Press Textbook of Substance Abuse Treatment. Washington, DC, American Psychiatric Press, 1994, pp 67–89.

55. Froehlich J, Zweifel M, Harts J, et al. Importance of delta opioid receptors in maintaining high alcohol drinking. Psychopharmacology 1991;103:467–472.

55a. Drummond DC, Thom B, Brown C, et al. Specialist versus general practitioner treatment of problem drinkers. Lancet 1990;336:915–918.

56. Merikangas KR. The genetic epidemiology of alcoholism. Psychol Med 1990;20:11–22.

56a. Bien TH, Miller WR, Tonigan JS. Brief interventions for alcohol problems: A review. Addiction 1993;88:315-336.

57. Mosier W. Alcohol addiction: Intervention strategies that work. Part II. JAAPA 1999;12:45–60.

57a. Charness ME. Brain lesions in alcoholics. Alcohol Clin Exp Res. 1993;17:2–11.

58. Virkkunen M, Linnoila M. Brain serotonin, type II alcoholism and impulsive violence. J Stud Alcohol (Suppl) 1993;11:163–169.

58a. Dube CE, Lewis DC, eds. Project ADEPT: Curriculum for Primary Care Physician Training. Providence, RI, Brown University, 1994.

59. World Health Organization Brief Intervention Study Group. A cross-national trial of brief interventions with heavy drinkers. Am J Public Health 1996;86:984–955.

60. Miller WR, Brown JM, Simpson TH, et al. What works? A methodological analysis. In Hester RK, Miller WR (eds), Handbook of Alcoholism Treatment Approaches: Effective Alternatives. New York, Guilford Press, 1995, pp 12–44.

61. Kushner MG, Sher KJ, Beitman BD. The relation between alcohol problems and the anxiety disorders. Am J Psychiatry 1990;174:685–695.

62. American Psychiatric Association. Practice Guidelines for Treatment of Patients with Substance Use Disorders: Alcohol, Cocaine, Opioids. Washington, DC, American Psychiatric Association, 1995.

63. Litten RZ, Allen JP. Pharmacotherapies for alcoholism: Promising agents and clinical issues. Alcohol Clin Exp Res 1991;15:620–633.

64. Lowinson JH, Ruiz P, Millman RB, Langrod JG. Substance Abuse: A Comprehensive Textbook, 3rd ed. Baltimore, Williams & Wilkins, 1997, pp 119–148.

65. Volpicelli JR, Alterman Al, Hayashida M, O'Brien CP. Naltrexone in the treatment of alcohol dependence. Arch Gen Psychiatry 1992;49:876–880.

66. O'Malley SS, Jaffe AJ, Chang G, et al. Naltrexone and coping skills

therapy for alcohol dependence. A controlled study. Arch Gen Psychiatry 1992;49:881–887.

67. American Society of Addiction Medicine. Patient Placement Criteria for the Treatment of Substance-Related Disorders, 2nd ed. Washington, DC, American Society of Addiction Medicine, 1996.

68. Maier W, Lichtermann D, Minges J. The relationship between alcoholism and unipolar depression: A controlled family study. J Psychiatr Res 1994;28:303–317.

69. Barnes HN, Aronson MD, Delbanco TH, eds. Alcoholism: A Guide for the Primary Care Physician. New York, Springer-Verlag, 1987.

70. Heather N, Kissoon-Singh J, Fenton GW. Assisted natural recovery from alcohol problems: Effects of a self-help manual with and without supplementary telephone contact. Br J Addict 1990;85:1177–1185.

71. Sobell LC, Sobell MB, Toneatto T, Leo GI. What triggers the resolution of alcohol problems without treatment? Alcohol Clin Exp Res 1993;17:217–224.

72. Morse RM, Flavin DK. The definition of alcoholism. JAMA 1992; 268:1012–1014.

73. American Medical Association, Council on Scientific Affairs. AMA Guidelines for Physician Involvement in the Care of Substance Abusing Patients. Chicago, American Medical Association, 1979.

74. Noble EP, Blum K, Ritchie T, et al. Allelic association of the D2 dopamine receptor gene with receptor-binding characteristics in alcoholism. Arch Gen Psychiatry 1991;48:648–654.

75. Babor TF, de la Fuente JR, Saunders J, Grant M. AUDIT: The Alcohol Use Disorders Identification Test: Guidelines for Use in Primary Health Care. Geneva, Switzerland, World Health Organization, 1992.

76. Mosier W. Alcohol Addiction: Identifying the patient who drinks. Part I. JAAPA 1999;12:24–42.

77. Winokur G, Cook B, Liskow B, Fowler R. Alcoholism in manic depressive (bipolar) patients. J Stud Alcohol 1993;54:574–756.

78. Persson J, Magnusson PH, Borg S. Serum gamma-glutamyl transferase (GGT) in a group of organized teetotalers. Alcohol 1990;7:87–89.

79. U.S. Department of Health and Human Services. The Health Benefits of Smoking Cessation: A Report of the Surgeon General (DHHS Publication no. CDC 9~841 6). U.S. Department of Health and Human Services, Public Health Service, 1990.

80. Fiore MC, Newcomb P, McBride P. Natural history and epidemiology of tobacco use and addiction. *In* Orleans CT, Slade J (eds), Nicotine Addiction: Principles and Management. New York, Oxford University Press, 1993.

81. Coldberg L, Bents R, Bosworth E, et al. Anabolic steroid education and adolescents: Do scare tactics work? Pediatrics 1991; 87:283–286.

82. Porcerelli JH, Sandier BA. Narcissism and empathy in steroid users. Am J Psychiatry 1995;152:1672–1674.

Resources Appendix

The Consumer Health Committee
of the Georgia Health Sciences
Library Association

* Chair: Jan LaBeause, MLS, AHIP, Interim Director, Medical Library and Peyton Anderson Learning Resources Center, Mercer University School of Medicine, Macon, GA (labeause.j@gain.mercer.edu)
* Carolyn M. Brown, MLS, AHIP, Reference Librarian, Health Sciences Center Library, Emory University School of Medicine, Atlanta, GA (librcb@emory.edu)
* Rebecca R. Fehrenbach, MLIS, SLIS, Head of Library Information Center, Robert B. Greenblatt M.D. Library, Medical College of Georgia, Augusta, GA (rfehrenb@mail.mcg.edu)
* Mary Fielder, MLS, AHIP, Outreach Librarian, Three Rivers Area Health Education Center, Columbus, GA (threeriversahec@mindspring.com)
* Pat Herndon, MLIS, Librarian, Noble Learning Resource Center, Shepherd Center, Atlanta, GA (Pat_Herndon@shepherd.org)
* Lee R. McCarley, MLIS, AHIP, Systems Librarian, Medical Library and Peyton Anderson Learning Resources Center, Mercer University School of Medicine, Macon, GA (mccarley.l@gain.mercer.edu)
* Roxanne M. Nelson, RN, MSLIS, Head of Public Services, Medical Library and Peyton Anderson Learning Resources Center, Mercer University School of Medicine, Macon, GA (nelson.r@gain.mercer.edu)
* Beth C. Poisson, MSLS, Branch Librarian, Multi-Media Center, Morehouse School of Medicine, Atlanta, GA (poissob@msm.edu)
* Annette J. Sheppard, MLIS, Health Sciences Librarian, Candler Campus of the St. Joseph's-Candler Health System, Savannah, GA (shepparda@st.josephs-candler.org)
* Lisa P. Smith, MLS, Outreach Librarian, Magnolia Coastlands Area Health Education Center, Statesboro, GA (lsmith@gsvms2.cc.gasou.edu)
* Rita B. Smith, MLIS, Rural Health Information Clearinghouse (RHIC) Librarian, Medical Library and Peyton Anderson Learning Resources Center, Mercer University School of Medicine, Macon, GA (smith.r@gain.mercer.edu)

* Kathy Torrente, MLS, AHIP, Head of Reference and Instructional Services, Health Sciences Center Library, Emory University School of Medicine, Atlanta, GA (libkjt@emory.edu)
* Linda Venis, AS, Library Services Manager, Kennestone Hospital Health Sciences Library and Cobb Hospital Medical Library, Well-Star Health System, Marietta, GA (Linda.venis@wellstar.org)
* Mia Sohn White, MILS, AHIP, Reference Librarian, Health Sciences Center Library, Emory University School of Medicine, Atlanta, GA (msohn01@emory.edu)
* Cathy Woolbright, MS/LIS, Director, Simon Schwob Medical Library, Columbus Regional Healthcare System, Columbus, GA (cathy.woolbright@crhs.net)

INTRODUCTION

Today's consumers are more curious and knowledgeable than in the past about personal health and the challenge of staying well. At the same time, increased access to the Internet and the subsequent explosion in publishing on the World Wide Web and commercialization of the web have made it more difficult than ever to keep up with accepted standards, new discoveries, and trends in health care.

Health care-related government agencies and reliable support organizations have been in existence for many years. Most of these groups have traditionally provided some patient education materials to consumers. Now the Internet has given these offices an additional outlet for educating the public and distributing information.

However, the Internet is also a place of business for thousands of self-styled "health care information providers." The lack of peer review and the absence of established standards for information distributed via the Internet have made it difficult for patients and consumers to separate fact from fiction. Recognizing *quality* health information becomes another challenge for the public and health care providers alike.

EVALUATING RESOURCES AND INFORMATION

Patients and consumers must be urged to evaluate all health care information they receive, whether in print or electronically. In evaluating any resource, the user must ask several basic questions:

* WHO is responsible for the content, and FOR WHOM is the information intended?
* WHEN was it published and how often is it updated?
* WHAT is the intent: Is it informational, educational, or commercial?

For a more in-depth discussion of guidelines and criteria, the reader is directed to the work of the Health Summit Working Group[1] and the document by Gale Dutcher from the National Library of Medicine.[2] In addition, the Health on the Net (HON) Foundation[3] is a resource dedicated to alerting Internet users to credible, reliable health information sites. Sites displaying the HON logo attest that the information provided is made available in accordance with the HON Foundation's HONcode principles. At the same time, Quackwatch, Inc.,[4] informs readers of resources offering questionable or fraudulent information.

Electronic Discussion Groups

Because the quality of health and wellness information shared through electronic discussions cannot be monitored or evaluated, specific on-line discussion or self-help resources have not been included in this Resources Appendix. Several reputable, well-established professional associations and support groups (e.g., Association of On-line Cancer Resources) sponsor discussion boards or patient forums at their web sites, and those are mentioned in the individual annotations for that group. In addition, there are a number of sites for locating public electronic discussions (Table Appendix–1). However, the public must remember to apply the same criteria for evaluating both printed materials and web sites. It is suggested that guidelines and archives be reviewed before joining a group and the following questions asked:

* WHO sponsors and/or monitors the group (professional health care association, self-help support organization, commercial enterprise), and FOR WHOM is it intended (see who provides information to the group, and, if health professionals participate, check their credentials)?
* WHEN have questions and responses been posted (is it an active group)?
* WHAT is the content and intent (does it address your needs)?

Search Services

The popularity of personal search services through an information broker seems to have waned as the Internet has become more user friendly. However, some consumers may express an interest in contacting a search service to prepare and deliver a package of information. Such services are available through a number of organizations. The reader is directed to an annotated list and discussion of these

Table Appendix–1. Web Sites for Locating Electronic
                    Discussion Groups

Another Net.
URL: http://www.another.net/

CataList. The Official Catalog of LISTSERV Lists.
URL: http://www.lsoft.com/lists/listref.html

DejaNews.
URL: http://www.dejanews.com

Egroups. Health.
URL: http://www.onelist.com/dir/Health/

HotBot. Usenet.
URL: http://www.hotbot.com/usenet/

List of Lists.
URL: http://catalog.com/vivian/interest-group-search.html

Liszt Select: Health.
URL: http://liszt.com/select/Health/

Lycos. Chat.
URL: http://clubs.lycos.com/live/ChatRooms/ChatHome.asp?Area=1

Webcrawler Health. Support Groups.
URL: http://www.webcrawler.com/health/support_groups/

Yahoo! Message Boards. Health & Wellness.
URL: http://messages.yahoo.com/yahoo/Health_Wellness/index.html

vendors in the *Consumer Health Information Source Book,* by Alan
M. Rees.[5]

RESOURCE COVERAGE

For each topic covered by a chapter in this handbook, a list of
resources for health care providers, patients, and consumers has been
compiled. Each subject area includes complete contact information
for recommended resources of three types:
1. Organizations, Associations, and Support Groups
2. Government Agencies and Offices
3. Other Web Sites (i.e., those sponsored by educational institutions
   or commercial enterprises)
   The United States government resources are usually divisions of
the Centers for Disease Control and Prevention (CDC), the National

Institutes of Health (NIH), the Department of Health and Human Services (DHHS) or the Health Resources and Services Administration (HRSA). The emphasis is on U.S. sites with free access, although some do require first-time users to register.

Disclaimer

All contact information and links were current at the time of publication. No direct recommendation, endorsement, or sponsorship of any of these sites is intended or implied. Patients and consumers should always consult their health care provider for information specific to their condition or question.

Acknowledgements

The researchers for each topic in this chapter were members of the Consumer Health Committee of the Georgia Health Sciences Library Association. The Committee thanks Beth M. Westcott, MLS, Network Access Coordinator at the National Network of Libraries of Medicine, Southeastern/Atlantic Region, located at the Health Sciences and Human Services Library at the University of Maryland, Baltimore, MD; Onnalee Henneberry, MS, Technical Information Specialist, CDC Information Center, Centers for Disease Control and Prevention, Atlanta, GA; Kay McCall, Librarian, Nicholas Davies Community Health Library, Piedmont Hospital, Atlanta, GA; and Katherine L. Tucker, Technical Information Specialist, CDC Information Center, Centers for Disease Control and Prevention, Atlanta, GA for their help.

GENERAL PREVENTIVE STRATEGIES
(Chapter I)

ORGANIZATIONS, ASSOCIATIONS, AND SUPPORT GROUPS

American Academy of Family Physicians (AAFP)
11400 Tomahawk Creek Parkway
Leawood, KS 66211-2672
Phone: (913) 906-6000
E-mail: fp@aafp.org
URL: http://familydoctor.org/
Familydoctor.org is AAFP's new patient education web site with Health Info

Handouts, AAFP Family Health Facts, and Self-Care Flowcharts excerpted from the AAFP *Family Health and Medical Guide*.

American Academy of Nurse Practitioners
P.O. Box 12846
Austin, TX 78711
(512) 442-4262
URL: http://www.aanp.org/
Addresses issues pertaining to nurse practitioner practice.

American Academy of Pediatrics (AAP)
141 Northwest Point Boulevard
P.O. Box 927
Elk Grove Village, IL 60009-0927
Phone: (847) 228-5005
URL: http://www.aap.org/family/
You and Your Family is AAP's consumer-oriented web site featuring information on car safety, immunization schedules, and SIDS prevention.

American Academy of Physician Assistants
950 N. Washington St.
Alexandria, VA 22314-1552
(703) 836-2272
URL: http://www.aapa.org/
Addresses issues pertaining to physician assistant practice.

American College of Nurse Practitioners
503 Capital Ct NE #300
Washington, DC
(202) 546-4825
URL: http://www.nurse.org/acnp/index.shtml
Addresses issues pertaining to nurse practitioner practice.

American Medical Association (AMA)
515 North State Street
Chicago, IL 60610
Phone: (312) 464-5000
URL: http://www.ama-assn.org/consumer.htm
Health Insight is AMA's on-line consumer health information for everyone in a searchable database with links to directories for locating physicians and hospitals.

American Nurses Association
600 Maryland Avenue, SW
Suite 100 West
Washington, DC 20024
(800) 274-4ANA
URL: http://www.nursingworld.org/
Addresses issues pertaining to the profession of nursing.

National Health Information Center (NHIC)
P.O. Box 1133
Washington, DC 20013-1133
Phone: (301) 565-4167 or (800) 336-4797
URL: http://nhic-nt.health.org

Helps public locate health information by referring questions to appropriate resource. Also prepares and distributes publications and directories on health promotion and disease prevention.

GOVERNMENT AGENCIES AND OFFICES

Centers for Disease Control and Prevention (CDC)
1600 Clifton Road NE
Atlanta, GA 30333
Phone: (800) 311-3435
URL: http://www.cdc.gov/
A wealth of information from statistics to travel to current health topics. Reliable site for health information and prevention guidelines with keyword search capability.

Federal Consumer Information Center
Department WWW
Pueblo, CO 81009
Phone: (719) 948-4000
Fax: (719) 948-9724
E-mail: catalog.pueblo@gsa.gov
URL: http://www.pueblo.gsa.gov/health.htm
Service of the U.S. General Services Administration that distributes full-text consumer information on health, exercise, nutrition, etc.

National Institutes of Health (NIH)
Bethesda, Maryland 20892
URL: http://www.nih.gov/health/consumer/
Although the primary NIH mission is focused on research, communicating research findings is also paramount to the purpose of the institutes. Most of the 25 separate institutes and centers under NIH provide public information for consumers and patients. The Consumer Health Information page is browseable by institute or subject.

OTHER WEB SITES

About.com: Health/Fitness
URL: http://home.about.com/health/index.htm
An ever-evolving index of useful Internet resources on health and fitness topics providing information and discussions for the consumer.

California Consumer HealthScope
URL: http://www.healthscope.org/hw/default.asp
Consumer information relating to health care from the Pacific Business Group on Health. This site offers information about preventive health care.

CAPHIS Web Sites You Can Trust
URL: http://caphis.njc.org/caphisconsumer.html
The Consumer and Patient Health Information Section (CAPHIS) of the Medical Library Association refers health care consumers to quality-filtered

links for health care information. Includes an annotated list of mega-web sites on a variety of topics.

Combined Health Information Database (CHID)

E-mail: chid@aerie.com

URL: http://chid.aerie.com/index.html

Database of health education materials including fact sheets, brochures, and audiovisual materials produced by health-related agencies of the federal government.

The Daily Apple. A Click a Day

URL: http://www.thedailyapple.com/

Free but requires registration. Wealth of information and services including "Family Health Records," "Health Checkup," and community boards for information and support.

Dr. Koop's Health and Wellness

URL: http://www.drkoop.com/wellness/

This section on Dr. Koop's page has many features and links to information on family health, conditions, and concerns, mental health, health tips, and many more. A good place to begin locating information on wellness.

Guide to Clinical Preventive Services

URL: http://odphp.osophs.dhhs.gov/pubs/guidecps/

This guide from the U.S. Preventive Services Task Force provides recommended preventive services for routine use. The second edition is available for downloading at this site as a text or PDF file. A link is also provided to the on-line searchable HSTAT (Health Services Technology Assessment Text) database at the National Library of Medicine, where this guide and many other documents are available.

HealthAtoZ

URL: http://www.healthatoz.com/

Searchable subject guide to Internet resources in health and medicine including web sites, mailing lists, and newsgroups.

Healthfinder

URL: http://www.healthfinder.gov/

Site hosted by U.S. Department of Health and Human Services that features keyword searching, hot topics, news, smart choices, and links to other databases. Some information is available in Spanish.

HealthGate

URL: http://www.healthgate.com/

Searchable web site for consumers that covers a variety of health topics. Includes an "Ask the expert column," a link to perform MEDLINE searches, JCAHO-approved patient education materials, and a link to Reuters Daily Health eLine.

Healthy Generations

URL: http://www.healthygenerations.com/

Site helps you establish a family medical record to better manage and understand your health and that of your family.

InteliHealth

URL: http://cgi.intelihealth.com/IH/

This joint venture of U.S. Aetna Healthcare and Johns Hopkins University distributes more than two million pages of branded, trustworthy, consumer-friendly health content covering hundreds of diseases and conditions. Major focus on prevention for consumers looking to better manage their health. Includes live forums and discussion boards.

Mayo Health Oasis
URL: http://www.mayohealth.org/index.htm
Well-known Mayo Clinic's consumer health web site. Includes news headlines, reference articles, drug information, age and topic specific links, and "Ask the Mayo Physician."

Medic Alert
2323 Colorado
Turlock, California 95381
800-432-5378
http://www.medicalert.org/
Information and ordering of Medic Alert bracelets.

Medical Matrix
URL: http://www.medmatrix.org
Requires free registration but provides professionally annotated links to medical information.

MEDLINE*plus*, Health Information
URL: http://www.medlineplus.gov
Consumer health database from the National Library of Medicine linked to selected full-text materials, association publications, dictionaries, and MEDLINE database.

NetWellness
URL: http://www.netwellness.org
Nonprofit consumer web site from the medical schools of Case Western Reserve University, the University of Cincinnati, and Ohio State University includes "Ask an Expert" service and the latest health news.

Stay Healthy
URL: http://www.stayhealthy.com
Site offers a diverse and comprehensive list of resources on health and wellness. Features links to daily and weekly health news headlines and stories. Contains "Centers" covering such topics as children's health, fitness, mental health, natural medicine, and many more. Site also provides drug information, keyword searches, calorie tracker, and tips to stay healthy.

Virtual Hospital
URL: http://www.vh.org/Patients/Patients.html
Service of the University of Iowa Health Care. Browseable and searchable Iowa Health Book of educational materials for patients and families with links to the library and other health sciences resources.

Wellness Web. The Patient's Network
URL: http://www.wellweb.com/
Membership required but free. Site provides a variety of topics listed in a master index with broad categories of conventional medicine, alternative/complementary medicine, fitness, nutrition, medical research, and more.

Wellness Web Community provides forum for exchange of information with other consumers and health professionals.

You First Health Risk Assessment
URL: http://www.youfirst.com/
Excellent 15-min assessment for creating your own health outlook. Tells how you can correct some at-risk problems, such as stress or high blood pressure.

ALTERNATIVE MEDICINE (Chapter 2)

See also Cultural Influence (Chapter 3).

ORGANIZATIONS, ASSOCIATIONS, AND SUPPORT GROUPS

American Holistic Health Association
P.O. Box 17400
Anaheim, CA 92817-7400
Phone: (714) 779-6152
URL: http://www.healthy.net/ahha/
Group for those seeking to enhance their health and well-being. Services include: help locating a holistic practitioner in your area, booklet on wellness, resource list of individuals, organizations and materials, self-help articles, and articles on holistic medicine.

Alternative Medicine Foundation
5411 West Cedar Lane, Suite 205-A
Bethesda, MD 20814
Phone: (301) 581-0116
Fax: (301) 581-0119
E-mail: amfi@amfoundation.org
URL: http://www.amfoundation.org/
Organization providing evidence-based research resources for health care professionals, and responsible, reliable information for patients and consumers. Includes HerbMed—an interactive, evidence-based herbal formulary, TibetMed—an information resource for Tibetan medicine, and Journal of Alternative and Complementary Medicine.

GOVERNMENT AGENCIES AND OFFICES

National Center for Complementary and Alternative Medicine
9000 Rockville Pike
Bethesda, MD 20892
URL: http://nccam.nih.gov/
Center within NIH that researches alternative medical treatments to determine their effectiveness and provides reliable information on those therapies.

Includes a site index, keyword search engine, and links to what is in the news. The Center also maintains the CAM Citation Index (extracted from NLM's MEDLINE database) and the Office of Alternative Medicine Clearinghouse, which disseminates fact sheets, information packages, and publications to improve public understanding.

OTHER WEB SITES

Alternative Health News On-line
URL: http://www.altmedicine.com
Directs readers to informative, credible sites on alternative (complementary) medicine, including nutrition. Advises readers to use critical thinking when interpreting information on alternative medicine.

The Alternative Medicine Homepage
URL: http://www.pitt.edu/~cbw/altm.html
Reputable sites ponsored by the University of Pittsburgh that promotes itself as a "jump station for sources of information on unconventional, unorthodox, unproven, or alternative, complementary, innovative, integrative therapies."

Ask Dr. Weil
URL: http://www.pathfinder.com/drweil/
Andrew Weil, a Harvard-trained doctor specializing in alternative medicine, mind/body interactions, and medical botany, offers a searchable consumer health information service at this site including an on-line 8-week program for improving one's health.

China-Med.net: Traditional Chinese Medicine
URL: http://www.china-med.net/research_center.html
Resource on traditional Chinese medicine including information on over 500 different herbs that can be searched in a number of ways.

HerbMed
URL: http://www.herbmed.org
An interactive, electronic herbal database of evidence-based information for professionals, researchers, and the general public.

The Natural Pharmacist
URL: http://www.tnp.com/home.asp
Science-based, easy to understand site for consumers and professionals covering conditions, herbs and supplements, drug interactions, answers from experts, and a list of resources.

Rosenthal Center for Complementary and Alternative Medicine
URL: http://cpmcnet.columbia.edu/dept/rosenthal/
Organization affiliated with Columbia University that researches the safety and effectiveness of alternative and complementary remedies and practices, and develops programs to promote wider knowledge, greater understanding, and credible scientific efforts in the field.

Your Spine
URL: http://www.yourspine.com/

Source for chiropractic resources on line, including basic information about chiropractic and what it entails. An interactive anatomy section provides consumers with information on parts of the body and problems that can occur. Other sections are geared to athletes, children, and nutrition.

CULTURAL INFLUENCES (Chapter 3)

Note: Includes consumer health and patient education materials in other languages. *See also* Alternative Medicine (Chapter 2).

ORGANIZATIONS, ASSOCIATIONS, AND SUPPORT GROUPS

National Alliance for Hispanic Health
1501 Sixteenth Street NW
Washington D.C. 20036-1401
Phone: (202) 387-5000
E-mail: alliance@hispanichealth.org
URL: http:// www.hispanichealth.org
The web site, Hispanic Health Link, focuses on the health, mental health, and human services needs of the diverse Hispanic communities.

GOVERNMENT AGENCIES AND OFFICES

Office of Minority Health. Resource Center
P.O. Box 37337
Washington, DC 20013-7337
Phone: (800) 444-6472
E-mail: info@omhrc.gov
URL: http://www.omhrc.gov/
Agency of the U.S. Department of Health and Human Services provides a national resource and referral service on minority health issues. Provides referrals and distributes multilingual materials.

OTHER WEB SITES

Ask NOAH. New York On-line Access to Health
URL: http://www.noah-health.org
Spanish and English site that provides high-quality full-text consumer health information that is accurate, timely, relevant, and unbiased.

Bilingual Patient Education Materials
URL: http://www.ncfh.org/pateduc/pateduc.html

A portfolio of low-literacy, bilingual presentations from the National Center for Farmworker Health, Inc.

The Black Health Network
URL: http://www.blackhealthnet.com/
A variety of minority health issues are addressed for African Americans. Includes a searchable database for locating health care providers.

Closing the Gap
URL: http://closing-the-gap.com/
On-line magazine dedicated to the exploration of multiethnic health care issues for a variety of populations; includes drug research and research on multiethnic health care, commentaries by experts in the field, and an event calendar.

Cultural Medicine
URL: http://medicine.ucsf.edu/resources/guidelines/culture.html
Very comprehensive, annotated links to cross-cultural sites as a part of the Primary Care Clinical Guidelines site targeted at the primary care physician.

CulturedMed
URL: http://www.sunyit.edu/library/culturedmed/
Resource center at SUNY Institute of Technology provides a resource of print materials and electronic databases dealing with culturally competent health care for refugees and immigrants. Contains links to relevant resources about refugees and immigrants for nursing students, health care providers, social workers, medical interpreters, and other interested people, and links to patient information in foreign languages.

EthnoMed
URL: http://www.hslib.washington.edu/clinical/ethnomed/
University of Washington site contains information about cultural beliefs and medical issues, as well as links to translated patient education materials.

Refugee Health
URL: http://www.baylor.edu/~Charles_Kemp/refugee_health.htm
Site sponsored by Baylor University contains information about health care beliefs and practices of recent Asian refugees to the U.S. The site addresses specific problems dealing with women's health, mental health, and religious issues.

Transcultural and Multicultural Health Links
URL: http://www.lib.iun.indiana.edu/trannurs.htm
Award-winning, annotated compilation of links by subject category including Government Offices, Religious Groups, Ethnic Groups, and Special Populations.

Transcultural Nursing. Diversity in Health and Illness
URL: http://www.megalink.net/~vic/
Site developed by two U.S. nurses to share their experiences and thoughts on the complexities involved in caring for people from diverse cultural backgrounds. Includes basic concepts and case studies.

DOMESTIC VIOLENCE (Chapter 4)

ORGANIZATIONS, ASSOCIATIONS, AND SUPPORT GROUPS

American Bar Association
Commission on Domestic Violence
740 15th Street NW, 9th Floor
Washington, DC 20005-1022
Phone: (800) 799-SAFE
URL: http://www.abanet.org/domviol/home.html
Provides referral information, technical assistance, violence statistics, and links to national agencies listing names and telephone numbers to call for assistance. This is a very comprehensive site and has a wealth of information.

Family Violence Prevention Fund
383 Rhode Island St., Ste. 304
San Francisco, CA 94103-5133
Phone: (415) 252-8900
Fax: (415) 252-8991
E-mail: fund@fvpf.org
URL: http://www.fvpf.org/
National nonprofit organization dedicated to the elimination (prevention) of domestic violence through public education, prevention campaigns, public policy reform, model training, advocacy programs, and organizing. Sponsors workshops and has publications for order.

National Clearinghouse on Child Abuse and Neglect
P.O. Box 1182
Washington, DC 20013
Phone: (703) 385-7565 or (800) FYI-3366
URL: http://www.calib.com/nccanch/
Consumer materials available on child abuse and neglect, sexual abuse, domestic violence, etc.

National Coalition Against Violence
P.O. Box 18749
Denver, CO 80218
Phone: (303) 839-1852 or (800) 799-7233
Fax: (303) 831-9251
URL: http://www.ncadv.org
A volunteer organization devoted to making every home a safe home. This site has information and programs on preventing domestic violence, along with links to other agencies and resources.

Prevent Child Abuse America
200 South Michigan Avenue
17th Floor
Chicago, IL 60604-2404
Phone: (312) 663-3520 or (800) CHILDREN
Fax: (312) 939-8962
URL: http://www.preventchildabuse.org/
Formerly the National Committee to Prevent Child Abuse, this organization's

programs consist of public awareness and education, national volunteer networks, technical and consultative services, primary prevention, and advocacy. Public awareness and education involve national media campaigns, publications, conferences, and workshops. Offers a variety of educational materials, including booklets, brochures, pamphlets, and bibliographies dealing with child abuse, neglect, and parenting. Some publications are available in Spanish.

Respond, Inc.
P.O. Box 555
Somerville, MA 02143
Phone: (617) 623-5900
URL: http:www2.shore.net/~respond/services.html
A not-for-profit organization that provides direct services to battered women and their children. The hotline is staffed 24 h a day by highly trained volunteers who speak Haitian, Creole, Spanish, Portuguese, and French. The staff provides information on legal issues, welfare rights, the courts, restraining orders, housing, and the names of other shelters.

GOVERNMENT AGENCIES AND OFFICES

Stop Violence Against Women
810 7th Street NW
Washington, DC 20531
Phone: (202) 616-8894
Fax: (202) 307-3911
URL: http://www.ojp.usdoj.gov/vawo/welcome.html
The Office of Justice Programs sponsors this site offering information on national laws and regulations that protect women from abuse and violence. Links to state hotlines, coalitions, and advocacy groups. Also provides model programs and information to communities and law enforcement to help fight violence.

OTHER WEB SITES

Domestic Violence, Family Violence, Child Abuse Page
URL: http://www.famvi.com
Site devoted to helping end all forms of family violence and to providing information about services available to families in need of assistance. Numerous links to local, regional, and national hotlines, including those for missing and exploited children.

Partnerships Against Violence Network
URL: http://www.pavnet.org
Maintains a virtual library of searchable information about violence and youth-at-risk, with data from seven federal government agencies to help reduce redundancy and provide one-stop shopping for states and local communities.

ENVIRONMENTAL HEALTH AND SANITATION
(Chapter 5)

ORGANIZATIONS, ASSOCIATIONS, AND SUPPORT GROUPS

American Environmental Health Foundation (AEHF)
8345 Walnut Hill Lane, Suite 225
Dallas, TX 75231
Phone: (214) 361-9515 or (800) 428-2343
Fax: (214) 361-2534
URL: http://www.aehf.com/
Nonprofit organization providing research and education into chemical sensitivity by providing information on environmental medicine to physicians, patients, and the general public. Also provides the public with access to environmentally safe products, and offers referral services to other sources of information.

Children's Environmental Health Network
California office:
5900 Hollis Street, Suite R3
Emeryville, CA 94608
Phone: (510) 597-1393
Fax: (510) 597-1399
District of Columbia office:
110 Maryland Avenue NE, Suite 511
Washington, DC 2002
Phone: (202) 543-4033
Fax: (202) 543-8797
E-mail: cehn@cehn.org
URL: http://www.cehn.org
Seeks to "promote a healthy environment and protect the fetus and the child from environmental health hazards," by educating health professionals, policy makers, and community members in preventive strategies, and raising public awareness of environmental hazards to children. Web site features *Resource Guide on Children's Environmental Health*, links to national and local organizations, sources of data and information on environmental hazards and health effects, and more.

National Safety Council Environmental Health Center
1025 Connecticut Avenue NW, Suite 1200
Washington, DC 20036
Phone: (202) 293-2270
Fax: (202) 293-0032
URL: http://www.nsc.org/ehc.htm
Goal is "to foster improved public understanding of significant health risks and challenges facing modern society." Web site provides resources for the general public, including information on air quality, climate change, lead poisoning, sun safety, and water issues.

GOVERNMENT AGENCIES AND OFFICES

Environmental Protection Agency (EPA)
Public Information Center, 3404 (PIC)
401 M Street SW
Washington, DC 20460
Phone: (202) 260-2080
Fax: (202) 260-6257
URL: http://www.epa.gov
Distributes nontechnical information to consumers and professionals on drinking water, pesticides, radon, indoor air quality, and recycling. Provides referrals to information resources and assists public with locating EPA technical documents. Some publications available in Spanish. Web site includes sections for concerned citizens, students, and teachers, as well as a "For Kids" section.

National Center for Environmental Health (NCEH)
Centers for Disease Control and Prevention
4770 Buford Highway NE, Mailstop F-29
Atlanta, GA 30341-3724
Phone: (770) 488-7000 or (888) 232-6789
Fax: (770) 488-7015
E-mail: ncehinfo@cdc.gov
URL: http://www.cdc.gov/nceh/
CDC component working to prevent illness, disability, and death from interactions between people and the environment, especially in populations that are particularly vulnerable to certain environmental hazards—children, the elderly, and people with disabilities. Web site includes links to fact sheets, brochures, and books, as well as the "NCEH Kids' Page." Spanish-language version of site is available.

National Institute of Environmental Health Sciences (NIEHS)
111 Alexander Drive
P.O. Box 12233
Research Triangle Park, NC 27709
Phone: (919) 541-3345 or (800) 643-4794
Fax: (919) 541-4395 or (919) 361-9408
URL: http://www.niehs.nih.gov/
Institute under NIH that conducts research on the health effects of environmental agents and the prevention of environmentally-related diseases, such as respiratory diseases, cancer, and lead poisoning. Provides an information clearinghouse for the public on the health effects of lead, radon, chemicals, electromagnetic fields, and other environmental conditions. Web site includes a map showing locations of NIEHS centers across the U.S., and links to on-line resources.

Toxicology and Environmental Health Information Program (TEHIP)
National Library of Medicine
Specialized Information Services Division
8600 Rockville Pike
Bethesda, MD 20894
Phone: (301) 496-6531 or (301) 496-1131
Fax: (301) 480-3537

E-mail: tehip@teh.nlm.nih.gov

URL: http://sis.nlm.nih.gov/tehip.cfm

Sponsors publications, responds to information queries, and develops interactive retrieval services in toxicology and environmental health. Web site has links to publications, tutorials, TEHIP databases, and other environmental health resources on the web.

OTHER WEB SITES

Airnow. Real Time Air Pollution Data

URL: http://www.epa.gov/airnow/

Site sponsored by the Office of Air Quality Planning and Standards with information about air pollution and what can be done about it.

Environmental Defense Scorecard. Health Effects

URL: http://www.scorecard.org/health-effects/

Lists chemicals that can cause cancer, harm the immune system, contribute to birth defects, or lead to other problems.

EPIDEMIOLOGY (Chapter 6)

GOVERNMENT AGENCIES AND OFFICES

National Center for Health Statistics

Division of Data Services

Hyattsville, MD 20782-2003

Phone: (301) 458-4636

URL: http://www.cdc.gov/nchs/

Premier site at the CDC for reliable health statistics, and the government's primary health statistics agency. Web site offers data on "health status, lifestyle and exposure to unhealthy influences, the onset and diagnosis of illness and disability, and the use of health care." On-line resources include information on "Top 10 Downloads," public use data files and documentation, state data, Healthy People 2000, and links to web sites of virtually every federal and nonfederal organization offering statistics about health care in the U.S. The "FASTATS A to Z" portion of the site provides brief statistical overviews and links to further statistics for over a hundred health topics.

OTHER WEB SITES

Health Statistics

URL: http://www.nlm.nih.gov/medlineplus/healthstatistics.html

This portion of the National Library of Medicine's MEDLINEPlus provides links to government resources, organizations, condition-specific statistics, and more.

EXERCISE (Chapter 7)

ORGANIZATIONS, ASSOCIATIONS, AND SUPPORT GROUPS

Exercise Research Associates
URL: http://www.exra.org/

Exercise Research Associates (ExRA) is a nonprofit research and consulting company that performs and disseminates the results of scientific research in the fields of health, fitness, sports medicine, and other related sport science and health disciplines. The primary area of focus is the epidemiology of sports injuries. This web site provides access to the results of research performed by ExRA staff, most of which has appeared in peer-reviewed professional publications. Articles are organized by topic or sport.

GOVERNMENT AGENCIES AND OFFICES

President's Council on Physical Fitness and Sports
200 Independence Avenue SW
Hubert H. Humphrey Building, Room 738H
Washington, DC 20201
Phone: (202) 690-9000
Fax: (202) 690-5211
URL: http://www.indiana.edu/~preschal/council.html

Program under the Office of Public Health and Science that promotes fitness and offers a number of publications, including *Fitness Fundamental: Guidelines for Personal Exercise Programs.*

OTHER WEB SITES

Exercise Site
URL: http://exercise.about.com/health/exercise/index.htm

This web site includes information on a variety of types of exercise for adults and children, exercise physiology, and the effect of nutrition on exercise. Learn to build a better exercise program. There is a forum where people can share their experiences and get support from others.

Fitness Jumpsite
URL: http://www.primusweb.com/fitnesspartner/

An annotated, categorized, and searchable directory of hundreds of fitness and health-related web pages and resources. There's also a library of full-text articles on topics including book reviews, managing weight, sports, martial arts, equipment for home gyms, resorts, and more. The Fitness Forum encourages interactive discussions of fitness topics.

Just Move
URL: http://www.justmove.org/home.cfm

American Heart Association site has fitness news and health facts, local and national fitness events, and an on-line forum for discussing fitness-related topics. You can also learn about your personal fitness level and use the on-line fitness diary to keep track of your own exercise activities.

Nutrio.com The Weight Loss Community
URL: http://www.nutrio.com/servlet/nutrio
In spite of the name, this web site includes a wealth of information on different types of exercise, including aerobics, walking, and sports such as basketball and golf. Each type of exercise has basic information about the sport, what muscles are used, helpful tips, how not to get hurt, and essential equipment needed. It has information on how to create an exercise program, cross training, and fat burning.

Workout.com
URL: http://www.workout.com/
This web site offers over 500 exercises with complete instructions including photos, tips, and video clips. It also has professionally designed training programs for general workouts as well as sports-specific regimens.

CLINICAL GENETICS (Chapter 8)

Note: Includes birth defects.

ORGANIZATIONS, ASSOCIATIONS, AND SUPPORT GROUPS

Genetic Alliance
4301 Connecticut Avenue NW, #404
Washington, DC 20008-2304
Phone: (202) 966-5557
Fax: (202) 966-8553 or (800) 336-GENE
E-mail: info@geneticalliance.org
URL: http://www.geneticalliance.org/
Builds partnerships to enhance lives of everyone impacted by genetics, is international in scope, links individuals to support groups, maintains a listserv, and puts out a newsletter.

March of Dimes—Birth Defects Foundation
1275 Mamaroneck Avenue
White Plains, NY 10605
Phone: (888) MODIMES (663-4637)
URL: http://www.modimes.org/
Maintains an on-line health library with information for consumers on having a healthy baby and an extensive list of fact sheets, including many on genetic disorders.

National Easter Seal Society
230 West Monroe
Chicago, IL 60606
Phone: (800) 221-6827
E-mail: info@easter-seals.org
URL: http://www.easter-seals.org/

This nonprofit, community-based health and human services provider is dedicated to helping children and adults with disabilities and special needs gain greater independence. The web site also includes information on early identification and intervention.

National Organization for Rare Disorders (NORD)
P.O. Box 8923
New Fairfield, CT 06812-8923
Phone: (203) 746-6518 or (800) 999-6673
E-mail: orphan@rarediseases.org
URL: http://www.rarediseases.org/
Nonprofit organization working toward the prevention, treatment, and cure of rare "orphan" diseases. Sponsors searchable databases of information about rare diseases, support organizations, orphan drugs, medical assistance programs, and grants.

GOVERNMENT AGENCIES AND OFFICES

Division of Birth Defects, Child Development, and Disability and Health
National Center for Environmental Health
Centers for Disease Control and Prevention
4770 Buford Highway NE, MS F-34
Atlanta, GA 30341-3724
Phone: (770) 488-7150
Fax: (770) 488-7156
E-mail: ncehinfo@cdc.gov
URL: http://www.cdc.gov/nceh/cddh/default.htm
Division of CDC's National Center for Environmental Health that seeks to promote optimal fetal, infant, and child development; prevent birth defects and childhood developmental disabilities; and enhance the quality of life and prevent secondary conditions among children, adolescents, and adults who are living with a disability. Branches of this division address birth defects and pediatric genetics, developmental disabilities, disability and health, and fetal alcohol syndrome. Maintains the Genetics Information Database, which provides current, on-line information on the impact of human genetic research on public health and disease prevention. Web site includes a site for children and bilingual materials.

National Center for Biotechnology Information (NCBI)
National Library of Medicine
Building 38A, Room 8N805
Bethesda, MD 20894
Phone: (301) 496-2475
Fax: (301) 480-9241
E-mail: info@ncbi.nlm.nih.gov
URL: http://www.ncbi.nlm.nih.gov/
Home of GenBank, a national resource for molecular biology information. Areas of emphasis include the Cancer Genome Anatomy Project, clusters of orthologous groups, Human Genome Resources, and Electronic PCR. The center creates public databases and conducts research in computational

biology, aiming at a better understanding of molecular processes affecting human health and disease.

National Human Genome Research Institute (NHGRI)
Education Coordinator
Office of Policy Coordination
National Human Genome Research Institute
National Institutes of Health
Building 31, Room 4B09
9000 Rockville Pike
Bethesda, Maryland 20892-2152
URL: http://www.nhgri.nih.gov/
Users' Guide to Genetics: The Medicine of the Future presents users with a new gene map of the human genome, with access to the Human Genome Project and an introduction to NHGRI. Includes a talking glossary of genetic terms and a special web resource for teachers, students, and anyone curious about genetics: *Learning Tools For Understanding Genetics and Genetic Research.*

OTHER WEB SITES

Genetics Resource Center
URL: http://www.pitt.edu/~edugene/resource/
On-line resource and starting point for genetic counseling-related information, including support and bereavement groups, and an extensive list of public information links.

Human Genetics
URL: http://www.who.int/ncd/hgn/index.htm
Human genetics guidelines from the World Health Organization (WHO) reside here and focus on ethical issues in medical genetics and genetic services, including criteria for screening and counseling. Includes news, publications, databases, country profiles, collaborating centers, and related sites.

Medical Genetics Brochure: What Is a Gene?
URL: http://www2.mc.duke.edu/depts/medicine/medgen/brochure.html
Duke University Medical Center publishes this easy-to-understand brochure for use by health professionals, allied health professionals, science students, and patients.

GERIATRICS (Chapter 9)

ORGANIZATIONS, ASSOCIATIONS, AND SUPPORT GROUPS

Alzheimer's Association
70 East Lake Street
Chicago, IL 60601

Phone: (800) 621-0379
URL: http://www.alz.org
Offers information, referrals, counseling assistance, help solving problems, and choosing care options.

American Association for Geriatric Psychiatry
7910 Woodmont Avenue, Suite 1050
Bethesda, MD 20814
Phone: (301) 654-7850
Fax: (301) 654-4137
URL: http://www.aagpgpa.org/
Provides a Consumer Corner with links to "What a Geriatric Psychiatrist Does," and "Mental Health Services and HMOs: 10 Key Questions." Brochures and referrals provided.

American Association of Retired Persons (AARP)
601 E Street NW
Washington, DC 20049
Phone: (800) 424-2277
URL: http://www.aarp.org
The AARP's site is loaded with information and links to address just about every need an older person may face. The site has many important links to health and wellness sites as well as links to legislative information regarding the elderly. The site also provides full-text access to the most current issues of *Modern Maturity* and the *AARP Bulletin*.

National Council on the Aging
409 3rd Street SW #200
Washington, DC 20024
Phone: (800) 424-9046
URL: http://www.ncoa.org/
A collaboration of organizations and professionals dedicated to promoting the dignity, self-determination, and well being of older persons. Information on advocacy and links to resources for senior citizens and their caregivers.

GOVERNMENT AGENCIES AND OFFICES

MEDICARE
Phone: (800) MEDICARE (633-4227)
URL: http://www.medicare.gov
The Health Care Financing Administration administers Medicare, the nation's largest health insurance program, providing health insurance to people age 65 and over and others with disabilities. The Official U.S. Government Site for Medicare Information is the searchable, consumer-oriented, multilingual site with large print and easy-to-read and understand information. The link to Health Information contains a wealth of information including a downloadable PDF document *Medicare Preventive Services to Help Keep You Healthy*.

National Institute on Aging
Information Center
P.O. Box 8057
Gaithersburg, MD 20898-8057

Phone: (800) 496-1752 or (800) 222-2225

URL: http://www.nih.gov/nia/

NIH agency that supplies publications (including Age Page fact sheets) on health topics of interest to older adults, the public, and health educators. Sponsors the Alzheimer's Disease Education and Referral Center (ADEAR), which indexes patient materials and supplies single copies.

OTHER WEB SITES

Aging Well Village

URL: http://agingwell.state.ny.us/

Health and wellness information (i.e., safety, nutrition, fitness, healing, medications) for those over age 50.

Geriatrics and Aging Online

URL: http://www.geriatricsandaging.com/ga_homepage.htm

This on-line journal is published in Canada, and though the primary focus is physicians who specialize in geriatrics, the articles are easily understood by the layperson. In addition, many colorful graphics help illustrate the articles' main points.

Merck Manual of Geriatrics

URL: http://www.merck.com/pubs/mm_geriatrics/

Published by Merck, the second edition of the manual is available free on the Internet and provides valuable information on etiology, diagnosis, and treatments in a searchable or browseable format.

SAFETY PRECAUTIONS IN AND AROUND THE HOME (Chapter 10)

See also Trauma (Chapter 14).

ORGANIZATIONS, ASSOCIATIONS, AND SUPPORT GROUPS

American Association of Poison Control Centers

3201 New Mexico Avenue, Suite 310

Washington, DC 20016

Phone: (202) 362-7217

E-mail: aapcc@poison.org

URL: http://www.aapcc.org/

Web site of this national organization of poison centers and interested individuals offers prevention tips and a directory of local poison control centers.

American Red Cross

Public Inquiry Office

431 18th Street NW

Washington, DC 20006

Phone: (202) 639-3520
E-mail: info@usa.redcross.org
URL: http://www.redcross.org/hss/tipgloss.html.
Offers health and safety tips on a variety of home safety topics.

National Fire Protection Association
1 Batterymarch Park
P.O. Box 9101
Quincy, MA 02269-9101
Phone: (617) 770-3000
E-mail: Public_affairs@nfpa.org
URL: http://www.nfpa.org
Nonprofit international organization dedicated to the protection of people, property, and the environment from devastating fires. Web site provides links to news, reports, safety tips for adults, and a children's fire safety site.

National Safety Council
1121 Spring Lake Drive
Itasca, IL 60143-3201
Phone: (630) 285-1121 or (800) 621-7615
E-mail: customerservice@nsc.org
URL: http://www.nsc.org/library.htm
Nonprofit organization dedicated to the prevention of unintentional injuries. The *On-line Resources* provides numerous consumer health fact sheets on topics such as crib safety, pesticides, and drowning prevention. Also an opportunity to join listservs.

GOVERNMENT AGENCIES AND OFFICES

National Center for Injury Prevention and Control (NCIPC)
4770 Buford Highway NE, MS K65
Atlanta, GA 30341-3724
Phone: (770) 488-1506
E-mail: OHCINFO@cdc.gov
URL: http://www.cdc.gov/ncipc/cmprfact.htm
Part of the CDC and the lead federal agency for injury prevention. Provides factsheets on injury prevention topics at this web site, as well as statistics, publications, and grant funding information.

United States Consumer Products Safety Commission
Washington, DC 20207-0001
Phone: (800) 638-2772
E-mail: info@cpsc.gov
URL: http://www.cpsc.gov
An independent federal regulatory agency that seeks to reduce the risk of injury or death from consumer products. See the Publications portion of the web site for consumer information on child safety, clothing safety, fire safety, holiday safety, and many other topics.

OTHER WEB SITES

Danger in the Home
URL: http://www.hud.gov/healthy/safehome.html

Web site from the U.S. Department of Housing and Urban Development provides short home safety checklists for each room in the house.

Kidd Safety
URL: http://www.cpsc.gov/kids/kidsafety/index.html
Points out prevention of injuries to children associated with consumer products.

National Crime Prevention Council
URL: http://www.ncpc.org
The National Crime Prevention Council strives to prevent crime and build safer communities. This site contains information on how to start neighborhood action plans, on-line safety tips, and other publications that can be accessed in English or in Spanish.

National SAFE KIDS Campaign
URL: http://www.safekids.org/fact.html.
Nonprofit organization dedicated to childhood injury prevention. Provides fact sheets on various safety topics.

Public Education Brochures
URL: http://www.acep.org/public/index.cfm/pid/13
Injury prevention and safety brochures from the American College of Emergency Physicians.

Safe at Home
URL: http://www.cdc.gov/safeusa/home/safehome.htm
SafeUSA is a nonprofit partnership of organizations and government agencies concerned with injury control. This portion of the web site provides numerous consumer health materials on prevention of falls, poisoning, and other home accidents.

Safe Within
URL: http://www.safewithin.com/index.cgi
Contains news and information relating to family safety, security, and health issues. Updated daily with top safety tips, it also includes hypertext links to resources and statistics on preventable deaths and injuries that occur in the home.

IMMUNIZATIONS (Chapter 11)

ORGANIZATIONS, ASSOCIATIONS, AND SUPPORT GROUPS

Immunization Action Coalition
1573 Selby Avenue, Suite 234
St. Paul, MN 55104
Phone: (651) 647-9009
Fax: (651) 647-9131

E-mail: admin@immunize.org

URL: http://www.immunize.org/

Promotes physician, community, and family awareness on immunizations of children and adults to prevent diseases. Contains free educational materials on child, adolescent, and adult immunizations and on hepatitis B that are available in different languages. *Needle Tips and the Hepatitis B Coalition News*, a semi-annual publication of this organization, is reviewed by the Centers for Disease Control and Prevention. Vaccine information statements are available in PDF format in 22 different languages, including English.

National Vaccine Information Center

512 West Maple Avenue, Suite 206

Vienna, VA 22180

Phone: (703) 938-DPT3 or (800) 909-SHOT

Fax: (703) 938-5768

E-mail: info@909shot.com

URL: http://www.909shot.com/

Nonprofit organization promotes and advocates changing the mass vaccination system in the U.S. Specifically for parents, site lists information on U.S. congressional hearings on vaccine safety and National Childhood Vaccine Injury Act of 1986.

GOVERNMENT AGENCIES AND OFFICES

The National Immunization Program (NIP)

Centers for Disease Control and Prevention

1600 Clifton Road, Mailstop E-05

Atlanta, Georgia 30333

Phone: (877) 394-8747

URL: http://www.cdc.gov/nip/

Part of the CDC that provides leadership in conducting, coordinating, and planning nationwide immunization activities. The web site contains a large number of educational materials and resources and lists the latest news in new immunization developments. Check the Information and Education Resource portion of the web site for consumer education materials on immunization and specific vaccines.

OTHER WEB SITES

All Kids Count

URL: http://www.allkidscount.org

A list of directories of vendors offering immunization registry software and support.

Allied Vaccine Group

URL: http://vaccine.org/

Composed of six web sites (Bill and Melinda Gates Children's Vaccine Program, Immunization Action Coalition, National Network for Immunization Information, Parents of Kids with Infectious Diseases [PKIDs], American Academy of Pediatrics, and The Vaccine Page) dedicated to providing unbiased scientific information on vaccines. This information is based on scientific evidence and can be used by the public or health professional. All members' web sites can be searched at one time.

Every Child By Two (ECBT). The Carter/Bumpers Campaign
URL: http://www.ecbt.org/
Nonprofit organization focused on timely immunizations to avoid infant mortality and to provide a systematic method of immunization for America's children by age 2.

The Immunization Gateway: Your Vaccine Fact-Finder
URL: http://www.immunofacts.com/
Authoritative site, sponsored by Facts and Comparisons and based on the book *ImmunoFacts: Vaccines and Immunologic Drugs*. Provides electronic links to sections of the book, and includes the lastest news on vaccines, vaccine information statements, state immunizations programs, grass roots, and professional support.

National Network for Immunization Information
URL: http://www.immunizationinfo.org
Sponsored by the Infectious Diseases Society of America, the Pediatric Infectious Diseases Society, the American Academy of Pediatrics, and the American Nurses Association. Mission is to provide scientific-based information on immunization issues for the public and the health professional.

Recommended Childhood Immunization Schedule
URL: http://www.aafp.org/exam/rep-520.html
A childhood immunization schedule for vaccines recommended by the American Academy of Family Physicians.

Vaccine Adverse Event Reporting System (VAERS)
Phone: (800) 835-4709 or (301) 827-1800
E-mail: octma@cber.fda.gov
URL: http://www.fda.gov/cber/vaers/vaers.htm
A cooperative safety vaccine program of the CDC and the United States Food and Drug Administration that collects information on adverse events from U.S. licensed drugs after their administration. This information can be reported by the public, pharmacists, doctors, and other health professionals.

Vaccine Page
URL: http://vaccines.org/
Provides very current news on vaccines and a searchable, annotated database of vaccine Internet sites divided into topics such as Adult, Practitioner, Parents, journals and organizations.

PATIENT EDUCATION AND LITERACY
(Chapter 12)

OTHER WEB SITES

Bilingual Patient Education Materials
URL: http://www.ncfh.org/pateduc.htm

A portfolio of low literacy, bilingual presentations from the National Center for Farmworker Health, Inc.

Easy-to-Read Publications
URL: http://www.fda.gov/opacom/lowlit/7lowlit.html
Bilingual, easy-to-read brochures on clinical trials, AIDS, child safety, nutrition, arthritis, heart disease, skin cancer, and other health concerns from the U.S. Food and Drug Administration. Viewable as HTML or PDF files.

Low-Literacy Patient Education Handouts
URL: http://itsa.ucsf.edu/~hclinic/handouts.dir/lowlit.dir/lowlit.html
Handouts from the University of California San Francisco Student Homeless Clinic cover wound dressing, STDs, teeth and gums, asthma, lice, and more. They are full-text, on-line, and easily modified for local conditions or organizations.

New Mexico AIDS InfoNet
URL: http://www.nmia.com/~hivcc/index.html
Bilingual AIDS and HIV fact sheets available at eighth or ninth grade reading level.

Patient Education Menu
URL: http://lib-sh.lsumc.edu/fammed/pted/pted.html
Extensive collection of on-line patient education materials from Louisiana State University Medical Center providing documents in 15 specialty areas for low and average literacy levels.

NUTRITION EDUCATION IN THE CLINICAL SETTING (Chapter 13)

ORGANIZATIONS, ASSOCIATIONS, AND SUPPORT GROUPS

American Dietetics Association
216 West Jackson Boulevard
Chicago, IL 60606-6995
Phone: (312) 899-0040
URL: http://www.eatright.org
Provides nutrition resources, daily nutrition tips, and a dietitian locater service.

GOVERNMENT AGENCIES AND OFFICES

United States Department of Agriculture
Center for Nutrition Policy and Promotion
1120 20th Street NW, Suite 200, North Lobby
Washington, DC 20036
Phone: (202) 418-2312
URL: http://www.usda.gov/cnpp
This site provides an interactive Healthy Eating Index, the 2000 Dietary

Guidelines for Americans, current and back issues of the newsletter *Nutrition Insights*, and information about the Food Guide Pyramid.

United States Food and Drug Administration
Center for Food Safety and Applied Nutrition
200 C Street SW
Washington, DC 20204
Phone: (202) 205-4850
URL: http://vm.cfsan.fda.gov/
Provides information on key topics including food labeling, food-borne illness, and disease-specific information. Also provides links to information from other federal government agencies.

OTHER WEB SITES

CyberDiet
URL: http://www.cyberdiet.com
Interactive site to identify the best diet for a "healthy lifestyle." Includes sections on nutrition, fast food, and recipes.

Delicious Decisions
URL: http://www.deliciousdecisions.org
Web site sponsored by the American Heart Association.

Kids Food Cyberclub
URL: http://www.kidfood.org
Designed to teach children about good food and nutrition with sections on growing food, recipes, and the food pyramid.

Nutrition Navigator
URL: http://navigator.tufts.edu
Tufts University nutritionists evaluate and rate nutrition web sites, including those especially for kids, parents, women, and those with special dietary needs.

ShapeUp America. Healthy Weight for Life
URL: http://www.shapeup.org/
Organization founded by C. Everett Koop, MD, includes information for the general public and health professionals about safe weight management and physical fitness.

TRAUMA (Chapter 14)

See also Safety Precautions in and Around the Home (Chapter 10).

ORGANIZATIONS, ASSOCIATIONS, AND SUPPORT GROUPS

American Trauma Society (ATS)
8903 Presidential Parkway, Suite 512

Upper Marlboro, MD 20772
Phone: (301) 420-4189 or (800) 556-7890
E-mail: info@amtrauma.org
URL: http://www.amtrauma.org/prevent/
Information on trauma prevention, education programs, and an excellent selection of related web addresses.

Brain Injury Association, Inc.
105 North Alfred Street
Alexandria, VA 22314
Phone: (703) 236-6000
Fax: (703) 236-6001
URL: http://www.biausa.org/index.html
Consumer-oriented site that promotes awareness, understanding, and prevention of brain injury through education, advocacy, research grants, and community support services that lead toward reduced incidence and improved outcomes of children and adults with brain injuries.

THINK FIRST Foundation
22 S. Washington Street
Park Ridge, IL 60068
Phone: (847) 692-2740 or (800) Think56
Fax: (847) 692-2394
URL: http://www.thinkfirst.org/
Mission is to prevent brain and spinal cord injuries through the education of individuals, community leaders, and the creators of public policy.

GOVERNMENT AGENCIES AND OFFICES

National Center for Injury Prevention and Control (NCIPC)
4770 Buford Highway NE, MS K65
Atlanta, GA 30341-3724
Phone: (770) 488-1506
E-mail: OHCINFO@cdc.gov
URL: http://www.cdc.gov/ncipc/cmprfact.htm
Part of the CDC and the lead federal agency for injury prevention. Provides fact sheets on injury prevention topics at this web site, as well as statistics, publications, and grant funding information.

National Institute for Occupational Safety and Health (NIOSH)
Hubert H. Humphrey Building, Room 715H
200 Independence Avenue SW
Washington, DC 20201
Phone: (800) 356-4674
Fax: (513) 533-8573
URL: http://www.cdc.gov/niosh/homepage.html
Division of the CDC responsible for conducting research and making recommendations for the prevention of work-related illnesses and injuries.

Occupational Safety and Health Administration (OSHA)
200 Constitution Avenue NW
Washington, D.C. 20210

Phone: (800) 321-OSHA (6742)
URL: http://www.osha.gov/
Office under the U.S. Department of Labor responsible for creating and enforcing workplace safety and health regulations.

OTHER WEB SITES

Computer Related Repetitive Strain Injury
URL: http://www.engr.unl.edu/eeshop/rsi.html
Includes section on prevention of repetitive strain injuries, with pictures showing the right and wrong ways to type or use a computer keyboard.

Information for Parents, Teachers, and Administrators
URL: http://www.nrahq.org/safety/eddie/info.shtml
Site sponsored by the National Rifle Association promoting gun safety through the Eddie Eagle program and offering a free brochure, *Parent's Guide to Gun Safety.*

Project Home Safe
URL: http://www.projecthomesafe.org
Sponsored by the National Shooting Sports Foundation, which distributes safety kits with free gun-locking devices for firearms owners in participating communities. Site provides links to safety information and education.

Public Education Brochures
URL: http://www.acep.org/public/index.cfm/pid/13
Injury prevention and safety brochures from the American College of Emergency Physicians.

SafeUSA
URL: http://www.cdc.gov/safeusa/
A nonprofit partnership of organizations and government agencies based at the CDC concerned with injury prevention and control at home, school, and work.

TIPP. The Injury Prevention Program
URL: http://www.aap.org/family/tippmain.htm
Injury prevention program sponsored by the American Academy of Pediatrics features a "TIPP of the Month" and a series of age-related safety sheets.

Trauma Org
URL: http://www.trauma.org/injury/index.html
Injury prevention site with links to international statistics, mailing lists, and a comprehensive list of U.S. injury prevention centers.

HEALTH PLANNING AND ILLNESS PREVENTION FOR INTERNATIONAL TRAVEL
(Chapter 15)

See also Immunizations (Chapter 11).

GOVERNMENT AGENCIES AND OFFICES

Traveler's Health
URL: http://www.cdc.gov/travel/
CDC site from the National Center for Infectious Diseases for U.S. travelers visiting another country. Contains information on recommended immunizations and basic preparations for safe travel. Includes other information on outbreak notices, traveling with children, and special needs travelers.

OTHER WEB SITES

Health. Pills, Ills, and Bellyaches
URL: http://www.lonelyplanet.com/health/
A humorous, irreverent site maintained by Lonely Planet with very useful links and helpful hints for travelers.

MedicinePlanet
URL: http://www.medicineplanet.com/home/
Dedicated to providing travelers worldwide with definitive, one-stop health resources before, during, and after any journey.

The Travel Clinic. On Your Return
URL: http://www.drwisetravel.com/return.html
Provides information on illnesses that may appear following travel.

Travel Medicine. MCW HealthLINK
URL: http://healthlink.mcw.edu/travel-medicine/
Medical College of Wisconsin's site addresses illnesses a traveler may encounter and the associated treatments. Licensed physicians dispense advice.

Traveler Health Concerns
URL: http://www.tripprep.com/concerns/index.html
Comprehensive index of consumer fact sheets on general concerns and travel illnesses maintained by Shoreland Travel Health On-line.

WOMEN'S HEALTH (Chapter 16)

ORGANIZATIONS, ASSOCIATIONS, AND SUPPORT GROUPS

American College of Obstetricians and Gynecologists
409 12th Street SW
P.O. Box 96920
Washington, DC 20090-6920
URL: http://www.acog.com
Premier professional group of women's health care physicians provides a number of consumer and patient education materials at its web site.

National Center for Education in Maternal and Child Health
2000 15th Street N, Suite 701
Arlington, VA 22201-2617
Phone: (703) 524-7802
Fax: (703) 524-9335
URL: http://www.ncemch.org/pubs/default.html
This research center at Georgetown University's Public Policy Institute provides a number of consumer-oriented materials on pregnancy and other aspects of maternal health.

National Osteoporosis Foundation
1232 22nd Street NW
Washington, DC 20037-1292
Phone: (202) 223-2226
URL: http://www.nof.org
Quality information on prevention and treatment for both health care professionals and consumers.

National Women's Health Resource Center
120 Albany Street, Suite 820
New Brunswick, NJ 08901
Phone: (877) 986-9472
URL: http://www.healthywomen.org
A nonprofit organization dedicated to helping women make informed health choices. It provides resources on dozens of health topics and includes information on disease prevention and wellness.

North American Menopause Society
P.O. Box 94527
Cleveland, OH 44101-4527
Phone: (440) 442-7550
URL: http://www.menopause.org
Nonprofit scientific organization devoted to promoting understanding of menopause and improving women's health through midlife and beyond. Web site includes extensive consumer resources, referral lists, news and educational events.

GOVERNMENT AGENCIES AND OFFICES

National Women's Health Information Center
200 Independence Avenue, Room 730B

Washington, DC 20201
Phone: (800) 994-9662
URL: http://4woman.gov/
Project of the Office of Women's Health of the U.S. Department of Health and Human Services. Site offers health statistics, access to on-line dictionaries and journals, information in Spanish, and a searchable database of organizations and publications on a variety of women's health conditions.

Office of Women's Health
1600 Clifton Road, NE
Atlanta, GA 30333
Phone: (404) 639-7230
URL: http://www.cdc.gov/od/owh/whhome.htm
Office at CDC that offers an overview of several women's health issues such as reproductive health, HIV/AIDS, violence, and tobacco use.

Osteoporosis and Related Bone Diseases National Resource Center
1150 17th Street NW #500
Washington, DC 20036
Phone: (800) 624-BONE or (202) 223-0344
URL: http://www.osteo.org
NIH information center sponsored by the National Institute of Arthritis and Musculoskeletal and Skin Diseases. Provides information to the public on osteoporosis, Paget's disease of the bone, osteogenesis imperfecta, and primary hyperparathyroidism.

OTHER WEB SITES

OBGYN.net—the "for women" section
URL: http://www.obgyn.net/women/women.htm
Commercial site with information on most aspects of women's health.

Women's Cancer Network
URL: http://www.wcn.org
Nonprofit organization sponsored by the Gynecologic Cancer Foundation that promotes preventing, detecting, and conquering cancer in women. Award-winning web site has a number of links to educational materials, scientific reports, and news.

Women's Health
URL: http://www.hrsa.dhhs.gov/WomensHealth/default.htm
From the Health Resources and Services Administration (HRSA).

Women's Health Issues
URL: http://feminist.com/health.htm
Comprehensive list of links to women's health pages from Feminist.com.

Women's Health Matters
URL: http://www.womenshealthmatters.ca
Canadian site sponsored by Sunnybrook and Women's College Health Sciences Centre to give women access to quality, timely, relevant health information. Includes support groups and on-line communities. Reader should be aware that site does include advertisements.

Women's Wellness
URL: http://www.womens-wellness.com/wellness.html
Site that addresses health issues of interest to women. The site has extensive information on breast and cervical cancers. Features include cancer research, discussion groups, inspirational stories, and e-mail for members.

MEN'S HEALTH (Chapter 17)

ORGANIZATIONS, ASSOCIATIONS, AND SUPPORT GROUPS

Men's Health Network
P.O. Box 75972
Washington, DC 20013
Phone: (202) 543-MHN1 (6461)
E-mail: info@menshealthnetwork.org
URL: http://www.menshealthnetwork.org
Promotes itself as "an informational and educational organization recognizing men's health as a specific social concern."

National Black Men's Health Network
250 Georgia Avenue, Suite 321
Atlanta, GA 30312
Phone: (404) 524-7237
Produces and disseminates educational materials, such as an educational brochure on AIDS titled "AIDS: You Can Protect Yourself" (available in English and Spanish).

National Prostate Cancer Coalition
1158 Fifteenth Street, NW
Washington, DC 20005
Phone: (202) 463-9455
E-mail: info@4npcc.org
URL: http://www.4npcc.org/
The National Prostate Cancer Coalition is an "alliance of prostate cancer patients and survivors, family members, medical groups, advocacy organizations, and caring individuals, dedicated to ensuring that adequate federal funds are allocated to help support promising prostate cancer research." Although not a medical organization, the NPCC web site provides links to cancer organizations, disease resources, U.S. government resources, and other related resources.

GOVERNMENT AGENCIES AND OFFICES

National Kidney and Urologic Diseases Information Clearinghouse
3 Information Way
Bethesda, MD 20892-3580

Phone: (301) 654-4415

URL: http://www.niddk.nih.gov/health/kidney/nkudic.htm

Collects and disseminates patient information on kidney and urologic diseases including kidney stones, incontinence, impotence, and prostate problems.

OTHER WEB SITES

Memorial Sloan-Kettering Cancer Center. Prostate Cancer

URL: http://www.mskcc.org/patients_n_public/about_cancer_and_treatment/cancer_information_by_type/genitourinary_cancers/prostate_cancers.html

Good overview of prostate cancer and provides answers to common questions, as well as diagnosis and treatment options.

National Men's Resource Center (Menstuff)

URL: http://www.menstuff.org/

Menstuff is an educational, nonprofit web site providing information on more than a hundred men's issues, including abuse, aging, circumcision, divorce, health, prostate, resources, sexuality, and more. An extensive collection of book reviews on topics of interest to men is available at the web site. The site has thousands of on-site men's book reviews and covers, men's resources and hyperlinks, and hundreds of men's events, periodicals, and groups.

New York Times Men's Health

URL: http://www.nytimes.com/library/national/science/menshealth/resources.html

Resources for a variety of specific health issues such as aging, AIDS, alcohol, arthritis, back pain, cholesterol, colorectal cancer, coronary artery disease, depression, diet and exercise, headache, prostate, smoking, sexually transmitted diseases, stress, and stroke.

PROACT. Prostate Action, Inc.

URL: http://www.prostateaction.org/

Provided as a public service to increase awareness about the early diagnosis and treatment of prostate disease.

Prostate Disease: Vital Information for Men Over 40

URL: http://www.afud.org/conditions/pd.html

Site sponsored by the American Foundation for Urologic Disease.

The Testicular Cancer Resource Center

URL: http://www.acor.org/diseases/TC/

A nonprofit organization devoted to providing information regarding testicular cancer to all interested parties. The web site offers a self-examination guide, lists of articles and on-line resources, questions to ask your physician, and more.

University of Pittsburgh Health Sciences Library. Men's Health

URL: http://www.hsls.pitt.edu/intres/internet_resources.html?page-18

Provides guide to sites on Internet for coverage of men's health issues.

Yale University Men's Health

URL: http://www.med.yale.edu/library/sir

Extensive listing of resources including associations, organizations, facts and information, magazines, and reference materials.

CARDIOLOGY (Chapter 18)

ORGANIZATIONS, ASSOCIATIONS, AND SUPPORT GROUPS

American Heart Association (AHA)
7272 Greenville Avenue
Dallas, TX 75231
Phone: (800) 242-8721
URL: http://www.americanheart.org
Offers a number of consumer-oriented fact sheets on diseases, conditions, treatments, recovery, and prevention (including the roles of nutrition and exercise). Addresses both heart disease and stroke.

GOVERNMENT AGENCIES AND OFFICES

National Heart, Lung, and Blood Institute Information Center (NHLBI)
Building 31, Room 4A-21
Bethesda, MD 20892
Phone: (301) 251-1222
E-mail: NHLBIinfo@rover.nhlbi.nih.gov
URL: http://www.nhlbi.nih.gov/
Branch of NIH that provides leadership in diseases of the heart, blood vessels, lung, and blood; blood resources; and sleep disorders. Web site includes a number of health information materials for patients and the general public.

OTHER WEB SITES

HeartPoint Home Page
URL: http://www.heartpoint.com/
Presents material for information, education, and entertainment. Designed to help the consumer understand the heart and heart disease. Contains health tips, news alerts, commentaries by health care professionals, and a guide to foods that are good for you.

Preventing Heart Disease
URL: http://www.acc.org/media/patient/chd/index.htm
Patient education site from the American College of Cardiology.

Recovering from Heart Problems Through Cardiac Rehabilitation
URL: http://text.nlm.nih.gov/ftrs/dbaccess/crpp
Site designed primarily for heart patients in rehabilitation that also has keys to heart health and risk factors for heart disease.

BONE AND JOINT DISORDERS (Chapter 19)

ORGANIZATIONS, ASSOCIATIONS, AND SUPPORT GROUPS

American Academy of Orthopaedic Surgeons
222 South Prospect Avenue
Park Ridge, IL 60068
URL: http://orthoinfo.aaos.org/
Your Orthopaedic Connection is a site specifically for public information and patient education. Includes fact sheets and brochures dedicated to specific areas such as the neck, shoulder, and foot. The articles give advice about how to prevent injury, how to alleviate pain, and how to prevent further aggravation of injuries. Some materials also available in Spanish.

American College of Rheumatology
1800 Century Place, Suite 250
Atlanta, GA 30345
Phone: (404) 633-3777
Fax: (404) 633-1870
E-mail: acr@rheumatology.org
URL: http://www.rheumatology.org/patients/factsheets.html
Patient-specific information from the ACR. Also includes links to support group information and maintains a research registry.

Arthritis Foundation
1330 West Peachtree Street
Atlanta, GA 30309
Phone: (800) 238-7800
URL: http://www.arthritis.org/
Contains valuable information about what the foundation is doing in terms of arthritis research and the latest developments in arthritis research. Many valuable health links are also available for the arthritis sufferer. For publications including those on fibromyalgia, call (800) 207-8633.

GOVERNMENT AGENCIES AND OFFICES

National Institute of Arthritis and Musculoskeletal and Skin Diseases. Health Information
31 Center Drive, MSC 2350
Bethesda, MD 20892-2380
Phone: (301) 495-4484 or (301) 496-8188
URL: http://www.nih.gov/niams/healthinfo/
An NIH Information Clearinghouse that serves the public, patients, and health care professionals by providing information, locating other information sources, creating health information materials, and participating in a national federal database on health information. Also sponsors the Osteoporosis and Related Bone Diseases National Resource Center that seeks to create an awareness of osteoporosis, Paget's disease, and osteogenesis imperfecta, and of the general possibilities for therapy. Includes some of the patient informa-

tion in Spanish. Maintains National Arthritis and Musculoskeletal and Skin Diseases Information Clearinghouse.

OTHER WEB SITES

Osteoporosis and Bone Physiology. Basic Prevention
URL: http://courses.washington.edu/bonephys/opprev.html
Site maintained by physician at the University of Washington "to educate physicians as well as patients about osteoporosis and bone physiology . . . that a patient is never too old to begin therapy aimed at decreasing the risk of osteoporotic fractures."

The Paget Foundation for Paget's Disease of Bone and Related Disorders
120 Wall Street, Suite 1602
New York, NY 1005
Phone: (212) 509-5335
Fax: (212) 509-8492
URL: www.healthanswers.com/Sources/nhc/homepages/pf/pf2.html
Serves patients with Paget's disease of bone, primary hyperparathyroidism, and other related disorders; and assists the medical community that treats these patients.

Southern California Orthopedic Institute
URL: http://www.scoi.com
Useful information about orthopedics for consumers with a major focus on patient education.

University of Washington Bone and Joint Sources
URL: http://www.orthop.washington.edu/
Public information for patients, families, students, physicians, scientists, and therapists, with links to informative articles and other orthopedic sites.

GASTROINTESTINAL DISORDERS (Chapter 20)

ORGANIZATIONS, ASSOCIATIONS, AND SUPPORT GROUPS

American College of Gastroenterology
4900 B South 31st Street
Arlington, VA 22206-1656
Phone: (703) 820-7400
Fax: (703) 931-4520
URL: http://www.acg.gi.org/acg-dev/patientinfo/index_patientinfo.html
Digest this! is the web site featuring patient education literature produced by the ACG.

American Gastroenterological Association Public Section
7910 Woodmont Avenue
Bethesda, MD 20814

URL: http://www.gastro.org/public.html

Patient education brochures, consumer magazine *Digestive Health and Nutrition,* directory of gastroenterologists, and links to other gastroenterologic information and news.

American Liver Foundation

75 Maiden Lane, Suite 603

New York, NY 10038

Phone: (800) GOLIVER (465-4837)

URL: http://www.liverfoundation.org

National, voluntary nonprofit health agency dedicated to preventing, treating, and curing liver diseases through research, education, and support groups.

Crohn's and Colitis Foundation of America, Inc.

386 Park Avenue South, 17th Floor

New York, New York 10016-8804

Phone: (212) 685-3440 or (800) 932-2423

Fax: (212) 779-4098

E-mail: info@ccfa.org

URL: http://www.ccfa.org/

Mission is to prevent and cure Crohn's disease and ulcerative colitis through research, and to improve the quality of life of persons affected by these diseases through education and support.

Helicobacter Foundation

P.O. Box 7965

Charlottesville, VA 22906-7965

URL: http://www.helico.com

Dedicated to providing the latest information about *Helicobacter pylori* and its diagnosis, treatment, and clinical correlations.

International Foundation for Functional Gastrointestinal Disorders

P.O. Box 17864

Milwaukee, WI 53217

Phone: (414) 964-1799 or (888) 964-2001

E-mail: iffgd@iffgd.org

URL: http://www.iffgd.org/

Nonprofit educational and research organization whose mission is to inform, assist, and support people affected by functional gastrointestinal disorders or bowel incontinence. Includes information on irritable bowel syndrome; functional diarrhea; functional constipation; bloating and gas; abdominal, pelvic floor, or anorectal pain; esophageal disorders and GERD; gastroduodenal disorders; biliary disorders; anorectal disorders and incontinence.

GOVERNMENT AGENCIES AND OFFICES

National Institute of Diabetes and Digestive and Kidney Diseases

31 Center Drive, MSC 2650

Bethesda, MD 20892-2560

Phone: (301) 654-3810

URL: http://www.niddk.nih.gov/health/digest/digest.htm

The NIDDK's health information section lists titles of lay-language and easy-to-read publications on topics covered by NIDDK. Maintains National Digestive Diseases Information Clearinghouse.

OTHER WEB SITES

Irritable Bowel Syndrome and Digestion Information
URL: http://www.digestioninfo.com/
Consumer information about the digestive system and diseases such as irritable bowel syndrome, acid reflux, and heartburn. Includes links to other GI resources.

Jackson Gastroenterology. Patient Education
URL: http://www.gicare.com/pated/e000001.htm
Site maintained by Jackson Gastroenterology Clinic of Camp Hill, PA. Emphasizes educating patients about their disorders with patient-friendly information on diseases, procedures, diets, and drugs. Adventurous individuals can review the "Gallery of Endoscopic Images," which shows and describes what the gastroenterologist sees in the GI tract.

INFECTIOUS DISEASE (Chapter 21)

See also Immunizations (Chapter 11).

ORGANIZATIONS, ASSOCIATIONS, AND SUPPORT GROUPS

Association for Professionals in Infection Control and Epidemiology, Inc. (APIC)
1275 K Street NW, Suite 1000
Washington, DC 20005-4006
Phone: (202) 789-1890
E-mail: APICinfo@apic.org
URL: http://www.apic.org
International nonprofit organization providing a consumer information site with information on various infectious disease topics for the public.

National Foundation for Infectious Diseases (NFID)
4733 Bethesda Avenue, Suite 750
Bethesda, MD 20814
Phone: (301) 656-0003
E-mail: info@nfid.org
URL: http://www.nfid.org/

Nonprofit organization supporting both professional and public education on infectious diseases. Includes fact sheets on prevention.

Parents of Kids with Infectious Diseases (PKIDS)
P.O. Box 5666
Vancouver, WA 9866
Phone: (360) 695-0293 or (877) 55-PKIDS
Fax: (360) 695-6941
E-mail: pkids@pkids.org
URL: http://pkids.org/pkidshome.htm
A group for parents who have children with infectious diseases for whom they try to find the best care and also offer preventive information so that other children will not develop these infectious diseases.

World Health Organization (WHO)
Avenue Appia 20
1211 Geneva 27
Switzerland
Phone: +00 4122 791 21 11
URL: http://www.who.int/health-topics/idindex.htm
World Health Organization page on infectious diseases.

GOVERNMENT AGENCIES AND OFFICES

National Center for Infectious Diseases (NCID)
1600 Clifton Road NE
Atlanta, GA 30333
E-mail: ncid@cdc.gov
URL: http://www.cdc.gov/ncidod/
Part of the CDC whose mission is to prevent illness, disability, and death caused by infectious diseases in the U.S. and around the world. Provide resources and information on specific diseases at their web site.

National Institute of Allergy and Infectious Diseases (NIAID)
Public Affairs Office
31 Center Drive, Room 7A03
Bethesda, MD 20892-2520
Phone: (301) 492-5717
URL: http://www.niaid.nih.gov/
Part of NIH that supports research in diagnosing, treating, and preventing infectious diseases. The Publications section of its web site provides fact sheets and links to resources on the most common infectious diseases.

National Prevention Information Network (NPIN)
P.O. Box 6003
Rockville, MD 20849-6003
Phone: (800) 458-5231
URL: http://www.cdcnpin.org

National reference service with assistance and current information on AIDS/ HIV, sexually transmitted diseases, and tuberculosis.

OTHER WEB SITES

Center for AIDS Prevention Studies. (CAPS)
URL: http://www.caps.ucsf.edu
Multilingual site based at the University of California San Francisco and committed to maintaining a focus on prevention of HIV disease, using the expertise of multiple disciplines, and an applied and community-based perspective within a university setting.

Communicable Disease Fact Sheets
URL: http://www.health.state.ny.us/nysdoh/consumer/commun.htm
Fact sheets on over 60 diseases from the New York State Department of Health.

HIV/AIDS Information on the Internet
URL: http://www.aegis.org
Promotes itself as the largest HIV/AIDS web site in the world and is updated hourly. Contains information on prevention, diagnosis, and treatment, as well as links to support groups. Sponsored by AEGIS (AIDS Education Global Information System) and funded by pharmaceutical companies and the National Library of Medicine.

Infectious Facts
URL: http://astdhpphe.org/infect
Fact sheets on many infectious diseases from the Association of State and Territorial Directors of Health Promotion and Public Health Education.

Kids Understanding AIDS
URL: http://www.westnet.com/~rickd/AIDS/AIDS1.html
AIDS handbook for middle school-aged children discussing prevention, transmission, symptoms, and treatment.

New Mexico AIDS InfoNet
URL: http://www.nmia.com/~hivcc/index.html
Bilingual AIDS and HIV factsheets available at an eighth or ninth grade reading level.

MENTAL HEALTH (Chapter 22)

See also Neurologic Disease (Chapter 25) and Substance Abuse (Chapter 26).

ORGANIZATIONS, ASSOCIATIONS, AND SUPPORT GROUPS

American Psychiatric Association
1400 K Street NW

Washington, DC 20005
Phone: (202) 682-6000
URL: http://www.psych.org/public_info/
Public Information site provides information on mental health issues including fact sheets, pamphlets, etc.

Center for Mental Health Services
Knowledge Exchange Network (KEN)
P.O. Box 42490
Washington, DC 20015
Phone: (800) 789-2647
Fax: (301) 984-8796
E-mail: ken@mentalhealth.org
URL: http://www.mentalhealth.org/
Site provided by the U.S. Department of Mental Health as part of the Substance Abuse and Mental Health Services Administration, the Center for Mental Health Services (CMHS) Knowledge Exchange Network (KEN) provides information about mental health via a toll-free telephone number, a web site, and more than 200 publications. Web site features a publications catalog, consumer/survivor information, Spanish-language resources, links to databases of mental health information, and resources for children.

Mental Health Net (MHN)
570 Metro Place North
Dublin, OH 43017
Phone: (614) 764-0143 or (800) 467-1482
Fax: (614) 764-0362
E-mail: Webmaster@cmhc.com
URL: http://www.mhnet.org/ or http://mentalhelp.net
Comprehensive guide to mental health on line, featuring three sections: Disorders and Treatments; Professional Resources; and a Reading Room, with articles from news sources, professional journals, and patient education materials. The site lists more than 3500 resources. MHN is directed by Mark Dombeck, PhD, a clinical psychologist. One of the oldest, most comprehensive sites, with behavioral health information on the web. This site includes basic information on disorders and treatments, links to professional organizations and associations, and full textbooks and articles on mental health. Includes chat rooms and support forums.

National Alliance for the Mentally Ill (NAMI)
Colonial Place Three
2107 Wilson Boulevard, Suite 300
Arlington, VA 22201-3042
Phone: (703) 524-7600 or (800) 950-NAMI (6264)
Fax: (703) 524-9094
URL: http://www.nami.org/
Mission is "to eradicate mental illness and improve the quality of life of those affected by these diseases." Maintains a directory of more than 1000 state and local affiliates. The helpline provides information, support, and referral services to persons who have questions about or are affected by mental illness. Web site features a book store, reviews of books on mental health topics, information about a free education program for families, and more.

National Center for PTSD
VA Medical Center, Room 116D
White River Junction, VT 05009
Phone: (802) 296-5132
Fax: (802) 296-5135
URL: http://www.ncptsd.org/
National Center for PTSD (posttraumatic stress disorder) is a program of the
U.S. Department of Veterans Affairs and conducts a range of activities in
research, training, and public information. Web site features information for
veterans and their families, trauma survivors, and women, among others. A
link to the PILOTS database, an index to the worldwide literature on
traumatic stress, is available from the site. The Center maintains a collection
of copies of every publication indexed in the PILOTS database.

National Mental Health Association (NMHA)
1021 Prince Street
Alexandria, VA 22314-2971
Phone: (703) 684-7722 or (800) 969-NMHA (6642)
Fax: (703) 684-5968
URL: http://www.nmha.org/
Goals are "spreading tolerance and awareness, improving mental health services, preventing mental illness, and promoting mental health." The organization provides mental health news, legislative alerts, pamphlets, books, news-
letters, free fact sheets, and other educational materials. The web site has a
searchable database that can be used to find the nearest affiliate, and
provides an information center of mental health resources.

GOVERNMENT AGENCIES AND OFFICES

National Institute of Mental Health (NIMH)
Public Inquiries
6001 Executive Boulevard, Room 8184, MSC 9663
Bethesda, MD 20892-9663
Phone: (301) 443-4513
Fax: (301) 443-4279
E-mail: nimhinfo@nih.gov
URL: http://www.nimh.nih.gov/
Part of NIH that provides information to help people better understand mental
health and mental disorders. Web site features a For the Public section that
has the latest information from NIMH about the symptoms, diagnosis, and
treatment of various mental illnesses. Included are brochures and informa-
tion sheets, reports, press releases, fact sheets, and other educational materials.

OTHER WEB SITES

Healthy People 2010 Resource Directory for Mental Health
URL: http://www.mentalhealth.org/information/resources.htm
Full-text directory of mental health resources by category.

Internet Mental Health
URL: http://www.mentalhealth.com/fr01.html
Free encyclopedia of behavioral health information. The site contains information on 52 of the most common mental disorders, diagnostic information, and information on 65 psychiatric medications.

Mental Health Consumer
URL: http://www.athealth.com/Consumer/Consumer.html
Sponsored by At He@lth.com and provides behavioral health care information about conditions and disorders, articles and important issues, and mental health medications, and focuses on promoting healthy behaviors and sound emotional health.

Psych Central: Dr. John Grohol's Mental Health Page
URL: http://psychcentral.com/
Maintained by Dr. John Grohol, PsyD, Psych Central is an annotated guide to the most useful web sites, newsgroups, and mailing lists on line today in mental health, psychology, social work, and psychiatry. More than 1200 resources are indexed by broad category.

METABOLIC CONDITIONS (Chapter 23)

ORGANIZATIONS, ASSOCIATIONS, AND SUPPORT GROUPS

American Association of Diabetes Educators
100 West Monroe Street
Fourth Floor
Chicago, IL 60603-1901
Phone: (312) 424-2426
http://www.aadenet.org/
The AADE is a multidisciplinary organization representing any and all health care professionals who provide diabetes education and care. Web site includes links to research.

American Diabetes Association
National Service Center
1660 Duke Street
Alexandria, VA 22314
Phone: (800) DIABETES
URL: http://www.diabetes.org/ada/diabetesinfo.asp
Information includes complications and treatment, living with diabetes, and advice for the newly diagnosed. Some Spanish language materials also.

American Foundation of Thyroid Patients
P.O. Box 820195
Houston, TX 77282-0195
Phone: (281) 496-4460 or (888) 996-4460
E-mail: thyroid@flash.net
URL: http://www.thyroidfoundation.org

Nonprofit organization for the awareness, education, and support of thyroid patients, their family members, health care providers, and interested parties. Features support/interest groups, low-cost public thyroid disease screenings, educational information/seminars, and thyroid physician referrals.

Cushing's Support and Research Foundation, Inc.
65 East India Row 22B
Boston, MA 02110
Phone: (617) 723-3824 or (617) 723-3674
URL: http://world.std.com/~csrf/
Provides information and support for patients along with expert medical advice from physicians.

Hypoglycemia Support Foundation, Inc.
3822 NW 122nd Terrace
Sunrise, FL 33323
Phone: (954) 742-3098
URL: http://www.hypoglycemia.org
Seeks to inform, support, and encourage people with hypoglycemia about diet and hypoglycemia.

National Adrenal Diseases Foundation
505 Northern Boulevard, Suite 200
Great Neck, NY 11021
Phone: (516) 487-4992
URL: http://medhelp.org/www/nadf.htm
Provides a national self-help network for educational and emotional support for patients and their families.

Thyroid Foundation of America, Inc.
Room 350, Ruth Sleeper Hall
40 Parkman Street
Boston, MA 02114-2698
Phone: (617) 726-8500 or 1-800-832-8321
E-mail: info@tsh.org
URL: http://www.tsh.org
Provides public education programs, patient information, and support.

The Thyroid Society for Education and Research
7515 South Main Street, Suite 545
Houston, TX 77030
Phone: (713) 799-9909 or (800) THYROID
URL: http://www.the-thyroid-society.org
Pursues the prevention, treatment, and cure of thyroid disease and engages in patient, physician, and community education.

GOVERNMENT AGENCIES AND OFFICES

National Institute of Diabetes and Digestive and Kidney Diseases (NIDDK)
31 Center Drive, MSC 2650
Bethesda, MD 20892-2560

Phone: (301) 654-3810
URL: http://www.niddk.nih.gov/health/health.htm
Patient information on diabetes, endocrine disorders, and metabolic diseases among others. Some Spanish language patient education also. Also includes links to statistics, organizations, and the National Diabetes Information Clearinghouse.

OTHER WEB SITES

Endocrine Web
URL: http://www.endocrineweb.com/
Web site devoted to thyroid, parathyroid, adrenal, and pancreas disorders, diabetes, and osteoporosis. The information is intended for the education of patients and their families. Pages are added approximately twice weekly and include information on endocrine disease, hormone problems, and treatment options, including all types of thyroid, parathyroid, and adrenal surgery.

Organizations for Endocrine and Metabolic Diseases
URL: http://www.niddk.nih.gov/health/endo/pubs/endorg/endorg.htm
Extensive list of information on nonprofit service, support, education, and advocacy groups that serve the public. Site is maintained by NIDDK.

Joslin Diabetes Center
URL: http://www.joslin.harvard.edu/education/library/index.html
General and nutritional information for diabetic patients and their families.

NEOPLASTIC CONDITIONS (Chapter 24)

ORGANIZATIONS, ASSOCIATIONS, AND SUPPORT GROUPS

American Cancer Society
1599 Clifton Road NE
Atlanta, GA 30329
Phone: (800) 227-2345
URL: http://www.cancer.org/
Highlights recent research, statistics, publications, and prevention, making it a good site for patients and families afflicted with cancer. An interactive bulletin board offers answers on prostate cancer. Includes link to Cancer Statistics. Spanish option available.

GOVERNMENT AGENCIES AND OFFICES

National Cancer Institute (NCI)
Office of Cancer Communications
9000 Rockville Pike

Building 31, Room 10A24
Bethesda, MD 20892
Phone: (800) 4-CANCER
URL: http://cancernet.nci.nih.gov/
Sponsored by the U.S. government's principal agency for cancer research and training information, CancerNet has information on types of cancer, treatment, testing for cancer, prevention, coping with cancer, supportive care, genetics, complementary and alternative medicine, and publications. Also links to related programs, e.g., Clinical Cancer Trials, CANCERLIT, and Cancer Genetics Services Directory.

OTHER WEB SITES

Association of Online Cancer Resources
URL: http://www.acor.org/
Pulls oncology resources together. Search or browse electronic mailing lists specifically designed to be public on-line support groups and a variety of unique web sites created by patients, their supporters, cancer advocacy organizations, or professional organizations.

Cancer Care, Inc.
URL: http://www.cancercare.org/
Extensive on-line and telephone resources for cancer care, including counseling and emotional support, information about cancer and treatment, referrals to support services, educational services and materials, financial support, and professional consultations and educational programs. Provides a special section with information on the major cancers, cancer-related pain and fatigue, and health policy advocacy. Users can listen to RealAudio educational programs through teleconference and participate in on-line or telephone support groups. Searchable by concepts or keywords. Index included. Spanish option available.

National Center for Complementary and Alternative Medicine (NCCAM)
Phone: (800) NIHNCAM
URL: http://NCCAM.NIH.gov/NCCAM/
NCCAM is dedicated to investigating the effectiveness of alternative/complementary therapies and includes a link to The Cancer Advisory Panel for Complementary and Alternative Medicine.

OncoLink
URL: http://cancer.med.upenn.edu/
Comprehensive resource from the University of Pennsylvania includes a well-maintained resource list on cancer causes, screening, and prevention.

University of Texas, M.D. Anderson Cancer Center
1515 Holcombe Blvd.
Houston, TX 77030
Phone: (800) 392-1611
713-792-6161
URL: www.mdanderson.org
Links to information on various cancer types. Includes information for professionals treating cancer patients, clinical trials, and prevention. Easy to navigate.

NEUROLOGIC DISEASE (Chapter 25)

ORGANIZATIONS, ASSOCIATIONS, AND SUPPORT GROUPS

American Academy of Neurology
1080 Montreal Avenue
St. Paul, MN 55116
Phone: (651) 695-1940
URL: http://www.aan.com/
Offers an A-Z library of Patient Information Guides for Neurology from acoustic neuroma to Wilson's disease.

American Association of Neurological Surgeons
22 South Washington Street
Park Ridge, IL 60068-4287
Phone: (847) 692-9500 or (888) 566-AANS
Fax: (847) 692-2589
URL: http://www.neurosurgery.org/health/patient/index.asp
Neurosurgery On-Call, the official web site, provides information for patients and professionals on neurologic topics.

American Council for Headache Education (ACHE)
19 Mantua Road
Mt. Royal, NJ 08061
Phone: (856) 423-0258
Fax: (856) 423-0082
URL: http://www.achenet.org/
A nonprofit patient-health professional partnership dedicated to advancing the treatment and management of headache and to raising the public awareness of headache as a valid, biologically based illness.

American Pain Foundation
111 South Calvert Street, Suite 2700
Baltimore, MD 21202
URL: http://www.painfoundation.org/
Nonprofit information resource and patient advocacy organization serving people with pain that seeks to improve the quality of life of people with pain by providing practical information for patients, raising public awareness and understanding of pain, and advocating against barriers to effective treatment.

National Parkinson Foundation, Inc.
1501 NW 9th Ave.
Miami, FL 33136
URL: http://www.parkinson.org/index.htm
Useful information for patients and clinicians. Research and trials included. Links to the Parkinson's web ring.

National Stroke Association
96 Inverness Drive East, Suite 1
Englewood, CO 80112-5311
Phone: (303) 649-9299 or (800) STROKES

Fax: (303) 649-1328
URL: http://www.stroke.org/
Promotes national awareness of stroke risk, supports and encourages stroke survivors and their families, builds a national network of community based chapters, and sponsors research.

GOVERNMENT AGENCIES AND OFFICES

National Institute of Neurological Disorders and Strokes
Office of Communications and Public Liaison
P.O. Box 5801
Bethesda, MD 20824
Phone: (800) 352-9424
URL: http://www.ninds.nih.gov/
Part of NIH that conducts, fosters, coordinates, and guides research on the causes, prevention, diagnosis, and treatment of neurologic disorders and stroke, and supports basic research in related scientific areas.

OTHER WEB SITES

Gateway to Neurology—MGH Neurology
URL: http://neuro-www.mgh.harvard.edu/
Provides access to web-based information for patients, including bulletin board discussions, chat rooms, and support and education about various neurologic conditions.

Headache Information Network
URL: http://www.htinet.com/hin.html
A 24-h interactive resource offering 90 min of recorded television talk show programs devoted to headache. Users may access and print the transcripts from the web site or click to listen to audio segments.

Neurology Channel
URL: http://www.neurologychannel.com/
Neurology Channel claims to be the Internet's most comprehensive resource for neurology-related consumer health care.

Neurology Webforums at Massachusetts General Hospital
URL: http://neuro-mancer.mgh.harvard.edu/cgi-bin/Ultimate.cgi
A continuing effort by the Department of Neurology at Massachusetts General Hospital to foster on-line discussions between patients, caregivers, and physicians about various neurology-related topics.

Stroke. An Easy to Understand Guide from Lifeclinic.com
URL: http://www.lifeclinic.com/focus/stroke/
Basic information about strokes, including prevention, diagnosis, treatment and rehabilitation.

SUBSTANCE ABUSE (Chapter 26)

See also Mental Health (Chapter 22).

ORGANIZATIONS, ASSOCIATIONS, AND SUPPORT GROUPS

Alcoholics Anonymous
AA World Services, Inc.
P.O. Box 459
New York, NY 10163
Phone: (212) 870-3400
URL: http://www.aa.org
Maintained by the Alcoholics Anonymous World Services, this web site offers assistance and support to individuals recovering from alcohol abuse. The information is presented in English, Spanish, and French, and covers the 12-step recovery program.

Narcotics Anonymous
P.O. Box 9999
Van Nuys, CA 91409
Phone: (818) 773-9999
URL: http://www.na.org
A sister organization to AA, Narcotics Anonymous is a worldwide support organization designed to help individuals recover from drug addiction. This site provides information about the organization, how to start a local group, and a worldwide directory of local NA telephone helplines.

National Clearinghouse for Alcohol and Drug Information (NCADI)
11426 Rockville Pike, Suite 200
P.O. Box 2345
Rockville, MD 20847-2345
Phone: (301) 468-2600 or (800) 729-6686
Fax: (301) 468-6433
URL: http://www.health.org
One of the Substance Abuse and Mental Health Services Administration's four clearinghouses, the NCADI services include an information services staff (English, Spanish, TDD capability) equipped to respond to the public's alcohol, tobacco, and drug (ATD) inquiries; the distribution of free or low-cost ATD materials, including fact sheets, brochures, pamphlets, monographs, posters, and video tapes from an inventory of over 1000 items; and access to the Prevention Materials Database (PMD), including over 8000 prevention-related materials and the Treatment Resources Database, available to the public in electronic form.

GOVERNMENT AGENCIES AND OFFICES

National Institute on Alcohol Abuse and Alcoholism (NIAAA)
6000 Executive Boulevard—Willco Building

Bethesda, Maryland 20892-7003
Phone: (301) 443-3860
Fax: (301) 443-6077
URL: http://www.niaaa.nih.gov/
Supports and conducts biomedical and behavioral research on the causes, consequences, treatment, and prevention of alcoholism and alcohol-related problems. Although primarily a research institute, publications include pamphlets and brochures for the public on a wide range of alcohol-related topics. Spanish-language materials are also available.

National Institute on Drug Abuse—Steroids
UTRL: http://www.steroidabuse.org/
Includes on line articles, medical news, and links related to anabolic steroid abuse.

Office on Smoking and Health
4770 Buford Highway NE
Atlanta, GA
Phone: (770) 488-5705 or (800) CDC-1311
URL: http://www.cdc.gov/tobacco/
CDC office under the National Center for Chronic Disease Prevention and Health Promotion, with consumer publications for distribution on smoking and teenagers, smoking and pregnancy, smoking cessation, and smoking and health. Web site is TIPS. Tobacco Information and Prevention Source.

Substance Abuse and Mental Health Services Administration (SAMHSA)
Room 12-105 Parklawn Building
5600 Fishers Lane
Rockville, MD 20857
Phone: (301) 443-4795
Fax: (301) 443-0284
E-mail: info@samhsa.gov
URL: http://www.samhsa.gov/
Federal agency under the Department of Health and Human Services, SAMHSA is charged with improving the quality and availability of resources geared toward the prevention, rehabilitation and treatment of substance abuse and mental illness. This site offers a directory of service providers and treatment facilities, telephone help line numbers, and four information clearinghouses.

OTHER WEB SITES

The National Center on Addiction and Substance Abuse at Columbia University
URL: http://www.casacolumbia.org
Centered at Columbia University, this site provides information on addiction and substance abuse for parents and teenagers. It provides links to other sites containing state and local resources.

Tips4Kids
URL: http://www.cdc.gov/tobacco/tips4youth.htm

Strong antismoking themes presented as advice of teen idols in tip sheets, artwork, and a special report from the surgeon general.

Web of Addictions
URL: http://www.well.com/user/woa/
The site contains fact sheets and valuable information about alcohol and drug addiction. The site also supplies hot line numbers and addresses of organizations and information on meetings and conferences on specific addictions.

REFERENCES

1. Health Summit Working Group. (Last revised 1999, May 4). Criteria for Assessing the Quality of Health Information on the Internet—Policy Paper. McClean, VA, Mitretek Systems. Retrieved June 19, 2000 from the World Wide Web: http://hitiweb.mitretek.org/docs/policy.html
2. Dutcher G. (Last revised 1999, June 1). Evaluating Internet Resources: Factors to Consider. Bethesda, MD, National Network of Libraries of Medicine. Retrieved June 19, 2000 from the World Wide Web: http://www.nnlm.nlm.nih.gov/partners/eval.html
3. Health on the Net Foundation. (Last revised 2000, January 25). HON Code of Conduct (HONcode) for Medical and Health Web Sites. Geneva, Switzerland, By the Author. Retrieved June 19, 2000 from the World Wide Web: http://www.hon.ch/HONcode
4. Barrett S. (Last revised 2000, June 12). Quackwatch, Inc.: Your Guide to Health Fraud, Quackery, and Intelligent Decisions. Retrieved June 19, 2000 from the World Wide Web: http://www.quackwatch.com
5. Rees AM. Consumer Health Information Source Book, 6th ed. Phoenix, AZ, Oryx Press, 1999, pp 51–52.

Index

Note: Page numbers in *italics* refer to illustrations. Page numbers followed by the letter b refer to boxed material; those followed by t refer to tables.

AAFP (American Academy of Family Physicians), 239
  childhood immunizations endorsed by, 240–244, *241*, 243t
AAP (American Academy of Pediatrics), 239
  childhood immunizations endorsed by, 240–244, *241*, 243t
ABCs, of depression, 573b
ABCDEs, of trauma care, 339–340
Abdominal cramps, in foodborne illness, 95t
Abortion, therapeutic, 377–378
Abstinence, as method of contraception, 375
Abuse, alcohol. See *Alcohol abuse.*
  anabolic steroid. See *Anabolic steroid abuse.*
  child, 71
    clinical indicators of, 71b
    sexual, 393–394
  elder, 71–72
    risk factors for, 70b, 200t
  laxative, 498
  nicotine. See *Nicotine abuse.*
  of women. See also *Domestic violence.*
    predisposing factors for, 70b
  substance. See *Substance abuse.*
Accidents, in home, 217
  risk of, in men, 412
Accreditation standards, imposition of, in assuring linguistic access to care, 283–284

Accuracy, in Pulitzer's formula for prize-winning writing, 280–281
Acetazolamide, for altitude sickness, 362
Achalasia, 495
ACIP (Advisory Committee on Immunization Practices), 239
  childhood immunizations endorsed by, 240–244, *241*, 243t
Acquired immunodeficiency syndrome (AIDS), 509–518
  CD T-lymphocyte count in, 510
  end-stage, neoplasms associated with, 627
  epidemiology of, 512
  frequent HIV-related problems in, 514t
  pathophysiology of, 509–512, *511*
  patient education about, 515–518
  prevention of, 518
  screening for, 518
  spread of, 510
  treatment of, 512–515
    approved medications in, 513–514, 516t
    combination therapy in, 517t
    highly active antiretroviral therapy in, 515
    prophylactic, indications for, 515t
    rationale for, 514–515
  virus causing, 510. See also *Human immunodeficiency virus (HIV).*
ACTH (adrenocorticotropic hormone), 595

ACTH (adrenocorticotropic hormone) *(Continued)*
    hypersecretion of, 618. See also *Cushing's syndrome.*
    inadequate secretion of, 621. See also *Addison's disease.*
Active (new) disease, diagnosis and treatment of, 6
Activities of daily living (ADL), cross-sectional study of, 131
    difficulties with, 190
    Fillenbaum instrumental assessment of, 197b
    health benefits of physical activity in, 152–153
    Katz index assessment of, 196b
Acupuncture, 25–26
Addison's disease, 620–623
    epidemiology of, 622
    pathophysiology of, 620–622
    prevention of, 623
    treatment of, 622
ADHD. See *Attention deficit hyperactivity disorder (ADHD).*
Adjusted rate(s), as measure of disease frequency, 122, 124–125
    direct method of, 124
    indirect method of, 125, 125t
ADL. See *Activities of daily living (ADL).*
Adolescent(s), anabolic steroid abuse in, 708
    body dysmorphic disorder in, 588
    caloric requirements of, 305
    competitive sports and, 227
    female, caring for, 388–394
        gynecologic examination of, 389–391, 390t
    male, use of tobacco products in, 411
    motor vehicle permit or license and, 226–227
    risk-taking by, 225–228
        counseling suggestions for, 227–228, 227b
    sexually transmitted disease in, 550–551, 550b
        prevention of, 560

Adolescent(s) *(Continued)*
    vaccine-preventable disease in, 259b–260b
Adolescent injury prevention guidance, 227b
Adrenal glands, 595–596
    disorder(s) of, 618–623
        Addison's disease as, 620–623
        Cushing's syndrome as, 618–620
Adrenocorticotropic hormone (ACTH), 595
    hypersecretion of, 618. See also *Cushing's syndrome.*
    inadequate secretion of, 621. See also *Addison's disease.*
Adult(s), literacy skills of, *3,* 267–269. See also *Hypoliteracy; Literacy.*
    older. See *Elderly.*
Advanced Trauma Life Support (ATLS), 338–341
Advisory Committee on Immunization Practices (ACIP), 239
    childhood immunizations endorsed by, 240–244, *241,* 243t
AFFIRM (Atrial Fibrillation Follow-up Investigation of Rhythm Management) trial, 429
AFP (alpha-fetoprotein), in hepatocellular cancer, 649
African American and African Caribbean communities, health and illness in, 56–58, 58b, 59b
Agency for Toxic Substances and Disease Registry (ATSDR), 81
Age-specific death rate, 122, 123t
Aging. See also *Elderly.*
    successful, definition of, 191
    with dignity, "five wishes" document in, 201b
Agoraphobia, 582t
Agricultural accidents, prevention of, 335, 338
AIDS. See *Acquired immunodeficiency syndrome (AIDS).*

Air pollution, classification of, 106

Air quality, 105–107
  health issues related to, 105

Aire de oido, as Mexican folk illness, 55b

Airway, management of, in trauma care, 339

Alcohol, oxidation of, biochemical changes due to, 697

Alcohol abuse, 411–412
  epidemiology of, 699
  pathophysiology of, 697–698
  patient education about, 703
  prevention of, 703
  screening for, 703–704
  trauma due to, prevention of, 330
  treatment of, 699–703, 700t

Alcohol Use Questionnaire (AUQ), 700t, 703–704

Alcohol withdrawal, signs of, 702b
  suppression of, 702

Alcoholism, 697. See also *Alcohol abuse.*
  family history of, 699

All terrain vehicle (ATV) accidents, prevention of, 331

Allergic symptoms, in foodborne illness, 96t

Allium sativum, 28

Aloe vera, 30

Alpha-1 antitrypsin deficiency, 497

Alpha-adrenergic agonists, for urinary incontinence, 212t

Alpha-2 adrenergic agonists, in suppression of alcohol withdrawal symptoms, 702

Alpha-adrenergic antagonists, for urinary incontinence, 212t

Alpha-blockers, for benign prostatic hypertrophy, 402

Alpha-fetoprotein (AFP), in hepatocellular cancer, 649

Alternative medicine, 23–44
  acupuncture as, 25–26
  aroma therapy as, 34–37
  biofeedback as, 39–40, 41b
  categories of, 23–25

Alternative medicine *(Continued)*
  Government Agencies and Offices for, 724–725
  herbal medicine as, 27–30, 31t
  homeopathy as, 26–27
  massage as, 38–39
  Organization, Associations, and Support Groups for, 724
  reflexology as, 37, *38*
  resources for, 41–44
  single nutrients in, 30, 32–34
  web sites for, 725–726

Altitude sickness, 362

Alzheimer's disease, 185–186, 207
  diagnostic criteria for, 666b
  early-onset of, 185
  epidemiology of, 667–668
  late-onset of, 185
  pathophysiology of, 665–667
  patient education about, 669–670
  prevention of, 670
  screening for, 670–671
  treatment of, 668–669

American Academy of Family Physicians (AAFP), 239
  childhood immunizations endorsed by, 240–244, *241,* 243t

American Academy of Pediatrics (AAP), 239
  childhood immunizations endorsed by, 240–244, *241,* 243t

American Cancer Society screening recommendations, for early detection of cancer, 631t

American Diabetes Association, physical activity recommended by, 152

American Heart Association (AHA) recommendations, for endocarditis prophylaxis, 526, 527t, 528t

American Public Health Association, 80

Amniocentesis, indications for, 171b

Amok, 52

Amoxicillin, prophylactic, for dental, oral, respiratory tract, or esophageal procedures, 527t
  for genitourinary and gastrointestinal procedures, 528t
Ampicillin, prophylactic, for dental, oral, respiratory tract, or esophageal procedures, 527t
  for genitourinary and gastrointestinal procedures, 528t
AMPLE mnemonic, in trauma care, 340
Amsterdam criteria, for hereditary nonpolyposis colorectal cancer, 184
Anabolic steroid abuse, epidemiology of, 708–709
  pathophysiology of, 707–708
  prevention of, 709
  screening for, 710
  treatment of, 709
Anal fissure, 501
Analysis, in epidemiologic studies, 140–141
Anaphylaxis, in foodborne illness, 96t
Anencephaly, prenatal screening for, 173–174
Angina, 430
Angiodysplasia, 497
Anorectal disease, 500–501
Anorexia nervosa, 572t
Antibiotics, for encephalitis, 521
  for meningitis, 543
  for traveler's diarrhea, 351–352, 352t
  resistance to, 509
Anticholinergics, for urinary incontinence, 212t
Anticonvulsants, for bipolar disorder, 580
Antidepressants, 576–577
Antioxidant vitamins, benefits of, 295
  for elderly, 206
Antiplatelet therapy, prophylactic, for stroke, 690

Antirheumatic drugs, disease-modifying, 456–457
Anxiety, effect of physical activity on, 155
Anxiety disorder(s), DSM-IV definitions of, 582t–583t
  epidemiology of, 584
  pathophysiology of, 581, 584
  patient education about, 585
  prevention of, 586
  treatment of, 584–585
Aortic stenosis, 445
  in children, 447
Apolipoprotein E 4 allele, in Alzheimer's disease, 185–186, 665–666
Appendicitis, 483–486
  pathophysiology of, 483–485
  treatment of, 485
Appendix, 483
Appreciation, in Pulitzer's formula for prize-winning writing, 278–280
Aroma therapy, 34–37
  clary sage in, 35–36
  eucalyptus in, 36
  lavender in, 36
  tea tree oil in, 36–37
  ylang-ylang in, 37
Arrhythmias. See *Cardiac arrhythmias.*
Arterial occlusion, 434
Arthritis, osteo-, 460–463. See also *Osteoarthritis.*
  rheumatoid, 453–457. See also *Rheumatoid arthritis.*
Arthropod(s), as agent/vector in disease, 86–87, 86b, 87t
Arthropod-borne disease(s), 352–356, 353t. See also specific disease, e.g., *Malaria.*
Asbestos, causing cancer, 628–629
Asian Americans, health and illness in, 54, 56, 57t
Asphyxiation deaths, caused by choking, in elderly, 334
Aspirin, prophylactic, for embolic stroke, 688

Assisted living, for elderly, 213–214
Atherosclerosis, 430, 433
 cerebrovascular, 685–686
 health benefits of physical activity in, 151
ATLS (Advanced Trauma Life Support), 338–341
Atraque de nervios, 52–53
Atrial fibrillation, embolic stroke related to, 686, 690
 treatment of, 428
Atrial Fibrillation Follow-up Investigation of Rhythm Management (AFFIRM) trial, 429
"Atrial kick," 428
Atrioventricular node, 424
ATSDR (Agency for Toxic Substances and Disease Registry), 81
Attention and calculation, in Folstein's mini-mental status examination, 193b
Attention deficit hyperactivity disorder (ADHD),
 epidemiology of, 590
 pathophysiology of, 589–590
 patient education and prevention of, 591
 screening for, 591
 treatment of, 590
ATV (all terrain vehicle) accidents, prevention of, 331
Auditory deficits, in elderly, 209
AUQ (Alcohol Use Questionnaire), 700t, 703–704
Aura, in migraine headache, 672
Awareness, cultural, 47
Azithromycin, prophylactic, for dental, oral, respiratory tract, or esophageal procedures, 527t

Bacille Calmette-Guérin (BCG) vaccine, 563
Bacillus cereus, in foodborne illness, 98t, 99t
Back pain, low, 661–665. See also *Low back pain.*

Balance, evaluation of, 209
Balloon angioplasty, transluminal, for peripheral vascular disease, 435
Barrett's esophagus, 473, 495
Barrier methods, of contraception, 374
Basal body temperature, measurement of, ovulation and, 369
Basal cell carcinoma, 655
Basal energy expenditure, measurement of, 303–304
Basilar migraine, 672. See also *Migraine headache.*
BCG (bacille Calmette-Guérin) vaccine, 563
Behavior, change in, theory of, 12–17
 consequences of, 226
 learned, in domestic violence, 68
 social, individual, 8
Behavior therapy, for anxiety, 585
Benign prostatic hypertrophy (BPH), screening for, 401, 402b
 symptoms of, 401
 treatment of, medical, 402
  surgical, 403
Beta blockers, in suppression of alcohol withdrawal symptoms, 702
Beverage(s), contaminated, 91–92
Bezoar, 495
Bias, definition of, 138
 in epidemiologic studies, 138–139
Bicultural providers, 50
Bicycle injuries, prevention of, 335
Bilingual providers, 50
Bilingual staff, recruitment and hiring of, 284
Bioelectromagnetics, in complementary medical practices, 25
Biofeedback, 39–40, 41b
Biofield systems, in complementary medical practices, 25
Biological weapons, 110

Biologically-based therapies, in complementary medical practices, 24
Bipolar disorder, 574t, 579–581
  pathophysiology of, 579–580
  prevention of, 580
  treatment of, 580
Bismuth subsalicylate, for traveler's diarrhea, 350–351, 351t, 352t
Black cohosh, 29
Bladder cancer, pathophysiology of, 633–634
  prevention and screening for, 635
  treatment of, 634
Bleeding disorder(s), epidemiology of, 437–438
  pathophysiology of, 436–437
  patient education about, 439
  prevention of, 439
  treatment of, 438
Blood, HIV-contaminated, exposure to, 510
Blood pressure, control of, role of physical activity in, 150–151
Blood transfusions, transmission of infection via, 509
Body dysmorphic disorder, pathophysiology of, 587–588
  patient education about, 589
  prevention of, 589
  treatment of, 588
Body fluids, HIV-contaminated, exposure to, 510
Body mass density, physical activity and, 153
Body mass index, 297
  nomogram for, *299*
Body mass index chart, *298*
Bone disorders, 453–468. See also specific disorder, e.g., *Osteoporosis.*
  Government Agencies and Offices for, 753–754
  Organizations, Associations, and Support Groups for, 753
  web sites for, 754
Bordetella pertussis, 246. See also *Pertussis.*
Botulism, 103t

Bowel, obstruction of, 499–500
Bowel disease, functional, pathophysiology of, 486–487
  treatment of, 487–488
  inflammatory, 490–494. See also *Inflammatory bowel disease.*
BPH (benign prostatic hypertrophy), screening for, 401, 402b
  symptoms of, 401
  treatment of, medical, 402
    surgical, 403
Bradycardia, treatment of, 427–428
"Brain attack." See *Stroke.*
Brain fag syndrome, 53
BRCA1 gene, 635
  mutations of, 182
BRCA2 gene, 635
  mutations of, 182–183
Breast cancer, American Cancer Society screening recommendations for, 631t
  hereditary, 180–183
    BRCA1 gene in, 181–182, 635
    BRCA2 gene in, 182–183, 635
  hormone-related, 630–631
  in men, 414
  pathophysiology of, 635–636
  patient education about, 637
  prevention of, 637
  screening for, 631t, 637
  treatment of, 636–637
Breast self-examination, 381–382, 637
  easy steps in, 382b–383b
Breathing, in trauma care, 339
Brevity, in Pulitzer's formula for prize-winning writing, 277
Briquet's syndrome (somatization disorder), 586
Bris, 60
Brudzinski's sign, 542
Bulimia nervosa, 572t
Bundle of His, 424
Burns, prevention of, 333–334
Bypass grafting, coronary artery, 432

Bypass grafting *(Continued)*
for peripheral vascular disease, 435

CABG (coronary artery bypass grafting), 432
CAH (congenital adrenal hyperplasia), 621
Caida de mollera, as Mexican folk illness, 55b
Calcium, 33
for osteoporosis, 459
in healthy diet, 295
supplemental, for elderly, 205
Caloric prescription(s), 300, 302–306
calorie adjustment in, 303
for adolescents, 305
for adults, Harris-Benedict equation in, 303–304
for children, 305
for infants, 304
for toddlers, 305
for weight gain, 302
for weight loss, 302
for weight maintenance, 302
formula A, 302–303
formula B, 303
formula C, 303
Calorie-specific prescription(s), circle pyramid guide in, 306, *308,* 309
sample meal plans in, 306, 309, 310t
special precautions in, 309–311, 312b–313b, 314
CAM (complementary and alternative medicine). See also *Alternative medicine.*
definition of, 23
Cameron-Myers vaginoscope, 393
Cancer, 180–184, 624–660. See also at anatomic site, e.g., *Breast cancer.*
cause(s) of, 627–631
asbestos as, 628–629
chemical, 628, 629t
hormonal factors as, 630–631
ionizing radiation as, 629–630
viral, 627, 628t

Cancer *(Continued)*
chemoprevention of, 633–634, 642
common types of, in men, 412
counseling patients about, 631–633
early detection of, American Cancer Society screening recommendations for, 631t
family medical history suggestive of, 181b
Government Agencies and Offices for, 763–764
metastatic, 626
new, leading sites of, 632t
Organizations, Associations, and Support Groups for, 763
prevention of, 625
web sites for, 764
Cancer deaths, by site and sex, 632t
Car safety, 234
Carbamazepine, in suppression of alcohol withdrawal symptoms, 702
Carbidopa, for Parkinson's disease, 684
Carcinogenesis, 624
agents implicated in, 624–625, 633
asbestos, mechanisms of, 628–629, 629t
steps in, 625, *626*
Carcinogens, chemical, 628, 629t
Cardiac. See also *Heart* entries.
Cardiac arrhythmias, epidemiology of, 427
pathophysiology of, 425–427
patient education about, 428–429
prevention of, 429
screening for, 429
treatment of, 427–428
Cardiac muscle, properties of, 425
Cardiac output, 425
Cardiac physiology, neural regulation in, 425
Cardiac rehabilitation, following myocardial infarction, 432

Cardiology, Government Agencies and Offices for, 752
  Organizations, Associations, and Support Groups for, 752
  web sites for, 752
Cardiovascular disease, health benefits of physical activity in, 149–150
  in women, 382–384
Cardiovascular fitness, measurement of, 151–152
Caregiver Strain Index, Gerontological Society of America's, 199b
Case-control study(ies), epidemiologic, 131–132
Cataracts, 209
Cause-specific death rate, 122, 123t
CD4 T-lymphocyte count, in HIV infection, 510
CD8 T-lymphocyte count, in HIV infection, 510
Cefazolin, prophylactic, for dental, oral, respiratory tract, or esophageal procedures, 527t
Ceftriaxone, for gonorrhea, 554
Centers for Disease Control and Prevention, 81
  immunization recommendations of, for women of reproductive age, 367
Cephalexin, prophylactic, for dental, oral, respiratory tract, or esophageal procedures, 527t
Cervical cancer, American Cancer Society screening recommendations for, 631t
  pathophysiology of, 638–639
  prevention of, 639
  screening for, 639–640
  treatment of, 639
Cervical cap, 374
Cervical spine, nerve root compression in, 662
  protection of, in trauma care, 339
Cervix, adolescent, examination of, 391
Chamomile tea, 30

Chancroids, pathophysiology of, 550
  treatment of, 557
Chemical(s), causing cancer, 628, 629t
Chemical leachates, in ground water, 104–105
Chemical weapons, lethal, 110
Chemoprevention, of cancer, 633–634
  colorectal, 642
Chemoprophylaxis, for malaria, 354, 355t, 356
Chickenpox. See *Varicella* entries.
Child(ren). See also *Infant(s); Toddler(s).*
  abuse of, 71
    clinical indicators of, 71b
    sexual, 393–394
  AIDS in, 510
  alcohol abuse in, 698
  anxiety disorder in, 581, 584
  appendicitis in, 484
  arrhythmias in, 426
  attention deficit hyperactivity disorder in, 589–591
  bipolar disorder in, 579
  bleeding disorders in, 436–437
  body dysmorphic disorder in, 587
  caloric requirements of, 305
  CMV mononucleosis in, 545–546
  congenital adrenal hyperplasia in, 621
  coronary artery disease in, 430
  cryptorchidism in, 657
  depression in, 573–574
  diabetes mellitus type I in, 608
  diabetes mellitus type II in, 611
  encephalitis in, 520
  encopresis in, 502
  failure to thrive in, 503
  gallbladder disease in, 479
  gastroenteritis in, 530
  GERD in, 473
  hyperlipidemia in, 614
  hyperparathyroidism in, 603
  hypoparathyroidism in, 605
  hypothyroidism in, 600

Child(ren) *(Continued)*
 in day care and school settings, risks for, 225
 infective endocarditis in, 523
 inguinal hernias in, 489
 meningitis in, 541–542
 migraine headaches in, 673
 nicotine abuse in, 704
 obesity in, prevalence of, 293
 pancreatitis in, 481–482
 prepubertal, gynecologic examination of, 391–393
 rectal prolapse in, 502
 rheumatoid arthritis in, 454
 seminomas and teratomas in, 657
 sexually transmitted disease in, 550–551, 550b
 systolic hypertension in, 443
 tuberculosis in, 561
 vaccine-preventable diseases in, 259b–261b
 valvular heart disease in, 446–447
Child safety seats, in trauma prevention, 330–331
Childproofing home, 221–223, 221b–222b
 counseling suggestions for, 223
Chills, in foodborne illness, 97t
Chinese remedies, traditional, 57t
Chlamydia, 378
 epidemiology of, 552
 in pregnancy, 551
 pathophysiology of, 548
 patient education about, 557
 treatment of, 553
Chlamydia trachomatis, 378, 548
Chloroquine, prophylactic, for malaria, 355t
Choking, asphyxiation deaths caused by, in elderly, 334
Cholecystectomy, 480
Cholecystitis, 479
 gallstones associated with, 481
Cholelithiasis, 479
Cholera, 94
 vaccine-preventable, in international traveler, 359–360
Cholesterol, 594–595, 617
Cholinergic agonists, for urinary incontinence, 212t

Cholinesterase inhibitors, for dementia, 668
Chondroitin, 34, 206
Chorionic villus sampling, indications for, 171b
Christmas disease (hemophilia B), 436–437
Chromium, 33
Chronic disease, in elderly, 211
 management of, 5–6
Chylomicrons, 595
Cigarette smoking. See also *Nicotine abuse.*
 in men, 411
 in women, 384
Ciguatera poisoning, 103t
Cimicifuga racemosa, 29
Ciprofloxacin, for traveler's diarrhea, 351t, 352t
Circle pyramid guide, in calorie plan, 306, *308,* 309
Circulation, with hemorrhage control, in trauma care, 340
Clarithromycin, prophylactic, for dental, oral, respiratory tract, or esophageal procedures, 527t
Clarity, in Pulitzer's formula for prize-winning writing, 278–280
Clary sage, in aroma therapy, 35–36
Clean Air Act (1970), 105
Clindamycin, prophylactic, for dental, oral, respiratory tract, or esophageal procedures, 527t
Clinical genetics. See *Genetics.*
Clinical trials, randomized, epidemiologic, 134–136
 types of error in, 135t
Clinicians' legal responsibility(ies), in assuring linguistic access to care, 281–284
 accreditation standards and, 283–284
 federal law and, 282–283
 liability for negligence and, 283
Clostridium botulinum, in foodborne illness, 103t

Clostridium difficile infection, pseudomembranous colitis associated with, 490–491

Clostridium perfringens, in foodborne illness, 99t, 529

Cluster sampling, in epidemiologic studies, 138

CMV (cytomegalovirus), associated with infectious mononucleosis, 544–545, 545t

c-myc oncogene, in endometrial cancer, 642

Cognitive decline, in multiple sclerosis, 679

Cohort study(ies), epidemiologic, 133–134
    prospective, 133–134
    retrospective, 134

Coitus interruptus (withdrawal), as method of contraception, 375, 416

Colic, in infants, 502

Colitis, ischemic, 499
    pseudomembranous, 490–491
        treatment of, 493–494
    ulcerative, 491
        treatment of, 493

Colon, conditions affecting, 497–500

Colonoscopy, 642

Colorectal cancer, American Cancer Society screening recommendations for, 631t
    health benefits of physical activity in, 154
    hereditary, 183–184
    pathophysiology of, 640–641
    prevention of, 641
    screening for, 642
    treatment of, 641

Comfort care issues, for elderly, 214

Communicable disease(s), arthropods as agents/vectors in, 86–87, 86b, 87t
    control of, 85–88
    rabies as, 88
    snakebites and, 87–88

Communication gap, bridging, with LEP patients, 284–285, 285b

Communication styles, 48–51, 48b, 49b, 50b

Community, moving about in, 234–235

Community culture, 61–62

Community health workers, 50

Community preplanning, for regional disasters, 108–109

Complementary and alternative medicine (CAM). See also *Alternative medicine.*
    definition of, 23

Complementary medical practices, categories of, 23–25

Compliance, as factor in nutritional therapy, 293

Condoms, 374, 415–416

Conduction system, of heart, 424–425

Condylomata, flat, 554–555, 554t

Condylomata acuminata, 554t

Confidence interval, in epidemiology, 128–129

Confidentiality, discussion of, with female adolescent, 388–389

Confounding, in epidemiology, 140–141

Confounding variable, 140

Congenital adrenal hyperplasia (CAH), 621

Congestive heart failure, 439–442. See also *Heart failure, congestive.*

Constipation, 497–499

Consumer Health Committee, of Georgia Health Sciences Library Association, 715–716

Contraception, 369–378
    barrier methods of, 374
    emergency, 375, 376t, 377
    hormonal, injectable and implantable forms of, 372–374
    intrauterine device in, 374
    male, 415–416
    oral, 370–372
        choice of, 371–372, 372b
        contraindications to, 370t
        noncontraceptive benefits of, 371

Contraception *(Continued)*
warning signs associated with, 371t
sterilization as method of, 375, 416
therapeutic abortion as method of, 377–378
withdrawal and abstinence as method of, 375
Conversion disorder, 587
Copycat behavior, consequences of, 226
Coronary artery(ies), 424
Coronary artery bypass grafting (CABG), 432
Coronary artery disease, 430–433
epidemiology of, 431
in men, 414
pathophysiology of, 430–431
patient education about, 432
physical inactivity as risk factor for, 151
prevention of, 433
screening for, 433
treatment of, 431–432
Corticosteroids, for encephalitis, 521
Cramps, abdominal, in foodborne illness, 95t
C-reactive protein, as predictor of myocardial infarction, 433
C-reactive protein test, for heart disease, 383
Creutzfeldt-Jakob disease, 667
Crohn's disease, 491–492
treatment of, 493
Cross-cultural environment, monolingual providers in, guidelines for, 48b
Cross-sectional studies, epidemiologic, 130–131
Crude rate, as measure of disease frequency, 122, 123t
Cryptorchidism, 657
Cryptosporidium parvum, in foodborne illness, 102t, 530
Cults, 60–61
Cultural awareness, 47
Cultural competence, 46–47
components of, 47–48
Cultural encounters, 47
Cultural folk condition(s), 54–62

Cultural folk condition(s) *(Continued)*
African American and African Caribbean, 56–58, 58b, 59b
Asian American, 54, 56, 57t
community and situational, 61–62
disabilities as, 61
Mexican American, 54, 55b
Native American, 54, 56t
religious, 58–61
sexual diversity as, 61
Cultural influence(s), 46–62
Government Agencies and Offices for, 726
Organizations, Associations, and Support Groups for, 726
resources for, 63–65
web sites for, 726–728
Cultural knowledge, 47
Cultural skill, 47
Culture-bound syndrome(s), 51–53
amok as, 52
atraque de nervios as, 52–53
brain fag as, 53
falling out as, 53
hwa-byung as, 52
koro as, 51–52
susto as, 53
Cumulative incidence, as measure of disease frequency, 121
Cushing's syndrome, epidemiology of, 619
pathophysiology of, 618–619
patient education about, 620
prevention and screening for, 620
treatment of, 619
Cutaneous ulcers, in peripheral vascular disease, 434
Cyclospora cayetanensis, in foodborne illness, 102t, 530
Cyclothymic disorder, 574t
Cylert (pemoline), for attention deficit hyperactivity disorder, 590
Cystic fibrosis, carrier testing for, 176–178
ethnic groups affected by, 178t

Cystic fibrosis *(Continued)*
  gene for, 176
  genetic counseling in, indications for, 177b
  risk of pancreatitis with, 481
Cytomegalovirus (CMV),
  associated with infectious
  mononucleosis, 544–545,
  545t

Dairy products, recall of, 91
Daredevil behavior, consequences
  of, 226
DASH (dietary approach to stop
  hypertension), 311
"Dawn phenomenon," in
  diabetes mellitus, 608
Day care, children in, risks for,
  225
Death, according to mechanism
  and intent, based on
  International Classification of
  Diseases, 322t–324t
  by asphyxiation, in elderly, 334
  leading causes of, for ages 1–4,
  318t
    for ages 5–14, 319t
    for ages 15–25, 319t–320t
    for ages 25–44, 320t
    for ages 45–64, 320t–321t
    for ages 65 and over, 321t
    for all ages, 318t
  sudden, during exercise, 156
Death rate, 122, 123t
  cancer, by site and sex, 632t
  for infectious diseases, *506*
Decision-making capacities, in
  elderly, 207
Deforestation, water degradation
  due to, 104
Dehydration, associated with
  gastroenteritis, 530
Delirium tremens (DTs), 702
Dementia, definition of, 665
  epidemiology of, 667–668
  of Alzheimer's type, diagnostic
  criteria for, 666b
  pathophysiology of, 665–667
  patient education about, 669–
  670
  prevention of, 670

Dementia *(Continued)*
  screening for, 670–671
  treatment of, 668–669
  types of, 665
Demyelination, in multiple
  sclerosis, 677, 678
Density, incidence, as measure of
  instantaneous rate, 121
Deoxyribonucleic acid. See *DNA*
  entries.
Depo-Provera
  (medroxyprogesterone
  acetate), 372–374
Depression, 573–579
  course of, 574t
  effect of physical activity on,
  155
  epidemiology of, 576
  in elderly, 207
  in men, 410–411
    risk factors for, 410
  pathophysiology of, 573–576,
  573b
  patient education about, 577
  postpartum, 574–575
  prevention of, 577–579
  screening for, 579
  treatment of, 576–577
    rationale for initiation of,
    578–579
Design method(s) and critical
  review, of epidemiologic
  studies, 136–144
  analysis in, 140–141
  bias in, 138–139
  conclusions in, 141–142
  effect modification in, 141
  presentation of findings in,
  140
    by media, interpretation of,
    142
  sampling in, 136–138
  screening in, 142–144, 143t
  study observations in, 139
Diabetes mellitus, 607–614
  education tips for, 311, 312b–
  313b
  insulin-dependent (type I), epidemiology of, 609
    health benefits of physical activity in, 152
  pathophysiology of, 607–609

Diabetes mellitus *(Continued)*
  patient education about, 610
  treatment of, 609–610
  non–insulin-dependent (type
    II), epidemiology of, 612
  health benefits of physical ac-
    tivity in, 151–152
  pathophysiology of, 611–612
  prevention and screening for,
    613–614
  treatment of, 612–613
Diabetic ketoacidosis, 607
Diabetic ulcers, in peripheral
  vascular disease, 434
Diagnostic and Statistical Manual
  of Mental Disorders (DSM-
  IV) criteria, for substance
  abuse, 695b
  for substance dependence,
    696b
Diaphragm, contraceptive, 374
DIAPPERS mnemonic, 210
Diarrhea, chronic, 497
  in foodborne illness, 95t, 99t–
    102t
  in waterborne illness, 99t–102t
  traveler's, 347–352
    causes of, 347t
    dietary advice for avoidance
      of, 348–350, 348t, 349b
    prevention and treatment of,
      350–352, 351t, 352t
    vs. dysentery, 348t, 350
Dietary advice, for avoidance of
  traveler's diarrhea, 348–350,
  348t, 349b
Dietary approach to stop
  hypertension (DASH), 311
Dietary fiber, benefits of, 295
Dietary restrictions, Islamic, 58
  Jewish, 59–60
Dietary supplements, for elderly,
  204–206
Digital rectal examination, for
  colorectal cancer, 642
  for prostate cancer, 655
Dignity, aging with, "five wishes"
  document in, 201b
Diphtheria, immunization for,
  247
  vaccine-preventable, in adoles-
    cence, 259b

Diphtheria *(Continued)*
  in childhood, 256b
Disability(ies), 61
  developmental, 167–170
    fragile X syndrome as, 168
    hemochromatosis as, 169–170
    Marfan's syndrome as, 168–
      169
  neurologic examination for, in
    trauma care, 340
Disaster(s), definition of, 107
  management of, 107–112
  manmade, 109–112
  natural, 107–109, 108t, 109b
    disease spread by, 89
  regional, community preplan-
    ning in, 108–109
Disease, communicable, 85–88
  emerging and re-emerging,
    88–90
    factors favoring, 90, 90b
  exposure and, association be-
    tween, *126,* 126–127
  prevention of, as national
    health policy, 3
  primary, 4–5
  secondary, 5
  vaccination and, 263
  vectors of, 87t
Disease frequency, measure(s) of,
  117–125
  adjusted rates as, 122, 124–
    125, 125t
  crude and specific rates as,
    122, 123t
  incidence as, 121
  morbidity rates as, 118, 120t
  prevalence as, 121–122
  proportion as, 118, 119t
  rate as, 118, 119t
  ratio as, 118, 119t
Disease-modifying antirheumatic
  drugs (DMARDs), 455–456
Displacement, mental health
  aspects of, 108
Disulfiram, in treatment of
  alcohol abuse, 702
Diverticulitis, 499
Diverticulosis, 499
DMARDs (disease-modifying
  antirheumatic drugs),
  455–456

DNA, alteration in, neoplasia and, 624, 627
  fetal, prenatal testing of, 170, 171b
  proviral, in HIV infection, 510
DNA fingerprinting, in postnatal parentage testing, 172
  in prenatal parentage testing, 171
DNA mismatch repair, 624
  hereditary nonpolyposis colorectal cancer caused by, 184
DNA molecule, genes in, 163
DNA testing, for cystic fibrosis gene, 176
Document literacy, 268
Domestic violence, 67–79
  assessment of, 72–73
  documentation of, 72
  etiology of, 68
  Government Agencies and Offices for, 729
  intervention in, 72, 75
  Organizations, Associations, and Support Groups for, 728–729
  phases of, 67–68
  presentation of, 71–72
  screening for, 68–70, 69b, 70b
  web sites for, 729
Domestic Violence Crisis Hotlines, by State, 75t
Domestic Violence Organizations, National, 74t
  State and Regional, 76t–78t
Dopamine agonists, for Parkinson's disease, 684
Dopaminergic activity, loss of, in Parkinson's disease, 683
Down syndrome (trisomy 21), prenatal screening for, 174–175
Doxycycline, prophylactic, for malaria, 355t
Drinking water, regulation of, 96, 104
Drowning, prevention of, 334
Drug(s). See also named drug or drug group.
  injury due to, prevention of, 330

Dry gangrene, 434
DTs (delirium tremens), 702
Duke's Older Americans Resources and Services (OARS) Multidimensional Functional Assessment Questionnaire, 198b
Dysentery, vs. traveler's diarrhea, 347t, 350
Dyskinesia, in Parkinson's disease, 684
Dyspepsia, non-ulcer, pathophysiology of, 486
  treatment of, 487–488
Dysthymia, 574t

Earthquake, effect of, on health, 108t
Eating disorders, 291
Ebstein's anomaly, associated with lithium use in pregnancy, 180
EBV (Epstein-Barr virus), associated with infectious mononucleosis, 544, 545t
  oncogenic potential of, 628t
Echinacea, 28–29
Ecological fallacy, 129
Ecological study(ies), epidemiologic, 129–130
Ecotourism, pathogens encountered through, 89
ED. See Erectile dysfunction (ED).
Education issue(s), safety as, 217, 218t
  sexually transmitted disease as, 379–380
Effect modification, in epidemiologic studies, 141
Ejaculation, premature, 409
Elastic stockings, for varicosities, 450
Elderly, 190–215
  abuse of, 71–72. See also Domestic violence.
    risk factors for, 70b, 200t
  AIDS in, 512
  alcohol abuse in, 698
  Alzheimer's disease in. See Alzheimer's disease.

Elderly *(Continued)*
anxiety disorder in, 584
appendicitis in, 484–485
arrhythmias in, 427
asphyxiation deaths in, caused by choking, 334
assisted living and long-term care for, 213–214
bleeding disorders in, 437
body dysmorphic disorder in, 588
chronic diseases in, 211
colorectal cancer in, 640–641
concept of health in, 191
coronary artery disease in, 431
depression in, 575–576
diabetes mellitus in, 609, 612
end-of-life concerns for, 214
exercise for, 206–207
falls by, 208–209
  cause of, 208t
  prevention of, 332–333
gallbladder disease in, 479
gastritis and peptic ulcer disease in, 476–477
gastroenteritis in, 531
Government Agencies and Offices for, 737–738
home safety checklist for, 230b–232b
hyperlipidemia in, 615
hyperparathyroidism in, 603
hyperthyroidism in, 597–598
hypothyroidism in, 601
incontinence and urinary retention in, 210–211, 212t
independence of, 206–207
infective endocarditis in, 524
low back pain in, 663
meningitis in, 542
mobility/immobility of, 207
nicotine abuse in, 705
nutritional, herbal, vitamin, or dietary supplements for, 204–206
Organizations, Associations, and Support Groups for, 736–737
Parkinson's disease in, 683
polypharmacy and iatrogenesis in, 211–213
problems requiring intervention in, 204–207

Elderly *(Continued)*
prostate cancer in, 653–654
quality of life for, 214
resources for, 215–216
screening and health assessment of, 191–204. See also *Health assessment, of elderly.*
screening for cervical cancer in, 638–639
senility, or decision-making capacities in, 207
sensory deficits in, 209
special precautions for, 228–229
  counseling suggestions in, 229
swallowing disorders in, 209–210
tuberculosis in, 562
web sites for, 738
WHO definition of, 190
Electronic discussion groups, 717
location of, web sites for, 718t
Embolus, origins of, 686
pulmonary, 438
Emergency contraception, postcoital, 375, 376t, 377
Emergency department visits, by selected characteristics of trauma, 328t
injury-related, by intent and mechanism of cause, 329t
Emergency telephone numbers, 220, 220b
Emerging and re-emerging disease(s), 88–90
factors favoring, 90, 90b
Emotional health, 8
Empacho, as Mexican folk illness, 55b
Empowering patients, concept of, 1
Encephalitis, 519–522
Japanese, vaccine-preventable, in international traveler, 361
pathophysiology of, 519–520, 519t
patient education about, 521–522
prevention of, 522
treatment of, 520–521

Encopresis, in children, 502
Encounters, cultural, 47
Endarterectomy, for peripheral vascular disease, 435
Endocarditis, infective, diagnosis of, 525t
  epidemiology of, 524
  pathophysiology of, 522–524
  patient education about, 526
  prevention of, 526, 527t, 528t
  treatment of, 524–526
End-of-life concerns, of elderly, 214
Endometrial cancer, hormone-related, 630
  pathophysiology of, 642
  prevention of, 644
  treatment of, 643
Entamoeba histolytica, in foodborne illness, 102t, 530
Enteritis, regional (Crohn's disease), 491–492
  treatment of, 493
Environment, humankind's impact on, 80
Environmental agent(s), exposure to, 83–84
  index of suspicion and clinical acumen in, 84–85
  symptoms following, 84
Environmental epidemiologists, 82–83
Environmental factors, in domestic violence, 68
Environmental health and sanitation, 80–112. See also *Health and sanitation, environmental.*
Environmental Protection Agency (EPA), 81
  air monitoring by, 105
Environmental services, 81–85
Environmental spills, 111
EPA (Environmental Protection Agency), 81
  air monitoring by, 105
Ephedrine compounds, for elderly, 206
Epidemiology, 115–144
  analytic, 125–127, *126*
  basic parameters used in, 115
  chance in results and, 128–129

Epidemiology *(Continued)*
  descriptive, 117
  design method(s) and critical review of, 136–144
    analysis in, 140–141
    bias in, 138–139
    conclusions in, 142
    effect modification in, 142
    presentation of findings in, 140
      by media, interpretation of, 142–143
    sampling in, 137–138
    screening in, 143–144, 143t, 144t
    study observations in, 139–140
  Government Agencies and Offices for, 732
  measures of disease frequency in, 117–125
  measures of effect in, 127
  resources for, 145
  study design(s) in, 129–136
    case-control, 131–132
    cohort, 133–134
    cross-sectional, 130–131
    ecological, 129–130
    randomized clinical trials in, 134–136, 135t
  study of prostate cancer in, 116t
  web sites for, 732
Epstein-Barr virus (EBV), associated with infectious mononucleosis, 544, 545t
  oncogenic potential of, 628t
Erectile dysfunction (ED), definition of, 403
  depression associated with, 405
  laboratory evaluation of, 405
  medical conditions causing, 404
  patient and partner education in, 409b
  patient guide to, 406b–407b
  psychogenic origin of, 404–405
  treatment of, 408–409
ERT (estrogen replacement therapy), osteoporosis and, 387–388
  postmenopausal, 385

Escherichia coli, in foodborne illness, 100t, 101t, 529

Esophageal cancer, pathophysiology of, 644–645
prevention and screening for, 645
treatment of, 645

Esophageal strictures, benign, 495

Essential oils, 34–35

Estrogen, for urinary incontinence, 212t

Estrogen replacement therapy (ERT), osteoporosis and, 387–388
postmenopausal, 385

Ethambutol, for pediatric tuberculosis, 561

Ethical issues, of human genome project, 165

Eucalyptus, in aroma therapy, 36

Exercise, 146–158. See also *Physical activity.*
as subset of physical activity, definition of, 147
Government Agencies and Offices for, 733
Organizations, Associations, and Support Groups for, 733
web sites for, 733–734

Exercise training, excessive vs. moderate, 154–155

Experience, role of, in literacy and health care, 274–275

Exposure, patient, in trauma care, 340

Facial flushing, in foodborne illness, 96t

Factor VIII deficiency, 436

Factor IX deficiency, 436–437

Failure to thrive, 503

Faith, issues of, 9–10

Fall(s), in elderly, 208–209
causes of, 208t
prevention of, 332–333

Fallacy, ecological, 129

Falling out disorder, 53

Family, as interpreters, 285, 285b

Farm accidents, prevention of, 335, 338

Fast-twitch muscle fibers, 153

FDA (Food and Drug Administration), 90

Fecal impaction, 497–498

Fecal occult blood testing, 642

Federal law, in assuring linguistic access to care, 282–283

Femoral hernia, 488

Fertility, and infertility, 368–369
and preconception counseling, 366–367
awareness of, as method of contraception, 375

Fever, in foodborne illness, 97t

Feverfew, 30

Fibrillation, atrial, embolic stroke related to, 686, 690
treatment of, 428
ventricular, treatment of, 428

Fibromyalgia, epidemiology of, 467
pathophysiology of, 466–467
patient education in, 467–468
treatment of, 467

Fillenbaum instrumental activities of daily living assessment, 197b

Fire, personal safety in case of, 233–234

Fire extinguishers, appropriate use of, 220
in home, 218

Firearm(s), in home, counseling about, 223

Firearm accidents, fatal, *332*
prevention of, 331–332, *332*

First aid kit, 220

Fish poisoning, scombroid, 103t

Fissure, anal, 501

Fistula-in-ano, 501

Fitz-Hugh–Curtis syndrome, 553

Flat condylomata, 554–555, 554t

Flooding, disease spread by, 89
effect of, on health, 108t

Fluoroquinolone, for gastroenteritis, 532–533
for traveler's diarrhea, 352t

Folic acid (folate), deficiency of, 295

Folic acid (folate) *(Continued)*
  for women planning pregnancy, 367
  prevention of neural tube defects with, 174
Folk illnesses, Mexican, 55b
Folstein mini-mental status examination, 192b–193b
Food(s), contamination of, 91–92
    sources of, 91b
  particular type of, diseases associated with, 103t
  safe handling of, 94
Food and Drug Administration (FDA), 90
Food choices, pyramid guide to, *307*
    calorie-specific, 306, *308,* 309
Foodborne illness, 90–96
  acute, compendium of, 98t–103t
  allergic symptoms in, 96t
  characteristics of, 93b
  contaminated food and beverage causing, 91–92
  epidemiology of, 531
  factors favoring, 90b
  gastrointestinal tract symptoms of, lower, 95t
    upper, 94t
  neurologic symptoms in, 96t, 97t
  organisms associated with, 92t
  outbreak of, suspected, 92, 93b
  pathophysiology of, 527–531
  patient education about, 533
  patient management of, 95b
  prevention of, 533–534
  safe food handling and, 94
  screening for, 534
  shellfish toxins causing, 97t
  treatment of, 532–533
Foodborne pathogens, emergence of, factors contributing to, 93b
FoodNet, 96
Foot reflexology chart, *38*
Fracture(s), hip, osteoporotic, 459
Fragile X syndrome, 168
Friends, as interpreters, 285, 285b

Functional competency levels, of literacy, *268,* 268–269
  skills in, 270b

Gait, evaluation of, 209
Gallbladder disease,
    pathophysiology of, 478–479
  prevention of, 480–481
  treatment of, 480
Gallstones, 478–479
  associated with cholecystitis, 481
  risk factors for, 480–481
Gangrene, 434
Garlic, 28, 206
Gastric cancer, pathophysiology of, 645
  prevention and screening for, 646–647
  treatment of, 646
Gastric disorder(s), 495–496
Gastritis, 475–478
  definition of, 475
Gastroenteritis, dehydration associated with, 530
  infectious, 529
  related to foodborne illness, 527. See also *Foodborne illness.*
Gastroesophageal reflux disease (GERD), epidemiology of, 473
  pathophysiology of, 472–473
  patient education about, 474
  prevention of, 474–475
  treatment of, 474
Gastrointestinal disease, 472–503. See also specific disease, e.g., *Inflammatory bowel disease.*
  Government Agencies and Offices for, 755–756
  Organizations, Associations, and Support Groups for, 754–755
  symptoms of, in foodborne illness, 94t, 95t. See also *Foodborne illness.*
  waterborne, compendium of, 98t–103t
  web sites for, 756

Gastrointestinal procedures, recommended prophylaxis for, 528t

Gastroparesis, 496

Gender-specific death rate, 122, 123t

Gene(s). See also specific gene, e.g., *BRCA1 gene.*
cystic fibrosis, 176
for Marfan's syndrome, 169
responsible for malignant transformation, 624
activation of, 625

Gene mapping, 163–164

Gene sequence, 164

Gene therapy, 165
types of, 166–167

Genetic counseling, in cystic fibrosis, indications for, 177b

Genetic traits, associated with testicular cancer, 658

Genetics, 163–186
and Alzheimer's disease, 184–186
and cancer, 180–184
and reproduction, 170–180. See also *Prenatal* entries.
Government Agencies and Offices for, 735–736
human genome project in, 163–165
in germline therapy, 167
in somatic cell therapy, 166–167
of developmental disabilities, 167–170. See also *Disability(ies), developmental.*
Organizations, Associations, and Support Groups for, 734–735
uses of genomic information in, 165–166
web sites for, 736

Genital herpes, 378–379, 548–549
epidemiology of, 552
in children, 550
in pregnancy, 551
patient education about, 557–558
treatment of, 553

Genitalia, female, examination of, 390

Genitourinary procedures, recommended prophylaxis for, 528t

Genome, human, mapping and sequencing of, 163–164
developing laboratory and computational tools in, 164
ethical, legal, and social implications of, 165
uses for information based on, 165–166
of other organisms, mapping and sequencing of, 164

Gentamicin, prophylactic, for genitourinary and gastrointestinal procedures, 528t

Georgia Health Sciences Library Association, Consumer Health Committee of, 715–716

Geriatric Depression Scale, Yesavage-Brink, 195b

Geriatrics. See *Elderly.*

German measles (rubella), immunization for, 245–246
preconception counseling about, 367
vaccine-preventable, in adolescence, 262b
in childhood, 261b

Germline therapy, 167

Gerontological Society of America's Caregiver Strain Index, 199b

Gestational diabetes. See also *Diabetes mellitus.*
screening for, 614

Giardia lamblia, in foodborne illness, 102t, 530

Gilbert's syndrome, 496

Ginkgo biloba, 29, 206

Ginseng, 30, 206

Glatiramer acetate, for multiple sclerosis, 680

Glaucoma, 209

Gliosis, in multiple sclerosis, 678

Glucagon, for hypoglycemic emergencies, 610

Glucosamine, 33–34, 206

Gonadal tissue, germline therapy affecting, 167
Gonorrhea, 378
  epidemiology of, 552
  in children, 551
  Neisseria gonorrhoeae in, 378, 549
  pathophysiology of, 549
  patient education about, 558
  treatment of, 554
Gout, epidemiology of, 464–465
  pathophysiology of, 463–464
  prevention of, 465
  treatment of, 465
Government Agencies and Offices, for alternative medicine, 724–725
  for bone and joint disorders, 753–754
  for cardiology, 752
  for cultural influence, 726
  for domestic violence, 729
  for elderly, 737–738
  for environmental health and sanitation, 731
  for epidemiology, 732
  for exercise, 733
  for gastrointestinal disorders, 755–756
  for genetics, 735–736
  for health planning and illness prevention for international travel, 747
  for immunizations, 741
  for infectious diseases, 757–758
  for men's health, 750–751
  for mental health, 760
  for metabolic conditions, 762–763
  for neoplastic conditions, 763–764
  for neurologic disease, 766
  for nutrition education, 743–744
  for preventive strategies, 721
  for safety precautions in home, 739
  for substance abuse, 767–768
  for trauma, 745–746
  for women's health, 748–749
Graves' disease, 596, 597, 599

Ground water, chemical leachates in, 104–105
Gynecologic examination, of prepubertal child, 391–393
  of young adolescent, 389–391, 390t

HAART (highly active antiretroviral therapy), for AIDS, 515
Haemophilus influenzae type b (Hib), vaccine-preventable, in childhood, 258b
Haemophilus influenzae type b (Hib) vaccine, *241, 242, 248*
Harris-Benedict equation, for adults' caloric requirements, 303–304
Hashimoto's thyroiditis, 601
HBM (Health Belief Model), 13–14
  concepts of, 14
HBV (hepatitis B virus), hepatocellular cancer associated with, 627, 628t
HDL (high-density lipoprotein), 594, 595, 615
  and atherosclerosis, 151
Headache(s), migraine, diagnostic criteria for, 671b
  epidemiology of, 674–675
  pathophysiology of, 671–674
  patient education about, 675, 677
  prevention and screening for, 677
  subtypes of, 672
  treatment of, 675, 676t
Health, effects of natural disasters on, 108t
  overall, improvement of, 7
  WHO definition of, 7
Health and illness, in African American and African Caribbean communities, 56–58, 58b, 59b
  in Asian American communities, 54, 56, 57t
  in Mexican American communities, 54, 55b

Health and sanitation, environmental, 80–112
air quality and, 105–107
control of communicable diseases and, 85–88
emerging and re-emerging diseases and, 88–90
foodborne illness and, 90–96, 94t, 95t, 96t, 97t, 98t–103t
Government Agencies and Offices for, 731–732
in disaster management, 107–112
Organizations, Associations, and Support Groups for, 730
resources for, 113–114
services in, 81–85
water quality and, 96, 104–105
web sites for, 732
Health assessment, of elderly, 191–204
physical examination in, 192–204
aging with dignity's "five wishes" document in, 201b
assessment of abuse risk in, 200t
Fillenbaum instrumental ADL assessment in, 197b
Folstein mini-mental status examination in, 192b–193b
Gerontological Society of America's Caregiver Strain Index in, 199b
Katz index in ADL assessment in, 196b
laboratory tests in, 202t–203t
OARS multidimensional functional assessment questionnaire in, 198b
paper bag or shoebox test in, 201b
preventive screening, counseling, and prophylaxis recommendations in, 194t

Health assessment *(Continued)*
Yesavage-Brink geriatric depression scale in, 195b
Health behavior theories, 13–15
Health belief(s), client's, 47–48
Health Belief Model (HBM), 13–14
concepts of, 14
Health benefit(s), of physical activity, 147
for atherosclerosis, 151
for cardiovascular disease, 149–150
for colon cancer, 154
for hypertension, 150–151
for immune system, 154–155
for insulin-dependent diabetes mellitus, 152
for mental well-being, 155
for non–insulin-dependent diabetes mellitus, 151–152
for obesity, 152
for osteoarthritis, 152–153
for osteoporosis, 153–154
for skeletal muscle strength, 152–153
in activities of daily living, 152–153
physiologic explanations for, 149–155
Health care, linguistic access to, 281–286
bridging communication gap with LEP patients in, 284–285, 285b
clinicians' legal responsibilities in, 281–284
qualified interpreters in, 285–286
literacy and, 272–275
differences in processing information in, 272–274, *273*
role of logic, language, and experience in, 274–275
mental. See *Mental health care.*
Health educators, tasks of, 18

Health literacy, concept of, 267
Health promotion, as national
    health policy, 3
Health Risk Appraisal (HRA), 12
Health workers, community, 50
Health-literacy connection,
    269–272. See also
    Hypoliteracy; Literacy.
  effects of, 272
  lifestyle practices and, 271
  poverty and, 270–271
  stress and, 271
Healthy People 2010, goals of,
    3–4
Heart. See also *Cardiac* entries.
  anatomy of, 424
  conduction system of, 424–425
Heart disease, in women,
    382–384
  valvular, 445–449
    epidemiology of, 447
    pathophysiology of, 445–447
    patient education about, 448
    prevention of, 448–449
    treatment of, 448
Heart failure, congestive,
    439–442
    definition of, 439
    epidemiology of, 441, 441t
    pathophysiology of, 439–440
    patient education about, 442
    prevention of, 442
    treatment of, 441–442
Heart rate, 425
Heavy metals, in foodborne
    illness, 98t
Height, calculation of weight
    based on, 297
Helicobacter pylori infection,
    associated with gastric
    cancer, 646
  associated with gastritis and du-
    odenal ulcers, 475, 476,
    478
  screening for, 647
Hemiplegic migraine, 672. See
    also *Migraine headache.*
Hemochromatosis, 169–170, 496
Hemophilia A, 436
Hemophilia B (Christmas
    disease), 436–437

Hemorrhagic stroke, 685, 686.
    See also *Stroke.*
Hemorrhoids, 500–501
Hepatic disorder(s), 496–497
Hepatitis, 496–497
  epidemiology, 537
  pathophysiology of, 534–536,
    535t
  patient education about, 538–
    539
  prevention of, 539–540
  treatment of, 537–538
Hepatitis A, 534, 535t
  vaccine-preventable, in adoles-
    cence, 262b
    in international traveler,
      358–359
Hepatitis A vaccine, *241,* 242,
    255–256
Hepatitis B, 379, 534, 535t
  vaccine-preventable, in adoles-
    cence, 262b
    in childhood, 261b
    in international traveler, 361
Hepatitis B vaccine, 240–241,
    241, 248–249, 539
  new, 256
Hepatitis B virus (HBV),
    associated with increased
    risk of hepatocellular cancer,
    627, 628t
Hepatitis C, 535, 535t, 536
Hepatitis D, 535, 535t, 536
Hepatitis E, 535, 535t
Hepatocellular cancer, hepatitis B
    virus associated with, 627,
    628t
  pathophysiology of, 647
  prevention and screening for,
    648–649
  treatment of, 648
Her-2/neu oncogene, in
    endometrial cancer, 642
Herbal medicine, 27–30, 31t
  black cohosh in, 29
  dangerous, 31t
  echinacea in, 28–29
  garlic in, 28, 395
  ginkgo biloba in, 29, 395
  ginseng in, 30, 395
  other common herbs in, 30
  saw palmetto berry in, 29, 395

Herbal medicine *(Continued)*
St. John's wort in, 28, 395
Hereditary nonpolyposis
colorectal cancer (HNPCC),
183–184, 640. See also
Colorectal cancer.
Hernia, definition of, 488
epidemiology of, 489
pathophysiology of, 488–489
treatment of, 490
Herniated disk, 663
Herpes simplex virus, 548. See
also *Genital herpes.*
High-density lipoprotein (HDL),
594, 595, 615
and atherosclerosis, 151
Highly active antiretroviral
therapy (HAART), for AIDS,
515
Hip fractures, osteoporotic, 459
HIV. See *Human
immunodeficiency virus
(HIV).*
HNPCC (hereditary nonpolyposis
colorectal cancer), 183–184,
640. See also *Colorectal
cancer.*
Home, safety precaution(s) in,
217–235
childproofing as, 221–223,
221b–222b
essentials for, 218–221, 220b
for elderly, 228–229, 230b–
232b
Government Agencies and Offices for, 739
hazards and, 224
Organizations, Associations,
and Support Groups for,
738–739
personal issues as, 233–235
resources for, 236–238
web sites for, 739–740
Home remedies, African
Caribbean, 57–58
Native American, 56t
Homeopathy, 26–27
Homosexual men, 416–418
health issues in, 417–418
Hormonal contraception,
injectable and implantable
forms of, 372–374

Hormonal factors, role of, in
cancer, 630–631
Hormone replacement therapy
(HRT), postmenopausal,
385–386
benefits associated with, 385t
initiation of, 386–387
osteoporosis and, 387–388,
388t
risks associated with, 386t
Hospitalized patient, nutrition
education of, guidelines for,
295–296
HPV. See *Human papillomavirus
(HPV).*
HRA (Health Risk Appraisal), 12
HRT. See *Hormone replacement
therapy (HRT).*
Hsueh, in acupuncture, 25
Huffman-Graves speculum, 390
Human genome project, goals of,
163–165
Human immunodeficiency virus
(HIV), exposure to, 510
global impact of, 512
infection with, 380–381. See
also *Acquired immunode-
ficiency syndrome (AIDS).*
at-risk groups for, education
of, 517–518
counseling following, 517
diagnosis of, 512
neoplasms associated with,
627
symptoms of, 512–513
transmission of, 515–516
rates of, 516
Human papillomavirus (HPV),
379
cervical cancer associated with,
627, 628t, 638
classification of, 554t
in pregnancy, 551
pathophysiology of, 549, 549t
patient education about, 558
treatment of, 554–555
Huntington's disease, 667
Hurricane, effect of, on health,
108t
Hwa-byung, 52

Hydrocortisone sodium
succinate, for Addison's
disease, 622
21-Hydroxylase deficiency, 619
17-Hydroxyprogesterone, 619
5-Hydroxytryptamine (5-HT)
receptors, in migraine
headaches, 673
Hypercoagulability, 437
Hyperglycemia, 607–608
in pregnancy, 609
Hypericum perforatum, 28
Hyperlipidemia, epidemiology of,
615
pathophysiology of, 614–615
patient education about, 616
prevention of, 616–617
screening for, 617–618
treatment of, 615–616, 616t
Hyperliteracy, 266, 272. See also
Literacy.
Hyperparathyroidism,
epidemiology of, 605
pathophysiology of, 604–605
prevention and screening for,
606
treatment of, 605–606
Hypertension, benefits of
physical activity on, 150–151
definition of, 442–443
epidemiology of, 444
essential, 443
pathophysiology of, 442–443
patient education about, 444
prevention and screening for,
445
treatment of, 444
Hyperthyroidism, epidemiology
of, 598
pathophysiology of, 596–598
patient education about, 598–
600
prevention of, 600
treatment of, 598
Hypochondriasis, 587
Hypoglycemia, in pregnancy, 608
Hypoliteracy, 266. See also
Literacy.
causes of, 268–269
direct impacts of, 270
lifestyle choices limited by, 271
NALS data on, 269

Hypoliteracy *(Continued)*
universal precautions for, 275–
281
accuracy in, 280–281
brevity in, 277
clarity and appreciation in,
278–280
picturesque in, 280
Pulitzer's formula in, 277–
281
Hypoparathyroidism,
epidemiology of, 606
pathophysiology of, 605–606
patient education for, 606
prevention of, 607
treatment of, 606
Hypothesis testing, in
epidemiology, 127–128
Hypothyroidism, epidemiology
of, 601
pathophysiology of, 599–600
patient education about, 601–
602
prevention of, 602
treatment of, 601

Idiopathic thrombocytic purpura
(ITP), in children, 436
Ileus, paralytic, 499–500
Illness. See also *Health and
illness.*
terminal, counseling patients
about, 631, 633–634
management of, 5
travel-related. See *Travel-related illness.*
Immobility, in elderly, 207
Immune system, health benefits
of physical activity for,
154–155
Immunization(s), 239–264
and disease, 263
bacille Calmette-Guérin, 563
childhood, 240–244, *241,* 243t
cost-benefit analysis of, 243t
epidemiology and rationale for,
240, 242, 243t, 244–250
for HIV-positive patients, 513
for infectious diseases, 508

Immunization(s) *(Continued)*
for international travelers, 357t
Government Agencies and Offices for, 741
Haemophilus influenzae type b, 248
hepatitis B, 248–249
measles-mumps-rubella, 244–246
missed, strategies to prevent, 250–253
newer, 253–256
for hepatitis, 263
for meningococcus, 262–263
for rotavirus, 262
for varicella, 254, 261
Organizations, Associations, and Support Groups for, 740–741
pertussis-diphtheria-tetanus, *241*, 242, 246–248
pneumococcal, 249–250
polio, 240, 242, 244
resources for, 264–265
things you need to know about, 254b–256b
web sites for, 741–742
Immunization schedules, current, 240, *241–242*
Immunosuppression therapy, for multiple sclerosis, 680
Inactivity, prolonged, 155–156
Incarcerated hernia, 489
Incidence, as measure of disease frequency, 121
Incidence density, as measure of instantaneous rate, 121
Incontinence, in elderly, 210–211
medications for, 212t
Independence, in elderly, 206–207
Infant(s). See also *Child(ren)*.
caloric requirements of, 304
colic in, 502
Infarction, myocardial, C-reactive protein as predictor of, 433
rehabilitation following, 432
pulmonary, 438
Infection(s), 505–565. See also specific infection, e.g., *Tuberculosis (TB)*.
antibiotic resistance and, 509

Infection(s) *(Continued)*
control of, public health strategies for, 508
death rate for, *506*
emergence of, factors contributing to, 508b
Institute of Medicine definition of, 507
foodborne. See *Foodborne illness*.
Government Agencies and Offices for, 757–758
immunizations for, 508
newly recognized pathogens causing, 507t
Organizations, Associations, and Support Groups for, 756–757
pathophysiology and etiology of, 505–506
transmission of, via blood transfusions, 509
web sites for, 758
Infectious mononucleosis, 544–548. See also *Mononucleosis, infectious*.
Infective endocarditis, 522–527, 527t, 528t. See also *Endocarditis, infective*.
Infertility, female, 368–369
causes of, 368
definition of, 368
male, 414–415
causes of, 415b
Inflammatory bowel disease, 490–494
Crohn's disease as, 491–492
epidemiology of, 492–493
patient education about, 494
prevention of, 494
pseudomembranous colitis as, 490–491
treatment of, 493–494
ulcerative colitis as, 491
Influenza, vaccine-preventable, in adolescence, 260b
Information, differences in processing, literacy and health care and, 272–274, *273*
Information bias, 139
Inguinal hernia, 488, 489

Inguinal hernia *(Continued)*
treatment of, 490
Injury. See *Trauma.*
Institute of Medicine, emerging
infections defined by, 507
Insulin, 594–595
Insulin therapy, for diabetes
mellitus type I, 609–610
Insulin-dependent diabetes
mellitus. See *Diabetes
mellitus, insulin-dependent
(type I).*
Intellectual health, 9
Interferon(s), for hepatitis B, 538
for hepatitis C, 538
for multiple sclerosis, 680
Intermittent claudication, in
peripheral vascular disease,
434
International Screening Prostate
Questionnaire, 402t
International travel, health
planning and illness
prevention for, 343–364.
See also *Travel-related
illness.*
Government Agencies and Offices for, 747
web sites for, 747
Internet, as resource for
alternative medicine, 41–42
patient education and, 18–19
Interpreter(s), 48–51, 48b, 49b,
50b
family and friends as, 285,
285b
language bank, 50
nonprofessional, 51
professional, 50–51
qualified, in linguistic access to
care, 285–286
Interpreter-dependent interviews,
language use in, guidelines
for, 50b
Interviewer bias, 139
Intestinal polyps, 500
Intimate relationships, abusive,
71. See also *Domestic
violence.*
Intrauterine device (IUD), 374
postcoital, as emergency contraception, 376t, 377

Ionizing radiation, causing
cancer, 629–630
Iron accumulation, in body,
169–170
Irritable bowel syndrome,
pathophysiology of, 486
treatment of, 487
Ischemic colitis, 499
Ischemic infarct, 686
Islam religion, 58–59
Isoniazid, for pediatric
tuberculosis, 561
Itching, in foodborne illness, 96t
ITP (idiopathic thrombocytic
purpura), in children, 436
IUD (intrauterine device), 374
postcoital, as emergency contra-
ception, 376t, 377

Janeway's lesions, in infective
endocarditis, 524
Japanese encephalitis, vaccine-
preventable, in international
traveler, 361
Jaundice, in pregnancy, 536
newborn, 502
Joint(s), healthy, physical activity
for, 153
Joint disorders, 453–471. See also
specific disorder, e.g.,
Rheumatoid arthritis.
Government Agencies and Offices for, 753–754
Organizations, Associations,
and Support Groups for, 753
web sites for, 754
Judaism, Orthodox, 59–60

Katz index, in, ADL assessment,
196b
Keratotic warts, 554t
Kernig's sign, 542
Ketoacidosis, diabetic, 607
Knowledge, cultural, 47
Koro, 51–52
Kosher, keeping, 60
Kussmaul's respiration, 607

Laboratory tests, for elderly,
202t–203t

Lacunar infarct, 686
Lamivudine, for hepatitis B, 538
Language, in Folstein's mini-mental status examination, 193b
　in interpreter-dependent interviews, guidelines for, 50b
　role of, in literacy and health care, 274–275
Language bank interpreter, 50
Lap belt(s), in trauma prevention, 330
Latter-Day Saints, 60
Lavandula species, 36
Lavender, in aroma therapy, 36
Law, requirements of, in trauma prevention, 326
Laxatives, abuse of, 498
LDL (low-density lipoprotein), 430, 594, 595, 614
　and atherosclerosis, 151
Lead poisoning, in home, 224
LEARN acronym, 47
Learned behavior, in domestic violence, 68
Legal issues, of human genome project, 165
Legal responsibility(ies), clinicians',
　in assuring linguistic access to care, 281–284
　　accreditation standards and, 283–284
　　federal law and, 282–283
　　liability for negligence and, 283
LEP. See *Limited English proficiency (LEP)*.
LES (lower esophageal sphincter), hypofunctioning of, 472–473
Lethal chemical weapons, 110
Levodopa, for Parkinson's disease, 684
Levofloxacin, for traveler's diarrhea, 351t, 352t
Levothyroxine, for hyperthyroidism, 598
Lewy body(ies), in Alzheimer's disease, 667
　in Parkinson's disease, 683
Lewy body disease, 667

Lhermitte's phenomenon, in multiple sclerosis, 678
Liability for negligence, in failure to overcome language barrier, 283
Lifestyle and disease prevention, in complementary medical practices, 24
Lifestyle practices, and literacy, 271
　high-risk, preconception counseling about, 366–367
Lighting, yard, 234
Limited English proficiency (LEP), 267
　patients with, bridging communication gap for, 284–285, 285b
Linguistic access, to care, 281–286
　bridging communication gap with LEP patients in, 284–285, 285b
　clinicians' legal responsibilities in, 281–284
　qualified interpreters in, 285–286
Lipid metabolism, 594–595
Lipoprotein(s), 594, 595, 614, 615
　levels of, in atherosclerosis, 151, 430
Listening comprehension, literacy skills in, 272–273
Listeria monocytogenes, in foodborne illness, 100t
Literacy, 266–286. See also *Hypoliteracy.*
　affecting health, 269–270
　definitions of, 266–267
　document, 268
　health, concept of, 267
　health care and, 272–275
　　differences in processing information in, 272–274, *273*
　　role of logic, language, and experience in, 274–275
　lifestyle practices and, 271
　NALS measurement of, functional competency levels in, *268,* 268–269
　skills in, 270b

Literacy *(Continued)*
poverty and, 270–271
prose, 268
quantitative (numeracy), 268
resources concerning, 288–290
stress and, 271
Literate, functionally, 267
Lithium use, in pregnancy, 180
Liver disease, chronic, 496–497
inflammatory. See *Hepatitis* entries.
neoplastic. See *Hepatocellular cancer.*
Logic, language, and experience (LLE), role of, in literacy and health care, 274–275
Long-term care, for elderly, 213–214
Loperamide, for traveler's diarrhea, 351, 352t
Low back pain, pathophysiology of, 661–663
prevention of, 664
screening for, 664–665
treatment of, 663–664
Low self-esteem, effect of physical activity on, 155
Low-density lipoprotein (LDL), 430, 594, 595, 614
and atherosclerosis, 151
Lower esophageal sphincter (LES), hypofunctioning of, 472–473
Lumbar spine, nerve root compression in, 662
Lung cancer, epidemiology of, 650
in women, 384
pathophysiology of, 649–650
prevention and screening for, 651
treatment of, 650
Lymph glands, swollen, in foodborne illness, 97t

Mal de ojo, as Mexican folk illness, 55b
Malabsorption, 497
Malaise, in foodborne illness, 97t
Malaria, 353–356

Malaria *(Continued)*
chemoprophylaxis for, 354, 355t, 356
Male menopause, 410
Mallory-Weiss tear, 495
Malnutrition, 294
Manic episode, 574t
Manipulative and body-based systems, in complementary medical practices, 24–25
Manmade disaster(s), 109–112
environmental spills as, 111
warfare as, 110–111
Mantoux test, 563
MAOIs (monoamine oxidase inhibitors), for anxiety, 585
for depression, 577
Marfan's syndrome, 168–169
Mass casualty incident, 107
Massage, 38–39
Maternal serum alpha-fetoprotein, elevated, prenatal screening for, 173
Maximal oxygen uptake (VO_{2max}), in cardiovascular fitness, 151–152
Meal plan(s), 1200 calorie sample, 306, 309, 310t
pyramid-based, 311
Measles, vaccine-preventable, in adolescence, 259b
in childhood, 257b
Measles-mumps-rubella (MMR) vaccine, *241*, 243, 244–246
for healthy women of reproductive age, 367
Measures of effect, in epidemiology, 127
Meat, recall of, 91
Media, presentation of findings in epidemiologic studies by, interpretation of, 142
Medicine knowledge, traditional and alternative, 11
Medroxyprogesterone acetate (Depo-Provera), 372–374
Mefloquine, prophylactic, for malaria, 355t
Megacolon, toxic, 500
Melaleuca species, 36
Melanoma, 655
treatment of, 656

Meningitis, pathophysiology of, 540–542
prevention of, 544
treatment of, 542–543
Meningococcus vaccine, 260b, 262–263
Menopause, hormone replacement therapy for, 385–386, 385t, 386t
initiation of, 386–387
osteoporosis and, 387–388, 388t
male, 410
support through, 384–385
Men's health issues, Government Agencies and Offices for, 750–751
Organizations, Associations, and Support Groups for, 750
web sites for, 751–752
Menses, cessation of, 384. See also *Menopause.*
Mental health, aspects of, displacement and shelter living as, 108
benefits of physical activity in, 155
delivery of care and, changes in, 569–570
Government Agencies and Offices for, 760
in primary care setting, 571–572
Organizations, Associations, and Support Groups for, 758–760
web sites for, 760–761
Mental health disorder(s), 569–591. See also specific disorder, e.g., *Depression.*
documented prevalence of, in U.S., 569
hospitalization in, 570–571
referral to specialist for, 570
specialty care for, 572t
treatment of, 570
Metabolic disorder(s), 593–623. See also specific disorder, e.g., *Diabetes mellitus.*
Government Agencies and Offices for, 762–763

Metabolic disorder(s) *(Continued)*
Organizations, Associations, and Support Groups for, 761–762
web sites for, 763
Metastasis, 626
Methylphenidate hydrochloride (Ritalin), for attention deficit hyperactivity disorder, 590
Methylprednisolone, for multiple sclerosis, 680
Mexican Americans, health and illness in, 54, 55b
Micronutrients, deficiency of, 294
role of, in disease prevention, 294–295
Mid-life crisis, male, 410–411
Migraine headache, diagnostic criteria for, 671b
epidemiology of, 674–675
pathophysiology of, 671–674
patient education about, 675, 677
prevention and screening for, 677
subtypes of, 672
treatment of, 675, 676t
Mind-body medicine, 23–24
Mini-mental status examination, Folstein's, 192b–193b
Minocycline, for rheumatoid arthritis, 456
Mismatch-repair genes, 624
Mitral regurgitation, 446, 447
Mitral stenosis, 445–446
Mitral valve prolapse, in children, 447
Mobility, in elderly, 207
reduced, 228
Monoamine oxidase inhibitors (MAOIs), for anxiety, 585
for depression, 577
Monolingual providers, in cross-cultural environment, guidelines for, 48b
Mononucleosis, infectious, 544–548
complications associated with, 545t
pathophysiology of, 544–546
patient education about, 547
prevention of, 548
treatment of, 546–547

Monospot test, for infectious mononucleosis, 547

Mood disorder(s), 573–586. See also under specific condition for details.
anxiety as, 581–586
bipolar, 579–581
classification of, 574t
depression as, 573–579

Morbidity rates, 120t, 121
standard, 125, 125t

Mormons, 60

Mortality rates, 123t
standard, 125, 125t

Motor vehicle(s), alterations to, in trauma prevention, 326–327
safety of, design features affecting, 226

Motor vehicle accident(s), as leading cause of death, 317
prevention of, 327, 330–331

Motorcycle accidents, prevention of, 331

Moxibustion, with acupuncture, 25

Mueller vaginoscope, 393

Multiple sclerosis, categories of, 679
epidemiology of, 680
pathophysiology of, 677–680
patient education about, 681
prevention and screening for, 681–682
treatment of, 680–681

Multivitamin supplements, 295. See also *Vitamin* entries.

Mumps, immunization for, 245
vaccine-preventable, in adolescence, 262b
in childhood, 260b

Münchausen's syndrome by proxy, suspicion of, 71

Muscle(s), types of, 153

Mushrooms, poisonous, 103t

Mycobacterium tuberculosis, 560. See also *Tuberculosis (TB).*

Myocardial infarction, C-reactive protein as predictor of, 433
rehabilitation following, 432

NALS (National Adult Literacy Survey), 267, *268,* 268–269

Naltrexone, in treatment of alcohol abuse, 702

National Adult Literacy Survey (NALS), 267, *268,* 268–269

National Center for Complementary and Alternative Medicine (NCCAM), 23

National Commission for Certification of Acupuncturists (NCCA), 26

National Domestic Violence Organizations, 74t

National Institute on Alcohol Abuse and Alcoholism (NIAAA), 701

National Literacy Act, 267

National Safety Council (NSC), actions and items recommended by, 219b

Native American communities, health and illness in, 54, 56t

Natural disasters, 107–109
disease spread by, 89
effects of, on health, 108t
postdisaster management and relief recommendations for, 109b

Nausea, in foodborne illness, 94t

NCCA (National Commission for Certification of Acupuncturists), 26

NCCAM (National Center for Complementary and Alternative Medicine), 23

Negligence, liability for, in failure to overcome language barrier, 283

Neisseria gonorrhoeae, 378, 549. See also *Gonorrhea.*

Neisseria meningitidis, 255

Neisseria meningitis, 540, 541. See also *Meningitis.*

Neoplasia. See *Cancer.*

Nerve root compression, in low back pain, 662

Neural tube defects, prenatal screening for, 173–174

Neuritic plaques, 665

Neurologic disease, 661–690. See also specific disease, e.g., *Multiple sclerosis.*
  Government Agencies and Offices for, 766
  Organizations, Associations, and Support Groups for, 765–766
  web sites for, 766
Neurologic symptoms, in foodborne illness, 96t, 97t
New York Heart Association (NYHA) Functional Classification, of congestive heart failure, 441, 441t
Newborn jaundice, 502
NIAAA (National Institute on Alcohol Abuse and Alcoholism), 701
Nicotine abuse, epidemiology of, 705
  pathophysiology of, 704–705
  patient education about, 706
  prevention of, 706–707
  screening for, 707
  treatment of, 705–706
NNRTIs (non-nucleoside reverse transcriptase inhibitors), for AIDS, 513, 517t
Non–insulin-dependent diabetes mellitus. See *Diabetes mellitus, non–insulin-dependent (type II).*
Non–intravenous drug use-related endocarditis, 523
Non-nucleoside reverse transcriptase inhibitors (NNRTIs), for AIDS, 513, 517t
Nonprofessional interpreter, 51
Nonseminomatous germ cell tumors, 657. See also *Testicular cancer.*
Nonsteroidal anti-inflammatory drugs (NSAIDs), for osteoarthritis, 462
  for rheumatoid arthritis, 455
  role of, in gastritis and peptic ulcer disease, 476
Non-ulcer dyspepsia, pathophysiology of, 486
  treatment of, 487–488

Norplant, 373–374
NRTIs (nucleoside reverse transcriptase inhibitors), for AIDS, 513, 517t
NSAIDs. See *Nonsteroidal anti-inflammatory drugs (NSAIDs).*
NSC (National Safety Council), actions and items recommended by, 219b
Nucleoside reverse transcriptase inhibitors (NRTIs), for AIDS, 513, 517t
Numeracy (quantitative literacy), 268
Nutraceuticals, for osteoarthritis, 462
Nutrient(s), single, in alternative medicine, 30, 32–34
Nutrition education, 291–314
  in clinical practice, Government Agencies and Offices for, 743–744
    Organizations, Associations, and Support Groups for, 743
    tool(s) for integration of, 296–314
      caloric prescriptions as, 12–16, 300
      caloric-specific, 306–314
      weight change intervention as, 296–300
    web sites for, 744
  micronutrients in, 294–295
  of hospitalized patient, guidelines for, 295–296
  patient assessment in, 291–292
  principles and purposes of, 292–294
Nutritional drinks, 206
Nutritional screening, preconception, 367
Nutritional supplements, for elderly, 204–206

Obesity, 291. See also *Nutrition education.*
  genetic tendency for, 293

Obesity *(Continued)*
  health benefits of physical activity in, 152
  in children, prevalence of, 293
Obsessive-compulsive disorder, 583t
Occupational health, 9
Occupational Safety and Health Administration (OSHA), 84
Odds ratio, as measure of effect in epidemiology, 127
Office intervention(s), 1–2
Ofloxacin, for traveler's diarrhea, 351t, 352t
Oil(s), essential, 34–35
  tea tree, 36–37
Older Americans Resources and Services (OARS) Multidimensional Functional Assessment Questionnaire, 198b
Oncogene(s), 624. See also *Gene(s);* specific oncogene.
  activation of, 625
Ophthalmorphic migraine, 672. See also *Migraine headache.*
Optic neuritis, in multiple sclerosis, 678
Oral contraceptive pill, 370–372
  choice of, 371–372, 372b
  contraindications to, 370t
  noncontraceptive benefits of, 371
  warning signs associated with, 371t
Organic compounds, volatile, in buildings, 107
Organizations, Associations, and Support Groups, for alternative medicine, 724
  for bone and joint disorders, 753
  for cardiology, 752
  for cultural influence, 726
  for domestic violence, 728–729
  for elderly, 736–737
  for environmental health and sanitation, 730
  for exercise, 733
  for gastrointestinal disorders, 754–755
  for genetics, 734–735

Organizations *(Continued)*
  for immunizations, 740–741
  for infectious diseases, 756–757
  for men's health, 750
  for mental health, 758–760
  for metabolic conditions, 761–762
  for neoplastic conditions, 763
  for neurologic disease, 765–766
  for nutrition education, 743
  for safety precautions in home, 738–739
  for substance abuse, 767
  for trauma, 744–745
  for women's health, 748
Orientation, in Folstein's mini-mental status examination, 192b
Orthodox Judaism, 59–60
OSHA (Occupational Safety and Health Administration), 84
Osler's nodes, in infective endocarditis, 524–525
Osteoarthritis, epidemiology of, 461–462
  health benefits of physical activity in, 152–153
  pathophysiology of, 460–461
  patient education in, 462–463
  prevention of, 463
  treatment of, 462
Osteoporosis, epidemiology of, 458–459
  health benefits of physical activity in, 153–154
  hormone replacement therapy and, 387–388
  pathophysiology of, 457–458
  patient education in, 459–460
  prevention of, 460
  risks for, 387
  screening for, 460
  secondary, 457–458
  treatment of, 459
  Type I, 457
  Type II, 457
  worsening, medications associated with, 388t
Ovarian cancer, hereditary, 180–183
  BRCA1 gene in, 181–182

Ovarian cancer *(Continued)*
  BRCA2 gene in, 182–183
  hormone-related, 630
Ovulation, laboratory
    documentation of, 369
  presumptive, determination of,
    368–369
Oxygen uptake, maximal (VO_{2max}),
    in cardiovascular fitness,
    151–152

p24 core antigen analysis, of HIV
    infection, 512
p53 tumor suppressor gene, in
    breast cancer, 636
Pad test, 211
Pain, 587
  low back. See *Low back pain.*
Paint, lead-based, 224
Panax ginseng, 30
Pancreas, endocrine, 594
Pancreatic cancer, 651–653
Pancreatitis, pathophysiology of,
    481–482
  treatment of, 482–483
Panic attacks, 582t
  treatment of, 585
Papanicolaou (Pap) smear, for
    cervical cancer, 640
  in adolescence, 391
Papaverine, self-injection of, for
    erectile dysfunction, 408
Paper bag test, of elderly, 201b
Papular warts, 554t
Paralysis, in foodborne illness,
    96t
Paralytic ileus, 499–500
Parathyroid gland, 594
  disorder(s) of, 602–607
    hyperparathyroidism as,
      602–605
    hypoparathyroidism as, 605–
      607
Parathyroid hormone (PTH), 594
  hypersecretion of, 602–603. See
    also *Hyperparathyroidism.*
Parathyroidectomy, for
    hyperparathyroidism, 604
Parentage, testing for, postnatal,
    172
  prenatal, 171–172

Parkinson's disease, dementia
    associated with, 667
  pathophysiology of, 682–683,
    683t
  prevention and screening for,
    685
  treatment of, 684–685
Parkinson's syndrome, 682
Paternity testing, postnatal, 172
  prenatal, 171–172
Pathogens, newly recognized,
    causing infection, 507t
Patient(s), counseling, about
    prognosis of malignancy,
    631, 633–634
  empowering, concept of, 1
  hospitalized, nutrition educa-
    tion of, guidelines for,
    295–296
  management of, with food-
    borne illness, 95b
Patient education, and Internet,
    18–19
  and literacy, 266–286. See also
    Hypoliteracy; Literacy.
    web sites for, 742–743
  concept of, 17–18
  follow-up in, 11–12
  levels in, 15
  materials in, translation of, 284
  medicine knowledge base in,
    traditional and alternative,
    11
  rationale and barriers for,
    10–18
  time commitment in, 11
  understanding and identifying
    risk factors in, 12
  understanding behavior change
    in, 12–17
PCP *(Pneumocystis carinii*
    pneumonia), 510
PCRs (polymerase chain
    reactions), in prenatal
    parentage testing, 172
PEI (pesticide exposure
    indicator), 130
Pelvic examination, of female
    adolescent, 389
Pelvic inflammatory disease
    (PID), 378
  epidemiology of, 552

Pelvic inflammatory disease (PID) *(Continued)*
  pathophysiology of, 549
  treatment of, 555–556
Pemoline (Cylert), for attention deficit hyperactivity disorder, 590
Penile prosthesis, implantation of, for erectile dysfunction, 409
Peptic ulcer disease, epidemiology of, 477
  pathophysiology of, 475–477
  patient education about, 478
  prevention of, 478
  treatment of, 477–478
Percutaneous transluminal coronary angioplasty (PTCA), 431
Period prevalence, as measure of disease frequency, 121–122
Peripheral vascular disease, 433–436. See also *Vascular disease, peripheral.*
Person, epidemiologic description of, 117
Personal protective devices (PPDs), in trauma care, 340
Personal safety, issues of, 233–235
  of international travelers, preventive measures for, 363b
Personality characteristics, domestic violence and, 68
Personality disorder(s), 572t
Persuasion, in trauma prevention, 326
Pertussis (whooping cough), immunization for, 246–247
  vaccine-preventable, in childhood, 257b
Pertussis-diphtheria-tetanus vaccine, *241,* 242, 246–248
Pesticide exposure indicator (PEI), 130
Pharmacogenetics, 165–166
Phenylketonuria, 167
Phlebotomy, for hemochromatosis, 170
Phobia(s), social, 583t
Physical activity. See also *Exercise.*

Physical activity *(Continued)*
  counseling about, approaches to, 157
    effectiveness of, 156–157
  definitions of, 147–148
  guidelines for, 146
  health benefits of, 147
    for atherosclerosis, 151
    for cardiovascular disease, 149–150
    for colon cancer, 154
    for hypertension, 150–151
    for immune system, 154–155
    for insulin-dependent diabetes mellitus, 152
    for mental well-being, 155
    for non–insulin-dependent diabetes mellitus, 151–152
    for obesity, 152
    for osteoarthritis, 152–153
    for osteoporosis, 153–154
    for skeletal muscle strength, 152–153
    in activities of daily living, 152–153
    physiologic explanations for, 149–155
  in elderly, 206–207
  intermittent bursts of, 148
  maintenance of, 155–156
  moderate, 148t
    examples of, 147–149
  patterns of, 146–147
  promotion of, for future generations, 158
  resources for, 160–161
  risks of, 156
  sudden cardiac death during, 156
Physical examination, of elderly, 192–204
  aging with dignity's "five wishes" document in, 201b
  assessment of abuse risk in, 200t
  Duke's OARS multidimensional functional assessment questionnaire in, 198b

Physical examination
  (Continued)
  Fillenbaum instrumental
      ADL assessment in, 197b
  Folstein mini-mental status
      examination in, 192b–
      193b
  Gerontological Society of
      America's Caregiver
      Strain Index in, 199b
  Katz index in, 196b
  laboratory tests in, 202t–203t
  paper bag or shoebox test in,
      201b
  preventive screening, coun-
      seling, and prophylaxis
      recommendations in,
      194t
  Yesavage-Brink geriatric de-
      pression scale in, 195b
Physical health, 8
Physical security, 233
Pick's disease, 667
Picturesque, in Pulitzer's formula
    for prize-winning writing,
    280
PID. See *Pelvic inflammatory
    disease (PID).*
Place, epidemiologic description
    of, 117
Plants, poisonous, 103t
Plasma lipid metabolism, 594–595
Plasmodium falciparum, 353. See
    also *Malaria.*
Plasmodium vivax, 353. See also
    Malaria.
Plummer-Vinson syndrome, 495
Pneumococcal vaccine, 249–250
  new, 256
Pneumococcus, vaccine-
    preventable, in adolescence,
    260b
Pneumocystis carinii pneumonia
    (PCP), 510
Poisoning, food, 103t. See also
    Foodborne illness.
  lead, in home, 224
  prevention of, 333
Polio (poliomyelitis), vaccine-
    preventable, in childhood,
    256b
  in international traveler, 360

Polio vaccine, 240, *241,* 242
  inactivated, 244
  oral, 244
Pollution, air, classification of,
    106
Polymerase chain reactions
    (PCRs), in prenatal parentage
    testing, 172
Polypharmacy, in elderly,
    211–213
Polyposis syndromes, 640
Polyps, intestinal, 500
Population x, age-adjusted death
    rate for, 124
Population y, age-adjusted death
    rate for, 124
Postcoital emergency
    contraception, 375, 376t, 377
Postinjury emergency care,
    improvement in, 327
Postpartum bipolar disorder, 577
Postpartum blues, 574
Postpartum psychosis, 574–575
Postpartum thyroiditis, 601
Posttraumatic stress disorder
    (PTSD), 581
  defined, 583t
Postvoiding residual test, 211
Potential disease, prevention of,
    6–7
Potentization, in homeopathic
    medicine, 26
Poultry, recall of, 91
Poverty, and literacy, 270–271
PPDs (personal protective
    devices), in trauma care, 340
Preconception counseling, for
    women, 366–367
Preeclampsia, 443
Pregnancy, Addison's disease
    during, 621–622
  adverse effects of teratogens
      during, 179–180, 179b
  alcohol abuse during, 698
  anxiety disorder during, 584
  appendicitis during, 484
  arrhythmias during, 426
  bleeding disorders during, 437
  carrier testing for cystic fibrosis
      during, 176–178. See also
      Cystic fibrosis.

Pregnancy *(Continued)*
  Cushing's syndrome in, 618–619
  diabetes mellitus type I in, 608–609
  diabetes mellitus type II in, 611–612
  diagnosis of breast cancer during, 636
  fibromyalgia in, 466–467
  gallstones during, 479
  gastroenteritis during, 531
  GERD during, 473
  hernias during, 489
  HIV-related disease in, course of, 511
  hyperparathyroidism in, 604–605
  hypertension during, 443
  hyperthyroidism in, 597
  hypothyroidism in, 600–601
  increased risk of stroke during, 687
  infective endocarditis during, 523–524
  inflammatory bowel disease during, 492
  migraine headaches during, 673–674, 674t
  multiple sclerosis and, 679
  nicotine abuse in, 705
  osteoporosis and, 458
  pancreatitis during, 482
  parentage in, postnatal testing for, 172
  prenatal testing for, 171–172
  prenatal diagnosis during, 170, 171b
  prenatal triple screening during, 172–176
    abnormal results in, evaluation of, 175–176
    for elevated maternal serum alpha-fetoprotein, 173
    for neural tube defects, 173–174
    for trisomy 18, 175
    for trisomy 21 (Down syndrome), 174–175
  rheumatoid arthritis and, 454–455
  sexually transmitted disease and, 551

Pregnancy *(Continued)*
  viral hepatitis during, 536
  voluntary interruption of, 377–378
Premature ejaculation, 409
Prenatal diagnosis, 170, 171b
Prenatal triple screening, 172–176
  abnormal results in, evaluation of, 175–176
  for elevated maternal serum alpha-fetoprotein, 173
  for neural tube defects, 173–174
  for trisomy 18, 175
  for trisomy 21 (Down syndrome), 174–175
Prepubertal child, gynecologic examination of, 391–393
Presentation of findings, in epidemiologic studies, 140
  by media, interpretation of, 142
Prevalence, as measure of disease frequency, 121–122
Preventive strategy(ies), 1–19
  Government Agencies and Offices for, 721
  introduction to, 1–7
  Organizations, Associations, and Support Groups for, 719–721
  patient education in, Internet and, 18–19
    rationale for and barriers to, 10–18
  resources for, 22
  understanding, 4–7
  web sites for, 721–724
  wellness as, 7–10
Primary prevention, of disease, 4–5
Prize-winning writing, Pulitzer's formula for, 277–281
Processing information, differences in, literacy and health care and, 272–274, *273*
Proctitis, 501
Professional interpreter, 50–51
Proportion, as measure of disease frequency, 118, 119t
Prose literacy, 268

Prosorbacol, for rheumatoid arthritis, 457

Prostaglandin E₁, self-injection of, for erectile dysfunction, 408

Prostaglandin F₂ synthesis, increased, exercise and, 154

Prostate cancer, American Cancer Society screening recommendations for, 631t
  basic sciences, clinical medicine, and epidemiology in, 116t
  fear of, 397
  hormone-related, 630
  pathophysiology of, 653–654
  patient education about, 654
  PSA screening for, 399, 654
    recommended, 400
  treatment of, 654

Prostate-specific antigen (PSA), 398–400, 654
  age-specific, 399, 399t
  elevation of, benign prostatic hypertrophy and, 401
  in screening for prostate cancer, 399, 655
    recommendations for, 400
  normal value of, 398

Prostate-specific antigen density (PSAD), calculation of, 399

Prostatitis, 400–401

Prostatodynia, 400–401

Prosthesis, implantation of, for erectile dysfunction, 409

Prostration, in foodborne illness, 97t

Protease inhibitors, for AIDS, 513–514, 517t

Provider-interpreter-patient interactions, guidelines for, 49b

PSA. See *Prostate-specific antigen (PSA).*

PSAD (prostate-specific antigen density), calculation of, 399

Pseudomembranous colitis, 490–491
  treatment of, 493–494

Psychosis, postpartum, 574–575

Psychotherapeutic approaches, to depression, 576

PTCA (percutaneous transluminal coronary angioplasty), 431

PTH (parathyroid hormone), 594
  hypersecretion of, 604. See also *Hyperparathyroidism.*

PTSD (posttraumatic stress disorder), 581
  defined, 583t

Public health, science of. See *Epidemiology.*

Public health strategies, for control of infections, 508

Pulitzer's formula, for prize-winning writing, 277–281
  accuracy in, 280–281
  brevity in, 277
  clarity in, 278–280
  picturesque in, 280

Pulmonary embolism, 438

Pulmonary infarction, 438

Pulmonary valvular disease, in children, 446

Purkinje system, 424

P-value, in epidemiology, 128

Pyramid guide, to food choices, calorie-specific, 306, *308,* 309
  to serving choices and sizes, *307*

Qualified interpreters, in linguistic access to care, 285–286

Quality of life, elderly and, 214

Quantitative literacy (numeracy), 268

Quick reactions, reduced capacity for, in elderly, 229

Rabies, 88
  vaccine-preventable, in traveler, 361

Race-specific death rate, 122, 123t

Radiation, ionizing, causing cancer, 629–630

Radiation therapy, risk of secondary malignancies associated with, 629

Radiculopathy, 661–665
Radon, in home, 224
  risk of lung cancer associated
    with, 630
Random sampling, in
    epidemiologic studies, 137
Randomized clinical trials,
    epidemiologic, 134–136
  types of error in, 135t
Rate(s), as measure of disease
    frequency, 118, 119t
  adjusted, 122, 124–125, 125t
    direct method of, 124
    indirect method of, 125,
      125t
  crude and specific, 122, 123t
Ratio, as measure of disease
    frequency, 118, 119t
Readability of materials, 279–280
Readers, skilled and unskilled,
    274. See also *Hypoliteracy;
    Literacy.*
Recall, in Folstein's mini-mental
    status examination, 193b
Recall bias, 139
Rectal prolapse, in children, 502
Red measles (rubeola),
    immunization for, 244–245
Reducible hernia, 488–489
Reflex disease, gastroesophageal.
    See *Gastroesophageal reflux
    disease (GERD).*
Reflexology, 37, *38*
Regional disasters, community
    preplanning for, 108–109
Regional enteritis (Crohn's
    disease), 491–492
  treatment of, 493
Registration, in Folstein's mini-
    mental status examination,
    193b
Regurgitation, 445
  mitral, 446, 447
Rehydration, for gastroenteritis,
    532
Relative risk, as measure of effect
    in epidemiology, 127
Relaxation technique, 41b
Reliability, of screening test, 143
Relief recommendations,
    postdisaster, 109b
Religious culture(s), 58–61

Religious culture(s) *(Continued)*
  cults as, 60–61
  expressions of spirituality as,
    60–61
  Islam as, 58–59
  Latter-Day Saints as, 60
  Mormons as, 60
  Orthodox Judaism as, 59–60
Reproduction. See *Pregnancy.*
Resource coverage, 718–719
Resources and Information,
    evaluation of, 716–717
Respiration, Kussmaul's, 607
Respiration biofeedback, 40
Restriction fragment length
    polymorphism (RFLP)
    analysis, in prenatal
    parentage testing, 171–172
Rheumatoid arthritis,
    epidemiology of, 455
  pathophysiology of, 453–455
  patient education in, 456
  prevention of, 456–457
  treatment of, 455–456
Rhythm method, of
    contraception, 375
Ribavirin, for hepatitis C, 538
Ritalin (methylphenidate
    hydrochloride), for attention
    deficit hyperactivity disorder,
    590
RNA molecule, genes in, 163
Rotavirus vaccine, 262
Rubella (German measles),
    immunization for, 245–246
  preconception counseling
    about, 367
  vaccine-preventable, in adoles-
    cence, 259b
  in childhood, 257b–258b
Rubeola (red measles),
    immunization for, 244–245
Rules, limited acceptance of,
    among elderly, 229

Safety, personal, issues of,
    233–235
  of international travelers, 363b
Safety education issues, 217, 218t
Safety essentials, in home,
    218–221

Safety essentials *(Continued)*
  counseling suggestions for,
    219–221, 220b
Safety plans, for domestic
  violence, 73
Safety precautions, in home,
  217–235, 217–238. See also
  *Home, safety precaution(s)
  in.*
Safety seats, vehicle, 223
SAGE (Systematic Assessment of
  Geriatric drug use via
  Epidemiology), 131
St. John's wort, 28, 206
Salmonella, in foodborne illness,
  99t
Salmonella enterica, in
  gastroenteritis, 531
Salvia sclarea, 35
Sample frame, 136
Sampling, in epidemiologic
    studies, 136–138
  cluster, 138
  simple random, 137
  stratified, 137
  systematic random, 137
Sanitation. See *Health and
  sanitation.*
SAST (Substance Abuse
  Screening Tool), 694t
Saw palmetto, 29, 206
Schatzki's ring, 495
Schizophrenia, 572t
School settings, children in, risks
  for, 225
Sclerotherapy, for varicosities,
  450–451
Scombroid fish poisoning, 103t
Screening tests, in epidemiologic
    studies, 143–144
  results of, 143t, 144t
  validity and reliability of,
    142–143
Search services, 717
Seat belt(s), in trauma
  prevention, 327, 330
Seat belt laws, 226
Secondary prevention, of disease,
  5
Selection bias, 138–139

Selective serotonin reuptake
  inhibitors (SSRIs), for
  anxiety, 585
  for depression, 576–577
Self-efficacy, definition of, 14
Self-esteem, low, effect of
  physical activity on, 155
Self-examination, of breast,
    381–382, 637
  easy steps in, 382b–383b
  of testicles, 412, 413b, 657
Self-sufficiency, loss of, in
  elderly, 228
Semen analysis, for infertility,
  368
Seminomatous germ cell tumors,
  657. See also *Testicular
  cancer.*
Senility, 207
Sensory deficits, in elderly, 209
Serenoa repens, 29
Serving choices and sizes,
  pyramid guide to, *307*
Serving guide, to foods and
  serving sizes, 309
Sexual abuse, of children,
  393–394
Sexual diversity, 61
Sexual dysfunction, 572t
  male, 403–410. See also *Erectile dysfunction (ED).*
Sexual history, questions
  concerning, 559b
Sexual maturity rating, in
  females, Tanner classification
  of, 390t
Sexually transmitted disease
  (STD), 362–363, 378–381,
  548–560. See also specific
  disease, e.g., *Syphilis.*
  counseling about, 381
  detection of, 380–381
  education about, 379–380
  epidemiology of, 552
  in abused child, 394
  pathophysiology of, 548–552
  patient education about, 557–
    558
  prevention of, 559–560, 559b
    condoms in, 416
  risk factors for, in adolescents,
    550b

Sexually transmitted disease (STD) *(Continued)*
  screening for, 560
  treatment of, 552–557
  vaginitis and vaginosis in, 381
Shellfish toxins, 97t
Shelter living, mental health aspects of, 108
Shigella, in foodborne illness, 101t
Shigellosis, 531
  in children, 530
Shoebox test, in elderly, 201b
Short bowel syndrome, 500
Shoulder belt(s), in trauma prevention, 330
Sick building syndrome, 106–107
Sickle cell disease, 437
Sickle cell trait, 437
Sigmoidoscopy, 642
Simple random sampling, in epidemiologic studies, 137
Sinus node, 424
Situational culture, 61–62
Skeletal muscle strength, health benefits of physical activity for, 152–153
Skill, cultural, 47
Skin cancer, American Cancer Society screening recommendations for, 631t
  pathophysiology of, 655–656
  prevention of, 656
  screening for, 656–657
  treatment of, 656
Slow-twitch muscle fibers, 153
Smoke detectors, 219
Smoking. See also *Nicotine abuse.*
  cigarette, in men, 411
  in women, 384
Snakebites, 87–88
Social behavior, individual, 8
Social factors, in domestic violence, 68
Social health, 8
Social issues, of human genome project, 165
Social phobia, 583t
Societal health, 8–9
Society, hypoliteracy and, 269
Sodium chloride, in diet, 295

Somatic cell therapy, 166–167
Somatin, 595
Somatization disorder (Briquet's syndrome), 586
Somatoform disorder(s), 586–589. See also specific disorder, e.g., *Body dysmorphic disorder.*
Somogyi phenomenon, in diabetes mellitus, 608
Specific rate, as measure of disease frequency, 122, 123t
Speculum, choice of, in adolescent gynecologic examination, 390–391
Spermicidal gels, 374
Spina bifida, prenatal screening for, 173–174
Spiritual health, 9–10
Spirituality, 9
  expressions of, 60–61
Splenomegaly, in infectious mononucleosis, 547
Sports injuries, 336t–337t
  prevention of, 335
Sports massage, 39
Squamous cell carcinoma, 655
SSRIs (selective serotonin reuptake inhibitors), for anxiety, 585
  for depression, 576–577
Staphylococcus aureus, in foodborne illness, 98t
  in postoperative meningitis, 541
State and Regional Domestic Violence Organizations, 76t–78t
State Domestic Violence Crisis Hotlines, 75t
STD. See *Sexually transmitted disease (STD).*
Stenosis, valvular, 445–446
Sterilization, as method of contraception, female, 375
  male, 416
Steroid abuse, anabolic, epidemiology of, 708–709
  pathophysiology of, 707–708
  prevention of, 709
  screening for, 710
  treatment of, 709

Stratified sampling, in
epidemiologic studies, 138
Streptococcus pneumoniae,
causing meningitis, 540, 541
Stress, and literacy, 271
Stroke, during pregnancy,
increased risk of, 687
epidemiology of, 687, 688t
hemorrhagic, 685, 686
in women, 382
increased risk factors for, 688t
pathophysiology of, 685–687
patient education about, 689
prevention of, 689–690
thrombus-induced, 685, 686
treatment of, 688–689
Stroke volume, 425
Study design(s), epidemiologic,
129–136
case-control, 131–132
cohort, 132–134
cross-sectional, 130–131
ecological, 129–130
randomized clinical trials in,
134–136, 135t
Study observations, in
epidemiologic studies, 139
Substance abuse, 572t, 693–710.
See also *Alcohol abuse;
Anabolic steroid abuse;
Nicotine abuse.*
chronic, 693–694
DSM-IV criteria for, 695b
environmental rewiring associated with, 693
Government Agencies and Offices for, 767–768
Organizations, Associations,
and Support Groups for,
767
psychologic disorders associated with, 694
screening for, 694–695, 694t
web sites for, 768–769
Substance Abuse Screening Tool
(SAST), 694t
Substance dependence, DSM-IV
criteria for, 696b
treatment of, effectiveness of
brief interventions in, 696–
697
readiness for, 695

Sucralfate suspension, for
gastritis and ulcers, 477
Sudden cardiac death, during
exercise, 156
Suk-yeong (koro), 51–52
Sulfasalazine, for inflammatory
bowel disease, 493
Susto, 53
Swallowing disorders, in elderly,
209–210
Swedish massage, 39
Syphilis, 378
epidemiology of, 552
in children, 551
in pregnancy, 551
pathophysiology of, 550
patient education about, 558
signs and symptoms of, 556t
treatment of, 556–557
Systematic Assessment of
Geriatric drug use via
Epidemiology (SAGE), 131
Systematic random sampling, in
epidemiologic studies, 137

Tachycardia, treatment of, 428
Tamoxifen, prophylactic, for
breast cancer, 637
Tanner classification, of sexual
maturity rating, in females,
390t
Tay-Sachs disease, carrier testing
for, 178
ethnic groups affected by, 178t
potential of germline therapy
in, 167
TB. See *Tuberculosis (TB).*
Tea tree oil, in aroma therapy,
36–37
Teen's right of passage, 226
Telephone numbers, emergency,
220, 220b
Teratogens, 179–180, 179b
Terminal illness, counseling
patients about, 631, 633–634
management of, 5
Tertiary prevention, of disease, 5
Testicular cancer, 412
epidemiology of, 658
pathophysiology of, 657–658
patient education about, 659

Testicular cancer *(Continued)*
  prevention of, 659
  screening for, 659
  self-examination for, 412, 413b,
    659
  treatment of, 658
Tetanus, immunization for,
    247–248
  vaccine-preventable, in adoles-
    cence, 259b
  in childhood, 256b–257b
Theory and practice, alternative
    medical systems of, 24. See
    also *Alternative medicine.*
Therapeutic abortion, 377–378
Thermal biofeedback, 40
Thiamine, in treatment of alcohol
    abuse, 701
Thrombocytopenia, 437–438
Thrombosis, venous, 438
Thrombus-induced stroke, 685,
    686. See also *Stroke.*
Thyroid function testing, in
    pregnancy, 597
Thyroid gland, 593
  disorder(s) of, 596–602
    hyperthyroidism as, 596–599
    hypothyroidism as, 599–602
Thyroiditis, Hashimoto's, 601
  postpartum, 600–601
Thyroid-stimulating hormone
    (TSH), 593
  screening for, in elderly, 597
Thyrotropin-releasing hormone
    (TRH), 593
Thyroxine (T₄), 593
TIA (transient ischemic attack),
    686. See also *Stroke.*
Time, epidemiologic description
    of, 117
Time commitment, in patient
    education, 11
Tingling, in foodborne illness,
    96t
Tissue plasminogen activator
    (TPA), for stroke, 688
Title VI of 1964 Civil Rights Act,
    282–283
Tobacco use. See also *Nicotine
    abuse.*
  in men, 411
  in women, 384

Toddler(s). See also *Child(ren).*
  caloric requirements of, 305
Toxic megacolon, 500
Toxins, shellfish, 97t
TPA (tissue plasminogen
    activator), for stroke, 688
Transfusions, blood, transmission
    of infection via, 509
Transient ischemic attack (TIA),
    686. See also *Stroke.*
Translation materials, written, 51
Transluminal balloon angioplasty,
    for peripheral vascular
    disease, 435
Transtheoretical Model or Stages
    of Change Theory, 14–15
Trauma, 317–341. See also
    specific trauma, e.g.,
    Fracture(s).
  definition and mechanism of,
    325–327
  emergency department visits
    due to, by intent and mech-
    anism of cause, 329t
    selected characteristics of,
      328t
  epidemiology of, 317, 318t–
    321t, 322t–324t
  Government Agencies and Of-
    fices for, 745–746
  Organizations, Associations,
    and Support Groups for,
    744–745
  prevention of, basic strategies
    in, 325–326
    counseling in, 327, 330–335,
      338
    improved postinjury care in,
      327
    in adolescence, guidance for,
      227b
    persuasion in, 326
    requirement of law in, 326
    vehicle and environmental al-
      terations in, 326–327
  web sites for, 746–747
Trauma care, ABCDEs of,
    339–340
Trauma Life Support, advanced,
    338–341
Travel medical kit, 345b

Travel risk, assessment of, 346–347, 346t

Traveler(s), living arrangements of, 344

personal safety of, preventive measures for, 363b

with special needs, 345b

Travel-related illness, diarrhea and other enteric diseases in, 347–352

dietary advice for avoidance of, 348–350, 348t, 349b

prevention and treatment of, 350–352, 351t, 352t

incidence of, 343

insect and arthropod vectors of disease in, 352–356, 353t. See also specific disease, e.g., *Malaria.*

pretravel assessment of, 344–347

patient interview and history in, 344–345, 345b

preparation in, 344

risk in, 4t, 346–347

prevention of, 343–364

miscellaneous measures in, 362–363, 363b

vaccine-preventable, 356–362, 357t

cholera as, 359–360

hepatitis A as, 358–359

hepatitis B as, 361

Japanese encephalitis as, 361

polio as, 360

rabies as, 361

typhoid fever as, 359

yellow fever as, 360

TRH (thyrotropin-releasing hormone), 593

Triage, 338

Trichomoniasis, 557

Trigger factors, in migraine headaches, 675, 676t

Triglycerides, 594–595

Triiodothyronine (T_3), 593

Trimethoprim/sulfamethoxazole, for traveler's diarrhea, 351–352, 351t, 352t

Trisomy 18, prenatal screening for, 175

Trisomy 21 (Down syndrome), prenatal screening for, 174–175

TSH (thyroid-stimulating hormone), 593

screening for, in elderly, 597

Tuberculin skin test, 563

Tuberculosis (TB), epidemiology of, 562

pathophysiology of, 560–562

patient education about, 563–564

prevention of, 564

screening for, 564–565

treatment of, 562–563

Tumor(s). See *Cancer.*

Tumor suppressor genes, 624. See also *Gene(s).*

Typhoid fever, vaccine-preventable, in international traveler, 359

Typhoon, effect of, on health, 108t

Tzanck's test, 553

Ulcer(s), in peripheral vascular disease, 434

peptic, 475–478

Ulcerative colitis, 491

treatment of, 493

Ultraviolet radiation, risk of skin cancer associated with, 630

United States Preventive Services Task Force (USPSTF), 3, 191–192

United States Public Health Service (USPHS), 80–81

Urate crystal deposits, in gout, 463

Urinary retention, in elderly, 210–211

USPHS (United States Public Health Service), 80–81

USPSTF (United States Preventive Services Task Force), 3, 191–192

Vaccine(s). See *Immunization(s).*

Vaccine-preventable disease(s), 243t

Vaccine-preventable disease(s)
(*Continued*)
  in adolescence, 259b–260b
  in childhood, 256b–258b
  travel-related, 356–362, 357t
    cholera as, 359–360
    hepatitis A as, 358–359
    hepatitis B as, 361
    Japanese encephalitis as, 361
    polio as, 360
    rabies as, 361
    typhoid fever as, 359
    yellow fever as, 360
Vaginitis, 381
Vaginosis, 381
Validity, of screening test,
    142–143
P-Value, in epidemiology, 128
Valve(s), cardiac, 424
Valvular heart disease, 445–449.
    See also *Heart disease,
    valvular.*
Vancomycin, prophylactic, for
    genitourinary and
    gastrointestinal procedures,
    528t
Varicella (chickenpox), vaccine-
    preventable, in
    adolescence, 259b
  in childhood, 258b
Varicella vaccine, *241*, 243
  new, 254, 261
Varicosities, 449–451
  epidemiology of, 450
  esophageal, 495
  pathophysiology of, 449–450
  patient education of, 451
  treatment of, 450–451
Vascular dementia, 667
Vascular disease, peripheral,
    433–436
    epidemiology of, 434–435
    pathophysiology of, 433–434
    patient education about, 435
    prevention of, 435–436
    screening for, 436
    treatment of, 435
Vasectomy, 416
Vehicle safety seats, 223
Vein(s), varicose, 449–451
Vein stripping, 451
Venous thrombosis, 438

Venous ulcers, in peripheral
    vascular disease, 434
Ventilation and oxygenation, in
    trauma care, 339
Ventricular fibrillation, treatment
    of, 428
Vertigo, in foodborne illness, 96t
Very-low-density lipoprotein
    (VLDL), 594, 595, 614
Viagra, for erectile dysfunction,
    408
Vibrio cholerae, 359. See also
    Cholera.
  in foodborne illness, 100t–101t
Vibrio parahaemolyticus, in
    foodborne illness, 99t
Violence, domestic, 67–79. See
    also *Domestic violence.*
  male, 412
Virus(es), causing cancer, 627,
    628t
  causing demyelination, 678
Visual deficits, in elderly, 209
Visual disturbances, in foodborne
    illness, 96t
Vitamin(s), antioxidant, benefits
    of, 295
  for elderly, 206
  for elderly, 205–206
Vitamin A, 32
Vitamin B$_{12}$ deficiency, in elderly,
    206
Vitamin C, 32
Vitamin D, for osteoporosis,
    459
Vitamin E, 32–33
  for dementia, 668–669
  for elderly, 205
Vitamin K deficiency, 438
VLDL (very-low-density
    lipoprotein), 594, 595, 614
Vo$_{2max}$ (maximal oxygen uptake),
    in cardiovascular fitness,
    151–152
VOCs (volatile organic
    compounds), in buildings,
    107
Volatile organic compounds
    (VOCs), in buildings, 107
Volcanic eruption, effect of, on
    health, 108t

Vomiting, foodborne and waterborne illness typified by, 98t
in foodborne illness, 94t
Von Willebrand's disease, 436
Voodoo, 57
symbols of, 58b

Waist measurement(s), for men, 296
for women, 297
Waist-hip ratio, 300, *301*
Warfare, 110–111
Warfarin, for bleeding disorders, 438
Wart(s), flat, 554–555, 554t
keratotic, 554t
papular, 554t
Water, drinking, regulation of, 96, 104
ground, chemical leachates in, 104–105
organisms in, 104
Water supply, potable, 96, 104–105
Waterborne gastrointestinal diseases, compendium of, 98t–103t
Weapons, in home, counseling about, 223
Weapons of mass destruction (WMD), 110
Web(s), esophageal, 495
Web sites, for alternative medicine, 725–726
for bone and joint disorders, 754
for cardiology, 752
for cultural influence, 726–727
for domestic violence, 728–729
for elderly, 738
for environmental health and sanitation, 732
for epidemiology, 732
for exercise, 733–734
for gastrointestinal disorders, 756
for genetics, 736
for health planning and illness prevention for international travel, 747

Web sites *(Continued)*
for immunizations, 741–742
for infectious diseases, 758
for locating electronic discussion groups, 718t
for men's health, 751–752
for mental health, 760–761
for metabolic conditions, 763
for neoplastic conditions, 764
for neurologic disease, 766
for nutrition education, 744
for patient education and literacy, 742–743
for preventive strategies, 721–724
for safety precautions in home, 739–740
for substance abuse, 768–769
for trauma, 746–747
for women's health, 749–750
Weight, calculation of, based on height, 297
Weight change intervention, tool(s) to determine need for, body mass index as, 297, *298–299*
waist measurement as, 296–297
waist-hip ratio as, 300, *301*
weight measurement as, 297, 300t
Weight chart, at-risk, 300t
Weight gain, caloric prescription for, 302
Weight loss, caloric prescription for, 302
exercise and, 152
long-term, 293–294
Weight maintenance, caloric prescription for, 302
Wellness, dimensions of, 7–8
guidelines for, 8
Whooping cough (pertussis), immunization for, 246–247
vaccine-preventable, in childhood, 260b
Withdrawal (coitus interruptus), as method of contraception, 375, 416
WMD (weapons of mass destruction), 110

Wolff-Parkinson-White syndrome, 427

Women, abuse of. See also *Domestic violence.*
  predisposing factors in, 70b
  breast self-examination by, 381–382, 382b–383b
  cardiovascular disease in, 382–384
  contraceptives for, 369–378. See also *Contraception.*
  fertility in, 366–369
  health of, 366–394
  low back pain in, 662
  menopause in, 384–388
  pediatric and young adolescent, caring for, 388–394
  sexually transmitted diseases in, 378–381
  smoking and lung cancer in, 384

Women's health issues, Government Agencies and Offices for, 748–749
  Organizations, Associations, and Support Groups for, 748
  web sites for, 749–750

World Health Organization (WHO) definition, of elderly, 190
  of health, 7

Writing, prize-winning, Pulitzer's formula for, 277–281

Written translation materials, 51

Yard lighting, 234

Yellow fever, vaccine-preventable, in international traveler, 360

Yersinia enterocolitica, in foodborne illness, 101t

Yesavage-Brink Geriatric Depression Scale, 195b

Yin and yang, as health and illness issue, in Asian American communities, 54, 56
  in acupuncture, 25

Ylang-ylang, in aroma therapy, 37

Yohimbine, for erectile dysfunction, 408

Zone therapy, 37. See also *Reflexology.*